Mathematical Constants

Famous mathematical constants include the ratio of circular circumference to diameter, $\pi = 3.14\ldots$, and the natural logarithmic base, $e = 2.178\ldots$. Students and professionals usually can name at most a few others, but there are many more buried in the literature and awaiting discovery.

How do such constants arise, and why are they important? Here Steven Finch provides 136 essays, each devoted to a mathematical constant or a class of constants, from the well known to the highly exotic. Topics covered include the statistics of continued fractions, chaos in nonlinear systems, prime numbers, sum-free sets, isoperimetric problems, approximation theory, self-avoiding walks and the Ising model (from statistical physics), binary and digital search trees (from theoretical computer science), the Prouhet–Thue–Morse sequence, complex analysis, geometric probability, and the traveling salesman problem. This book will be helpful both to readers seeking information about a specific constant and to readers who desire a panoramic view of all constants coming from a particular field, for example, combinatorial enumeration or geometric optimization. Unsolved problems appear virtually everywhere as well. This is an outstanding scholarly attempt to bring together all significant mathematical constants in one place.

Steven R. Finch studied at Oberlin College and the University of Illinois in Urbana-Champaign, and held positions at TASC, MIT Lincoln Laboratory, and MathSoft Inc. He is presently a freelance mathematician in the Boston area. He is also a composer and has released a CD entitled "An Apple Gathering" devoted to his vocal and choral music.

ENCYCLOPEDIA OF MATHEMATICS AND ITS APPLICATIONS

FOUNDING EDITOR GIAN-CARLO ROTA
Editorial Board
R. Doran, P. Flajolet, M. Ismail, T.-Y. Lam, E. Lutwak,
Volume 94

ENCYCLOPEDIA OF MATHEMATICS AND ITS APPLICATIONS

Mathematical Constants

STEVEN R. FINCH

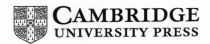

CAMBRIDGE
UNIVERSITY PRESS

PUBLISHED BY THE PRESS SYNDICATE OF THE UNIVERSITY OF CAMBRIDGE
The Pitt Building, Trumpington Street, Cambridge, United Kingdom

CAMBRIDGE UNIVERSITY PRESS
The Edinburgh Building, Cambridge CB2 2RU, UK
40 West 20th Street, New York, NY 10011-4211, USA
477 Williamstown Road, Port Melbourne, VIC 3207, Australia
Ruiz de Alarcón 13, 28014 Madrid, Spain
Dock House, The Waterfront, Cape Town 8001, South Africa

http://www.cambridge.org

First published 2003

Printed in the United States of America

Typeface Times New Roman PS 10/12.5 pt.   *System* LaTeX 2$_\varepsilon$ [TB]

A catalog record for this book is available from the British Library.

Library of Congress Cataloging in Publication Data
Finch, Steven R., 1959–
Mathematical constants / Steven R. Finch.
p.   cm. – (Encyclopedia of mathematics and its applications; v. 94)
Includes bibliographical references and index.
ISBN 0-521-81805-2
I. Mathematical constants.   I. Title.   II. Series.
QA41 .F54   2003
513 – dc21   2002074058

ISBN 0 521 81805 2 hardback

For Nancy Armstrong, the one constant

Contents

Preface

All numbers are not created equal. The fact that certain constants appear at all and then echo throughout mathematics, in seemingly independent ways, is a source of fascination. Formulas involving φ, e, π, or γ understandably fill a considerable portion of this book.

There are also many constants whose purposes are more specialized. Often such exotic quantities have been buried in the literature, known only to the experts of a narrow field, and invisible to the wider public. In some cases, the constants are easily computable; in other cases, they may be known to only one decimal digit of precision (or worse, none at all). Even rigorous proofs of existence might be unavailable.

My belief is that these latter constants are not as isolated as they may seem. The associated branches of research (unlike those involving φ, e, π, or γ) might simply require more time to develop the languages, functions, symmetries, etc., to express the constants more naturally. That is, if we work and listen hard enough, the echoes will become audible.

An elaborate taxonomy of mathematical constants has not yet been achieved; hence the organization of this book (by discipline) is necessarily subjective. A table of decimal approximations at the end gives an alternative organizational strategy (if ascending numerical order is helpful). The emphasis for me is not on the decimal expansions, but rather on the mathematical origins of the constants and their interrelationships. In short, the stories, not the table, tie the book together.

Material about well-known constants appears early and carefully, for the sake of readers without much mathematical background. Deeper into the text, however, I necessarily become more terse. My intended audience is advanced undergraduates and beyond (so I may assume readers have had calculus, matrix theory, differential equations, probability, some abstract algebra, and analysis). My aim is always to be clear and complete, to motivate why a particular constant or idea is important, and to indicate exactly where in the literature one should look for rigorous proofs and further elaboration.

I have incorporated Richard Guy's use of the ampersand (&) to denote joint work. For example, phrases like " ... follows from the work of Hardy & Ramanujan and

Rademacher" are unambiguous when presented as here. The notation [3, 7] means references 3 and 7, whereas [3.7] refers to Section 3.7 of this book. The presence of a comma or decimal point is clearly crucial.

Many people have speculated on the role of the Internet in education and research. I have no question about the longstanding impact of the Web as a whole, but I remain skeptical that any specific Web address I might give here will exist in a mere five years. Of all mathematical Web sites available today, I expect that at least the following three will survive the passage of time:

- the ArXiv preprint server at Los Alamos National Laboratory (the meaning of a pointer to "math.CA/9910045" or to "solv-int/9801008" should be apparent to all ArXiv visitors),
- MathSciNet, established by the American Mathematical Society (subscribers to this service will be acquainted with *Mathematical Reviews* and the meaning of "MR 3,270e," "MR 33 #3320," or "MR 87h:51043"), and
- the On-Line Encyclopedia of Integer Sequences, created by Neil Sloane (a sequence identifier such as "A000688" will likewise suffice),

but not many more will outlive us. Even those that persist will be moved to various new locations and the old addresses will eventually fail. I have therefore chosen not to include Web URLs in this book. When I cite a Web site (e.g., "Numbers, Constants and Computation," "Prime Pages," "MathPages," "Plouffe's Tables," or "Geometry Junkyard"), the reference will be by name only.

A project of this magnitude cannot possibly be the work of one person. These pages are filled with innumerable acts of kindness by friends. To express my appreciation to all would considerably lengthen this preface; hence I will not attempt this. Special thanks are due to Philippe Flajolet, my mentor, who provided valuable encouragement from the very beginning. I am grateful to Victor Adamchik, Christian Bower, Anthony Guttmann, Joe Keane, Pieter Moree, Gerhard Niklasch, Simon Plouffe, Pascal Sebah, Craig Tracy, John Wetzel, and Paul Zimmermann. I am also indebted to MathSoft Inc.,* the Algorithms Group at INRIA, and CECM at Simon Fraser University for providing Web sites for my online research notes – my window to the world! – and to Cambridge University Press for undertaking this publishing venture with me.

Comments, corrections, and suggestions from readers are always welcome. Please send electronic mail to *Steven.Finch@inria.fr*. Thank you.

---

* Portions of this book are © 2000–2003 MathSoft Engineering & Education, Inc. and are reprinted with permission.

Notation

$\lfloor x \rfloor$	*floor function:* largest integer $\leq x$
$\lceil x \rceil$	*ceiling function:* smallest integer $\geq x$
$\{x\}$	*fractional part:* $x - \lfloor x \rfloor$
$\ln x$	*natural logarithm:* $\log_e x$
$\dbinom{n}{k}$	*binomial coefficient:* $\dfrac{n!}{k!(n-k)!}$
$b_0 + \dfrac{a_1 \vert}{\vert b_1} + \dfrac{a_2 \vert}{\vert b_2} + \dfrac{a_3 \vert}{\vert b_3} + \cdots$	*continued fraction:* $b_0 + \cfrac{a_1}{b_1 + \cfrac{a_2}{b_2 + \cfrac{a_3}{b_3 + \cdots}}}$
$f(x) = O(g(x))$	*big O:* $\vert f(x)/g(x) \vert$ is bounded from above as $x \to x_0$
$f(x) = o(g(x))$	*little o:* $f(x)/g(x) \to 0$ as $x \to x_0$
$f(x) \sim g(x)$	*asymptotic equivalence:* $f(x)/g(x) \to 1$ as $x \to x_0$
$\displaystyle\sum_p$	summation over all prime numbers $p = 2, 3, 5, 7, 11, \ldots$ (only when the letter p is used)
$\displaystyle\prod_p$	same as $\sum_p$, with addition replaced by multiplication
$f(x)^n$	*power:* $(f(x))^n$, where n is an integer
$f^n(x)$	*iterate:* $\underbrace{f(f(\cdots f\,(x)\ldots))}_{n \text{ times}}$ where $n \geq 0$ is an integer

1

Well-Known Constants

1.1 Pythagoras' Constant, $\sqrt{2}$

The diagonal of a unit square has length $\sqrt{2} = 1.4142135623\ldots$. A theory, proposed by the Pythagorean school of philosophy, maintained that all geometric magnitudes could be expressed by rational numbers. The sides of a square were expected to be commensurable with its diagonals, in the sense that certain integer multiples of one would be equivalent to integer multiples of the other. This theory was shattered by the discovery that $\sqrt{2}$ is irrational [1–4].

Here are two proofs of the irrationality of $\sqrt{2}$, the first based on divisibility properties of the integers and the second using well ordering.

- If $\sqrt{2}$ were rational, then the equation $p^2 = 2q^2$ would be solvable in integers p and q, which are assumed to be in lowest terms. Since p^2 is even, p itself must be even and so has the form $p = 2r$. This leads to $2q^2 = 4r^2$ and thus q must also be even. But this contradicts the assumption that p and q were in lowest terms.
- If $\sqrt{2}$ were rational, then there would be a least positive integer s such that $s\sqrt{2}$ is an integer. Since $1 < 2$, it follows that $1 < \sqrt{2}$ and thus $t = s \cdot (\sqrt{2} - 1)$ is a positive integer. Also $t\sqrt{2} = s \cdot (\sqrt{2} - 1)\sqrt{2} = 2s - s\sqrt{2}$ is an integer and clearly $t < s$. But this contradicts the assumption that s was the smallest such integer.

Newton's method for solving equations gives rise to the following first-order recurrence, which is very fast and often implemented:

$$x_0 = 1, \qquad x_k = \frac{x_{k-1}}{2} + \frac{1}{x_{k-1}} \quad \text{for } k \geq 1, \qquad \lim_{k \to \infty} x_k = \sqrt{2}.$$

Another first-order recurrence [5] yields the reciprocal of $\sqrt{2}$:

$$y_0 = \frac{1}{2}, \qquad y_k = y_{k-1}\left(\frac{3}{2} - y_{k-1}^2\right) \quad \text{for } k \geq 1, \qquad \lim_{k \to \infty} y_k = \frac{1}{\sqrt{2}}.$$

The binomial series, also due to Newton, provides two interesting summations [6]:

$$1 + \sum_{n=1}^{\infty} \frac{(-1)^{n-1}}{2^{2n}(2n-1)} \binom{2n}{n} = 1 + \frac{1}{2} - \frac{1}{2 \cdot 4} + \frac{1 \cdot 3}{2 \cdot 4 \cdot 6} - + \cdots = \sqrt{2},$$

$$1 + \sum_{n=1}^{\infty} \frac{(-1)^{n}}{2^{2n}} \binom{2n}{n} = 1 - \frac{1}{2} + \frac{1 \cdot 3}{2 \cdot 4} - \frac{1 \cdot 3 \cdot 5}{2 \cdot 4 \cdot 6} + - \cdots = \frac{1}{\sqrt{2}}.$$

The latter is extended in [1.5.4]. We mention two beautiful infinite products [5, 7, 8]

$$\prod_{n=1}^{\infty} \left(1 + \frac{(-1)^{n+1}}{2n-1} \right) = \left(1 + \frac{1}{1} \right) \left(1 - \frac{1}{3} \right) \left(1 + \frac{1}{5} \right) \left(1 - \frac{1}{7} \right) \cdots = \sqrt{2},$$

$$\prod_{n=1}^{\infty} \left(1 - \frac{1}{4(2n-1)^2} \right) = \frac{1 \cdot 3}{2 \cdot 2} \cdot \frac{5 \cdot 7}{6 \cdot 6} \cdot \frac{9 \cdot 11}{10 \cdot 10} \cdot \frac{13 \cdot 15}{14 \cdot 14} \cdots = \frac{1}{\sqrt{2}}$$

and the regular continued fraction [9]

$$2 + \cfrac{1}{2 + \cfrac{1}{2 + \cfrac{1}{2 + \cdots}}} = 2 + \frac{1|}{|2} + \frac{1|}{|2} + \frac{1|}{|2} + \cdots = 1 + \sqrt{2} = (-1 + \sqrt{2})^{-1},$$

which is related to **Pell's sequence**

$$a_0 = 0, \qquad a_1 = 1, \qquad a_n = 2a_{n-1} + a_{n-2} \quad \text{for } n \geq 2$$

via the limiting formula

$$\lim_{n \to \infty} \frac{a_{n+1}}{a_n} = 1 + \sqrt{2}.$$

This is completely analogous to the famous connection between the Golden mean φ and Fibonacci's sequence [1.2]. See also Figure 1.1.

Viète's remarkable product for Archimedes' constant π [1.4.2] involves only the number 2 and repeated square-root extractions. Another expression connecting π and radicals appears in [1.4.5].

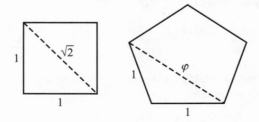

Figure 1.1. The diagonal of a regular unit pentagon, connecting any two nonadjacent corners, has length given by the Golden mean φ (rather than by Pythagoras' constant).

We return finally to irrationality issues: There obviously exist rationals x and y such that x^y is irrational (just take $x = 2$ and $y = 1/2$). Do there exist *irrationals* x and y such that x^y is *rational*? The answer to this is very striking. Let

$$z = \sqrt{2}^{\sqrt{2}}.$$

If z is rational, then take $x = y = \sqrt{2}$. If z is irrational, then take $x = z$ and $y = \sqrt{2}$, and clearly $x^y = 2$. Thus we have answered the question ("yes") without addressing the actual arithmetical nature of z. In fact, z is transcendental by the Gel'fond–Schneider theorem [10], proved in 1934, and hence is irrational. There are many unsolved problems in this area of mathematics; for example, we do not know whether

$$\sqrt{2}^z = \sqrt{2}^{\sqrt{2}^{\sqrt{2}}}$$

is irrational (let alone transcendental).

1.1.1 Generalized Continued Fractions

It is well known that any quadratic irrational possesses a periodic regular continued fraction expansion and vice versa. Comparatively few people have examined the generalized continued fraction [11–17]

$$w(p, q) = q + \cfrac{p + \cfrac{1}{q + \cfrac{p + \cdots}{q + \cdots}}}{q + \cfrac{p + \cfrac{1 + \cdots}{q + \cdots}}{q + \cfrac{p + \cdots}{q + \cdots}}},$$

which exhibits a fractal-like construction. Each *new* term in a particular generation (i.e., in a partial convergent) is replaced according to the rules

$$p \to p + \frac{1}{q}, \qquad q \to q + \frac{p}{q}$$

in the next generation. Clearly

$$w = q + \cfrac{p + \cfrac{1}{w}}{w}; \qquad \text{that is,} \quad w^3 - qw^2 - pw - 1 = 0.$$

In the special case $p = q = 3$, the higher-order continued fraction converges to $(-1 + \sqrt[3]{2})^{-1}$. It is conjectured that regular continued fractions for cubic irrationals behave like those for almost all real numbers [18–21], and no patterns are evident. The ordinary replacement rule

$$r \to r + \frac{1}{r}$$

is sufficient for the study of quadratic irrationals, but requires extension for broader classes of algebraic numbers.

Two alternative representations of $\sqrt[3]{2}$ are as follows [22]:

$$\sqrt[3]{2} = 1 + \cfrac{1}{3 + \cfrac{3}{a} + \cfrac{1}{b}}, \qquad \text{where} \quad a = 3 + \frac{3}{a} + \frac{1}{b}, \qquad b = 12 + \frac{10}{a} + \frac{3}{b}$$

and [23]

$$\sqrt[3]{2} = 1 + \frac{1|}{|3} + \frac{2|}{|2} + \frac{4|}{|9} + \frac{5|}{|2} + \frac{7|}{|15} + \frac{8|}{|2} + \frac{10|}{|21} + \frac{11|}{|2} + \cdots .$$

Other usages of the phrase "generalized continued fractions" include those in [24], with application to simultaneous Diophantine approximation, and in [25], with a geometric interpretation involving the boundaries of convex hulls.

1.1.2 Radical Denestings

We mention two striking radical denestings due to Ramanujan:

$$\sqrt[3]{\sqrt[3]{2} - 1} = \sqrt[3]{\frac{1}{9}} - \sqrt[3]{\frac{2}{9}} + \sqrt[3]{\frac{4}{9}}, \qquad \sqrt[2]{\sqrt[3]{5} - \sqrt[3]{4}} = \tfrac{1}{3}\left(\sqrt[3]{2} + \sqrt[3]{20} - \sqrt[3]{25} \right).$$

Such simplifications are an important part of computer algebra systems [26].

[1]   G. H. Hardy and E. M. Wright, *An Introduction to the Theory of Numbers*, 5th ed., Oxford Univ. Press, 1985, pp. 38–45; MR 81i:10002.

[2]   F. J. Papp, $\sqrt{2}$ is irrational, *Int. J. Math. Educ. Sci. Technol.* 25 (1994) 61–67; MR 94k:11081.

[3]   O. Toeplitz, *The Calculus: A Genetic Approach*, Univ. of Chicago Press, 1981, pp. 1–6; MR 11,584e.

[4]   K. S. Brown, Gauss' lemma without explicit divisibility arguments (MathPages).

[5]   X. Gourdon and P. Sebah, The square root of 2 (Numbers, Constants and Computation).

[6]   K. Knopp, *Theory and Application of Infinite Series*, Hafner, 1951, pp. 208–211, 257–258; MR 18,30c.

[7]   I. S. Gradshteyn and I. M. Ryzhik, *Tables of Integrals, Series and Products*, Academic Press, 1980, p. 12; MR 97c:00014.

[8]   F. L. Bauer, An infinite product for square-rooting with cubic convergence, *Math. Intellig.* 20 (1998) 12–13, 38.

[9]   L. Lorentzen and H. Waadeland, *Continued Fractions with Applications*, North-Holland, 1992, pp. 10–16, 564–565; MR 93g:30007.

[10] C. L. Siegel, *Transcendental Numbers*, Princeton Univ. Press, 1949, pp. 75–84; MR 11,330c.

[11] D. Gómez Morin, *La Quinta Operación Aritmética: Revolución del Número*, 2000.

[12] A. K. Gupta and A. K. Mittal, Bifurcating continued fractions, math.GM/0002227.

[13] A. K. Mittal and A. K. Gupta, Bifurcating continued fractions II, math.GM/0008060.

[14] G. Berzsenyi, Nonstandardly continued fractions, *Quantum Mag.* (Jan./Feb. 1996) 39.

[15] E. O. Buchman, Problem 4/21, *Math. Informatics Quart.*, v. 7 (1997) n. 1, 53.

[16] A. Dorito and K. Ekblaw, Solution of problem 2261, *Crux Math.*, v. 24 (1998) n. 7, 430–431.

[17] W. Janous and N. Derigiades, Solution of problem 2363, *Crux Math.*, v. 25 (1999) n. 6, 376–377.

[18] J. von Neumann and B. Tuckerman, Continued fraction expansion of $2^{1/3}$, *Math. Tables Other Aids Comput.* 9 (1955) 23–24; MR 16,961d.
[19] R. D. Richtmyer, M. Devaney, and N. Metropolis, Continued fraction expansions of algebraic numbers, *Numer. Math.* 4 (1962) 68–84; MR 25 #44.
[20] A. D. Brjuno, The expansion of algebraic numbers into continued fractions (in Russian), *Zh. Vychisl. Mat. Mat. Fiz.* 4 (1964) 211–221; Engl. transl. in *USSR Comput. Math. Math. Phys.*, v. 4 (1964) n. 2, 1–15; MR 29 #1183.
[21] S. Lange and H. Trotter, Continued fractions for some algebraic numbers, *J. Reine Angew. Math.* 255 (1972) 112–134; addendum 267 (1974) 219–220; MR 46 #5258 and MR 50 #2086.
[22] F. O. Pasicnjak, Decomposition of a cubic algebraic irrationality into branching continued fractions (in Ukrainian), *Dopovidi Akad. Nauk Ukrain. RSR Ser. A* (1971) 511–514, 573; MR 45 #6765.
[23] G. S. Smith, Expression of irrationals of any degree as regular continued fractions with integral components, *Amer. Math. Monthly* 64 (1957) 86–88; MR 18,635d.
[24] W. F. Lunnon, Multi-dimensional continued fractions and their applications, *Computers in Mathematical Research*, Proc. 1986 Cardiff conf., ed. N. M. Stephens and M. P. Thorne, Clarendon Press, 1988, pp. 41–56; MR 89c:00032.
[25] V. I. Arnold, Higher-dimensional continued fractions, *Regular Chaotic Dynamics* 3 (1998) 10–17; MR 2000h:11012.
[26] S. Landau, Simplification of nested radicals, *SIAM J. Comput.* 21 (1992) 81–110; MR 92k:12008.

1.2 The Golden Mean, φ

Consider a line segment:

What is the most "pleasing" division of this line segment into two parts? Some people might say at the halfway point:

----------------- • -----------------

Others might say at the one-quarter or three-quarters point. The "correct answer" is, however, none of these, and is supposedly found in Western art from the ancient Greeks onward (aestheticians speak of it as the principle of "dynamic symmetry"):

---------------------- • -----------

If the right-hand portion is of length $v = 1$, then the left-hand portion is of length $u = 1.618\ldots$. A line segment partitioned as such is said to be divided in Golden or Divine section. What is the justification for endowing this particular division with such elevated status? The length u, as drawn, is to the whole length $u + v$, as the length v is to u:

$$\frac{u}{u+v} = \frac{v}{u}.$$

Letting $\varphi = u/v$, solve for φ via the observation that

$$1 + \frac{1}{\varphi} = 1 + \frac{v}{u} = \frac{u+v}{u} = \frac{u}{v} = \varphi.$$

The positive root of the resulting quadratic equation $\varphi^2 - \varphi - 1 = 0$ is

$$\varphi = \frac{1 + \sqrt{5}}{2} = 1.6180339887\ldots,$$

which is called the **Golden mean** or **Divine proportion** [1, 2].

The constant φ is intricately related to **Fibonacci's sequence**

$$f_0 = 0, \qquad f_1 = 1, \qquad f_n = f_{n-1} + f_{n-2} \quad \text{for } n \geq 2.$$

This sequence models (in a naive way) the growth of a rabbit population. Rabbits are assumed to start having bunnies once a month after they are two months old; they always give birth to twins (one male bunny and one female bunny), they never die, and they never stop propagating. The number of rabbit pairs after n months is f_n.

What can φ possibly have in common with $\{f_n\}$? This is one of the most remarkable ideas in all of mathematics. The partial convergents leading up to the regular continued fraction representation of φ,

$$\varphi = 1 + \cfrac{1}{1 + \cfrac{1}{1 + \cfrac{1}{1 + \cdots}}} = 1 + \frac{1|}{|1} + \frac{1|}{|1} + \frac{1|}{|1} + \cdots,$$

are all ratios of successive Fibonacci numbers; hence

$$\lim_{n \to \infty} \frac{f_{n+1}}{f_n} = \varphi.$$

This result is also true for arbitrary sequences satisfying the same recursion $f_n = f_{n-1} + f_{n-2}$, assuming that the initial terms f_0 and f_1 are distinct [3, 4].

The rich geometric connection between the Golden mean and Fibonacci's sequence is seen in Figure 1.2. Starting with a single Golden rectangle (of length φ and width 1), there is a natural sequence of nested Golden rectangles obtained by removing the leftmost square from the first rectangle, the topmost square from the second rectangle, etc. The length and width of the nth Golden rectangle can be written as linear expressions $a + b\varphi$, where the coefficients a and b are always Fibonacci numbers. These Golden rectangles can be inscribed in a logarithmic spiral as pictured. Assume that the lower left corner of the first rectangle is the origin of an xy-coordinate system.

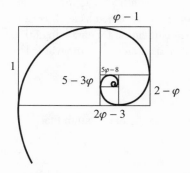

Figure 1.2. The Golden spiral circumscribes the sequence of Golden rectangles.

The accumulation point for the spiral can be proved to be $(\frac{1}{5}(1 + 3\varphi), \frac{1}{5}(3 - \varphi))$. Such logarithmic spirals are "equiangular" in the sense that every line through (x_∞, y_∞) cuts across the spiral at a constant angle ξ. In this way, logarithmic spirals generalize ordinary circles (for which $\xi = 90°$). The logarithmic spiral pictured gives rise to the constant angle $\xi = \text{arccot}(\frac{2}{\pi} \ln(\varphi)) = 72.968\ldots°$. Logarithmic spirals are evidently found throughout nature; for example, the shell of a chambered nautilus, the tusks of an elephant, and patterns in sunflowers and pine cones [4–6].

Another geometric application of the Golden mean arises when inscribing a regular pentagon within a given circle by ruler and compass. This is related to the fact that

$$2\cos\left(\frac{\pi}{5}\right) = \varphi, \qquad 2\sin\left(\frac{\pi}{5}\right) = \sqrt{3 - \varphi}.$$

The Golden mean, just as it has a simple regular continued fraction expansion, also has a simple radical expansion [7]

$$\varphi = \sqrt{1 + \sqrt{1 + \sqrt{1 + \sqrt{1 + \sqrt{1 + \cdots}}}}}.$$

The manner in which this expansion converges to φ is discussed in [1.2.1]. Like Pythagoras' constant [1.1], the Golden mean is irrational and simple proofs are given in [8,9].

Here is a series [10] involving φ:

$$\frac{2\sqrt{5}}{5} \ln(\varphi) = \left(1 - \frac{1}{2} - \frac{1}{3} + \frac{1}{4}\right) + \left(\frac{1}{6} - \frac{1}{7} - \frac{1}{8} + \frac{1}{9}\right)$$
$$+ \left(\frac{1}{11} - \frac{1}{12} - \frac{1}{13} + \frac{1}{14}\right) + \cdots,$$

which reminds us of certain series connected with Archimedes' constant [1.4.1]. A direct expression for φ as a sum can be obtained from the Taylor series for the square root function, expanded about 4. The Fibonacci numbers appear in yet another representation [11] of φ:

$$4 - \varphi = \sum_{n=0}^{\infty} \frac{1}{f_{2^n}} = \frac{1}{f_1} + \frac{1}{f_2} + \frac{1}{f_4} + \frac{1}{f_8} + \cdots.$$

Among many other possible formulas involving φ, we mention the four Rogers–Ramanujan continued fractions

$$\frac{1}{\alpha - \varphi} \exp\left(-\frac{2\pi}{5}\right) = 1 + \frac{e^{-2\pi}}{|1} + \frac{e^{-4\pi}}{|1} + \frac{e^{-6\pi}}{|1} + \frac{e^{-8\pi}}{|1} + \cdots,$$

$$\frac{1}{\beta - \varphi} \exp\left(-\frac{2\pi}{\sqrt{5}}\right) = 1 + \frac{e^{-2\pi\sqrt{5}}}{|1} + \frac{e^{-4\pi\sqrt{5}}}{|1} + \frac{e^{-6\pi\sqrt{5}}}{|1} + \frac{e^{-8\pi\sqrt{5}}}{|1} + \cdots,$$

$$\frac{1}{\kappa - (\varphi - 1)} \exp\left(-\frac{\pi}{5}\right) = 1 - \frac{e^{-\pi}}{|1} + \frac{e^{-2\pi}}{|1} - \frac{e^{-3\pi}}{|1} + \frac{e^{-4\pi}}{|1} - + \cdots,$$

$$\frac{1}{\lambda - (\varphi - 1)} \exp\left(-\frac{\pi}{\sqrt{5}}\right) = 1 - \frac{e^{-\pi\sqrt{5}}}{|1} + \frac{e^{-2\pi\sqrt{5}}}{|1} - \frac{e^{-3\pi\sqrt{5}}}{|1} + \frac{e^{-4\pi\sqrt{5}}}{|1} - + \cdots,$$

where

$$\alpha = \left(\varphi\sqrt{5}\right)^{\frac{1}{2}}, \qquad \alpha' = \frac{1}{\sqrt{5}}\left((\varphi-1)\sqrt{5}\right)^{\frac{5}{2}}, \qquad \beta = \frac{\sqrt{5}}{1+\sqrt[5]{\alpha'-1}},$$

$$\kappa = \left((\varphi-1)\sqrt{5}\right)^{\frac{1}{2}}, \qquad \kappa' = \frac{1}{\sqrt{5}}\left(\varphi\sqrt{5}\right)^{\frac{5}{2}}, \qquad \lambda = \frac{\sqrt{5}}{1+\sqrt[5]{\kappa'-1}}.$$

The fourth evaluation is due to Ramanathan [9, 12–16].

1.2.1 Analysis of a Radical Expansion

The radical expansion [1.2] for φ can be rewritten as a sequence $\{\varphi_n\}$:

$$\varphi_1 = 1, \qquad \varphi_n = \sqrt{1+\varphi_{n-1}} \quad \text{for } n \geq 2.$$

Paris [17] proved that the rate in which φ_n approaches the limit φ is given by

$$\varphi - \varphi_n \sim \frac{2C}{(2\varphi)^n} \quad \text{as } n \to \infty,$$

where $C = 1.0986419643\ldots$ is a new constant. Here is an exact characterization of C. Let $F(x)$ be the analytic solution of the functional equation

$$F(x) = 2\varphi F(\varphi - \sqrt{\varphi^2 - x}), \qquad |x| < \varphi^2,$$

subject to the initial conditions $F(0) = 0$ and $F'(0) = 1$. Then $C = \varphi F(1/\varphi)$. A power-series technique can be used to evaluate C numerically from these formulas. It is simpler, however, to use the following product:

$$C = \prod_{n=2}^{\infty} \frac{2\varphi}{\varphi + \varphi_n},$$

which is stable and converges quickly [18].

Another interesting constant is defined via the radical expression [7, 19]

$$\sqrt{1 + \sqrt{2 + \sqrt{3 + \sqrt{4 + \sqrt{5 + \cdots}}}}} = 1.7579327566\ldots,$$

but no expression of this in terms of other constants is known.

1.2.2 Cubic Variations of the Golden Mean

Perrin's sequence is defined by

$$g_0 = 3, \qquad g_1 = 0, \qquad g_2 = 2, \qquad g_n = g_{n-2} + g_{n-3} \quad \text{for } n \geq 3$$

and has the property that $n > 1$ divides g_n if n is prime [20, 21]. The limit of ratios of successive Perrin numbers

$$\psi = \lim_{n \to \infty} \frac{g_{n+1}}{g_n}$$

satisfies $\psi^3 - \psi - 1 = 0$ and is given by

$$\psi = \left(\tfrac{1}{2} + \tfrac{\sqrt{69}}{18}\right)^{\frac{1}{3}} + \tfrac{1}{3}\left(\tfrac{1}{2} + \tfrac{\sqrt{69}}{18}\right)^{-\frac{1}{3}} = \tfrac{2\sqrt{3}}{3}\cos\left(\tfrac{1}{3}\arccos\left(\tfrac{3\sqrt{3}}{2}\right)\right)$$
$$= 1.3247179572\ldots.$$

This also has the radical expansion

$$\psi = \sqrt[3]{1 + \sqrt[3]{1 + \sqrt[3]{1 + \sqrt[3]{1 + \sqrt[3]{1 + \cdots}}}}}.$$

An amusing account of ψ is given in [20], where it is referred to as the Plastic constant (to contrast against the Golden constant). See also [2.30].

The so-called **Tribonacci sequence** [22, 23]

$$h_0 = 0, \qquad h_1 = 0, \qquad h_2 = 1, \qquad h_n = h_{n-1} + h_{n-2} + h_{n-3} \qquad \text{for } n \geq 3$$

has an analogous limiting ratio

$$\chi = \left(\tfrac{19}{27} + \tfrac{\sqrt{33}}{9}\right)^{\frac{1}{3}} + \tfrac{4}{9}\left(\tfrac{19}{27} + \tfrac{\sqrt{33}}{9}\right)^{-\frac{1}{3}} + \tfrac{1}{3} = \tfrac{4}{3}\cos\left(\tfrac{1}{3}\arccos\left(\tfrac{19}{8}\right)\right) + \tfrac{1}{3}$$
$$= 1.8392867552\ldots,$$

that is, the real solution of $\chi^3 - \chi^2 - \chi - 1 = 0$. See [1.2.3]. Consider also the **four-numbers game**: Start with a 4-vector (a, b, c, d) of nonnegative real numbers and determine the cyclic absolute differences $(|b - a|, |c - b|, |d - c|, |a - d|)$. Iterate indefinitely. Under most circumstances (e.g., if a, b, c, d are each positive integers), the process terminates with the zero 4-vector after only a finite number of steps. Is this always true? No. It is known [24] that $v = (1, \chi, \chi^2, \chi^3)$ is a counterexample, as well as any positive scalar multiple of v, or linear combination with the 4-vector $(1, 1, 1, 1)$. Also, $w = (\chi^3, \chi^2 + \chi, \chi^2, 0)$ is a counterexample, as well as any positive scalar multiple of w, or linear combination with the 4-vector $(1, 1, 1, 1)$. These encompass all the possible exceptions. Note that, starting with w, one obtains v after one step.

1.2.3 Generalized Continued Fractions

Recall from [1.1.1] that generalized continued fractions are constructed via the replacement rule

$$p \to p + \frac{1}{q}, \qquad q \to q + \frac{p}{q}$$

applied to each new term in a particular generation. In particular, if $p = q = 1$, the partial convergents are equal to ratios of successive terms of the Tribonacci sequence, and hence converge to χ. By way of contrast, the replacement rule [25, 26]

$$r \to r + \cfrac{1}{r + \cfrac{1}{r}}$$

is associated with a root of $x^3 - rx^2 - r = 0$. If $r = 1$, the limiting value is

$$\left(\frac{29}{54} + \frac{\sqrt{93}}{18}\right)^{\frac{1}{3}} + \frac{1}{9}\left(\frac{29}{54} + \frac{\sqrt{93}}{18}\right)^{-\frac{1}{3}} + \frac{1}{3} = \frac{2}{3}\cos\left(\frac{1}{3}\arccos\left(\frac{29}{2}\right)\right) + \frac{1}{3}$$
$$= 1.4655712318\ldots.$$

Other higher-order analogs of the Golden mean are offered in [27–29].

1.2.4 Random Fibonacci Sequences

Consider the sequence of random variables

$$x_0 = 1, \qquad x_1 = 1, \qquad x_n = \pm x_{n-1} \pm x_{n-2} \quad \text{for } n \geq 2,$$

where the signs are equiprobable and independent. Viswanath [30–32] proved the surprising result that

$$\lim_{n\to\infty} \sqrt[n]{|x_n|} = 1.13198824\ldots$$

with probability 1. Embree & Trefethen [33] proved that generalized random linear recurrences of the form

$$x_n = x_{n-1} \pm \beta x_{n-2}$$

decay exponentially with probability 1 if $0 < \beta < 0.70258\ldots$ and grow exponentially with probability 1 if $\beta > 0.70258\ldots.$

1.2.5 Fibonacci Factorials

We mention the asymptotic result $\prod_{k=1}^{n} f_k \sim c \cdot \varphi^{n(n+1)/2} \cdot 5^{-n/2}$ as $n \to \infty$, where [34, 35]

$$c = \prod_{n=1}^{\infty}\left(1 - \frac{(-1)^n}{\varphi^{2n}}\right) = 1.2267420107\ldots.$$

See the related expression in [5.14].

[1] H. E. Huntley, *The Divine Proportion: A Study in Mathematical Beauty*, Dover, 1970.
[2] G. Markowsky, Misconceptions about the Golden ratio, *College Math. J.* 23 (1992) 2–19.
[3] S. Vajda, *Fibonacci and Lucas numbers, and the Golden Section: Theory and Applications*, Halsted Press, 1989; MR 90h:11014.
[4] C. S. Ogilvy, *Excursions in Geometry*, Dover, 1969, pp. 122–134.
[5] E. Maor, *e: The Story of a Number*, Princeton Univ. Press, 1994, pp. 121–125, 134–139, 205–207; MR 95a:01002.
[6] J. D. Lawrence, *A Catalog of Special Plane Curves*, Dover, 1972, pp. 184–186.
[7] R. Honsberger, *More Mathematical Morsels*, Math. Assoc. Amer., 1991, pp. 140–144.
[8] J. Shallit, A simple proof that phi is irrational, *Fibonacci Quart.* 13 (1975) 32, 198.
[9] G. H. Hardy and E. M. Wright, *An Introduction to the Theory of Numbers*, 5th ed., Oxford Univ. Press, 1985, pp. 44–45, 290–295; MR 81i:10002.

[10] G. E. Andrews, R. Askey, and R. Roy, *Special Functions*, Cambridge Univ. Press, 1999, p. 58, ex. 52; MR 2000g:33001.

[11] R. Honsberger, *Mathematical Gems III*, Math. Assoc. Amer., 1985, pp. 102–138.

[12] K. G. Ramanathan, On Ramanujan's continued fraction, *Acta Arith.* 43 (1984) 209–226; MR 85d:11012.

[13] J. M. Borwein and P. B. Borwein, *Pi and the AGM: A Study in Analytic Number Theory and Computational Complexity*, Wiley, 1987, pp. 78–81; MR 99h:11147.

[14] B. C. Berndt, H. H. Chan, S.-S. Huang, S.-Y. Kang, J. Sohn, and S. H. Son, The Rogers-Ramanujan continued fraction, *J. Comput. Appl. Math.* 105 (1999) 9–24; MR 2000b:11009.

[15] H. H. Chan and V. Tan, On the explicit evaluations of the Rogers-Ramanujan continued fraction, *Continued Fractions: From Analytic Number Theory to Constructive Approximation*, Proc. 1998 Univ. of Missouri conf., ed. B. C. Berndt and F. Gesztesy, Amer. Math. Soc., 1999, pp. 127–136; MR 2000e:11161.

[16] S.-Y. Kang, Ramanujan's formulas for the explicit evaluation of the Rogers-Ramanujan continued fraction and theta-functions, *Acta Arith.* 90 (1999) 49–68; MR 2000f:11047.

[17] R. B. Paris, An asymptotic approximation connected with the Golden number, *Amer. Math. Monthly* 94 (1987) 272–278; MR 88d:39014.

[18] S. Plouffe, The Paris constant (Plouffe's Tables).

[19] J. M. Borwein and G. de Barra, Nested radicals, *Amer. Math. Monthly* 98 (1991) 735–739; MR 92i:11011.

[20] I. Stewart, Tales of a neglected number, *Sci. Amer.*, v. 274 (1996) n. 7, 102–103; v. 275 (1996) n. 11, 118.

[21] K. S. Brown, Perrin's sequence (MathPages).

[22] S. Plouffe, The Tribonacci constant (Plouffe's Tables).

[23] N. J. A. Sloane, On-Line Encyclopedia of Integer Sequences, A000073.

[24] E. R. Berlekamp, The design of slowly shrinking labelled squares, *Math. Comp.* 29 (1975) 25–27; MR 51 #10133.

[25] G. A. Moore, A Fibonacci polynomial sequence defined by multidimensional continued fractions and higher-order golden ratios, *Fibonacci Quart.* 31 (1993) 354–364; MR 94g:11014.

[26] G. A. Moore, The limit of the golden numbers is 3/2, *Fibonacci Quart.* 32 (1994) 211–217; MR 95f:11008.

[27] P. G. Anderson, Multidimensional Golden means, *Applications of Fibonacci Numbers*, v. 5, Proc. 1992 St. Andrews conf., ed. G. E. Bergum, A. N. Philippou, and A. F. Horadam, Kluwer, 1993, pp. 1–9; MR 95a:11004.

[28] E. I. Korkina, The simplest 2-dimensional continued fraction (in Russian), *Itogi Nauki Tekh. Ser. Sovrem. Mat. Prilozh. Temat. Obz.*, v. 20, *Topologiya*-3, 1994; Engl. transl. in *J. Math. Sci.* 82 (1996) 3680–3685; MR 97j:11032.

[29] E. I. Korkina, Two-dimensional continued fractions: The simplest examples, *Singularities of Smooth Mappings with Additional Structures* (in Russian), ed. V. I. Arnold, *Trudy Mat. Inst. Steklov.* 209 (1995) 143–166; Engl. transl. in *Proc. Steklov Inst. Math.* 209 (1995) 124–144; MR 97k:11104.

[30] D. Viswanath, Random Fibonacci sequences and the number 1.13198824..., *Math. Comp.* 69 (2000) 1131–1155; MR 2000j:15040.

[31] B. Hayes, The Vibonacci numbers, *Amer. Scientist,* v. 87 (1999) n. 4, 296–301.

[32] I. Peterson, Fibonacci at random: Uncovering a new mathematical constant, *Science News* 155 (1999) 376.

[33] M. Embree and L. N. Trefethen, Growth and decay of random Fibonacci sequences, *Proc. Royal Soc. London A* 455 (1999) 2471–2485; MR 2001i:11098.

[34] R. L. Graham, D. E. Knuth, and O. Patashnik, *Concrete Mathematics*, Addison-Wesley, 1989, pp. 478, 571; MR 97d:68003.

[35] S. Plouffe, The Fibonacci factorial constant (Plouffe's Tables).

[36] *The Fibonacci Quarterly* (virtually any issue).

1.3 The Natural Logarithmic Base, e

It is not known who first determined

$$\lim_{x \to 0} (1 + x)^{\frac{1}{x}} = e = 2.7182818284\ldots.$$

We see in this limit the outcome of a fierce tug-of-war. On the one side, the exponent explodes to infinity. On the other side, $1 + x$ rushes toward the multiplicative identity 1. It is interesting that the additive equivalent of this limit

$$\lim_{x \to 0} x \cdot \frac{1}{x} = 1$$

is trivial. A geometric characterization of e is as follows: e is the unique positive root x of the equation

$$\int_{1}^{x} \frac{1}{u} du = 1,$$

which is responsible for e being employed as the natural logarithmic base. In words, e is the unique positive number exceeding 1 for which the planar region bounded by the curves $v = 1/u$, $v = 0$, $u = 1$, and $u = e$ has unit area.

The definition of e implies that

$$\frac{d}{dx} (c \cdot e^x) = c \cdot e^x$$

and, further, that any solution of the first-order differential equation

$$\frac{dy}{dx} = y(x)$$

must be of this form. Applications include problems in population growth and radioactive decay. Solutions of the second-order differential equation

$$\frac{d^2 y}{dx^2} = y(x)$$

are necessarily of the form $y(x) = a \cdot e^x + b \cdot e^{-x}$. The special case $y(x) = \cosh(x)$ (i.e., $a = b = 1/2$) is called a catenary and is the shape assumed by a certain uniform flexible cable hanging under its own weight. Moreover, if one revolves part of a catenary around the x-axis, the resulting surface area is smaller than that of any other curve with the same endpoints [1,2].

The series

$$e = \sum_{k=0}^{\infty} \frac{1}{k!} = 1 + \frac{1}{1} + \frac{1}{1 \cdot 2} + \frac{1}{1 \cdot 2 \cdot 3} + \cdots$$

is rapidly convergent – ordinary summation of the terms as listed is very quick for all practical purposes – so it may be surprising to learn that a more efficient means for computing the nth partial sum is possible [3,4]. Define two functions $p(a, b)$ and

$q(a, b)$ recursively as follows:

$$\begin{pmatrix} p(a, b) \\ q(a, b) \end{pmatrix} = \begin{cases} \begin{pmatrix} 1 \\ b \end{pmatrix} & \text{if } b = a + 1, \\ \begin{pmatrix} p(a, m)q(m, b) + p(m, b) \\ q(a, m)q(m, b) \end{pmatrix} & \text{otherwise, where} \\ & m = \left\lfloor \frac{a+b}{2} \right\rfloor. \end{cases}$$

Then it is not difficult to show that $1 + p(0, n)/q(0, n)$ gives the desired partial sum. Such a **binary splitting** approach to computing e has fewer single-digit arithmetic operations (i.e., reduced bit complexity) than the usual approach. Accelerated methods like this grew out of [5–7]. When coupled with FFT-based integer multiplication, this algorithm is asymptotically as fast as any known.

The factorial series gives the following matching problem solution [8]. Let $P(n)$ denote the probability that a randomly chosen one-to-one function $f : \{1, 2, 3, \ldots, n\} \to \{1, 2, 3, \ldots, n\}$ has at least one fixed point; that is, at least one integer k for which $f(k) = k$, $1 \le k \le n$. Then

$$\lim_{n \to \infty} P(n) = \sum_{k=1}^{\infty} \frac{(-1)^k}{k!} = 1 - \frac{1}{e} = 0.6321205588\ldots.$$

See Figure 1.3; a generalization appears in [5.4]. Also, let $X_1, X_2, X_3, \ldots$ be independent random variables, each uniformly distributed on the interval $[0, 1]$. Define an integer N by

$$N = \min \left\{ n : \sum_{k=1}^{n} X_k > 1 \right\};$$

then the expected value $E(N) = e$. In the language of stochastics, a renewal process with uniform interarrival times X_k has a mean renewal count involving the natural logarithmic base [9].

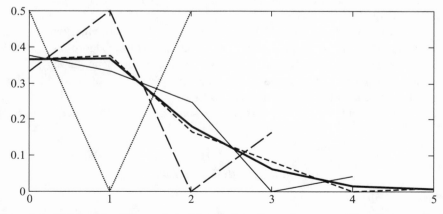

Figure 1.3. Distribution of the number of fixed points of a random permutation f on n symbols, tending to Poisson(1) as $n \to \infty$.

Break a stick of length r into m equal parts [10]. The integer m such that the product of the lengths of the parts is maximized is $\lfloor r/e \rfloor$ or $\lfloor r/e \rfloor + 1$. See [5.15] for information on a related application known as the secretary problem.

There are several Wallis-like infinite products [4, 11]

$$e = \frac{2}{1} \cdot \left(\frac{4}{3}\right)^{\frac{1}{2}} \cdot \left(\frac{6 \cdot 8}{5 \cdot 7}\right)^{\frac{1}{4}} \cdot \left(\frac{10 \cdot 12 \cdot 14 \cdot 16}{9 \cdot 11 \cdot 13 \cdot 15}\right)^{\frac{1}{8}} \cdots,$$

$$\frac{e}{2} = \left(\frac{2}{1}\right)^{\frac{1}{2}} \cdot \left(\frac{2 \cdot 4}{3 \cdot 3}\right)^{\frac{1}{4}} \cdot \left(\frac{4 \cdot 6 \cdot 6 \cdot 8}{5 \cdot 5 \cdot 7 \cdot 7}\right)^{\frac{1}{8}} \cdots$$

and continued fractions [1.3.2] as well as the following fascinating connection to prime number theory [12]. If we define

$$n? = \prod_{\substack{p \leq n \\ p \text{ prime}}} p, \qquad \text{then} \qquad \lim_{n \to \infty} (n?)^{\frac{1}{n}} = e,$$

which is a consequence of the Prime Number Theorem. Equally fascinating is the fact that

$$\lim_{n \to \infty} \frac{(n!)^{\frac{1}{n}}}{n} = \frac{1}{e}$$

by Stirling's formula; thus the growth of $n!$ exceeds that of $n?$ by an order of magnitude. We also have [13–15]

$$\lim_{n \to \infty} (n!)^{\frac{1}{n}} - ((n-1)!)^{\frac{1}{n-1}} = \frac{1}{e}, \qquad \lim_{n \to \infty} \prod_{k=1}^{n} (n^2 + k)(n^2 - k)^{-1} = e.$$

The irrationality of e was proved by Euler and its transcendence by Hermite; that is, the natural logarithmic base e cannot be a zero of a polynomial with integer coefficients [4, 16–18].

An unusual procedure for calculating e, known as the spigot algorithm, was first publicized in [19]. Here the intrigue lies not in the speed of the algorithm (it is slow) but in other characteristics: It is entirely based on integer arithmetic, for example.

Some people call e *Euler's constant*, but the same phrase is so often used to refer to the Euler–Mascheroni constant γ that confusion would be inevitable. Napier came very close to discovering e in 1614; consequently, some people call e *Napier's constant* [1].

1.3.1 Analysis of a Limit

The Maclaurin series

$$\frac{1}{e}(1 + x)^{\frac{1}{x}} = 1 - \frac{1}{2}x + \frac{11}{24}x^2 - \frac{7}{16}x^3 + \frac{2447}{5760}x^4 - \frac{959}{2304}x^5 + O(x^6)$$

describes more fully what happens in the limiting definition of e; for example,

$$\lim_{x \to 0} \frac{(1+x)^{\frac{1}{x}} - e}{x} = -\frac{1}{2}e, \qquad \lim_{x \to 0} \frac{\frac{(1+x)^{\frac{1}{x}} - e}{x} + \frac{1}{2}e}{x} = \frac{11}{24}e.$$

Quicker convergence is obtained by the formulas [20–24]:

$$\lim_{x \to 0} \left(\frac{2+x}{2-x} \right)^{\frac{1}{x}} = e, \qquad \lim_{n \to \infty} \frac{(n+1)^{n+1}}{n^n} - \frac{n^n}{(n-1)^{n-1}} = e.$$

To illustrate, the first terms in the corresponding asymptotic expansions are $1 + x^2/12$ and $1 + 1/(24n^2)$. Further improvements are possible.

1.3.2 Continued Fractions

The regular continued fraction for e,

$$e = 2 + \frac{1|}{|1} + \frac{1|}{|2} + \frac{1|}{|1} + \frac{1|}{|1} + \frac{1|}{|4} + \frac{1|}{|1} + \frac{1|}{|1} + \frac{1|}{|6} + \frac{1|}{|1} + \cdots,$$

is (after suitable transformation) one of a family of continued fractions [25–28]:

$$\coth\left(\frac{1}{m}\right) = \frac{e^{2/m} + 1}{e^{2/m} - 1} = m + \frac{1|}{|3m} + \frac{1|}{|5m} + \frac{1|}{|7m} + \frac{1|}{|9m} + \cdots,$$

where m is any positive integer. Davison [29] obtained an algorithm for computing quotients of $\coth(3/2)$ and $\coth(2)$, for example, but no patterns can be found. Other continued fractions include [1, 26, 30, 31]

$$e - 1 = 1 + \frac{2|}{|2} + \frac{3|}{|3} + \frac{4|}{|4} + \frac{5|}{|5} + \cdots, \qquad \frac{1}{e-2} = 1 + \frac{1|}{|2} + \frac{2|}{|3} + \frac{3|}{|4} + \frac{4|}{|5} + \cdots,$$

and still more can be found in [32, 33].

1.3.3 The Logarithm of Two

Finally, let us say a few words [34] about the closely related constant $\ln(2)$,

$$\ln(2) = \int_0^1 \frac{1}{1+t} dt = \lim_{n \to \infty} \sum_{k=1}^{n} \frac{1}{n+k} = 0.6931471805\ldots,$$

which has limiting expressions similar to that for e:

$$\lim_{x \to 0} \frac{2^x - 1}{x} = \ln(2) = \lim_{x \to 0} \frac{2^x - 2^{-x}}{2x}.$$

Well-known summations include the Maclaurin series for $\ln(1 + x)$ evaluated at $x = 1$ and $x = -1/2$,

$$\ln(2) = \sum_{k=1}^{\infty} \frac{(-1)^{k-1}}{k} = \sum_{k=1}^{\infty} \frac{1}{k2^k}.$$

A binary digit extraction algorithm can be based on the series

$$\ln(2) = \sum_{k=1}^{\infty} \left(\frac{1}{8k+8} + \frac{1}{4k+2} \right) \frac{1}{4^k},$$

which enables us to calculate the dth bit of $\ln(2)$ without being forced to calculate all the preceding $d - 1$ bits. See also [2.1], [6.2], and [7.2].

[1]   E. Maor, *e: The Story of a Number*, Princeton Univ. Press, 1994; MR 95a:01002.
[2]   G. F. Simmons, *Differential Equations with Applications and Historical Notes*, McGraw-Hill, 1972, pp. 14–19, 52–54, 361–363; MR 58 #17258.
[3]   X. Gourdon and P. Sebah, Binary splitting method (Numbers, Constants and Computation).
[4]   J. M. Borwein and P. B. Borwein, *Pi and the AGM: A Study in Analytic Number Theory and Computational Complexity*, Wiley, 1987, pp. 329–300, 343, 347–362; MR 99h: 11147.
[5]   R. P. Brent, The complexity of multiple-precision arithmetic, *Complexity of Computational Problem Solving*, Proc. 1974 Austral. Nat. Univ. conf., ed. R. S. Anderssen and R. P. Brent, Univ. of Queensland Press, 1976, pp. 126–165.
[6]   R. P. Brent, Fast multiple-precision evaluation of elementary functions, *J. ACM* 23 (1976) 242–251; MR 52 #16111.
[7]   E. A. Karatsuba, Fast evaluation of transcendental functions (in Russian), *Problemy Peredachi Informatsii* 27 (1991) 76–99; Engl. transl. in *Problems Information Transmission* 27 (1991) 339–360; MR 93c:65027.
[8]   M. H. DeGroot, *Probability and Statistics*, Addison-Wesley, 1975, pp. 36–37.
[9]   W. Feller, On the integral equation of renewal theory, *Annals of Math. Statist.* 12 (1941) 243–267; MR 3,151c.
[10] N. Shklov and C. E. Miller, Maximizing a certain product, *Amer. Math. Monthly* 61 (1954) 196–197.
[11] I. S. Gradshteyn and I. M. Ryzhik, *Table of Integrals, Series and Products*, Academic Press, 1980, p. 12; MR 97c:00014.
[12] T. Nagell, *Introduction to Number Theory*, Chelsea, 1981, pp. 38, 60–64; MR 30 #4714.
[13] J. Sandor, On the gamma function. II, *Publ. Centre Rech. Math. Pures* 28 (1997) 10–12.
[14] G. Pólya and G. Szegö, *Problems and Theorems in Analysis*, v. 1, Springer-Verlag, 1972, ex. 55; MR 81e:00002.
[15] Z. Sasvári and W. F. Trench, A Pólya-Szegö exercise revisited, *Amer. Math. Monthly* 106 (1999) 781–782.
[16] J. A. Nathan, The irrationality of exp(x) for nonzero rational x, *Amer. Math. Monthly* 105 (1998) 762–763; MR 99e:11096.
[17] G. H. Hardy and E. M. Wright, *An Introduction to the Theory of Numbers*, 5th ed., Oxford Univ. Press, 1985, pp. 46–47; MR 81i:10002.
[18] I. N. Herstein, *Topics in Algebra*, 2nd ed., Wiley, 1975, pp. 216–219; MR 50 #9456.
[19] A. H. J. Sale, The calculation of e to many significant digits, *Computer J.* 11 (1968) 229–230.
[20] L. F. Richardson and J. A. Gaunt, The deferred approach to the limit, *Philos. Trans. Royal Soc. London Ser. A* 226 (1927) 299–361.
[21] H. J. Brothers and J. A. Knox, New closed-form approximations to the logarithmic constant e, *Math. Intellig.*, v. 20 (1998) n. 4, 25–29; MR 2000c:11209.
[22] J. A. Knox and H. J. Brothers, Novel series-based approximations to e, *College Math. J.* 30 (1999) 269–275; MR 2000i:11198.
[23] J. Sandor, On certain limits related to the number e, *Libertas Math.* 20 (2000) 155–159; MR 2001k:26034.
[24] X. Gourdon and P. Sebah, The constant e (Numbers, Constants and Computation).

[25] L. Euler, De fractionibus continuis dissertatio, 1744, *Opera Omnia Ser. I*, v. 14, Lipsiae, 1911, pp. 187–215; Engl. transl. in *Math. Systems Theory* 18 (1985) 295–328; MR 87d:01011b.

[26] L. Lorentzen and H. Waadeland, *Continued Fractions with Applications*, North-Holland, 1992, pp. 561–562; MR 93g:30007.

[27] P. Ribenboim, *My Numbers, My Friends*, Springer-Verlag, 2000, pp. 292–294; MR 2002d:11001.

[28] C. D. Olds, The simple continued fraction expansion of *e*, *Amer. Math. Monthly* 77 (1970) 968–974.

[29] J. L. Davison, An algorithm for the continued fraction of $e^{l/m}$, *Proc. 8th Manitoba Conf. on Numerical Mathematics and Computing*, Winnipeg, 1978, ed. D. McCarthy and H. C. Williams, Congr. Numer. 22, Utilitas Math., 1979, pp. 169–179; MR 80j:10012.

[30] L. Euler, *Introduction to Analysis of the Infinite. Book I*, 1748, transl. J. D. Blanton, Springer-Verlag, 1988, pp. 303–314; MR 89g:01067.

[31] H. Darmon and J. McKay, A continued fraction and permutations with fixed points, *Amer. Math. Monthly* 98 (1991) 25–27; MR 92a:05003.

[32] J. Minkus and J. Anglesio, A continued fraction, *Amer. Math. Monthly* 103 (1996) 605–606.

[33] M. J. Knight and W. O. Egerland, $F_n = (n+2)F_{n-1} - (n-1)F_{n-2}$, *Amer. Math. Monthly* 81 (1974) 675–676.

[34] X. Gourdon and P. Sebah, The logarithm constant log(2) (Numbers, Constants and Computation).

1.4 Archimedes' Constant, π

Any brief treatment of π, the most famous of the transcendental constants, is necessarily incomplete [1–5]. Its innumerable appearances throughout mathematics stagger the mind.

The area enclosed by a circle of radius 1 is

$$A = \pi = 4 \int_0^1 \sqrt{1 - x^2}\,dx = \lim_{n \to \infty} \frac{4}{n^2} \sum_{k=0}^n \sqrt{n^2 - k^2} = 3.1415926535\ldots$$

while its circumference is

$$C = 2\pi = 4 \int_0^1 \frac{1}{\sqrt{1 - x^2}}\,dx = 4 \int_0^1 \sqrt{1 + \left(\frac{d}{dx}\sqrt{1 - x^2}\right)^2}\,dx.$$

The formula for A is based on the definition of area in terms of a Riemann integral, that is, a limit of Riemann sums. The formula for C uses the definition of arclength, given a continuously differentiable curve. How is it that the same mysterious π appears in both formulas? A simple integration by parts provides the answer, with no trigonometry required [6].

In the third century B.C., Archimedes considered inscribed and circumscribed regular polygons of 96 sides and deduced that $3\frac{10}{71} < \pi < 3\frac{1}{7}$. The recursion

$$a_0 = 2\sqrt{3}, \qquad b_0 = 3,$$
$$a_{n+1} = \frac{2a_n b_n}{a_n + b_n}, \qquad b_{n+1} = \sqrt{a_{n+1} b_n} \qquad \text{for } n \geq 0$$

(often called the Borchardt–Pfaff algorithm) essentially gives Archimedes' estimate on the fourth iteration [7–11]. It is only linearly convergent (meaning that the number of iterations is roughly proportional to the number of correct digits). It resembles the arithmetic-geometric-mean (AGM) recursion discussed with regard to Gauss' lemniscate constant [6.1].

The utility of π is not restricted to planar geometry. The volume enclosed by a sphere of radius 1 in n-dimensional Euclidean space is

$$
V = \begin{cases}
\dfrac{\pi^k}{k!} & \text{if } n = 2k, \\[2ex]
2^{2k+1}\dfrac{k!}{(2k+1)!}\pi^k & \text{if } n = 2k+1,
\end{cases}
$$

while its surface area is

$$
S = \begin{cases}
\dfrac{2\pi^k}{(k-1)!} & \text{if } n = 2k, \\[2ex]
2^{2k+1}\dfrac{k!}{(2k)!}\pi^k & \text{if } n = 2k+1.
\end{cases}
$$

These formulas are often expressed in terms of the gamma function, which we discuss in [1.5.4]. The planar case (a circle) corresponds to $n = 2$.

Another connection between geometry and π arises in Buffon's needle problem [1, 12–15]. Suppose a needle of length 1 is thrown at random on a plane marked by parallel lines of distance 1 apart. What is the probability that the needle will intersect one of the lines? The answer is $2/\pi = 0.6366197723\ldots$.

Here is a completely different probabilistic interpretation [16, 17] of π. Suppose two integers are chosen at random. What is the probability that they are coprime, that is, have no common factor exceeding 1? The answer is $6/\pi^2 = 0.6079271018\ldots$ (in the limit over large intervals). Equivalently, let $R(N)$ be the number of *distinct* rational numbers a/b with integers a, b satisfying $0 < a, b < N$. The total number of ordered pairs (a, b) is N^2, but $R(N)$ is strictly less than this since many fractions are not in lowest terms. More precisely, by preceding statements, $R(N) \sim 6N^2/\pi^2$.

Among the most famous limits in mathematics is Stirling's formula [18]:

$$
\lim_{n \to \infty} \frac{n!}{e^{-n}n^{n+1/2}} = \sqrt{2\pi} = 2.5066282746\ldots .
$$

Archimedes' constant has many other representations too, some of which are given later. It was proved to be irrational by Lambert and transcendental by Lindemann [2, 16, 19]. The first truly attractive formula for computing decimal digits of π was found by Machin [1, 13]:

$$
\frac{\pi}{4} = 4\arctan\left(\frac{1}{5}\right) - \arctan\left(\frac{1}{239}\right)
$$

$$
= 4\sum_{k=0}^{\infty} \frac{(-1)^k}{(2k+1)\cdot 5^{2k+1}} - \sum_{k=0}^{\infty} \frac{(-1)^k}{(2k+1)\cdot 239^{2k+1}} .
$$

The advantage of this formula is that the second term converges very rapidly and the first is nice for decimal arithmetic. In 1706, Machin became the first individual to correctly compute 100 digits of π.

We skip over many years of history and discuss one other significant algorithm due to Salamin and Brent [2, 20–23]. Define a recursion by

$$a_0 = 1, \qquad b_0 = 1/\sqrt{2}, \qquad c_0 = 1/2, \qquad s_0 = 1/2,$$

$$a_{n+1} = \frac{a_n + b_n}{2}, \quad b_{n+1} = \sqrt{a_n b_n}, \quad c_{n+1} = \left(\frac{c_n}{4a_{n+1}}\right)^2, \quad s_{n+1} = s_n - 2^{n+1}c_{n+1}$$

for $n \geq 0$. Then the ratio $2a_n^2/s_n$ converges quadratically to π (meaning that each iteration approximately doubles the number of correct digits). Even faster cubic and quartic algorithms were obtained by Borwein & Borwein [2, 22, 24, 25]; these draw upon Ramanujan's work on modular equations. These are each a far cry computationally from Archimedes' approach. Using techniques like these, Kanada computed close to a trillion digits of π.

There is a spigot algorithm for calculating π just as for e [26]. Far more important, however, is the digit-extraction algorithm discovered by Bailey, Borwein & Plouffe [27–29] based on the formula

$$\pi = \sum_{k=0}^{\infty} \frac{1}{16^k}$$
$$\times \left(\frac{4 + 8r}{8k + 1} - \frac{8r}{8k + 2} - \frac{4r}{8k + 3} - \frac{2 + 8r}{8k + 4} - \frac{1 + 2r}{8k + 5} - \frac{1 + 2r}{8k + 6} + \frac{r}{8k + 7}\right)$$

(for $r = 0$) and requiring virtually no memory. (The extension to complex $r \neq 0$ is due to Adamchik & Wagon [30, 31].) A consequence of this breakthrough is that we now know the quadrillionth digit in the binary expansion for π, thanks largely to Bellard and Percival. An analogous base-3 formula was found by Broadhurst [32].

Some people call π *Ludolph's constant* after the mathematician Ludolph van Ceulen who devoted most of his life to computing π to 35 decimal places.

The formulas in this essay have a qualitatively different character than those for the natural logarithmic base e. Wimp [33] elaborated on this: What he called "e-mathematics" is linear, explicit, and easily capable of abstraction, whereas "π-mathematics" is nonlinear, mysterious, and generalized usually with difficulty. Cloitre [34], however, gave formulas suggesting a certain symmetry between e and π: If $u_1 = v_1 = 0$, $u_2 = v_2 = 1$ and

$$u_{n+2} = u_{n+1} + \frac{u_n}{n}, \quad v_{n+2} = \frac{v_{n+1}}{n} + v_n, \quad n \geq 0,$$

then $\lim_{n \to \infty} n/u_n = e$ whereas $\lim_{n \to \infty} 2n/v_n^2 = \pi$.

1.4.1 Infinite Series

Over five hundred years ago, the Indian mathematician Madhava discovered the formula [35–38]

$$\frac{\pi}{4} = \sum_{n=0}^{\infty} \frac{(-1)^n}{2n+1} = 1 - \frac{1}{3} + \frac{1}{5} - \frac{1}{7} + \frac{1}{9} - \frac{1}{11} + - \cdots,$$

which was independently found by Gregory [39] and Leibniz [40]. This infinite series is conditionally convergent; hence its terms may be rearranged to produce a series that has any desired sum or even diverges to $+\infty$ or $-\infty$. The same is also true for the alternating harmonic series [1.3.3]. For example, we have

$$\frac{1}{4}\ln(2) + \frac{\pi}{4} = 1 + \frac{1}{5} - \frac{1}{3} + \frac{1}{9} + \frac{1}{13} - \frac{1}{7} + \frac{1}{17} + \frac{1}{21} - \frac{1}{11} + + - \cdots$$

(two positive terms for each negative term). Generalization is possible.

Changing the pattern of plus and minus signs in the Gregory–Leibniz series, for example, gives [41, 42]

$$\frac{\pi}{4}\sqrt{2} = 1 + \frac{1}{3} - \frac{1}{5} - \frac{1}{7} + \frac{1}{9} + \frac{1}{11} - \frac{1}{13} - \frac{1}{15} + + - - \cdots$$

or extracting a subseries gives [43]

$$\frac{\pi}{8}(1 + \sqrt{2}) = 1 - \frac{1}{7} + \frac{1}{9} - \frac{1}{15} + \frac{1}{17} - \frac{1}{23} + \frac{1}{25} - \frac{1}{31} + - \cdots.$$

We defer discussion of Euler's famous series

$$\sum_{n=1}^{\infty} \frac{1}{n^2} = \frac{\pi^2}{6}, \qquad \sum_{n=1}^{\infty} \frac{(-1)^{n+1}}{(2n-1)^3} = \frac{\pi^3}{32}$$

until [1.6] and [1.7]. Among many other series of his, there is [1, 44]

$$\frac{\pi}{2} = \sum_{n=0}^{\infty} \frac{2^n}{(2n+1)\binom{2n}{n}} = 1 + \frac{1}{3} + \frac{1 \cdot 2}{3 \cdot 5} + \frac{1 \cdot 2 \cdot 3}{3 \cdot 5 \cdot 7} + \cdots.$$

We note that [2, 45]

$$\sum_{n=1}^{\infty} \frac{1}{n^2 \binom{2n}{n}} = \frac{\pi^2}{18}, \qquad \sum_{n=1}^{\infty} \frac{(-1)^{n+1}}{n^2 \binom{2n}{n}} = 2\ln(\varphi)^2$$

and wonder in what other ways π and the Golden mean φ [1.2] can be so intricately linked.

Ramanujan [23, 24, 46] and Chudnovsky & Chudnovsky [47–50] discovered series at the foundation of some of the fastest known algorithms for computing π.

1.4.2 Infinite Products

Viète [51] gave the first known analytical expression for π:

$$\frac{2}{\pi} = \frac{\sqrt{2}}{2} \cdot \frac{\sqrt{2+\sqrt{2}}}{2} \cdot \frac{\sqrt{2+\sqrt{2+\sqrt{2}}}}{2} \cdot \frac{\sqrt{2+\sqrt{2+\sqrt{2+\sqrt{2}}}}}{2} \cdots,$$

which he obtained by considering a limit of areas of Archimedean polygons, and Wallis [52] derived the formula

$$\frac{\pi}{2} = \frac{2}{1} \cdot \frac{2}{3} \cdot \frac{4}{3} \cdot \frac{4}{5} \cdot \frac{6}{5} \cdot \frac{6}{7} \cdot \frac{8}{7} \cdot \frac{8}{9} \cdots = \lim_{n \to \infty} \frac{2^{4n}}{(2n+1)\binom{2n}{n}^2}.$$

These products are, in fact, children of the same parent [53]. We might prove their truth in many different ways [54]. One line of reasoning involves what some regard as the definition of sine and cosine. The following infinite polynomial factorizations hold [55]:

$$\sin(x) = x \prod_{n=1}^{\infty} \left(1 - \frac{x^2}{n^2\pi^2}\right), \qquad \cos(x) = \prod_{n=1}^{\infty} \left(1 - \frac{4x^2}{(2n-1)^2\pi^2}\right).$$

The sine and cosine functions form the basis for trigonometry and the study of periodic phenomena in mathematics. Applications include the undamped simple oscillations of a mechanical or electrical system, the orbital motion of planets around the sun, and much more [56]. It is well known that

$$\frac{d^2}{dx^2}(a \cdot \sin(x) + b \cdot \cos(x)) + (a \cdot \sin(x) + b \cdot \cos(x)) = 0$$

and, further, that any solution of the second-order differential equation

$$\frac{d^2y}{dx^2} + y(x) = 0$$

must be of this form. The constant π plays the same role in determining sine and cosine as the natural logarithmic base e plays in determining the exponential function. That these two processes are interrelated is captured by Euler's formula $e^{i\pi} + 1 = 0$, where i is the imaginary unit.

Famous products relating π and prime numbers appear in [1.6] and [1.7], as a consequence of the theory of the zeta function. One such product, due to Euler, is [57]

$$\frac{\pi}{2} = \prod_{p \text{ odd}} \frac{p}{p + (-1)^{(p-1)/2}} = \frac{3}{2} \cdot \frac{5}{6} \cdot \frac{7}{6} \cdot \frac{11}{10} \cdot \frac{13}{14} \cdot \frac{17}{18} \cdot \frac{19}{18} \cdots,$$

where the numerators are the odd primes and the denominators are the closest integers of the form $4n + 2$. See also [2.1]. A different appearance of π in number theory is the asymptotic expression

$$p(n) \sim \frac{1}{4\sqrt{3}n} \exp\left(\pi\sqrt{\frac{2n}{3}}\right)$$

due to Hardy & Ramanujan [58], where $p(n)$ is the number of unrestricted partitions of the positive integer n (order being immaterial). Hardy & Ramanujan [58] and Rademacher [59] proved an *exact* analytical formula for $p(n)$ [60, 61], which is too far afield for us to discuss here.

1.4.3 Definite Integrals

The most famous integrals include [62, 63]

$$\int_0^\infty e^{-x^2} dx = \frac{\sqrt{\pi}}{2} \qquad \text{(Gaussian probability density integral),}$$

$$\int_0^\infty \frac{1}{1+x^2} dx = \frac{\pi}{2} \qquad \text{(limiting value of arctangent),}$$

$$\int_0^\infty \sin(x^2) dx = \int_0^\infty \cos(x^2) dx = \frac{\pi\sqrt{2}}{4} \qquad \text{(Fresnel integrals),}$$

$$\int_0^{\frac{\pi}{2}} \ln(\sin(x)) dx = \int_0^{\frac{\pi}{2}} \ln(\cos(x)) dx = -\frac{\pi}{2} \ln(2),$$

$$\int_0^1 \sqrt{\ln\left(\frac{1}{x}\right)} dx = \frac{\sqrt{\pi}}{2}.$$

It is curious that

$$\int_0^\infty \frac{\cos(x)}{1+x^2} dx = \frac{\pi}{2e}, \qquad \int_0^\infty \frac{x \sin(x)}{1+x^2} dx = \frac{\pi}{2e}$$

have simple expressions, but interchanging $\cos(x)$ and $\sin(x)$ give complicated results. See [6.2] for details.

Also, consider the following sequence:

$$s_n = \int_0^\infty \left(\frac{\sin(x)}{x}\right)^n dx, \qquad n = 1, 2, 3, \ldots.$$

The first several values are $s_1 = s_2 = \pi/2$, $s_3 = 3\pi/8$, $s_4 = \pi/3$, $s_5 = 115\pi/384$, and $s_6 = 11\pi/40$. An exact formula for s_n, valid for all n, is found in [64].

1.4.4 Continued Fractions

Starting with Wallis's formula, Brouncker [1, 2, 52] discovered the continued fraction

$$1 + \frac{4}{\pi} = 2 + \frac{1^2|}{|2} + \frac{3^2|}{|2} + \frac{5^2|}{|2} + \frac{7^2|}{|2} + \frac{9^2|}{|2} + \cdots,$$

which was subsequently proved by Euler [41]. It is fascinating to compare this with other related expansions, for example [65–67],

$$\frac{4}{\pi} = 1 + \frac{1^2|}{|3} + \frac{2^2|}{|5} + \frac{3^2|}{|7} + \frac{4^2|}{|9} + \frac{5^2|}{|11} + \cdots,$$

$$\frac{6}{\pi^2 - 6} = 1 + \frac{1^2|}{|1} + \frac{1 \cdot 2|}{|1} + \frac{2^2|}{|1} + \frac{2 \cdot 3|}{|1} + \frac{3^2|}{|1} + \frac{3 \cdot 4|}{|1} + \frac{4^2|}{|1} + \cdots,$$

$$\frac{2}{\pi - 2} = 1 + \frac{1 \cdot 2|}{|1} + \frac{2 \cdot 3|}{|1} + \frac{3 \cdot 4|}{|1} + \frac{4 \cdot 5|}{|1} + \frac{5 \cdot 6|}{|1} + \frac{6 \cdot 7|}{|1} + \cdots,$$

$$\frac{12}{\pi^2} = 1 + \frac{1^4|}{|3} + \frac{2^4|}{|5} + \frac{3^4|}{|7} + \frac{4^4|}{|9} + \frac{5^4|}{|11} + \cdots,$$

$$\pi + 3 = 6 + \frac{1^2|}{|6} + \frac{3^2|}{|6} + \frac{5^2|}{|6} + \frac{7^2|}{|6} + \frac{9^2|}{|6} + \cdots.$$

1.4.5 Infinite Radical

Let S_n denote the length of a side of a regular polygon of 2^{n+1} sides inscribed in a unit circle. Clearly $S_1 = \sqrt{2}$ and, more generally, $S_n = 2\sin(\pi/2^{n+1})$. Hence, by the half-angle formula,

$$S_n = \sqrt{2 - \sqrt{4 - S_{n-1}^2}}.$$

(A purely geometric argument for this recursion is given in [68, 69].) The circumference of the 2^{n+1}-gon is $2^{n+1} S_n$ and tends to 2π as $n \to \infty$. Therefore

$$\pi = \lim_{n \to \infty} 2^n S_n = \lim_{n \to \infty} 2^n \sqrt{2 - \sqrt{2 + \sqrt{2 + \sqrt{2 + \sqrt{2 + \cdots \sqrt{2}}}}}},$$

where the right-hand side has n square roots.

Although attractive, this radical expression for π is numerically sound only for a few iterations. It is a classic illustration of the loss of floating-point precision that occurs when subtracting two nearly equal quantities. There are many ways to approximate π: This is not one of them!

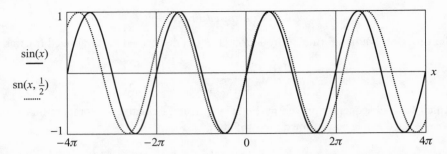

Figure 1.4. The circular function $\sin(x)$ has period $2\pi \approx 6.28$, while the elliptic function $\operatorname{sn}(x, 1/2)$ has (real) period $4K(1/2) \approx 6.74$.

1.4.6 Elliptic Functions

Consider an ellipse with semimajor axis length 1 and semiminor axis length $0 < r \leq 1$. The area enclosed by the ellipse is πr while its circumference is $4E\left(\sqrt{1 - r^2}\right)$, where

$$K(x) = \int_0^{\frac{\pi}{2}} \frac{1}{\sqrt{1 - x^2 \sin(\theta)^2}}\, d\theta = \int_0^1 \frac{1}{\sqrt{(1 - t^2)(1 - x^2 t^2)}}\, dt,$$

$$E(x) = \int_0^{\frac{\pi}{2}} \sqrt{1 - x^2 \sin(\theta)^2}\, d\theta = \int_0^1 \sqrt{\frac{1 - x^2 t^2}{1 - t^2}}\, dt$$

are **complete elliptic integrals** of the first and second kind. (One's first encounter with $K(x)$ is often with regard to computing the period of a physical pendulum [56].) The analog of the sine function is the **Jacobi elliptic function** $\operatorname{sn}(x, y)$, defined by

$$x = \int_0^{\operatorname{sn}(x,y)} \frac{1}{\sqrt{(1 - t^2)(1 - y^2 t^2)}}\, dt \quad \text{for } 0 \leq y \leq 1.$$

See Figure 1.4. Clearly we have $\operatorname{sn}(x, 0) = \sin(x)$ for $-\pi/2 \leq x \leq \pi/2$ and $\operatorname{sn}(x, 1) = \tanh(x)$. An assortment of extended trigonometric identities involving sn and its counterparts cn and dn can be proved. For fixed $0 < y < 1$, the function $\operatorname{sn}(x, y)$ can be analytically continued over the whole complex plane to a doubly periodic meromorphic function. Just as $\sin(z) = \sin(z + 2\pi)$ for all complex z, we have $\operatorname{sn}(z) = \operatorname{sn}\left(z + 4K(y) + 2iK\left(\sqrt{1 - y^2}\right)\right)$. Hence the constants $K(y)$ and $K\left(\sqrt{1 - y^2}\right)$ play roles for elliptic functions analogous to the role π plays for circular functions [2, 70].

1.4.7 Unexpected Appearances

A fascinating number-theoretic function $f(n)$ is described in [71–77]. Take any positive integer n, round it up to the nearest multiple of $n - 1$, then round this result up to the nearest multiple of $n - 2$, and then (more generally) round the kth result up to the nearest multiple of $n - k - 1$. Stop when $k = n - 1$ and let $f(n)$ be the final value. For example, $f(10) = 34$ since

$$10 \to 18 \to 24 \to 28 \to 30 \to 30 \to 32 \to 33 \to 34 \to 34.$$

The ratio $n^2/f(n)$ approaches π as n increases without bound. In the same spirit, Matiyasevich & Guy [78] obtained

$$\pi = \lim_{m \to \infty} \sqrt{\frac{6 \cdot \ln(f_1 \cdot f_2 \cdot f_3 \cdots f_m)}{\ln(\mathrm{lcm}(f_1, f_2, f_3, \ldots, f_m))}},$$

where $f_1, f_2, f_3, \ldots$ is Fibonacci's sequence [1.2] and lcm denotes least common multiple. It turns out that Fibonacci's sequence may be replaced by many other second-order, linear recurring sequences without changing the limiting value π.

In [1.4.1] and [1.4.2], we saw expressions resembling $\binom{2n}{n}/(n+1)$. These are known as **Catalan numbers** and are important in combinatorics, for example, when enumerating strictly binary trees with $2n + 1$ vertices. The average height h_n of such trees satisfies

$$\lim_{n \to \infty} \frac{h_n}{\sqrt{n}} = 2\sqrt{\pi}$$

by a theorem of Flajolet & Odlyzko [79, 80] (we introduce the language of trees in [5.6]). This is yet another unexpected appearance of the constant π.

[1] P. Beckmann, *A History of* π, St. Martin's Press, 1971; MR 56 #8261.
[2] J. M. Borwein and P. B. Borwein, *Pi and the AGM: A Study in Analytic Number Theory and Computational Complexity*, Wiley, 1987, pp. 46–52, 169–177, 337–362, 385–386; MR 99h:11147.
[3] D. Blatner, *The Joy of Pi*, Walker, 1997.
[4] P. Eymard and J.-P. Lafon, *Autour du nombre* π, Hermann, 1999; MR 2001a:11001.
[5] X. Gourdon and P. Sebah, The constant pi (Numbers, Constants and Computation).
[6] E. F. Assmus, Pi, *Amer. Math. Monthly* 92 (1985) 213–214.
[7] Archimedes, Measurement of a circle, 250 BC, in *Pi: A Source Book*, 2nd ed., ed. L. Berggren, J. M. Borwein, and P. B. Borwein, Springer-Verlag, 2000, pp. 7–14; MR 98f:01001.
[8] O. Toeplitz, *The Calculus: A Genetic Approach*, Univ. of Chicago Press, 1981, pp. 18–22; MR 11,584e.
[9] G. M. Phillips, Archimedes the numerical analyst, *Amer. Math. Monthly* 88 (1981) 165-169; also in *Pi: A Source Book*, pp. 15–19; MR 83e:01005.
[10] G. Miel, Of calculations past and present: The Archimedean algorithm, *Amer. Math. Monthly* 90 (1983) 17–35; MR 85a:01006.
[11] G. M. Phillips, Archimedes and the complex plane, *Amer. Math. Monthly* 91 (1984) 108–114; MR 85h:40003.
[12] S. D. Dubey, Statistical determination of certain mathematical constants and functions using computers, *J. ACM* 13 (1966) 511–525; MR 34 #2149.
[13] H. Dörrie, *100 Great Problems of Elementary Mathematics: Their History and Solution*, Dover, 1965, pp. 73–77; MR 84b:00001.
[14] E. Waymire, Buffon noodles, *Amer. Math. Monthly* 101 (1994) 550–559; addendum 101 (1994) 791; MR 95g:60021a and MR 95g:60021b.
[15] E. Wegert and L. N. Trefethen, From the Buffon needle problem to the Kreiss matrix theorem, *Amer. Math. Monthly* 101 (1994) 132–139; MR 95b:30036.

[16] G. H. Hardy and E. M. Wright, *An Introduction to the Theory of Numbers*, 5th ed., Oxford Univ. Press, 1985, pp. 47, 268–269; MR 81i:10002.
[17] A. M. Yaglom and I. M. Yaglom, *Challenging Mathematical Problems with Elementary Solutions*, v. I, Holden-Day, 1964, ex. 92–93; MR 88m:00012a.
[18] A. E. Taylor and R. Mann, *Advanced Calculus*, 2nd ed., Wiley, 1972, pp. 740–745; MR 83m:26001.
[19] T. Nagell, *Introduction to Number Theory*, Chelsea, 1981, pp. 38, 60–64; MR 30 #4714.
[20] R. P. Brent, Fast multiple-precision evaluation of elementary functions, *J. ACM* 23 (1976) 242–251; MR 52 #16111.
[21] E. Salamin, Computation of π using arithmetic-geometric mean, *Math. Comp.* 30 (1976) 565–570; MR 53 #7928.
[22] D. C. van Leijenhorst, Algorithms for the approximation of π, *Nieuw Arch. Wisk.* 14 (1996) 255–274; MR 98b:11130.
[23] G. Almkvist and B. Berndt, Gauss, Landen, Ramanujan, the arithmetic-geometric mean, ellipses, π, and the Ladies Diary, *Amer. Math. Monthly* 95 (1988) 585–608; MR 89j:01028.
[24] J. M. Borwein, P. B. Borwein, and D. H. Bailey, Ramanujan, modular equations, and approximations to pi, or how to compute one billion digits of pi, *Amer. Math. Monthly* 96 (1989) 201–219; also in *Organic Mathematics*, Proc. 1995 Burnaby workshop, ed. J. Borwein, P. Borwein, L. Jörgenson, and R. Corless, Amer. Math. Soc., 1997, pp. 35–71; MR 90d:11143.
[25] J. M. Borwein and F. G. Garvan, Approximations to pi via the Dedekind eta function, *Organic Mathematics*, Proc. 1995 Burnaby workshop, Amer. Math. Soc., 1997, pp. 89–115; MR 98j:11030.
[26] S. Rabinowitz and S. Wagon, A spigot algorithm for the digits of π, *Amer. Math. Monthly* 102 (1995) 195–203; MR 96a:11152.
[27] D. Bailey, P. Borwein, and S. Plouffe, On the rapid computation of various polylogarithmic constants, *Math. Comp.* 66 (1997) 903–913; MR 98d:11165.
[28] D. H. Bailey, J. M. Borwein, P. B. Borwein, and S. Plouffe, The quest for pi, *Math. Intellig.* 19 (1997) 50–57; CECM preprint 96:070; MR 98b:01045.
[29] M. D. Hirschhorn, A new formula for π, *Austral. Math. Soc. Gazette* 25 (1998) 82–83; MR 99d:01046.
[30] V. S. Adamchik and S. Wagon, π: A 2000-year-old search changes direction, *Mathematica Educ. Res.* 5 (1996) 11–19.
[31] V. S. Adamchik and S. Wagon, A simple formula for π, *Amer. Math. Monthly* 104 (1997) 852–854; MR 98h:11166.
[32] D. J. Broadhurst, Massive 3-loop Feynman diagrams reducible to SC* primitives of algebras of the sixth root of unity, *Europ. Phys. J. C Part. Fields* 8 (1999) 313–333; hep-th/9803091; MR 2002a:81180.
[33] J. Wimp, Book review of "Pi and the AGM," *SIAM Rev.* 30 (1988) 530–533.
[34] B. Cloitre, *e* and π in a mirror, unpublished note (2002).
[35] Madhava, The power series for arctan and π, 1400, in *Pi: A Source Book*, pp. 45–50.
[36] R. Roy, The discovery of the series formula for π by Leibniz, Gregory and Nilakantha, *Math. Mag.* 63 (1990) 291–306; also in *Pi: A Source Book*, pp. 92–107; MR 92a:01029.
[37] J. M. Borwein, P. B. Borwein, and K. Dilcher, Pi, Euler numbers, and asymptotic expansions, *Amer. Math. Monthly* 96 (1989) 681–687; MR 91c:40002.
[38] G. Almkvist, Many correct digits of π, revisited, *Amer. Math. Monthly* 104 (1997) 351–353; MR 98a:11189.
[39] J. Gregory, correspondence with J. Collins, 1671, in *Pi: A Source Book*, pp. 87–91.
[40] G. W. Leibniz, Schediasma de serierum summis, et seriebus quadraticibus, 1674, in J. M. Child, *The Early Mathematical Manuscripts of Leibniz*, transl. from texts published by C. I. Gerhardt, Open Court Publishing, 1920, pp. 60–61.
[41] L. Euler, *Introduction to Analysis of the Infinite. Book I*, 1748, transl. J. D. Blanton, Springer-Verlag, 1988, pp. 137–153, 311–312; MR 89g:01067.
[42] G. E. Andrews, R. Askey, and R. Roy, *Special Functions*, Cambridge Univ. Press, 1999, p. 58, ex. 52; MR 2000g:33001.

[43] L. B. W. Jolley, *Summation of Series*, 2nd rev. ed., Dover, 1961, pp. 14–17; MR 24 #B511.

[44] M. Beeler, R. W. Gosper, and R. Schroeppel, Series acceleration technique, HAKMEM, MIT AI Memo 239, 1972, item 120.

[45] G. Almkvist and A. Granville, Borwein and Bradley's Apéry-like formulae for $\zeta(4n + 3)$, *Experim. Math.* 8 (1999) 197–203; MR 2000h:11126.

[46] S. Ramanujan, Modular equations and approximations to π, *Quart. J. Math.* 45 (1914) 350–72.

[47] D. V. Chudnovsky and G. V. Chudnovsky, The computation of classical constants, *Proc. Nat. Acad. Sci. USA* 86 (1989) 8178–8182; MR 90m:11206.

[48] D. V. Chudnovsky and G. V. Chudnovsky, Classical constants and functions: Computations and continued fraction expansions, *Number Theory: New York Seminar 1989-1990*, ed. D. V. Chudnovsky, G. V. Chudnovsky, H. Cohn, and M. B. Nathanson, Springer-Verlag, 1991, pp. 13–74; MR 93c:11118.

[49] J. M. Borwein and P. B. Borwein, More Ramanujan-type series for $1/\pi$, *Ramanujan Revisited*, Proc. 1987 Urbana conf., ed. G. E. Andrews, R. A. Askey, B. C. Berndt, K. G. Ramanathan, and R. A. Rankin, Academic Press, 1988, pp. 375–472; MR 89d: 11118.

[50] D. V. Chudnovsky and G. V. Chudnovsky, Approximations and complex multiplication according to Ramanujan, *Ramanujan Revisited*, Proc. 1987 Urbana conf., Academic Press, 1988, pp. 375–472; MR 89f:11099.

[51] F. Viète, Variorum de Rebus Mathematicis Reponsorum Liber VIII, 1593, in *Pi: A Source Book*, pp. 53–56, 690–706.

[52] J. Wallis, Computation of π by successive interpolations, Arithmetica Infinitorum, 1655, in *Pi: A Source Book*, pp. 68–80.

[53] T. J. Osler, The union of Vieta's and Wallis's products for pi, *Amer. Math. Monthly* 106 (1999) 774–776.

[54] A. M. Yaglom and I. M. Yaglom, *Challenging Mathematical Problems with Elementary Solutions*, v. II, Holden-Day, 1967, ex. 139–147; MR 88m:00012b.

[55] J. B. Conway, *Functions of One Complex Variable*, 2nd ed. Springer-Verlag, 1978; MR 80c:30003.

[56] G. F. Simmons, *Differential Equations with Applications and Historical Notes*, McGraw-Hill, 1972, pp. 21–25, 83–86, 93–107; MR 58 #17258.

[57] A. Weil, *Number Theory: An Approach Through History from Hammurapi to Legendre*, Birkhäuser, 1984, p. 266; MR 85c:01004.

[58] G. H. Hardy and S. Ramanujan, Asymptotic formulae in combinatory analysis, *Proc. London Math. Soc.* 17 (1918) 75–115; also in *Collected Papers of G. H. Hardy*, v. 1, Oxford Univ. Press, 1966, pp. 306–339.

[59] H. Rademacher, On the partition function $p(n)$, *Proc. London Math. Soc.* 43 (1937) 241–254.

[60] G. E. Andrews, *The Theory of Partitions*, Addison-Wesley, 1976; MR 99c:11126.

[61] G. Almkvist and H. S. Wilf, On the coefficients in the Hardy-Ramanujan-Rademacher formula for $p(n)$, *J. Number Theory* 50 (1995) 329–334; MR 96e:11129.

[62] I. S. Gradshteyn and I. M. Ryzhik, *Table of Integrals, Series and Products*, 5th ed., Academic Press, 1980, pp. 342, 956; MR 97c:00014.

[63] M. Abramowitz and I. A. Stegun, *Handbook of Mathematical Functions*, Dover, 1972, pp. 78, 230, 302; MR 94b:00012.

[64] R. Butler, On the evaluation of $\int_0^\infty (\sin^m t)/t^m dt$ by the trapezoidal rule, *Amer. Math. Monthly* 67 (1960) 566–569; MR 22 #4841.

[65] L. Lorentzen and H. Waadeland, *Continued Fractions with Applications*, North-Holland, 1992, pp. 561–562; MR 93g:30007.

[66] M. A. Stern, Theorie der Kettenbrüche und ihre Anwendung. III, *J. Reine Angew. Math.* 10 (1833) 241–274.

[67] L. J. Lange, An elegant continued fraction for π, *Amer. Math. Monthly* 106 (1999) 456–458.

[68] R. Courant and H. Robbins, *What is Mathematics?*, Oxford Univ. Press, 1941, pp. 123–125, 299; MR 93k:00002.

[69] G. L. Cohen and A. G. Shannon, John Ward's method for the calculation of pi, *Historia Math.* 8 (1981) 133–144; MR 83d:01021.

[70] G. D. Anderson, M. K. Vamanamurthy, and M. Vuorinen, *Conformal Invariants, Inequalities, and Quasiconformal Maps*, Wiley, 1997, pp. 108–117; MR 98h:30033.

[71] K. Brown, Rounding up to pi (MathPages).

[72] P. Erdös and E. Jabotinsky, On sequences of integers generated by a sieving process, *Proc. Konink. Nederl. Akad. Wetensch. Ser. A* 61 (1958) 115–128; *Indag. Math.* 20 (1958) 115–128; MR 21 #2628.

[73] D. Betten, Kalahari and the sequence "Sloane No. 377," *Combinatorics '86*, Proc. 1986 Trento conf., ed. A. Barlotti, M. Marchi, and G. Tallini, Annals of Discrete Math. 37, North-Holland, 1988, pp. 51–58; MR 89f:05010.

[74] N. J. A. Sloane, On-Line Encyclopedia of Integer Sequences, A002491.

[75] Y. David, On a sequence generated by a sieving process, *Riveon Lematematika* 11 (1957) 26–31; MR 21 #2627.

[76] D. M. Broline and D. E. Loeb, The combinatorics of Mancala-type games: Ayo, Tchoukaitlon, and $1/\pi$, *UMAP J.* 16 (1995) 21–36.

[77] N. J. A. Sloane, My favorite integer sequences, *Sequences and Their Applications (SETA)*, Proc. 1998 Singapore conf., ed. C. Ding, T. Helleseth, and H. Niederreiter, Springer-Verlag, 1999, pp. 103–130; math.CO/0207175.

[78] Y. V. Matiyasevich and R. K. Guy, A new formula for π, *Amer. Math. Monthly* 93 (1986) 631–635; MR 2000i:11199.

[79] P. Flajolet and A. Odlyzko, The average height of binary trees and other simple trees, *J. Comput. Sys. Sci.* 25 (1982) 171–213; MR 84a:68056.

[80] A. M. Odlyzko, Asymptotic enumeration methods, *Handbook of Combinatorics*, v. II, ed. R. L. Graham, M. Grötschel, and L. Lovász, MIT Press, 1995, pp. 1063–1229; MR 97b:05012.

1.5 Euler–Mascheroni Constant, γ

The Euler–Mascheroni constant, γ, is defined by the limit [1–8]

$$\gamma = \lim_{n \to \infty} \left(\sum_{k=1}^{n} \frac{1}{k} - \ln(n) \right) = 0.5772156649\ldots.$$

In words, γ measures the amount by which the partial sums of the harmonic series (the simplest divergent series) differ from the logarithmic function (its approximating integral). It is an important constant, shadowed only by π and e in significance. It appears naturally whenever estimates of $\sum_{k=1}^{n} 1/k$ are required. For example, let $X_1, X_2, \ldots, X_n$ be a sequence of independent and identically distributed random variables with continuous distribution function. Define R_n to be the number of **upper records** in the sequence [9–12], that is, the count of times that $X_k > \max\{X_1, X_2, \ldots, X_{k-1}\}$. By convention, X_1 is included. The random variable R_n has expectation $E(R_n)$ satisfying $\lim_{n \to \infty}(E(R_n) - \ln(n)) = \gamma$. As another example, let the set $C = \{1, 2, \ldots, n\}$ of **coupons** be sampled repeatedly with replacement [13–15], and let S_n denote the number of trials needed to collect all of C. Then $\lim_{n \to \infty}((E(S_n) - n\ln(n))/n) = \gamma$.

There are certain applications, however, where γ appears quite mysteriously. Suppose we wish to factor a random permutation π on n symbols into disjoint cycles. For example, the permutation π on $\{0, 1, 2, \ldots, 8\}$ defined by $\pi(x) = 2x \bmod 9$ has cycle structure $\pi = (0)(124875)(36)$. What is the probability that no two cycles of π possess the same length, as $n \to \infty$? The answer to the question is $e^{-\gamma} = 0.5614594835 \ldots$. More about random permutations is found in [5.4]. Suppose instead that we wish to factor a random integer polynomial $F(x)$ of degree n, modulo a prime p. What is the probability that no two irreducible factors of $F(x)$ possess the same degree, as $p \to \infty$ and $n \to \infty$? The same answer $e^{-\gamma}$ applies [16–21], but proving this is complicated by the double limit.

Euler's constant appears frequently in number theory, for example, in connection with the Euler totient function [2.7]. Here are more applications. If $d(n)$ denotes the number of distinct divisors of n, then the average value of the divisor function satisfies [22–24]

$$\lim_{n \to \infty} \left(\frac{1}{n} \sum_{k=1}^{n} d(k) - \ln(n) \right) = 2\gamma - 1 = 0.1544313298 \ldots.$$

We discuss this again in [2.10]. A surprising result, due to de la Vallée Poussin [25–28], is

$$\lim_{n \to \infty} \frac{1}{n} \sum_{k=1}^{n} \left\{ \frac{n}{k} \right\} = 1 - \gamma = 0.4227843351 \ldots,$$

where $\{x\}$ denotes the fractional part of x. In words, if a large integer n is divided by each integer $1 \leq k \leq n$, then the average fraction by which the quotient n/k falls short of the next integer is not $1/2$, but γ! One can also restrict n to being all terms of an arithmetic sequence, or even to being all terms of the sequence of primes, and obtain the same mean value. Also, let $M(n)$ denote the number of primes p, not exceeding n, for which $2^p - 1$ is prime. It has been suggested [29–32] that $M(n) \to \infty$ at approximately the same rate as $\ln(n)$ and, moreover, $\lim_{n \to \infty} M(n)/\ln(n) = e^\gamma / \ln(2) = 2.5695443449 \ldots$. The empirical data supporting this claim is quite thin: There are only 39 known Mersenne primes [33]. Other number-theoretic applications include [34–37].

Calculating Euler's constant has not attracted the same public intrigue as calculating π, but it has still inspired the dedication of a few. The evaluation of γ is difficult and only several hundred million digits are known. For π, we have the Borweins' *quartically convergent* algorithm: Each successive iteration approximately quadruples the number of correct digits. By contrast, for γ, not even a quadratically convergent algorithm is known [38–40].

The definition of γ converges too slowly to be numerically useful. This fact is illustrated by the following inequality [41, 42]:

$$\frac{1}{2(n+1)} < \sum_{k=1}^{n} \frac{1}{k} - \ln(n) - \gamma < \frac{1}{2n},$$

which serves as a double-edged sword. On the one hand, if we wish K digits of accuracy (after truncation), then $n \geq 10^{K+1}$ suffices in the summation. On the other hand, $n < 10^K$ will not be large enough. Some alternative estimates and inequalities were reported in [43, 44]. The best-known technique, called Euler–Maclaurin summation, gives an improved family of estimates, including

$$\gamma = \sum_{k=1}^{n} \frac{1}{k} - \ln(n) - \frac{1}{2n} + \frac{1}{12n^2} - \frac{1}{120n^4} + \frac{1}{252n^6} - \frac{1}{240n^8} + \frac{1}{132n^{10}}$$

$$- \frac{691}{32760n^{12}} + O\left(\frac{1}{n^{14}}\right).$$

Euler correctly obtained γ to 15 digits using $n = 10$ in this formula [45–48]. Fast algorithms like Karatsuba's FEE method [49, 50] and Brent's binary splitting method [51] were essential in the latest computations [52–55]. Papanikolaou calculated the first 475006 partial quotients in the regular continued fraction expansion for γ (using results in [56]) and deduced that if γ is a rational number, then its denominator must exceed 10^{244663}. This is compelling evidence that Euler's constant is not rational. A *proof* of irrationality (let alone transcendence) is still beyond our reach [57]. See two invalid attempts in [58, 59].

Here are two other unanswered questions, the first related to the harmonic series and the second similar to the coupon collector problem. Given a positive integer k, let n_k be the unique integer n satisfying $\sum_{j=1}^{n-1} 1/j < k < \sum_{j=1}^{n} 1/j$. Is n_k equal to the integer nearest $e^{k-\gamma}$ always [60–65]? Suppose instead we are given a binary sequence B, generated by independent fair coin tosses, and a positive integer n. What is the waiting time T_n for all 2^n possible different patterns of length n to occur (as subwords of B)? It might be conjectured (on the basis of [66, 67]) that the mean waiting time satisfies $\lim_{n \to \infty} ((E(T_n) - 2^n n \ln(2))/2^n) = \gamma$, but this remains open. However, the minimum possible waiting time is only $2^n + n - 1$, as a consequence of known results concerning what are called de Bruijn sequences [68].

1.5.1 Series and Products

The following series is a trivial restatement of the definition of γ:

$$\gamma = \sum_{k=1}^{\infty} \left(\frac{1}{k} - \ln\left(1 + \frac{1}{k}\right) \right).$$

Other formulas involving γ include two more due to Euler [1],

$$\gamma = \frac{1}{2} \cdot \left(1 + \frac{1}{2^2} + \frac{1}{3^2} + \cdots\right) - \frac{1}{3} \cdot \left(1 + \frac{1}{2^3} + \frac{1}{3^3} + \cdots\right)$$

$$+ \frac{1}{4} \cdot \left(1 + \frac{1}{2^4} + \frac{1}{3^4} + \cdots\right) - + \cdots,$$

$$\gamma = \frac{1}{2} \cdot \left(\frac{1}{2^2} + \frac{1}{3^2} + \frac{1}{4^2} + \cdots\right) + \frac{2}{3} \cdot \left(\frac{1}{2^3} + \frac{1}{3^3} + \frac{1}{4^3} + \cdots\right)$$

$$+ \frac{3}{4} \cdot \left(\frac{1}{2^4} + \frac{1}{3^4} + \frac{1}{4^4} + \cdots\right) + \cdots,$$

one due to Vacca [69–75],

$$\gamma = \frac{1}{2} - \frac{1}{3} + 2 \cdot \left(\frac{1}{4} - \frac{1}{5} + \frac{1}{6} - \frac{1}{7}\right) + 3 \cdot \left(\frac{1}{8} - \frac{1}{9} + \cdots - \frac{1}{15}\right)$$
$$+ 4 \cdot \left(\frac{1}{16} - \frac{1}{17} + \cdots - \frac{1}{31}\right) + \cdots,$$

one due to Pólya [26, 76],

$$\gamma = 1 - \left(\frac{1}{2} + \frac{1}{3}\right) + \frac{3}{4} - \left(\frac{1}{5} + \frac{1}{6} + \frac{1}{7} + \frac{1}{8}\right) + \frac{5}{9} - \left(\frac{1}{10} + \frac{1}{11} + \cdots + \frac{1}{15}\right)$$
$$+ \frac{7}{16} - + \cdots,$$

and two due to Mertens [22, 77],

$$e^{\gamma} = \lim_{n \to \infty} \frac{1}{\ln(n)} \cdot \prod_{p \leq n} \frac{p}{p-1}, \qquad \frac{6e^{\gamma}}{\pi^2} = \lim_{n \to \infty} \frac{1}{\ln(n)} \cdot \prod_{p \leq n} \frac{p+1}{p},$$

where both products are taken over all primes p not exceeding n. Mertens' first formula may be rewritten as [55]

$$\gamma = \lim_{n \to \infty} \left(\sum_{p \leq n} \ln\left(\frac{p}{p-1}\right) - \ln(\ln(n)) \right).$$

If, in this series, the expression $\ln(p/(p-1))$ is replaced by its asymptotic equivalent $1/p$, then a different constant arises [2.2]. Other series and products appear in [78–95].

1.5.2 Integrals

There are many integrals that involve Euler's constant, including

$$\int_0^{\infty} e^{-x} \ln(x) dx = -\gamma, \qquad \int_0^{\infty} e^{-x^2} \ln(x) dx = -\frac{\sqrt{\pi}}{4}(\gamma + 2\ln(2)),$$

$$\int_0^{\infty} e^{-x} \ln(x)^2 dx = \frac{\pi^2}{6} + \gamma^2, \qquad \int_0^1 \ln\left(\ln\left(\frac{1}{x}\right)\right) dx = -\gamma,$$

$$\int_0^{\infty} \frac{e^{-x^a} - e^{-x^b}}{x} dx = \frac{a-b}{ab}\gamma, \qquad \int_0^{\infty} \frac{x}{1+x^2} \cdot \frac{1}{e^{2\pi x} - 1} dx = \frac{1}{4}(2\gamma - 1),$$

$$\int_0^1 \left(\frac{1}{\ln(x)} + \frac{1}{1-x}\right) dx = \gamma, \qquad \int_0^1 \frac{1}{1+x} \left(\sum_{k=1}^{\infty} x^{2^k}\right) dx = 1 - \gamma,$$

to mention a few [55,75,96,97]. It is assumed here that the two parameters a and b satisfy $a > 0$ and $b > 0$. If $\{x\}$ denotes the fractional part of x, then [22,24]

$$\int\limits_{1}^{\infty} \frac{\{x\}}{x^2}dx = \int\limits_{0}^{1} \left\{\frac{1}{y}\right\} dy = 1 - \gamma$$

and similar integrals appear in [1.6.5], [1.8], and [2.21]. See also [98–101].

1.5.3 Generalized Euler Constants

Boas [102–104] wondered why the original Euler constant has attracted attention but other types of constants of the form

$$\gamma(m, f) = \lim_{n\to\infty} \left(\sum_{k=m}^{n} f(k) - \int\limits_{m}^{n} f(x)dx \right)$$

have been comparatively neglected. The case $f(x) = x^{-q}$, where $0 < q < 1$, gives the constant $\zeta(q) + 1/(1 - q)$ involving a zeta function value [1.6] and the case $f(x) = \ln(x)^r/x$, where $r \geq 0$, gives the Stieltjes constant γ_r [2.21]. We give some sample numerical results in Table 1.1. Briggs [105] and Lehmer [106] studied the analog of γ corresponding to the arithmetic progression $a, a + b, a + 2b, a + 3b, \ldots$:

$$\gamma_{a,b} = \lim_{n\to\infty} \left(\sum_{\substack{0<k\leq n \\ k\equiv a \bmod b}} \frac{1}{k} - \frac{1}{b} \ln(n) \right).$$

For example, $\gamma_{0,b} = (\gamma - \ln(b))/b$, $\sum_{a=0}^{b-1} \gamma_{a,b} = \gamma$, and

$$\gamma_{1,3} = \frac{1}{3}\gamma + \frac{\sqrt{3}}{18}\pi + \frac{1}{6} \ln(3), \quad \gamma_{1,4} = \frac{1}{4}\gamma + \frac{1}{8}\pi + \frac{1}{4} \ln(2).$$

See also [107, 108]. A two-dimensional version of Euler's constant appears in [7.2] and a (different) n-dimensional lattice sum version is discussed in [1.10].

Table 1.1. *Generalized Euler Constants*

m	$f(x)$	$\gamma(m, f)$
1	$1/x$	$0.5772156649\ldots = \gamma_0$
2	$1/\ln(x)$	$0.8019254372\ldots$
2	$1/(x \cdot \ln(x))$	$0.4281657248\ldots$
1	$1/\sqrt{x}$	$0.5396454911\ldots = \zeta(1/2) + 2$
1	$\ln(x)/x$	$-0.0728158454\ldots = \gamma_1$

1.5.4 Gamma Function

For complex z, the Euler gamma function $\Gamma(z)$ is often defined by

$$\Gamma(z) = \lim_{n\to\infty} \frac{n! \cdot n^z}{\displaystyle\prod_{k=0}^{n}(z+k)}$$

and is analytic over the whole complex plane except for simple poles at the nonpositive integers. For real $x > 0$, this simplifies to the integral formula

$$\Gamma(x) = \int_0^\infty s^{x-1}e^{-s}ds = \int_0^1 \left(\ln\left(\frac{1}{t}\right)\right)^{x-1} dt$$

and, if n is a positive integer, $\Gamma(n) = (n-1)!$ This is the reason we sometimes see the expression

$$\left(-\frac{1}{2}\right)! = \sqrt{\pi} = 1.7724538509\ldots$$

since $\Gamma(1/2)$ transforms, by change of variable, to the well-known Gaussian probability density integral.

The Bohr–Mollerup theorem [109, 110] maintains that $\Gamma(z)$ is the most natural possible extension of the factorial function (among infinitely many possible extensions) to the complex plane.

For what argument values is the gamma function known to be transcendental? Chudnovsky [111–114] showed in 1975 that $\Gamma(1/6)$, $\Gamma(1/4)$, $\Gamma(1/3)$, $\Gamma(2/3)$, $\Gamma(3/4)$, and $\Gamma(5/6)$ are each transcendental and that each is algebraically independent from π. (It is curious [115, 116] that we have known $\Gamma(1/4)^4/\pi$ and $\Gamma(1/3)^2/\pi$ to be transcendental for many more years.) Nesterenko [117–121] proved in 1996 that π, e^π, and $\Gamma(1/4) = 3.6256099082\ldots$ are algebraically independent. The constant $\Gamma(1/4)$ appears in [3.2], [6.1], and [7.2]. Nesterenko also proved that π, $e^{\pi\sqrt{3}}$, and $\Gamma(1/3) = 2.6789385347\ldots$ are algebraically independent. A similarly strong result has not yet been proved for $\Gamma(1/6) = 5.5663160017\ldots$, nor has $\Gamma(1/5) = 4.5908437119\ldots$ even been demonstrated to be irrational. The reflection formula provides that

$$\Gamma\left(\tfrac{1}{4}\right)\Gamma\left(\tfrac{3}{4}\right) = \pi\sqrt{2}, \qquad \Gamma\left(\tfrac{1}{3}\right)\Gamma\left(\tfrac{2}{3}\right) = \tfrac{2}{3}\pi\sqrt{3},$$

$$\Gamma\left(\tfrac{1}{6}\right)\Gamma\left(\tfrac{5}{6}\right) = 2\pi, \quad \Gamma\left(\tfrac{1}{5}\right)\Gamma\left(\tfrac{4}{5}\right) = \tfrac{2}{5}\pi\sqrt{5}\sqrt{2+\varphi},$$

where φ is the Golden mean [1.2]. Furthermore [122, 123],

$$\Gamma\left(\tfrac{1}{4}\right) = 2^{\frac{1}{2}}\pi^{\frac{3}{4}}h_1^{\frac{1}{2}}, \quad \Gamma\left(\tfrac{1}{3}\right) = 2^{\frac{4}{9}}3^{-\frac{1}{12}}\pi^{\frac{1}{3}}h_3^{\frac{1}{3}}, \quad \Gamma\left(\tfrac{1}{6}\right) = 2^{\frac{5}{9}}3^{\frac{1}{3}}\pi^{\frac{5}{6}}h_3^{\frac{2}{3}},$$

where

$$h_1 = \tfrac{2}{\pi} K\left(\tfrac{\sqrt{2}}{2}\right) = \left(\sum_{n=-\infty}^{\infty} e^{-n^2\pi}\right)^2 = 1.1803405990\ldots,$$

$$h_3 = \tfrac{2}{\pi} K\left(\tfrac{\sqrt{2}}{4}(\sqrt{3}-1)\right) = \left(\sum_{n=-\infty}^{\infty} e^{-n^2\sqrt{3}\pi}\right)^2 = 1.0174087975\ldots,$$

and $K(x)$ is the complete elliptic integral of the first kind [1.4.6].

When plotting the gamma function $y = \Gamma(x)$, the minimum point in the upper right quadrant has xy-coordinates $(x_{\min}, \Gamma(x_{\min})) = (1.4616321449\ldots, 0.8856031944\ldots)$. If θ is the unique positive root of the equation

$$\frac{d}{dx}\ln(\Gamma(x))\bigg|_{x=\theta} = \ln(\pi)$$

then $d_s = 2\theta = 7.2569464048\ldots$ and $d_s = 2(\theta-1) = 5.2569464048\ldots$ are the fractional dimensions at which d-dimensional spherical surface area and volume, respectively, are maximized [124].

Several relevant series appear in [125–129]. Two series due to Ramanujan, for example [130–132], are

$$\sum_{n=0}^{\infty} \frac{(-1)^n}{2^{4n}}\binom{2n}{n}^2 = (2\pi)^{-\frac{3}{2}}\Gamma\left(\tfrac{1}{4}\right)^2, \quad \sum_{n=0}^{\infty} \frac{(-1)^n}{2^{6n}}\binom{2n}{n}^3 = \left(\frac{\Gamma\left(\tfrac{9}{8}\right)}{\Gamma\left(\tfrac{5}{4}\right)\Gamma\left(\tfrac{7}{8}\right)}\right)^2,$$

which extend a series mentioned in [1.1]. Two products [96, 133] are

$$\prod_{n=1}^{\infty}\left(1 - \frac{1}{(4n+1)^2}\right) = \frac{4\cdot 6}{5\cdot 5}\cdot\frac{8\cdot 10}{9\cdot 9}\cdot\frac{12\cdot 14}{13\cdot 13}\cdot\frac{16\cdot 18}{17\cdot 17}\cdots = \frac{1}{8\sqrt{\pi}}\Gamma\left(\tfrac{1}{4}\right)^2,$$

$$\prod_{n=1}^{\infty}\left(1 - \frac{1}{(2n+1)^2}\right)^{(-1)^n} = \frac{3^2}{3^2-1}\cdot\frac{5^2-1}{5^2}\cdot\frac{7^2}{7^2-1}\cdot\frac{9^2-1}{9^2}\cdots = \frac{1}{16\pi^2}\Gamma\left(\tfrac{1}{4}\right)^4.$$

A sample integral, with real parameters $u > 0$ and $v > 0$, is [96, 134, 135]

$$\int_0^{\frac{\pi}{2}} \sin(x)^{u-1}\cos(x)^{v-1}dx = \int_0^1 y^{u-1}(1-y^2)^{\frac{v}{2}-1}dy = \frac{1}{2}\frac{\Gamma(\tfrac{u}{2})\Gamma(\tfrac{v}{2})}{\Gamma(\tfrac{u+v}{2})}.$$

The significance of Euler's constant to Euler's gamma function is best summarized by the formula $\psi(1) = -\gamma$, where [90]

$$\psi(x) = \frac{d}{dx}\ln(\Gamma(x)) = -\gamma - \sum_{n=0}^{\infty}\left(\frac{1}{x+n} - \frac{1}{n+1}\right)$$

is the digamma function. Higher-order derivatives at $x = 1$ involve zeta function values [1.6]. Information on such derivatives (polygamma functions) is found in [134, 136].

[1] J. W. L. Glaisher, On the history of Euler's constant, *Messenger of Math.* 1 (1872) 25–30.

[2] R. Johnsonbaugh, The trapezoid rule, Stirling's formula, and Euler's constant, *Amer. Math. Monthly* 88 (1981) 696–698; MR 83a:26006.

[3] C. W. Barnes, Euler's constant and e, *Amer. Math. Monthly* 91 (1984) 428–430.

[4] D. Bushaw and S. C. Saunders, The third constant, *Northwest Sci.* 59 (1985) 147–158.

[5] J. Nunemacher, On computing Euler's constant, *Math. Mag.* 65 (1992) 313–322; MR 93j:65042.

[6] R. Barshinger, Calculus II and Euler also (with a nod to series integral remainder bounds), *Amer. Math. Monthly* 101 (1994) 244–249; MR 94k:26003.

[7] J. Sondow, An antisymmetric formula for Euler's constant, *Math. Mag.* 71 (1998) 219–220.

[8] T. M. Apostol, An elementary view of Euler's summation formula, *Amer. Math. Monthly* 106 (1999) 409–418.

[9] F. G. Foster and A. Stuart, Distribution-free tests in time-series based on the breaking of records, *J. Royal Stat. Soc. Ser. B* 16 (1954) 1–22; MR 16,385i.

[10] D. E. Knuth, *The Art of Computer Programming: Fundamental Algorithms*, v. 1, 2nd ed., Addison-Wesley, 1973, pp. 73–77, 94–99; MR 51 #14624.

[11] W. Katzenbeisser, On the joint distribution of the number of upper and lower records and the number of inversions in a random sequence, *Adv. Appl. Probab.* 22 (1990) 957–960; MR 92a:60046.

[12] B. C. Arnold, N. Balakrishnan, and H. N. Nagaraja, *Records*, Wiley, 1998, pp. 22–25; MR 2000b:60127.

[13] B. Dawkins, Siobhan's problem: The coupon collector revisited, *Amer. Statist.* 45 (1991) 76–82.

[14] B. Levin, Regarding "Siobhan's problem: The coupon collector revisited," *Amer. Statist.* 46 (1992) 76.

[15] R. Sedgewick and P. Flajolet, *Introduction to the Analysis of Algorithms*, Addison-Wesley, 1996, pp. 425–427.

[16] D. H. Lehmer, On reciprocally weighted partitions, *Acta Arith.* 21 (1972) 379–388; MR 46 #3437.

[17] D. E. Knuth, *The Art of Computer Programming: Seminumerical Algorithms*, v. 2, 2nd ed., Addison-Wesley, 1981, pp. 439, 629; MR 44 #3531.

[18] D. H. Greene and D. E. Knuth, *Mathematics for the Analysis of Algorithms*, 3rd ed., Birkhäuser, 1990, pp. 48–54, 95–98; MR 92c:68067.

[19] A. Knopfmacher and R. Warlimont, Distinct degree factorizations for polynomials over a finite field, *Trans. Amer. Math. Soc.* 347 (1995) 2235–2243; MR 95i:11144.

[20] P. Flajolet, X. Gourdon, and D. Panario, Random polynomials and polynomial factorization, *Proc. 1996 Int. Colloq. on Automata, Languages and Programming (ICALP)*, Paderborn, ed. F. Meyer auf der Heide and B. Monien, Lect. Notes in Comp. Sci. 1099, Springer-Verlag, 1996, pp. 232–243; MR 98e:68123.

[21] P. Flajolet, X. Gourdon, and D. Panario, The complete analysis of a polynomial factorization algorithm over finite fields, *J. Algorithms* 40 (2001) 37–81; INRIA preprint RR3370; MR 2002f:68193.

[22] G. H. Hardy and E. M. Wright, *An Introduction to the Theory of Numbers*, 5th ed., Oxford Univ. Press, 1985, pp. 264–265, 347, 351; MR 81i:10002.

[23] M. R. Schroeder, *Number Theory in Science and Communication: With Applications in Cryptography, Physics, Digital Information, Computing and Self-Similarity*, 2nd ed., Springer-Verlag, 1986, pp. 127–131; MR 99c:11165.

[24] T. M. Apostol, *Introduction to Analytic Number Theory*, Springer-Verlag, 1998, pp. 52–59; MR 55 #7892.

[25] Ch. de la Vallée Poussin, Sur les valeurs moyennes de certaines fonctions arithmétiques, *Annales de la Societe Scientifique de Bruxelles* 22 (1898) 84–90.

[26] G. Pólya and G. Szegö, *Problems and Theorems in Analysis*, v. 1, Springer-Verlag 1998, problems 18, 19, 32, 42; MR 81e:00002.

[27] L. E. Dickson, *History of the Theory of Numbers*, v. 1, *Divisibility and Primality*, Chelsea, 1971; pp. 134, 136, 294, 317, 320, 328, and 330; MR 39 #6807.

[28] J. H. Conway and R. K. Guy, *The Book of Numbers*, Springer-Verlag, 1996, p. 260; MR 98g:00004.

[29] S. S. Wagstaff, Divisors of Mersenne numbers, *Math. Comp.* 40 (1983) 385–397; MR 84j:10052.

[30] R. K. Guy, *Unsolved Problems in Number Theory*, 2nd ed., Springer-Verlag, 1994, sect. A3; MR 96e:11002.

[31] P. Ribenboim, *The New Book of Prime Number Records*, 3rd ed., Springer-Verlag, 1996, pp. 411–413; MR 96k:11112.

[32] R. Crandall and C. Pomerance, *Prime Numbers: A Computational Perspective*, Springer-Verlag, 2001, pp. 20–24; MR 2002a:11007.

[33] C. Caldwell, Mersenne Primes: History, Theorems and Lists (Prime Pages).

[34] P. Erdös and A. Ivić, Estimates for sums involving the largest prime factor of an integer and certain related additive functions, *Studia Sci. Math. Hungar.* 15 (1980) 183–199; MR 84a:10046.

[35] V. Sita Ramaiah and M. V. Subbarao, The maximal order of certain arithmetic functions, *Indian J. Pure Appl. Math.* 24 (1993) 347–355; MR 94i:11075.

[36] A. Knopfmacher and J. N. Ridley, Reciprocal sums over partitions and compositions, *SIAM J. Discrete Math.* 6 (1993) 388–399; MR 94g:11111.

[37] R. Warlimont, Permutations with roots, *Arch. Math. (Basel)* 67 (1996) 23–34; MR 97h:11109.

[38] D. H. Bailey, Numerical results on the transcendence of constants involving π, e and Euler's constant, *Math. Comp.* 50 (1988) 275–281; MR 88m:11056.

[39] D. H. Bailey and H. R. P. Ferguson, Numerical results on relations between fundamental constants using a new algorithm, *Math. Comp.* 53 (1989) 649–656; MR 90e:11191.

[40] J. M. Borwein and P. B. Borwein, On the complexity of familiar functions and numbers, *SIAM Rev.* 30 (1988) 589–601; MR 89k:68061.

[41] S. R. Tims and J. A. Tyrrell, Approximate evaluation of Euler's constant, *Math. Gazette* 55 (1971) 65–67.

[42] R. M. Young, Euler's constant, *Math. Gazette* 75 (1991) 187–190.

[43] D. W. DeTemple, A quicker convergence to Euler's constant, *Amer. Math. Monthly* 100 (1993) 468–470; MR 94e:11146.

[44] T. Negoi, A faster convergence to Euler's constant (in Romanian), *Gazeta Mat.* 15 (1997) 111–113; Engl. transl. in *Math. Gazette* 83 (1999) 487–489.

[45] D. E. Knuth, Euler's constant to 1271 places, *Math. Comp.* 16 (1962) 275–281; MR 26 #5763.

[46] D. W. Sweeney, On the computation of Euler's constant, *Math. Comp.* 17 (1963) 170–178; corrigenda 17 (1963) 488; MR 28 #3522.

[47] W. A. Beyer and M. S. Waterman, Error analysis of a computation of Euler's constant, *Math. Comp.* 28 (1974) 599–604; MR 49 #6555.

[48] C. Elsner, On a sequence transformation with integral coefficients for Euler's constant, *Proc. Amer. Math. Soc.* 123 (1995) 1537–1541; MR 95f:11111.

[49] E. A. Karatsuba, Fast evaluation of transcendental functions (in Russian), *Problemy Peredachi Informatsii* 27 (1991) 76–99; Engl. transl. in *Problems Information Transmission* 27 (1991) 339–360; MR 93c:65027.

[50] E. A. Karatsuba, On the computation of the Euler constant γ, *Numer. Algorithms* 24 (2000) 83–97; Univ. of Helsinki Math. Report 226 (1999); MR 2002f:33004.

[51] R. P. Brent, Fast multiple-precision evaluation of elementary functions, *J. ACM* 23 (1976) 242–251; MR 52 #16111.

[52] R. P. Brent, Computation of the regular continued fraction for Euler's constant, *Math. Comp.* 31 (1977) 771–777; MR 55 #9490.

[53] R. P. Brent and E. M. McMillan, Some new algorithms for high-precision computation of Euler's constant, *Math. Comp.* 34 (1980) 305–312; MR 82g:10002.

[54] B. Haible and T. Papanikolaou, Fast multiprecision evaluation of series of rational numbers, *Proc. 1998 Algorithmic Number Theory Sympos. (ANTS-III)*, Portland, ed. J. P. Buhler, Lect. Notes in Comp. Sci. 1423, Springer-Verlag, 1998, pp. 338–350; MR 2000i:11197.

[55] X. Gourdon and P. Sebah, The Euler constant gamma (Numbers, Constants and Computation).

[56] R. P. Brent, A. J. van der Poorten, and H. J. J. te Riele, A comparative study of algorithms for computing continued fractions of algebraic numbers, *Proc. 1996 Algorithmic Number Theory Sympos. (ANTS-II)*, Talence, ed. H. Cohen, Lect. Notes in Comp. Sci. 1122, Springer-Verlag, 1996, pp. 37–49; MR 98c:11144.

[57] J. Sondow, Criteria for irrationality of Euler's constant, math.NT/0209070.

[58] A. Froda, La constante d'Euler est irrationnelle, *Atti Accad. Naz. Lincei Rend. Cl. Sci. Fis. Mat. Natur.* 38 (1965) 338–344; MR 32 #5599.

[59] R. G. Ayoub, Partial triumph or total failure?, *Math. Intellig.*, v. 7 (1985) n. 2, 55–58; MR 86i:01001.

[60] S. M. Zemyan, On two conjectures concerning the partial sums of the harmonic series, *Proc. Amer. Math. Soc.* 95 (1985) 83–86; MR 86m:40002.

[61] L. Comtet, About $\sum 1/n$, *Amer. Math. Monthly* 74 (1967) 209.

[62] R. P. Boas and J. W. Wrench, Partial sums of the harmonic series, *Amer. Math. Monthly* 78 (1971) 864–870; MR 44 #7179.

[63] R. P. Boas, An integer sequence from the harmonic series, *Amer. Math. Monthly* 83 (1976) 748–749.

[64] G. Pólya and G. Szegö, *Problems and Theorems in Analysis*, v. 2, Springer-Verlag 1976, problems 249–251, 260; MR 57 #5529.

[65] K. T. Atanassov, Remark on the harmonic series, *C. R. Acad. Bulgare Sci.*, v. 40 (1987) n. 5, 25–28; MR 88m:40004.

[66] A. Benczur, On the expected time of the first occurrence of every k bit long patterns in the symmetric Bernoulli process, *Acta Math. Hungar.* 47 (1986) 233–286; MR 87m:60029.

[67] T. F. Móri, On the expectation of the maximum waiting time, *Annales Univ. Sci. Budapest Sect. Comput.* 7 (1987) 111–115; MR 90e:60048.

[68] N. G. de Bruijn, A combinatorial problem, *Proc. Konink. Nederl. Akad. Wetensch. Sci. Sect.* 49 (1946) 758–764; *Indag. Math.* 8 (1946) 461–467; MR 8,247d.

[69] G. Vacca, A new series for the Eulerian constant, *Quart. J. Pure. Appl. Math.* 41 (1910) 363–368.

[70] H. F. Sandham and D. F. Barrow, Problem/Solution 4353, *Amer. Math. Monthly* 58 (1951) 116–117.

[71] A. W. Addison, A series representation for Euler's constant, *Amer. Math. Monthly* 74 (1967) 823–824; MR 36 #1397.

[72] I. Gerst, Some series for Euler's constant, *Amer. Math. Monthly* 76 (1969) 273–275; MR 39 #3181.

[73] M. Beeler, R. W. Gosper, and R. Schroeppel, Series acceleration technique, HAKMEM, MIT AI Memo 239, 1972, item 120.

[74] J. Sandor, On the irrationality of some alternating series, *Studia Univ. Babes-Bolyai Math.* 33 (1988) 8–12; MR 91c:40003.

[75] B. C. Berndt and D. C. Bowman, Ramanujan's short unpublished manuscript on integrals and series related to Euler's constant, *Constructive, Experimental, and Nonlinear Analysis*, Proc. 1999 Limoges conf., ed. M. Théra, Amer. Math. Soc., 2000, pp. 19–27; MR 2002d:33001.

[76] G. Pólya, A series for Euler's constant, *Research Papers in Statistics (J. Neyman Festschift)*, Wiley, 1966, pp. 259–261; also in *Collected Papers*, v. 3, ed. J. Hersch and G.-C. Rota, MIT Press, 1984, pp. 475–477; MR 34 #8026.

[77] G. Tenenbaum, *Introduction to Analytic and Probabilistic Number Theory*, Cambridge Univ. Press, 1995, pp. 14–18; MR 97e:11005b.

[78] A. M. Glicksman, Euler's constant, *Amer. Math. Monthly* 50 (1943) 575.

[79] O. Dunkel, Euler's constant, *Amer. Math. Monthly* 51 (1944) 99–102.

[80] F. Supnick, A geometric facet of the Eulerian constant, *Amer. Math. Monthly* 69 (1962) 208–209.

[81] V. P. Burlachenko, Representation of some constants by double series (in Ukrainian), *Dopovidi Akad. Nauk Ukrain. RSR A* 4 (1970) 303–305, 380; MR 43 #5204.

[82] D. P. Verma and A. Kaur, Summation of some series involving Riemann zeta function, *Indian J. Math.* 25 (1983) 181–184; MR 87a:11077.

[83] J. Choi and H. M. Srivastava, Sums associated with the zeta function, *J. Math. Anal. Appl.* 206 (1997) 103–120; MR 97i:11092.

[84] M. Hata, Farey fractions and sums over coprime pairs, *Acta Arith.* 70 (1995) 149–159; MR 96c:11022.

[85] G. Xiong, On a kind of the best estimates for the Euler constant γ, *Acta Math. Scientia: English Ed.* 16 (1996) 458–468; MR 97m:11162.

[86] S. Ramanujan, A series for Euler's constant γ, *Messenger of Math.* 46 (1917) 73–80; also in *Collected Papers*, ed. G. H. Hardy, P. V. Seshu Aiyar, and B. M. Wilson, Cambridge Univ. Press, 1927, pp. 163–168, 325.

[87] B. C. Berndt, *Ramanujan's Notebooks: Part I*, Springer-Verlag, 1985, pp. 98–99, 196; MR 86c:01062.

[88] R. P. Brent, An asymptotic expansion inspired by Ramanujan, *Austral. Math. Soc. Gazette* 20 (1993) 149–155; MR 95b:33006.

[89] R. P. Brent, Ramanujan and Euler's constant, *Mathematics of Computation 1943-1993: A Half-Century of Computational Mathematics*, Proc. 1993 Vancouver conf., ed. W. Gautschi, Amer. Math. Soc. 1994, pp. 541–545; MR 95k:01022.

[90] D. Bradley, Ramanujan's formula for the logarithmic derivative of the gamma function, *Math. Proc. Cambridge Philos. Soc.* 120 (1996) 391–401; MR 97a:11132.

[91] H. S. Wilf and D. A. Darling, An infinite product, *Amer. Math. Monthly* 105 (1998) 376.

[92] F. K. Kenter, A matrix representation for Euler's constant, γ, *Amer. Math. Monthly* 106 (1999) 452–454.

[93] F. Pittnauer, Eine Darstellung der Eulerschen Konstanten, *Math. Semesterber* 31 (1984) 26–27; MR 85j:11017.

[94] H. G. Killingbergtø and C. P. Kirkebø, A new(?) formula for computing γ (in Norwegian), *Normat* 41 (1993) 120–124, 136; MR 94g:11117.

[95] P. Flajolet and I. Vardi, Zeta function expansions of classical constants, unpublished note (1996).

[96] I. S. Gradshteyn and I. M Ryzhik, *Tables of Integrals, Series and Products*, Academic Press, 1980; MR 97c:00014.

[97] J.-M. Arnaudiès, *Problèmes de préparation à l'Agrégation de Mathématiques*, v. 4, *Analyse, Intégrale, séries de Fourier, équations différentielles*, Edition Ellipses, 1998, pp. 63–80.

[98] S. K. Lakshmana Rao, On the sequence for Euler's constant, *Amer. Math. Monthly* 63 (1956) 572–573; also in *A Century of Calculus*, v. 1, ed. T. M. Apostol, H. E. Chrestenson, C. S. Ogilvy, D. E. Richmond, and N. J. Schoonmaker, Math. Assoc. Amer., 1992, pp. 389–390.

[99] J. Anglesio and D. A. Darling, An integral giving Euler's constant, *Amer. Math. Monthly* 104 (1997) 881.

[100] J. Anglesio, The integrals are Euler's constant, *Amer. Math. Monthly* 105 (1998) 278–279.

[101] J. Choi and T. Y. Seo, Integral formulas for Euler's constant, *Commun. Korean Math. Soc.* 13 (1998) 683–689; MR 2000i:11196.

[102] R. P. Boas, Growth of partial sums of divergent series, *Math. Comp.* 31 (1977) 257–264; MR 55 #13730.

[103] R. P. Boas, Partial sums of infinite series, and how they grow, *Amer. Math. Monthly* 84 (1977) 237–258; MR 55 #13118.

[104] J. V. Baxley, Euler's constant, Taylor's formula, and slowly converging series, *Math. Mag.* 65 (1992) 302–313; MR 93j:40001.

[105] W. E. Briggs, The irrationality of γ or of sets of similar constants, *Norske Vid. Selsk. Forh. (Trondheim)* 34 (1961) 25–28; MR 25 #3011.

[106] D. H. Lehmer, Euler constants for arithmetical progressions, *Acta Arith.* 27 (1975) 125–142; MR 51 #5468.

[107] W. Leighton, Remarks on certain Eulerian constants, *Amer. Math. Monthly* 75 (1968) 283–285; MR 37 #3235.

[108] T. Tasaka, Note on the generalized Euler constants, *Math. J. Okayama Univ.* 36 (1994) 29–34; MR 96k:11157.

[109] J. B. Conway, *Functions of One Complex Variable*, 2nd ed., Springer-Verlag, 1978, pp. 176–187; MR 80c:30003.

[110] W. Rudin, *Principles of Mathematical Analysis*, 3rd ed., McGraw-Hill, 1976, pp. 192–195; MR 52 #5893.

[111] G. V. Chudnovsky, Algebraic independence of constants connected with exponential and elliptic functions (in Russian), *Dokl. Akad. Nauk Ukrain. SSR Ser. A* 8 (1976) 698–701, 767; MR 54 #12670.

[112] M. Waldschmidt, Les travaux de G. V. Cudnovskii sur les nombres transcendants, *Séminaire Bourbaki: 1975/76*, Lect. Notes in Math. 567, Springer-Verlag, pp. 274–292; MR 55 #12650.

[113] G. V. Chudnovsky, *Contributions to the Theory of Transcendental Numbers*, Amer. Math. Soc., 1984; MR 87a:11004.

[114] M. Waldschmidt, Algebraic independence of transcendental numbers: Gel'fond's method and its developments, *Perspectives in Mathematics: Anniversary of Oberwolfach*, ed. W. Jäger, J. Moser, and R. Remmert, Birkhäuser, 1984, pp. 551–571; MR 86f:11054.

[115] P. J. Davis, Leonhard Euler's integral: A historical profile of the Gamma function, *Amer. Math. Monthly* 66 (1959) 849–869; MR 21 #5540.

[116] C. L. Siegel, *Transcendental Numbers*, Princeton Univ. Press, 1949, pp. 95–100; MR 11,330c.

[117] Yu. V. Nesterenko, Algebraic independence of π and e^π, *Number Theory and Its Applications*, Proc. 1996 Ankara conf., ed. C. Y. Yildirim and S. A. Stepanov, Dekker, 1999, pp. 121–149; MR 99k:11113.

[118] Yu. V. Nesterenko, Modular functions and transcendence problems, *C. R. Acad. Sci. Paris Sér. I Math.* 322 (1996) 909–914; MR 97g:11080.

[119] M. Waldschmidt, Algebraic independence of transcendental numbers: A survey, *Number Theory*, ed. R. P. Bambah, V. C. Dumir, and R. J. Hans Gill, Birkhäuser, 2000, pp. 497–527.

[120] M. Waldschmidt, Sur la nature arithmétique des valeurs des fonctions modulaires, *Séminaire Bourbaki*, 49ème année 1996–97, #824; MR 99g:11089.

[121] F. Gramain, Quelques résultats d'indépendance algébrique, *International Congress of Mathematicians*, v. 2, Proc. 1998 Berlin conf., *Documenta Mathematica* Extra Volume II (1998) 173–182; MR 99h:11079.

[122] J. M. Borwein and I. J. Zucker, Fast evaluation of the gamma function for small rational fractions using complete elliptic integrals of the first kind, *IMA J. Numer. Anal.* 12 (1992) 519–529; MR 93g:65028.

[123] A. Eagle, *The Elliptic Functions as They Should Be*, Galloway and Porter, 1958; MR 20 #123 and MR 55 #6767.

[124] D. Wells, *The Penguin Dictionary of Curious and Interesting Numbers*, Penguin, 1986, p. 6.

[125] G. H. Hardy, Srinivasa Ramanujan obituary notice, *Proc. London Math. Soc.* 19 (1921) xl–lviii.

[126] S. Ramanujan, On question 330 of Professor Sanjana, *J. Indian Math. Soc.* 4 (1912) 59–61; also in *Collected Papers*, ed. G. H. Hardy, P. V. Seshu Aiyar, and B. M. Wilson, Cambridge Univ. Press, 1927, pp. 15–17.

[127] W. D. Fryer and M. S. Klamkin, Comment on problem 612, *Math. Mag.* 40 (1967) 52–53.

[128] G. N. Watson, Theorems stated by Ramanujan. XI, *J. London Math. Soc.* 6 (1931) 59–65.

[129] E. R. Hansen, *A Table of Series and Products*, Prentice-Hall, 1975.

[130] B. C. Berndt, *Ramanujan's Notebooks: Part II*, Springer-Verlag, 1989, pp. 11, 24, 41; MR 90b:01039.

[131] G. H. Hardy, Some formulae of Ramanujan, *Proc. London Math. Soc.* 22 (1924) xii–xiii; also in *Collected Papers*, v. 4, Oxford Univ. Press, 1966, pp. 517–518.

[132] J. Todd, The lemniscate constants, *Commun. ACM* 18 (1975) 14–19, 462; MR 51 #11935.
[133] W. Magnus and F. Oberhettinger, *Formulas and Theorems for the Special Functions of Mathematical Physics*, Chelsea, 1949.
[134] A. Erdélyi, W. Magnus, F. Oberhettinger, and F. G. Tricomi, *Higher Transcendental Functions*, v. 1, McGraw-Hill, 1953, pp. 1–55; MR 15,419i.
[135] J. Choi and H. M. Srivastava, Gamma function representation for some definite integrals, *Kyungpook Math. J.* 37 (1997) 205–209; MR 98g:33002.
[136] X. Gourdon and P. Sebah, The Gamma function (Numbers, Constants and Computation).

1.6 Apéry's Constant, $\zeta(3)$

Apéry's constant, $\zeta(3)$, is defined to be the value of **Riemann's zeta function**

$$\zeta(x) = \sum_{n=1}^{\infty} \frac{1}{n^x}, \quad x > 1,$$

when $x = 3$. This designation of $\zeta(3)$ as Apéry's constant is new but well deserved. In 1979, Apéry stunned the mathematical world with a miraculous proof that $\zeta(3) = 1.2020569031\ldots$ is irrational [1–10]. We will return to this after a brief discussion of Riemann's function.

The zeta function can be evaluated exactly [11–14] at positive even integer values of x,

$$\zeta(2k) = \frac{(-1)^{k-1}(2\pi)^{2k} B_{2k}}{2(2k)!},$$

where $\{B_n\}$ denotes the **Bernoulli numbers** [1.6.1]. For example,

$$\zeta(2) = \frac{\pi^2}{6}, \quad \zeta(4) = \frac{\pi^4}{90}, \quad \zeta(6) = \frac{\pi^6}{945}.$$

Clearly $\zeta(1)$ cannot be defined, at least by means of our definition of $\zeta(x)$, since the harmonic series diverges. The zeta function can be analytically continued over the whole complex plane via the functional equation [15–19]:

$$\zeta(1 - z) = \frac{2}{(2\pi)^z} \cos\left(\frac{\pi z}{2}\right) \Gamma(z)\zeta(z)$$

with just one singularity, a simple pole, at $z = 1$. Here $\Gamma(z) = (z - 1)!$ is the gamma function [1.5.4]. The connection between $\zeta(x)$ and prime number theory is best summarized by the two formulas

$$\zeta(x) = \prod_{p \text{ prime}} \left(1 - \frac{1}{p^x}\right)^{-1}, \quad \frac{\zeta(2x)}{\zeta(x)} = \prod_{p \text{ prime}} \left(1 + \frac{1}{p^x}\right)^{-1}.$$

If the famous Riemann hypothesis [1.6.2] can someday be proved, more information about the distribution of prime numbers will become available.

A closely associated function is [20–22]

$$\eta(x) = \sum_{n=1}^{\infty} \frac{(-1)^{n-1}}{n^x}, \quad x > 0,$$

which equals $(1 - 2^{1-x})\zeta(x)$ for $x \neq 1$. For example,

$$\eta(1) = \ln(2), \quad \eta(2) = \frac{\pi^2}{12}, \quad \eta(4) = \frac{7\pi^4}{720}.$$

The constant $\zeta(3)$ has a probabilistic interpretation [23,24]: Given three random integers, the probability that no factor exceeding 1 divides them all is $1/\zeta(3) = 0.8319073725\ldots$ (in the limit over large intervals). By way of contrast, the probability that the three integers are pairwise coprime is only $0.2867474284\ldots$; see the formulation in [2.5]. If n is a power of 2, define $c(n)$ to be the number of positive integer solutions (i, j, p) with p prime of the equation $n = p + ij$ [25,26]. Then $\lim_{n\to\infty} c(n)/n = 105\zeta(3)/(2\pi^4)$. Other occurrences of $\zeta(3)$ in number theory are discussed in [2.7] and [27–30]. It also appears in random graph theory with regard to minimum spanning tree lengths [8.5].

A generalization of Apéry's work to $\zeta(2k + 1)$ for any $k > 1$ remains, as van der Poorten wrote, "a mystery wrapped in an enigma" [2]. It remains open whether $\zeta(3)$ is transcendental, or even whether $\zeta(3)/\pi^3$ is irrational. Rivoal [31,32] recently proved that there are infinitely many integers k such that $\zeta(2k + 1)$ is irrational, and Zudilin [33,34] further showed that at least one of the numbers $\zeta(5)$, $\zeta(7)$, $\zeta(9)$, $\zeta(11)$ is irrational. This is the most dramatic piece of relevant news since Apéry's irrationality proof of $\zeta(3)$.

1.6.1 Bernoulli Numbers

Define $\{B_n\}$, the Bernoulli numbers, by the generating function [7, 19–22]

$$\frac{x}{e^x - 1} = \sum_{k=0}^{\infty} B_k \frac{x^k}{k!}.$$

From this, it follows that $B_0 = 1$, $B_1 = -1/2$, $B_2 = 1/6$, $B_4 = -1/30$, $B_6 = 1/42$, and $B_{2n+1} = 0$ for $n > 0$.

(There is, unfortunately, an alternative definition of the Bernoulli numbers to confuse matters. Under this alternative definition, the subscripting is somewhat different and all the numbers are positive. One must be careful when reading any paper to establish which definition has been used.)

The Bernoulli numbers also arise in certain other series expansions, such as

$$\tan(x) = \sum_{k=1}^{\infty} \frac{(-1)^{k+1}2^{2k}(2^{2k} - 1)B_{2k}}{(2k)!}x^{2k-1}.$$

1.6.2 The Riemann Hypothesis

With Wiles' recent proof of Fermat's Last Theorem now confirmed, the most notorious unsolved problem in mathematics becomes the Riemann hypothesis. This conjecture states that all the zeros of $\zeta(z)$ in the strip $0 \leq \mathrm{Re}(z) \leq 1$ lie on the central line $\mathrm{Re}(z) = 1/2$.

Here is a completely elementary restatement of the Riemann hypothesis [35]. Define a positive square-free integer to be **red** if it is the product of an even number of distinct primes, and **blue** if it is the product of an odd number of distinct primes. Let $R(n)$ be the number of red integers not exceeding n, and let $B(n)$ be the number of blue integers not exceeding n. The Riemann hypothesis is equivalent to the following statement: For any $\varepsilon > 0$, there exists an integer N such that for all $n > N$,

$$|R(n) - B(n)| < n^{\frac{1}{2}+\varepsilon}.$$

This is usually stated in terms of the Möbius mu function [2.2]. It turns out that setting $\varepsilon = 0$ is impossible; what is known as the Mertens hypothesis is false!

Another restatement (among several [36, 37]) is as follows. The Riemann hypothesis is true if and only if [38]

$$\int\limits_0^\infty \int\limits_{\frac{1}{2}}^\infty \frac{1 - 12y^2}{(1 + 4y^2)^3} \ln |\zeta(x + iy)| \, dx \, dy = \frac{3 - \gamma}{32}\pi,$$

where γ is the Euler–Mascheroni constant [1.5]. It is interesting to compare this conditional equality with formulas we know to be unconditionally true. For example, if Z denotes the set of all zeros ρ in the critical strip, then [39–41]

$$\sum_{\rho \varepsilon Z} \frac{1}{\rho} = \frac{1}{2}\gamma + 1 - \ln(2) - \frac{1}{2}\ln(\pi) = 0.0230957089\ldots.$$

That is, although the zero locations remain a mystery, we know enough about them to exactly compute their reciprocal sum. Care is needed: $\sum_\rho |\rho|^{-1}$ diverges, but $\sum_\rho \rho^{-1}$ converges provided that we group together conjugate terms.

One consequence of Riemann's hypothesis (among many [17]) is mentioned in [2.13]. Our knowledge of the distribution of prime numbers will be much deeper if a successful proof is someday found. The essay on the de Bruijn–Newman constant [2.32] has details of a computational approach. A deeper hypothesis, called the Gaussian unitary ensemble hypothesis [2.15.3], governs the vertical spacing distribution between the zeros.

1.6.3 Series

Summing over certain arithmetic progressions gives slight variations [42, 43]:

$$\lambda(3) = \sum_{k=0}^\infty \frac{1}{(2k + 1)^3} = \frac{7}{8}\zeta(3), \quad \sum_{k=0}^\infty \frac{1}{(3k + 1)^3} = \frac{2\pi^3}{81\sqrt{3}} + \frac{13}{27}\zeta(3),$$

$$\sum_{k=0}^\infty \frac{1}{(4k + 1)^3} = \frac{\pi^3}{64} + \frac{7}{16}\zeta(3), \quad \sum_{k=0}^\infty \frac{1}{(6k + 1)^3} = \frac{\pi^3}{36\sqrt{3}} + \frac{91}{216}\zeta(3).$$

We will discuss $\lambda(x)$ later in [1.7]. Two formulas involving central binomial sums are [42, 44–47]

$$\sum_{k=1}^{\infty} \frac{(-1)^{k+1}}{k^3 \binom{2k}{k}} = \frac{2}{5}\zeta(3), \quad \sum_{k=1}^{\infty} \frac{30k-11}{(2k-1)k^3\binom{2k}{k}^2} = 4\zeta(3),$$

the former of which has become famous because of Apéry's work.

What is the analog for $\zeta(2n+1)$ of the exact formula for $\zeta(2n)$? No one knows, but series obtained by Grosswald [48–51],

$$\zeta(3) = \frac{7}{180}\pi^3 - 2\sum_{k=1}^{\infty} \frac{1}{k^3\left(e^{2\pi k}-1\right)}, \quad \zeta(7) = \frac{19}{56700}\pi^7 - 2\sum_{k=1}^{\infty} \frac{1}{k^7\left(e^{2\pi k}-1\right)},$$

and by Plouffe [52] and Borwein [26, 53],

$$\zeta(5) = \frac{1}{294}\pi^5 - \frac{72}{35}\sum_{k=1}^{\infty} \frac{1}{k^5\left(e^{2\pi k}-1\right)} - \frac{2}{35}\sum_{k=1}^{\infty} \frac{1}{k^5\left(e^{2\pi k}+1\right)},$$

might be regarded as leading candidates. The formulas were inspired by certain entries in Ramanujan's notebooks [54].

Some multiple series appearing in [55–62] include

$$\sum_{i=1}^{\infty}\sum_{j=1}^{\infty} \frac{1}{ij(i+j)} = 2\zeta(3), \quad \sum_{i=1}^{\infty}\sum_{j=1}^{\infty} \frac{(-1)^{i-1}}{ij(i+j)} = \frac{5}{8}\zeta(3),$$

$$\sum_{i=1}^{\infty}\sum_{j=1}^{\infty} \frac{(-1)^{i+j}}{ij(i+j)} = \frac{1}{4}\zeta(3), \quad \sum_{i=2}^{\infty}\sum_{j=1}^{i-1} \frac{1}{i^2 j} = \zeta(3),$$

$$\sum_{i=3}^{\infty}\sum_{j=2}^{i-1}\sum_{k=1}^{j-1} \frac{1}{i^3 j^2 k} = -\frac{29}{6480}\pi^6 + 3\zeta(3)^2,$$

and many more such evaluations (of arbitrary depth) are known [63–75].

If $0 < x < 1$, then the following is true [19]:

$$\lim_{n\to\infty} \left(\sum_{k=1}^{n} \frac{1}{k^x} - \frac{n^{1-x}}{1-x}\right) = \zeta(x) = \left(1 - 2^{1-x}\right)^{-1} \eta(x) = \frac{-1}{2^{1-x}-1} \sum_{k=1}^{\infty} \frac{(-1)^{k-1}}{k^x}.$$

For example, when $x = 1/2$, the limiting value is [76]

$$\lim_{n\to\infty} \left(1 + \tfrac{1}{\sqrt{2}} + \cdots + \tfrac{1}{\sqrt{n}} - 2\sqrt{n}\right) = -\left(\sqrt{2}+1\right)\left(1 - \tfrac{1}{\sqrt{2}} + \tfrac{1}{\sqrt{3}} - + \cdots\right)$$
$$= -1.4603545088\ldots$$

as mentioned with regard to Euler's constant [1.5.3]. Recall too from [1.5.1] that

$$\gamma = \sum_{k=2}^{\infty}(-1)^k \frac{\zeta(k)}{k}, \quad 1 - \gamma = \sum_{k=2}^{\infty} \frac{\zeta(k)-1}{k}.$$

A notable family of series involving zeta function values is [77, 78]

$$S(n) = \sum_{k=1}^{\infty} \frac{\zeta(2k)}{(2k+n)2^{2k-1}}, \quad n = 0, 1, 2, \ldots.$$

For example [79–83],

$$S(0) = \ln(\pi) - \ln(2), \quad S(1) = -\ln(2) + 1, \quad S(2) = \frac{7}{2\pi^2}\zeta(3) - \ln(2) + \frac{1}{2},$$

$$S(3) = \frac{9}{2\pi^2}\zeta(3) - \ln(2) + \frac{1}{3}, \quad S(4) = -\frac{93}{2\pi^4}\zeta(5) + \frac{9}{\pi^2}\zeta(3) - \ln(2) + \frac{1}{4}.$$

These can be combined in various ways (via partial fractions) to obtain more rapidly convergent series, for example,

$$\sum_{k=1}^{\infty} \frac{\zeta(2k)}{(2k+1)(2k+2)2^{2k}} = -\frac{7}{4\pi^2}\zeta(3) + \frac{1}{4}$$

due to Euler [84–89] and

$$\sum_{k=1}^{\infty} \frac{\zeta(2k)}{k(k+1)(2k+1)(2k+3)2^{2k}} = \frac{2}{\pi^2}\zeta(3) - \frac{11}{18} + \frac{1}{3}\ln(\pi)$$

due to Wilton [90–92]. Many more series exist [93–102].

Broadhurst [103] determined digit-extraction algorithms for $\zeta(3)$ and $\zeta(5)$ similar to the Bailey–Borwein–Plouffe algorithm for π. The corresponding series for $\zeta(3)$ is

$$\zeta(3) = \frac{48}{7} \sum_{k=0}^{\infty} \frac{1}{2 \cdot 16^k} \left(\frac{1}{(8k+1)^3} - \frac{7}{(8k+2)^3} - \frac{1}{2(8k+3)^3} + \frac{10}{2(8k+4)^3} - \frac{1}{2^2(8k+5)^3} - \frac{7}{2^2(8k+6)^3} \right.$$

$$+ \frac{1}{2^3(8k+7)^3} \right) + \frac{32}{7} \sum_{k=0}^{\infty} \frac{1}{8 \cdot 16^{3k}} \left(\frac{1}{(8k+1)^3} + \frac{1}{2(8k+2)^3} - \frac{1}{2^3(8k+3)^3} - \frac{2}{2^4(8k+4)^3} \right.$$

$$\left. - \frac{1}{2^6(8k+5)^3} + \frac{1}{2^7(8k+6)^3} + \frac{1}{2^9(8k+7)^3} \right).$$

Amdeberhan, Zeilberger and Wilf [104–106] discovered extremely fast series for computing $\zeta(3)$, which presently is known to several hundred million decimal digits. See also [107–110]. We mention [111–114]

$$\sum_{k=1}^{\infty} \frac{(-1)^k}{k^3(k+1)^3} = 10 - \frac{3}{2}\zeta(3) - 12\ln(2),$$

$$\text{Li}_3\left(\frac{1}{2}\right) = \frac{7}{8}\zeta(3) + \frac{\pi^2}{12}\ln\left(\frac{1}{2}\right) - \frac{1}{6}\ln\left(\frac{1}{2}\right)^3,$$

$$\text{Li}_3(2-\varphi) = \frac{4}{5}\zeta(3) + \frac{\pi^2}{15}\ln(2-\varphi) - \frac{1}{12}\ln(2-\varphi)^3,$$

where Li_3 denotes the trilogarithm function [1.6.8] and φ denotes the Golden mean [1.2].

Finally, the generating function for $\zeta(4n+3)$ [115, 116]

$$\sum_{n=0}^{\infty} \zeta(4n+3)x^n = \frac{5}{2} \sum_{i=1}^{\infty} \frac{(-1)^{i+1}}{i^3\binom{2i}{i}} \frac{1}{1-\frac{x}{i^4}} \prod_{j=1}^{i-1} \frac{j^4+4x}{j^4-x}, \quad |x| < 1,$$

includes the Apéry series in the special case $x = 0$. If we differentiate both sides with respect to x and then set $x = 0$, a fast series for $\zeta(7)$ emerges:

$$\zeta(7) = \frac{5}{2} \sum_{k=1}^{\infty} \frac{(-1)^{k+1}}{k^7 \binom{2k}{k}} + \frac{25}{2} \sum_{k=1}^{\infty} \frac{(-1)^{k+1}}{k^3 \binom{2k}{k}} \sum_{m=1}^{k-1} \frac{1}{m^4}$$

and likewise for larger n. No analogous generating function is known for $\zeta(4n + 1)$. How can the series [117]

$$\zeta(5) = 2 \sum_{k=1}^{\infty} \frac{(-1)^{k+1}}{k^5 \binom{2k}{k}} - \frac{5}{2} \sum_{k=1}^{\infty} \frac{(-1)^{k+1}}{k^3 \binom{2k}{k}} \sum_{m=1}^{k-1} \frac{1}{m^2}$$

be correspondingly extended?

1.6.4 Products

There is a striking family of matrix products due to Gosper [118]. The simplest case is

$$\prod_{k=1}^{\infty} \begin{pmatrix} -\frac{k}{2(2k+1)} & \frac{5}{4k^2} \\ 0 & 1 \end{pmatrix} = \begin{pmatrix} 0 & \zeta(3) \\ 0 & 1 \end{pmatrix},$$

which is equivalent to a central binomial sum given earlier. The general case involves $(n + 1) \times (n + 1)$ upper-triangular matrices, where $n \geq 2$:

$$\prod_{k=1}^{\infty} \begin{pmatrix} -\frac{k}{2(2k+1)} & \frac{1}{2k(2k+1)} & 0 & \cdots & 0 & \frac{1}{k^{2n}} \\ 0 & -\frac{k}{2(2k+1)} & \frac{1}{2k(2k+1)} & \cdots & 0 & \frac{1}{k^{2n-2}} \\ \vdots & \vdots & \vdots & & \vdots & \vdots \\ 0 & 0 & 0 & \cdots & \frac{1}{2k(2k+1)} & \frac{1}{k^4} \\ 0 & 0 & 0 & \cdots & -\frac{k}{2(2k+1)} & \frac{5}{4k^2} \\ 0 & 0 & 0 & \cdots & 0 & 1 \end{pmatrix} = \begin{pmatrix} 0 & \cdots & 0 & \zeta(2n+1) \\ 0 & \cdots & 0 & \zeta(2n-1) \\ \vdots & \vdots & & \vdots \\ 0 & \cdots & 0 & \zeta(5) \\ 0 & \cdots & 0 & \zeta(3) \\ 0 & \cdots & 0 & 1 \end{pmatrix},$$

where the diagonal and superdiagonal are extended (by repetition) as indicated, the rightmost column contains reciprocals of k^{2m}, and all remaining entries are zero.

1.6.5 Integrals

Riemann's zeta function has an alternative expression [17] for $x > 1$:

$$\zeta(x) = \frac{1}{\Gamma(x)} \int_0^{\infty} \frac{t^{x-1}}{e^t - 1} dt.$$

If $\{t\}$ denotes the fractional part of t, then [18, 19]

$$\int_1^{\infty} \frac{\{t\}}{t^{x+1}} dt = \begin{cases} \frac{1}{x-1} - \frac{\zeta(x)}{x} & \text{if } 0 < x < 1 \text{ or } x > 1, \\ 1 - \gamma & \text{if } x = 1. \end{cases}$$

For all remaining x the integral is divergent. A quick adjustment is, however, possible over a subinterval:

$$\int_1^\infty \frac{\{t\} - \frac{1}{2}}{t^{x+1}} dt = \begin{cases} \dfrac{1}{x-1} - \dfrac{1}{2x} - \dfrac{\zeta(x)}{x} & \text{if } -1 < x < 0, \\[2mm] \dfrac{1}{2}\ln(2\pi) - 1 & \text{if } x = 0. \end{cases}$$

Munthe Hjortnaes [119] proved that

$$\zeta(3) = 10 \int_0^{\ln(\varphi)} x^2 \coth(x)\, dx = 10 \int_0^{\frac{1}{2}} \frac{\operatorname{arcsinh}(y)^2}{y}\, dy,$$

which, after integration by parts, gives [120]

$$\zeta(3) = -5 \int_0^{2\ln(\varphi)} \theta \ln\left(2 \sinh\left(\frac{\theta}{2}\right)\right) d\theta.$$

Starting with an integral of Euler's [84, 121],

$$4 \int_0^\pi \theta \ln\left(\sin\left(\frac{\theta}{2}\right)\right) d\theta = 7\zeta(3) - 2\pi^2 \ln(2),$$

the same reasoning can be applied as before (but in reverse) to obtain [80, 81]

$$-8 \int_0^1 \frac{\arcsin(y)^2}{y}\, dy = -8 \int_0^{\frac{\pi}{2}} x^2 \cot(x)\, dx = 7\zeta(3) - 2\pi^2 \ln(2).$$

1.6.6 Continued Fractions

Stieltjes [122] and Ramanujan [54] discovered the continued fraction expansion

$$\zeta(3) = 1 + \frac{1|}{|2 \cdot 2} + \frac{1^3|}{|1} + \frac{1^3|}{|6 \cdot 2} + \frac{2^3|}{|1} + \frac{2^3|}{|10 \cdot 2} + \frac{3^3|}{|1} + \frac{3^3|}{|14 \cdot 2} + \cdots.$$

If we group terms together in a pairwise manner, we obtain

$$\zeta(3) = 1 + \frac{1|}{|5} - \frac{1^6|}{|21} - \frac{2^6|}{|55} - \frac{3^6|}{|119} - \frac{4^6|}{|225} - \frac{5^6|}{|385} - \cdots,$$

where the partial denominators are generated according to the polynomial $2n^3 + 3n^2 + 11n + 5$. The convergence rate of this expansion is not fast enough to demonstrate the irrationality of $\zeta(3)$. Apéry succeeded in accelerating the convergence to

$$\zeta(3) = \frac{6|}{|5} - \frac{1^6|}{|117} - \frac{2^6|}{|535} - \frac{3^6|}{|1463} - \frac{4^6|}{|3105} - \frac{5^6|}{|5665} - \cdots,$$

where the partial denominators are generated according to the polynomial $34n^3 + 51n^2 + 27n + 5$.

1.6.7 Stirling Cycle Numbers

Define $s_{n,m}$ to be the number of permutations of n symbols that have exactly m cycles [123]. The quantity $s_{n,m}$ is called the **Stirling number of the first kind** and satisfies the recurrence

$$s_{n,0} = \begin{cases} 1 & \text{if } n = 0, \\ 0 & \text{if } n \geq 1, \end{cases}$$

$$s_{n,m} = (n-1)s_{n-1,m} + s_{n-1,m-1} \quad \text{if } n \geq m \geq 1.$$

For example, $s_{3,1} = 2$ since (123) and (321) are distinct permutations. More generally, $s_{n,1} = (n-1)!$ and $s_{n,2} = (n-1)! \sum_{k=1}^{n-1} 1/k$. Similar complicated formulas involving higher-order harmonic sums apply for $m \geq 3$. Consequently [124],

$$\sum_{n=1}^{\infty} \frac{s_{n,m}}{n!n} = \zeta(m+1)$$

for $m \geq 1$. The case for $m = 2$ follows from one of the earlier multiple series (due to Euler [67]). The asymptotics of $s_{n,m}$ as $n \to \infty$ are found in [125].

1.6.8 Polylogarithms

Before defining the polylogarithm function Li_n, let us ask a question. It is known that

$$(-1)^k k! \zeta(k+1) = \int_0^1 \frac{\ln(x)^k}{1-x} dx, \quad k = 1, 2, 3, \dots.$$

What happens if the interval of integration is changed from $[0, 1]$ to $[1, 2]$? Ramanujan [42] showed that, if

$$a_k = \int_1^2 \frac{\ln(x)^k}{1-x} dx,$$

then $a_1 = \zeta(2)/2 = \pi^2/6$ and $a_2 = \zeta(3)/4$. We would expect the pattern to persist and for a_k to be a rational multiple of $\zeta(k+1)$ for all $k \geq 1$. This does not appear to be true, however, even for $k = 3$.

Define $\text{Li}_1(x) = -\ln(1-x)$ and [113, 114]

$$\text{Li}_n(x) = \sum_{k=1}^{\infty} \frac{x^k}{k^n} = \int_0^x \frac{\text{Li}_{n-1}(t)}{t} dt \quad \text{for any integer } n \geq 2, \text{ where } |x| \leq 1.$$

Clearly $\text{Li}_n(1) = \zeta(n)$. We mentioned special values, due to Landen, of the trilogarithm Li_3 earlier. Not much is known about the tetralogarithm Li_4, but Levin [126] demonstrated that

$$a_3 = \frac{\pi^4}{15} + \frac{\pi^2 \ln(2)^2}{4} - \frac{\ln(2)^4}{4} - \frac{21 \ln(2)}{4} \zeta(3) - 6 \text{Li}_4\left(\frac{1}{2}\right)$$

and more. To fully answer our question, therefore, requires an understanding of the arithmetic nature of $\text{Li}_n(1/2)$. Further details on polylogarithms are found in [127–131].

[1] R. Apéry, Irrationalité de $\zeta(2)$ et $\zeta(3)$, *Astérisque* 61 (1979) 11–13.
[2] A. van der Poorten, A proof that Euler missed... Apéry's proof of the irrationality of $\zeta(3)$, *Math. Intellig.* 1 (1979) 196–203; MR 80i:10054.
[3] A. van der Poorten, Some wonderful formulae... footnotes to Apéry's proof of the irrationality of $\zeta(3)$, *Séminaire Delange-Pisot-Poitu (Théorie des nombres)*, 20e année, 1978/79, n. 29, pp. 1–7; MR 82a:10037.
[4] A. van der Poorten, Some wonderful formulas... an introduction to polylogarithms, *Queen's Papers in Pure and Applied Mathematics*, n. 54, Proc. 1979 Queen's Number Theory Conf., ed. P. Ribenboim, 1980, pp. 269–286; MR 83b:10043.
[5] F. Beukers, A note on the irrationality of $\zeta(2)$ and $\zeta(3)$, *Bull. London Math. Soc.* 11 (1979) 268–272; MR 81j:10045.
[6] M. Prévost, A new proof of the irrationality of $\zeta(3)$ using Padé approximants, *J. Comput. Appl. Math.* 67 (1996) 219–235; MR 97f:11056.
[7] J. M. Borwein and P. B. Borwein, *Pi and the AGM: A Study in Analytic Number Theory and Computational Complexity*, Wiley, 1987, pp. 362–386; MR 99h:11147.
[8] P. Borwein and T. Erdélyi, *Polynomials and Polynomial Inequalities*, Springer-Verlag, 1995, pp. 372–381; MR 97e:41001.
[9] G. E. Andrews, R. Askey, and R. Roy, *Special Functions*, Cambridge Univ. Press, 1999, pp. 391–394; MR 2000g:33001.
[10] D. Huylebrouck, Similarities in irrationality proofs for π, $\ln(2)$, $\zeta(2)$, and $\zeta(3)$, *Amer. Math. Monthly* 108 (2001) 222–231; MR 2002b:11095.
[11] B. C. Berndt, Elementary evaluation of $\zeta(2n)$, *Math. Mag.* 48 (1975) 148–153; MR 51 #3078.
[12] F. Beukers, J. A. C. Kolk, and E. Calabi, Sums of generalized harmonic series and volumes, *Nieuw Arch. Wisk.* 4 (1993) 217–224; MR 94j:11022.
[13] R. Chapman, Evaluating $\zeta(2)$, unpublished note (1998).
[14] N. D. Elkies, On the sums $\sum_{k=-\infty}^{\infty}(4k+1)^{-n}$, math.CA/0101168.
[15] J. B. Conway, *Functions of One Complex Variable*, 2nd ed., Springer-Verlag, 1978, pp. 187–194; MR 80c:30003.
[16] W. Ellison and F. Ellison, *Prime Numbers*, Wiley, 1985, pp. 147–152; MR 87a:11082.
[17] E. C. Titchmarsh, *The Theory of the Riemann Zeta Function*, 2nd ed., rev. by D. R. Heath-Brown, Oxford Univ. Press, 1986, pp. 18–19, 282–328; MR 88c:11049.
[18] A. Ivić, *The Riemann Zeta-Function*, Wiley, 1985, pp. 1–12; MR 87d:11062.
[19] T. M. Apostol, *Introduction to Analytic Number Theory*, Springer-Verlag, 1976, pp. 55–56, 249–267; MR 55 #7892.
[20] M. Abramowitz and I. A. Stegun, *Handbook of Mathematical Functions*, Dover, 1972, pp. 807–808; MR 94b:00012.
[21] J. Spanier and K. B. Oldham, *An Atlas of Functions*, Hemisphere, 1987, pp. 25–33.
[22] I. S. Gradshteyn and I. M Ryzhik, *Tables of Integrals, Series and Products*, Academic Press, 1980; MR 97c:00014.
[23] J. E. Nymann, On the probability that k positive integers are relatively prime, *J. Number Theory* 4 (1972) 469–473; MR 46 #3478.
[24] P. Moree, Counting carefree couples, unpublished note (1999).
[25] B. M. Bredihin, Applications of the dispersion method in binary additive problems (in Russian), *Dokl. Akad. Nauk SSSR* 149 (1963) 9–11; MR 26 #2419.
[26] J. M. Borwein, D. M. Bradley, and R. E. Crandall, Computational strategies for the Riemann zeta function, *J. Comput. Appl. Math.* 121 (2000) 247–296; CECM preprint 98:118; MR 2001h:11110.
[27] S. Akiyama, A new type of inclusion exclusion principle for sequences and asymptotic formulas for $\zeta(k)$, *J. Number Theory* 45 (1993) 200–214; MR 94k:11027.

[28] S. Akiyama, A criterion to estimate the least common multiple of sequences and asymptotic formulas for $\zeta(3)$ arising from recurrence relation of an elliptic function, *Japan. J. Math.* 22 (1996) 129–146; MR 97f:11021.

[29] V. Strehl, Recurrences and Legendre transform, *Sémin. Lothar. Combin.* 29 (1992) B29b; MR 96m:11017.

[30] Y. Lan, A limit formula for $\zeta(2k + 1)$, *J. Number Theory* 78 (1999) 271–286; MR 2000f:11102.

[31] T. Rivoal, La fonction zêta de Riemann prend une infinité de valeurs irrationnelles aux entiers impairs, *C. R. Acad. Sci. Paris* 331 (2000) 267–270; math.NT/0008051; MR 2001k:11138.

[32] T. Rivoal, Irrationalité d'au moins un des neuf nombres $\zeta(5)$, $\zeta(7)$, ..., $\zeta(21)$, *Acta Arith.* 103 (2002) 157–167; math.NT/0104221.

[33] W. Zudilin, On the irrationality of the values of the zeta function at odd points (in Russian), *Uspekhi Mat. Nauk* 56 (2001) 215–216; Engl. transl. in *Russian Math. Surveys* 56 (2001) 423–424.

[34] W. Zudilin, One of the numbers $\zeta(5)$, $\zeta(7)$, $\zeta(9)$, $\zeta(11)$ is irrational (in Russian), *Uspekhi Mat. Nauk* 56 (2001) 149–150; Engl. transl. in *Russian Math. Surveys* 56 (2001) 774–776; MR 2002g:11098.

[35] H. S. Wilf, A greeting; and a view of Riemann's hypothesis, *Amer. Math. Monthly* 94 (1987) 3–6; MR 88a:11082.

[36] F. T. Wang, A note on the Riemann zeta-function, *Bull. Amer. Math. Soc.* 52 (1946) 319–321; MR 7,417a.

[37] M. Balazard, E. Saias, and M. Yor, Notes sur la fonction ζ de Riemann. II, *Adv. Math.* 143 (1999) 284–287; MR 2000c:11140.

[38] V. V. Volchkov, On an equality equivalent to the Riemann hypothesis (in Ukrainian), *Ukrain. Math. Zh.* 47 (1995) 422–423; Engl. transl. in *Ukrainian Math. J.* 47 (1995) 491–493; MR 96g:11111.

[39] H. M. Edwards, *Riemann's Zeta Function*, Academic Press, 1974, pp. 67, 159–160; MR 57 #5922.

[40] H. Davenport, *Multiplicative Number Theory*, 2nd ed., rev. by H. L. Montgomery, Springer-Verlag, 1980, pp. 79–83; MR 82m:10001.

[41] S. J. Patterson, *An Introduction to the Theory of the Riemann Zeta Function*, Cambridge Univ. Press, 1988, pp. 33–34; MR 89d:11072.

[42] B. C. Berndt, *Ramanujan's Notebooks: Part I*, Springer-Verlag, 1985, pp. 163–164, 232, 290–293; MR 86c:01062.

[43] E. R. Hansen, *A Table of Series and Products*, Prentice-Hall, 1975.

[44] J. M. Borwein, D. J. Broadhurst, and J. Kamnitzer, Central binomial sums, multiple Clausen values and zeta values, hep-th/0004153.

[45] S. Plouffe, The art of inspired guessing, unpublished note (1998).

[46] R. W. Gosper, A calculus of series rearrangements, *Algorithms and Complexity: New Directions and Recent Results*, Proc. 1976 Carnegie-Mellon conf., ed. J. F. Traub, Academic Press, 1976, pp. 121–151; MR 56 #9899.

[47] R. W. Gosper, Strip mining in the abandoned orefields of nineteenth century mathematics, *Computers in Mathematics*, Proc. 1986 Stanford Univ. conf., ed. D. V. Chudnovsky and R. D. Jenks, Dekker, 1990, pp. 261–284; MR 91h:11154.

[48] E. Grosswald, Die Werte der Riemannschen Zetafunktion an ungeraden Argumentstellen, *Nachr. Akad. Wiss. Göttingen, Math.-Phys. Klasse* 2 (1970) 9–13; MR 42 #7606.

[49] D. Shanks, Calculation and applications of Epstein zeta functions, *Math. Comp.* 29 (1975) 271–287; corrigenda 29 (1975) 1167 and 30 (1976) 900; MR 53 #13114a-c.

[50] D. H. Bailey, J. M. Borwein, and R. E. Crandall, On the Khintchine constant, *Math. Comp.* 66 (1997) 417–431; CECM preprint 95:036; MR 97c:11119.

[51] H. Cohen, High precision computation of Hardy-Littlewood constants, unpublished note (1999).

[52] S. Plouffe, Identities inspired from Ramanujan Notebooks. II, unpublished note (1998).

[53] J. M. Borwein, Experimental mathematics: Insight from computation, presentation at *AMS/MAA Joint Meetings*, San Antonio, 1999.

[54] B. C. Berndt, *Ramanujan's Notebooks: Part II*, Springer-Verlag, 1989, pp. 153–155, 275–276, 293; MR 90b:01039.

[55] W. E. Briggs, S. Chowla, A. J. Kempner, and W. E. Mientka, On some infinite series, *Scripta Math.* 21 (1955) 28–30; MR 16,1014d.

[56] L. J. Mordell, On the evaluation of some multiple series, *J. London Math. Soc.* 33 (1958) 368–371; MR 20 #6615.

[57] R. Sitaramachandrarao and A. Sivaramasarma, Some identities involving the Riemann zeta function, *Indian J. Pure Appl. Math.* 10 (1979) 602–607; MR 80h:10047.

[58] M. V. Subbarao and R. Sitaramachandrarao, On some infinite series of L. J. Mordell and their analogues, *Pacific J. Math.* 119 (1985) 245–255; MR 87c:11091.

[59] R. Sitaramachandrarao, A formula of S. Ramanujan, *J. Number Theory* 25 (1987) 1–19; MR 88c:11048.

[60] M. E. Hoffman, Multiple harmonic series, *Pacific J. Math.* 152 (1992) 275–290; MR 92i:11089.

[61] C. Markett, Triple sums and the Riemann zeta function, *J. Number Theory* 48 (1994) 113–132; MR 95f:11067.

[62] M. E. Hoffman and C. Moen, Sums of triple harmonic series, *J. Number Theory* 60 (1996) 329–331; MR 98a:11113.

[63] D. Zagier, Values of zeta functions and their applications, *First European Congress of Mathematics*, v. 2, Paris, 1992, ed. A. Joseph, F. Mignot, F. Murat, B. Prum, and R. Rentschler, Birkhäuser, 1994, pp. 497–512; MR 96k:11110.

[64] D. Borwein and J. Borwein, On an intriguing integral and some series related to $\zeta(4)$, *Proc. Amer. Math. Soc.* 123 (1995) 1191–1198; MR 95e:11137.

[65] D. H. Bailey, J. M. Borwein, and R. Girgensohn, Experimental evaluation of Euler sums, *Experim. Math.* 3 (1994) 17–30; MR 96e:11168.

[66] D. Borwein, J. M. Borwein, and R. Girgensohn, Explicit evaluation of Euler sums, *Proc. Edinburgh Math. Soc.* 38 (1995) 277–294; MR 96f:11106.

[67] P. Flajolet and B. Salvy, Euler sums and contour integral representations, *Experim. Math.* 7 (1998) 15–35; MR 99c:11110.

[68] J. M. Borwein and R. Girgensohn, Evaluation of triple Euler sums, *Elec. J. Combin.* 3 (1996) R23; MR 97d:11137.

[69] J. M. Borwein, D. M. Bradley, and D. J. Broadhurst, Evaluations of k-fold Euler/Zagier sums: A compendium of results for arbitrary k, *Elec. J. Combin.* 4 (1997) R5; MR 98b:11091.

[70] J. M. Borwein, D. M. Bradley, D. J. Broadhurst, and P. Lisonek, Combinatorial aspects of multiple zeta values, *Elec. J. Combin.* 5 (1998) R38; math.NT/9812020; MR 99g:11100.

[71] J. M. Borwein, D. M. Bradley, D. J. Broadhurst, and P. Lisonek, Special values of multidimensional polylogarithms, *Trans. Amer. Math. Soc.* 353 (2001) 907–941; math.CA/9910045; CECM preprint 98:106.

[72] N. R. Farnum and A. Tissier, Apéry's constant, *Amer. Math. Monthly* 106 (1999) 965–966.

[73] A. Granville, A decomposition of Riemann's zeta-function, *Analytic Number Theory*, Proc. 1996 Kyoto conf., ed. Y. Motohashi, Cambridge Univ. Press, 1997, pp. 95–101; MR 2000c:11134.

[74] O. M. Ogreid and P. Osland, Summing one- and two-dimensional series related to the Euler series, *J. Comput. Appl. Math.* 98 (1998) 245–271; hep-th/9801168; MR 99m:40003.

[75] O. M. Ogreid and P. Osland, More series related to the Euler series, hep-th/9904206.

[76] S. Ramanujan, On the sum of the square roots of the first n natural numbers, *J. Indian Math. Soc.* 7 (1915) 173–175; also in *Collected Papers*, ed. G. H. Hardy, P. V. Seshu Aiyar, and B. M. Wilson, Cambridge Univ. Press, 1927, pp. 47–49, 337.

[77] N.-Y. Zhang and K. S. Williams, Some series representations for $\zeta(2n + 1)$, *Rocky Mount. J. Math.* 23 (1993) 1581–1592; MR 94m:11099.

[78] N.-Y. Zhang and K. S. Williams, Some infinite series involving the Riemann zeta function, *Analysis, Geometry and Groups: A Riemann Legacy Volume*, ed. H. M. Srivastava and T. M. Rassias, Hadronic Press, 1993, pp. 691–712; MR 96a:11084.

[79] M. L. Glasser, Some integrals of the arctangent function, *Math. Comp.* 22 (1968) 445–447.

[80] C. Nash and D. J. O'Connor, Determinants of Laplacians, the Ray-Singer torsion on lens spaces and the Riemann zeta function, *J. Math. Phys.* 36 (1995) 1462–1505; erratum 36 (1995) 4549; MR 95k:58173.

[81] A. Dabrowski, A note on the values of the Riemann zeta function at odd positive integers, *Nieuw Arch. Wisk.* 14 (1996) 199–207; MR 97g:11142.

[82] M.-P. Chen and H. M. Srivastava, Some familes of series representations for the Riemann $\zeta(3)$, *Resultate Math.* 33 (1998) 179–197; MR 99b:11095.

[83] H. M. Srivastava, M. L. Glasser, and V. S. Adamchik, Some definite integrals associated with the Riemann zeta function, *Z. Anal. Anwendungen* 19 (2000) 831–846; MR 2001g:11136.

[84] L. Euler, Exercitationes Analyticae, 1772, *Opera Omnia Ser. I*, v. 15, Lipsiae, 1911, pp. 131–167.

[85] V. Ramaswami, Notes on Riemann's ζ-function, *J. London Math. Soc.* 9 (1934) 165–169.

[86] A. Terras, Some formulas for the Riemann zeta function at odd integer argument resulting from Fourier expansions of the Epstein zeta function, *Acta Arith.* 29 (1976) 181–189; MR 53 #299.

[87] J. A. Ewell, A new series representation for $\zeta(3)$, *Amer. Math. Monthly* 97 (1990) 219–220; MR 91d:11103.

[88] J. A. Ewell, On values of the Riemann zeta function at integral arguments, *Canad. Math. Bull.* 34 (1991) 60–66; MR 92c:11087.

[89] J. A. Ewell, On the zeta function values $\zeta(2k+1)$, $k = 1, 2, \ldots$, *Rocky Mount. J. Math.* 25 (1995) 1003–1012; MR 97i:11093.

[90] J. R. Wilton, A proof of Burnside's formula for $\log(\Gamma(x+1))$ and certain allied properties of Riemann's ξ-function, *Messenger of Math.* 52 (1922) 90–93.

[91] D. Cvijovic and J. Klinowski, New rapidly convergent series representations for $\zeta(2n+1)$, *Proc. Amer. Math. Soc.* 125 (1997) 1263–1271; MR 97g:11090.

[92] M. Katsurada, Rapidly convergent series representations for $\zeta(2n+1)$ and their χ-analogue, *Acta Arith.* 90 (1999) 79–89; MR 2000f:11101.

[93] U. Balakrishnan, A series for $\zeta(s)$, *Proc. Edinburgh Math. Soc.* 31 (1988) 205–210; MR 90g:11123.

[94] P. L. Butzer, C. Markett, and M. Schmidt, Stirling numbers, central factorial numbers, and representations of the Riemann zeta function, *Resultate Math.* 19 (1991) 257–274; MR 92a:11095.

[95] P. L. Butzer and M. Hauss, Riemann zeta function: rapidly converging series and integral representations, *Appl. Math. Lett.*, v. 5 (1992) n. 2, 83–88; MR 93b:11106.

[96] J. Choi, H. M. Srivastava, and J. R. Quine, Some series involving the zeta function, *Bull. Austral. Math. Soc.* 51 (1995) 383–393; MR 96d:11090.

[97] J. Choi and H. M. Srivastava, Sums associated with the zeta function, *J. Math. Anal. Appl.* 206 (1997) 103–120; MR 97i:11092.

[98] V. S. Adamchik and H. M. Srivastava, Some series of the zeta and related functions, *Analysis* 18 (1998) 131–144; MR 99d:11096.

[99] H. M. Srivastava, Further series representations for $\zeta(2n+1)$, *Appl. Math. Comput.* 97 (1998) 1–15; MR 99h:11148.

[100] H. M. Srivastava, Some rapidly converging series for $\zeta(2n+1)$, *Proc. Amer. Math. Soc.* 127 (1999) 385–396; MR 99c:11164.

[101] J. Choi, A. K. Rathie, and H. M. Srivastava, Some hypergeometric and other evaluations of $\zeta(2)$ and allied series, *Appl. Math. Comput.* 104 (1999) 101–108; MR 2000e:11104.

[102] J. Choi and H. M. Srivastava, Certain classes of series involving the zeta function, *J. Math. Anal. Appl.* 231 (1999) 91–117; MR 2000c:11143.

[103] D. J. Broadhurst, Polylogarithmic ladders, hypergeometric series and the ten millionth digits of $\zeta(3)$ and $\zeta(5)$, math.CA/9803067.

[104] T. Amdeberhan, Faster and faster convergent series for $\zeta(3)$, *Elec. J. Combin.* 3 (1996) R13; MR 97b:11154.

[105] T. Amdeberhan and D. Zeilberger, Hypergeometric series acceleration via the WZ method, *Elec. J. Combin.* 4 (1997) R3; MR 99e:33018.

[106] H. Wilf, Accelerated series for universal constants, by the WZ method, *Discrete Math. Theoret. Comput. Sci.* 3 (1999) 155–158.

[107] E. A. Karatsuba, Fast evaluation of $\zeta(3)$ (in Russian), *Problemy Peredachi Informatsii* 29 (1993) 68–73; Engl. transl. in *Problems Information Transmission* 29 (1993) 58–62; MR 94e:11145.

[108] E. A. Karatsuba, Fast evaluation of the Riemann zeta function $\zeta(s)$ for integer values of the argument s (in Russian), *Problemy Peredachi Informatsii* 31 (1995) 69–80; Engl. transl. in *Problems Information Transmission* 31 (1995) 353–362; MR 96k:11155.

[109] X. Gourdon and P. Sebah, The Apéry constant (Numbers, Constants and Computation).

[110] B. Gourevitch, Une formule BBP pour $\zeta(3)$, unpublished note (2000).

[111] J. W. L. Glaisher, Summations of certain numerical series, *Messenger of Math.* 42 (1912) 19–34.

[112] P. Kesava Menon, Summation of certain series, *J. Indian Math. Soc.* 25 (1961) 121–128; MR 26 #2761.

[113] L. Lewin, *Polylogarithms and Associated Functions*, North-Holland, 1981, pp. 153–156; MR 83b:33019.

[114] L. Lewin, ed., *Structural Properties of Polylogarithms*, Amer. Math. Soc., 1991; MR 93b:11158.

[115] J. Borwein and D. Bradley, Empirically determined Apéry-like formulae for $\zeta(4n + 3)$, *Experim. Math.* 6 (1997) 181–194; MR 98m:11142.

[116] G. Almkvist and A. Granville, Borwein and Bradley's Apéry-like formulae for $\zeta(4n + 3)$, *Experim. Math.* 8 (1999) 197–203; MR 2000h:11126.

[117] M. Koecher, Letter, *Math. Intellig.* 2 (1980) 62–64.

[118] R. W. Gosper, Analytic identities from path invariant matrix multiplication, unpublished manuscript (1976).

[119] M. Munthe Hjortnaes, Transformation of the series $\sum_{k=1}^{\infty} 1/k^3$ to a definite integral (in Norwegian), *Tolfte Skandinaviska Matematikerkongressen*, Proc. 1953 Lunds conf., Lunds Univ. Mat. Instit., 1954, pp. 211–213; MR 16,343a.

[120] N.-Y. Zhang and K. S. Williams, Values of the Riemann zeta function and integrals involving $\log(2\sinh(\theta/2))$ and $\log(2\sin(\theta/2))$, *Pacific J. Math.* 168 (1995) 271–289; MR 96f:11170.

[121] R. Ayoub, Euler and the zeta function, *Amer. Math. Monthly* 71 (1974) 1067–1086; MR 50 #12566.

[122] P. Flajolet, B. Vallée, and I. Vardi, Continued fractions from Euclid to the present day, École Polytechnique preprint (2000).

[123] L. Lovász, *Combinatorial Problems and Exercises*, 2nd ed., North-Holland, 1993; MR 94m:05001.

[124] V. S. Adamchik, On Stirling numbers and Euler sums, *J. Comput. Appl. Math.* 79 (1997) 119–130; MR 97m:11025.

[125] H. S. Wilf, The asymptotic behavior of the Stirling numbers of the first kind, *J. Combin. Theory Ser. A* 64 (1993) 344–349; MR 94m:11025.

[126] V. I. Levin, About a problem of S. Ramanujan (in Russian), *Uspekhi Mat. Nauk*, v. 5 (1950) n. 3, 161–166.

[127] N. Nielsen, Der Eulersche Dilogarithmus und seine Verallgemeinerungen, *Nova Acta Leopoldina, Abhandlungen der Kaiserlich Leopoldinisch-Carolinischen Deutschen Akademie der Naturforscher* 90 (1909) 121–212.

[128] K. S. Kölbig, Nielsen's generalized polylogarithms, *SIAM J. Math. Anal.* 17 (1986) 1232–1258; MR 88a:33028.

[129] M. J. Levine, E. Remiddi, and R. Roskies, Analytic contributions to the g factor of the electron in sixth order, *Phys. Rev. D* 20 (1979) 2068–2076.
[130] R. Gastmans and W. Troost, On the evaluation of polylogarithmic integrals, *Simon Stevin* 55 (1981) 205–219; MR 83c:65028.
[131] P. J. de Doelder, On some series containing $\psi(x) - \psi(y)$ and $(\psi(x) - \psi(y))^2$ for certain values of x and y, *J. Comput. Appl. Math.* 37 (1991) 125–141; MR 92m:40002.

1.7 Catalan's Constant, G

Catalan's constant, G, is defined by

$$G = \sum_{n=0}^{\infty} \frac{(-1)^n}{(2n+1)^2} = 0.9159655941\ldots.$$

Our discussion parallels that of Apéry's constant [1.6] and a comparison of the two is worthwhile. Here we work with **Dirichlet's beta function**

$$\beta(x) = \sum_{n=0}^{\infty} \frac{(-1)^n}{(2n+1)^x}, \quad x > 0$$

(also referred to as Dirichlet's L-series for the nonprincipal character modulo 4) and observe that $G = \beta(2)$.

The beta function can be evaluated exactly [1–3] at positive odd integer values of x:

$$\beta(2k+1) = \frac{(-1)^k E_{2k}}{2(2k)!} \left(\frac{\pi}{2}\right)^{2k+1},$$

where $\{E_n\}$ denote the **Euler numbers** [1.7.1]. For example,

$$\beta(1) = \frac{\pi}{4}, \quad \beta(3) = \frac{\pi^3}{32}, \quad \beta(5) = \frac{5\pi^5}{1536}.$$

Like the zeta function [1.6], $\beta(x)$ can be analytically continued over the whole complex plane via the functional equation [4–6]:

$$\beta(1-z) = \left(\frac{2}{\pi}\right)^z \sin\left(\frac{\pi z}{2}\right) \Gamma(z)\beta(z),$$

where $\Gamma(z) = (z-1)!$ is the gamma function [1.5.4]. Dirichlet's function, unlike Riemann's function, is defined everywhere and has no singularities. Its connection to prime number theory is best summarized by the formula [7]

$$\beta(x) = \prod_{\substack{p \text{ prime} \\ p \equiv 1 \bmod 4}} \left(1 - \frac{1}{p^x}\right)^{-1} \cdot \prod_{\substack{p \text{ prime} \\ p \equiv 3 \bmod 4}} \left(1 + \frac{1}{p^x}\right)^{-1} = \prod_{\substack{p \text{ odd} \\ \text{prime}}} \left(1 - \frac{(-1)^{\frac{p-1}{2}}}{p^x}\right)^{-1},$$

and the rearrangement of factors is justified by absolute convergence. A closely associated function is [8–10]

$$\lambda(x) = \sum_{n=0}^{\infty} \frac{1}{(2n+1)^x} = \left(1 - \frac{1}{2^x}\right)\zeta(x), \quad x > 1,$$

with sample values

$$\lambda(2) = \frac{\pi^2}{8}, \quad \lambda(4) = \frac{\pi^4}{96}, \quad \lambda(6) = \frac{\pi^6}{960}.$$

Unlike Apéry's constant, it is unknown whether G is irrational [11, 12]. We also know nothing about the arithmetic character of G/π^2. In statistical mechanics, G/π arises as part of the exact solution of the dimer problem [5.23]. Schmidt [13] pointed out a curious coincidence:

$$\frac{\pi^2}{12\ln(2)} = \left(1 - \frac{1}{2^2} + \frac{1}{3^2} - \frac{1}{4^2} + -\cdots\right)\left(1 - \frac{1}{2} + \frac{1}{3} - \frac{1}{4} + -\cdots\right)^{-1},$$

$$\frac{4G}{\pi} = \left(1 - \frac{1}{3^2} + \frac{1}{5^2} - \frac{1}{7^2} + -\cdots\right)\left(1 - \frac{1}{3} + \frac{1}{5} - \frac{1}{7} + -\cdots\right)^{-1},$$

where the former expression (Lévy's constant) is important in continued fraction asymptotics [1.8]. A variation of this,

$$\frac{8G}{\pi^2} = \left(1 - \frac{1}{3^2} + \frac{1}{5^2} - \frac{1}{7^2} + -\cdots\right)\left(1 + \frac{1}{3^2} + \frac{1}{5^2} + \frac{1}{7^2} + \cdots\right)^{-1},$$

occurs as the best coefficient for which a certain conjugate function inequality [7.7] is valid. The constant $2G/(\pi\ln(2))$ also appears as the average root bifurcation ratio of binary trees [5.6].

1.7.1 Euler Numbers

Define $\{E_n\}$, the Euler numbers, by the generating function [1, 8–10]

$$\text{sech}(x) = \frac{2e^x}{e^{2x} + 1} = \sum_{k=0}^{\infty} E_k \frac{x^k}{k!}.$$

It can be shown that all Euler numbers are integers: $E_0 = 1$, $E_2 = -1$, $E_4 = 5$, $E_6 = -61, \ldots$ and $E_{2n-1} = 0$ for $n > 0$.

(There is, unfortunately, an alternative definition of the Euler numbers to confuse matters. Under this alternative definition, the subscripting is somewhat different and all the numbers are positive. One must be careful when reading any paper to establish which definition has been used.)

The Euler numbers also arise in certain other series expansions, such as

$$\sec(x) = \sum_{k=0}^{\infty} \frac{(-1)^k E_{2k}}{(2k)!} x^{2k}.$$

1.7.2 Series

Summing over certain arithmetic progressions gives slight variations [14–16]:

$$\sum_{k=0}^{\infty} \frac{1}{(4k+1)^2} = \frac{1}{16}\pi^2 + \frac{1}{2}G, \quad \sum_{k=0}^{\infty} \frac{1}{(4k+3)^2} = \frac{1}{16}\pi^2 - \frac{1}{2}G.$$

Four formulas involving central binomial sums are [1, 17–19]

$$\sum_{k=0}^{\infty} \frac{2^{2k}}{(2k+1)^2\binom{2k}{k}} = 2G, \quad \sum_{k=0}^{\infty} \frac{1}{2^{3k}(2k+1)^2}\binom{2k}{k} = \frac{\pi}{4\sqrt{2}}\ln(2) + \frac{1}{\sqrt{2}}G,$$

$$\sum_{k=0}^{\infty} \frac{1}{(2k+1)^2\binom{2k}{k}} = \frac{8}{3}G - \frac{\pi}{3}\ln(2+\sqrt{3}),$$

$$\sum_{k=0}^{\infty} \frac{2^{4k}}{(k+1)(2k+1)^2\binom{2k}{k}^2} = 2\pi G - \frac{7}{2}\zeta(3).$$

As Berndt [17] remarked, it is interesting that the first of these is reminiscent of the famous Apéry series [1.6.3], yet it was discovered many years earlier. A family of related series is [20, 21, 23]

$$R(n) = \sum_{k=0}^{\infty} \frac{1}{2^{4k}(2k+n)}\binom{2k}{k}^2, \quad n = 0, 1, 2, \ldots,$$

which can be proved to satisfy the recurrence [1, 22, 24]

$$R(0) = 2\ln(2) - \frac{4G}{\pi}, \quad R(1) = \frac{4G}{\pi},$$

$$(n-1)^2 R(n) = (n-2)^2 R(n-2) + \frac{2}{\pi} \quad \text{for } n \geq 2.$$

What is the analog for $\beta(2n)$ of the exact formula for $\beta(2n+1)$? No one knows, but the series obtained by Ramanujan [16, 25],

$$G = \frac{5}{48}\pi^2 - 2\sum_{k=0}^{\infty} \frac{(-1)^k}{(2k+1)^2(e^{\pi(2k+1)}-1)} - \frac{1}{4}\sum_{k=1}^{\infty} \frac{\operatorname{sech}(\pi k)}{k^2},$$

might provide a starting point for research.

Some multiple series include [16, 17, 26–28]

$$\sum_{n=1}^{\infty} \frac{(-1)^{n+1}}{n}\sum_{k=0}^{n-1} \frac{(-1)^k}{2k+1} = G, \quad \sum_{n=0}^{\infty} \frac{(-1)^n}{2n+1}\sum_{k=1}^{n} \frac{1}{k} = G - \frac{\pi}{2}\ln(2),$$

$$\sum_{n=0}^{\infty} \frac{(-1)^n}{2n+1}\sum_{k=0}^{n-1} \frac{1}{2k+1} = \frac{\pi}{8}\ln(2) - \frac{1}{2}G, \quad \sum_{n=1}^{\infty} \frac{(-1)^{n+1}}{n^2}\sum_{k=0}^{n-1} \frac{1}{2k+1} = \pi G - \frac{7}{4}\zeta(3),$$

$$\sum_{n=1}^{\infty} \frac{(-1)^{n+1}}{n^2}\sum_{k=1}^{n} \frac{1}{k+n} = \pi G - \frac{33}{16}\zeta(3), \quad \sum_{n=0}^{\infty} \frac{2^n}{(2n+1)\binom{2n}{n}}\sum_{k=0}^{n} \frac{1}{2k+1} = 2G.$$

Two series involving zeta function values are [29–31]

$$\sum_{n=1}^{\infty} \frac{n\zeta(2n+1)}{2^{4n}} = 1 - G, \quad \sum_{n=1}^{\infty} \frac{\zeta(2n)}{2^{4n}(2n+1)} = \frac{1}{2} - \frac{1}{4}\ln(2) - \frac{1}{\pi}G.$$

Broadhurst [32–34] determined a digit-extraction algorithm for G via the following series:

$$G = 3\sum_{k=0}^{\infty} \frac{1}{2\cdot16^k}\left(\frac{1}{(8k+1)^2} - \frac{1}{(8k+2)^2} + \frac{1}{2(8k+3)^2} - \frac{1}{2^2(8k+5)^2} + \frac{1}{2^2(8k+6)^2} - \frac{1}{2^3(8k+7)^2}\right)$$

$$- 2\sum_{k=0}^{\infty} \frac{1}{8\cdot16^{3k}}\left(\frac{1}{(8k+1)^2} + \frac{1}{2(8k+2)^2} + \frac{1}{2^3(8k+3)^2} - \frac{1}{2^6(8k+5)^2} - \frac{1}{2^7(8k+6)^2} - \frac{1}{2^9(8k+7)^2}\right).$$

1.7.3 Products

As with values of the zeta function at odd integers [1.6.4], Gosper [35] found an infinite matrix product that gives beta function values at even integers. We exhibit the 4×4 case only:

$$\prod_{k=1}^{\infty}\begin{pmatrix} \frac{4k^2}{(4k-1)(4k+1)} & \frac{-1}{(4k-1)(4k+1)} & 0 & \frac{1}{(2k-1)^5} \\ 0 & \frac{4k^2}{(4k-1)(4k+1)} & \frac{-1}{(4k-1)(4k+1)} & \frac{1}{(2k-1)^3} \\ 0 & 0 & \frac{4k^2}{(4k-1)(4k+1)} & \frac{6k-1}{2(2k-1)(4k-1)} \\ 0 & 0 & 0 & 1 \end{pmatrix} = \begin{pmatrix} 0 & 0 & 0 & \beta(6) \\ 0 & 0 & 0 & \beta(4) \\ 0 & 0 & 0 & \beta(2) \\ 0 & 0 & 0 & 1 \end{pmatrix}.$$

The extension to the $(n+1) \times (n+1)$ case and to $\beta(2n)$ follows the same pattern as before.

1.7.4 Integrals

The beta function has an alternative expression [4] for $x > 0$:

$$\beta(x) = \frac{1}{2\Gamma(x)}\int_0^{\infty} \frac{t^{x-1}}{\cosh(t)}dt.$$

There are many integrals involving Catalan's constant [10, 15, 16, 36, 37], including

$$2\int_0^1 \frac{\arctan(x)}{x}dx = \int_0^{\frac{\pi}{2}} \frac{x}{\sin(x)}dx = 2G, \quad \frac{1}{2}\int_0^1 K(x)dx = \int_0^1 E(x)dx - \frac{1}{2} = G,$$

$$\int_0^1 \frac{\ln(x)}{1+x^2}dx = -\int_1^{\infty} \frac{\ln(x)}{1+x^2}dx = -G,$$

$$\int_0^{\frac{\pi}{4}} \ln(2\cos(x))dx = -\int_0^{\frac{\pi}{4}} \ln(2\sin(x))dx = \frac{1}{2}G,$$

$$4\int_0^1 \frac{\arctan(x)^2}{x}dx = \int_0^{\frac{\pi}{2}} \frac{x^2}{\sin(x)}dx = 2\pi G - \frac{7}{2}\zeta(3),$$

$$\int_0^{\frac{\pi}{2}} \operatorname{arcsinh}(\sin(x))dx = \int_0^{\frac{\pi}{2}} \operatorname{arcsinh}(\cos(x))dx = G,$$

where $K(x)$ and $E(x)$ are complete elliptic integrals [1.4.6]. See also [1.7.6].

1.7.5 Continued Fractions

The following expansions are due to Stieltjes [38], Rogers [39], and Ramanujan [40]:

$$2G = 2 - \frac{1|}{|3} + \frac{2^2|}{|1} + \frac{2^2|}{|3} + \frac{4^2|}{|1} + \frac{4^2|}{|3} + \frac{6^2|}{|1} + \frac{6^2|}{|3} + \cdots,$$

$$2G = 1 + \frac{1|}{|\frac{1}{2}} + \frac{1^2|}{|\frac{1}{2}} + \frac{1\cdot 2|}{|\frac{1}{2}} + \frac{2^2|}{|\frac{1}{2}} + \frac{2\cdot 3|}{|\frac{1}{2}} + \frac{3^2|}{|\frac{1}{2}} + \frac{3\cdot 4|}{|\frac{1}{2}} + \frac{4^2|}{|\frac{1}{2}} + \cdots.$$

1.7.6 Inverse Tangent Integral

Define $\mathrm{Ti}_1(x) = \arctan(x)$ and [41]

$$\mathrm{Ti}_n(x) = \sum_{k=0}^{\infty} \frac{(-1)^k}{(2k+1)^n} x^{2k+1}$$

$$= \int_0^x \frac{\mathrm{Ti}_{n-1}(s)}{s}ds, \text{ for any integer } n \geq 2, \text{ where } |x| \leq 1.$$

Clearly $\mathrm{Ti}_n(1) = \beta(n)$. The special case $n = 2$ is called the **inverse tangent integral**. It has alternative expressions

$$\mathrm{Ti}_2(\tan(\theta)) = \frac{1}{2}\int_0^{2\theta} \frac{t}{\sin(t)}dt = \theta \ln(\tan(\theta)) - \int_0^{\theta} \ln(2\sin(t))dt + \int_0^{\theta} \ln(2\cos(t))dt$$

for $0 < \theta < \pi/2$, and sample values [21, 41]

$$\mathrm{Ti}_2(2 - \sqrt{3}) = \frac{2}{3}G + \frac{\pi}{12}\ln(2 - \sqrt{3}), \quad \mathrm{Ti}_2(2 + \sqrt{3}) = \frac{2}{3}G + \frac{5\pi}{12}\ln(2 + \sqrt{3}).$$

In the latter formula, we use the integral expression (since the series diverges for $x > 1$, but the integral converges). Very little is known about $\mathrm{Ti}_n(x)$ for $n > 2$.

[1] J. M. Borwein and P. B. Borwein, *Pi and the AGM: A Study in Analytic Number Theory and Computational Complexity*, Wiley, 1987, pp. 198–199, 383–386; MR 99h:11147.

[2]   F. Beukers, J. A. C. Kolk, and E. Calabi, Sums of generalized harmonic series and volumes, *Nieuw Arch. Wisk.* 4 (1993) 217–224; MR 94j:11022.

[3]   N. D. Elkies, On the sums $\sum_{k=-\infty}^{\infty}(4k+1)^{-n}$, math.CA/0101168.

[4]   A. Erdélyi, W. Magnus, F. Oberhettinger, and F. G. Tricomi, *Higher Transcendental Functions*, v. 1, McGraw-Hill, 1953, pp. 27–35; MR 15,419i.

[5]   W. Ellison and F. Ellison, *Prime Numbers*, Wiley, 1985, p. 180; MR 87a:11082.

[6]   T. M. Apostol, *Introduction to Analytic Number Theory*, Springer-Verlag, 1976, pp. 249–263; MR 55 #7892.

[7]   P. Moree and J. Cazaran, On a claim of Ramanujan in his first letter to Hardy, *Expos. Math* 17 (1999) 289–312; MR 2001c:11103.

[8]   M. Abramowitz and I. A. Stegun, *Handbook of Mathematical Functions*, Dover, 1972, pp. 807–808; MR 94b:00012.

[9]   J. Spanier and K. B. Oldham, *An Atlas of Functions*, Hemisphere, 1987, pp. 25–33.

[10] I. S. Gradshteyn and I. M Ryzhik, *Tables of Integrals, Series and Products*, Academic Press, 1980; MR 97c:00014.

[11] W. Zudilin, Apéry-like difference equation for Catalan's constant, math.NT/0201024.

[12] T. Rivoal and W. Zudilin, Diophantine properties of numbers related to Catalan's constant, UMR preprint 317 (2002), l'Institut de Mathématiques de Jussieu.

[13] A. L. Schmidt, Ergodic theory of complex continued fractions, *Number Theory with an Emphasis on the Markoff Spectrum*, Proc. 1991 Provo conf., ed. A. D. Pollington and W. Moran, Dekker, 1993, pp. 215–226; MR 95f:11055.

[14] K. S. Kölbig, The polygamma function $\psi^{(k)}(x)$ for $x = 1/4$ and $x = 3/4$, *J. Comput. Appl. Math.* 75 (1996) 43–46; MR 98d:33001.

[15] V. S. Adamchik, 33 representations for the Catalan constant, unpublished note (1997).

[16] D. M. Bradley, Representations of Catalan's constant, unpublished note (2001).

[17] B. C. Berndt, *Ramanujan's Notebooks: Part I*, Springer-Verlag, 1985, pp. 264–267, 289–290, 293–294; MR 86c:01062.

[18] D. Bradley, A class of series acceleration formulae for Catalan's constant, *Ramanujan J.* 3 (1999) 159–173; MR 2000f:11163.

[19] R. W. Gosper, A calculus of series rearrangements, *Algorithms and Complexity: New Directions and Recent Results*, Proc. 1976 Carnegie-Mellon conf., ed. J. F. Traub, Academic Press, 1976, pp. 121–151; MR 56 #9899.

[20] E. P. Adams and R. L. Hippisley, *Smithsonian Mathematical Formulae and Tables of Elliptic Functions*, Smithsonian Institute, 1922, p. 142.

[21] E. R. Hansen, *A Table of Series and Products*, Prentice-Hall, 1975.

[22] J. Dutka, Two results of Ramanujan, *SIAM J. Math. Anal.* 12 (1981) 471; MR 83a:05010.

[23] S. Yang, Some properties of Catalan's constant G, *Int. J. Math. Educ. Sci. Technol.* 23 (1992) 549–556; MR 93j:11058.

[24] V. S. Adamchik, A certain series associated with Catalan's constant, unpublished note (2000).

[25] S. Ramanujan, On the integral $\int_0^x \tan^{-1}(t)\, dt/t$, *J. Indian Math. Soc.* 7 (1915) 93–96; also in *Collected Papers*, ed. G. H. Hardy, P. V. Seshu Aiyar, and B. M. Wilson, Cambridge Univ. Press, 1927, pp. 40–43, 336–337.

[26] O. Espinosa and V. H. Moll, On some definite integrals involving the Hurwitz zeta function, *Ramanujan J.* 6 (2002) 159–188; math.CA/0012078.

[27] R. Sitaramachandrarao, A formula of S. Ramanujan, *J. Number Theory* 25 (1987) 1–19; MR 88c:11048.

[28] G. J. Fee, Computation of Catalan's constant using Ramanujan's formula, *Proc. 1990 Int. Symp. Symbolic and Algebraic Computation (ISSAC)*, ed. S. Watanabe and M. Nagata, Tokyo, ACM, 1990, pp. 157–160.

[29] J. W. L. Glaisher, Numerical values of the series $1 - 1/3^n + 1/5^n - 1/7^n + 1/9^n - \cdots$, *Messenger of Math.* 42 (1913) 35–58.

[30] M.-P. Chen and H. M. Srivastava, Some familes of series representations for the Riemann
      $\zeta(3)$, *Resultate Math.* 33 (1998) 179–197; MR 99b:11095.
[31] J. Choi, The Catalan's constant and series involving the zeta function, *Commun. Korean
      Math. Soc.* 13 (1998) 435–443; MR 2000h:11091.
[32] D. J. Broadhurst, Polylogarithmic ladders, hypergeometric series and the ten millionth digits
      of $\zeta(3)$ and $\zeta(5)$, math.CA/9803067.
[33] J. M. Borwein, Experimental mathematics: Insight from computation, presentation at
      AMS/MAA Joint Meetings, San Antonio, 1999.
[34] J. M. Borwein and R. M. Corless, Emerging tools for experimental mathematics, *Amer.
      Math. Monthly* 106 (1999) 889–909; MR 2000m:68186.
[35] R. W. Gosper, Analytic identities from path invariant matrix multiplication, unpublished
      manuscript (1976).
[36] H. M. Srivastava and E. A. Miller, A simple reducible case of double hypergeometric series
      involving Catalan's constant and Riemann's zeta function, *Int. J. Math. Educ. Sci. Technol.*
      21 (1990) 375–377; MR 91d:33032.
[37] I. J. Zucker, G. S. Joyce, and R. T. Delves, On the evaluation of the integral
      $\int_0^{\pi/4} \ln(\cos^{m/n} \theta \pm \sin^{m/n} \theta) d\theta$, *Ramanujan J.* 2 (1998) 317–326; MR 99g:26019.
[38] T. J. Stieltjes, Recherches sur les fractions continues, *Annales Faculté Sciences Toulouse*
      8 (1894) J1–J122; 9 (1895) A1–A47; also in *Oeuvres Complètes*, t. 2, ed. W. Kapteyn
      and J. C. Kluyver, Noordhoff, 1918, pp. 402–566; Engl. transl. in *Collected Papers*, v. 2,
      ed. G. van Dijk, Springer-Verlag, 1993, pp. 406–570, 609–745; MR 95g:01033.
[39] L. J. Rogers, Supplementary note on the representation of certain asymptotic series as
      convergent continued fractions, *Proc. London Math. Soc.* 4 (1907) 393–395.
[40] B. C. Berndt, *Ramanujan's Notebooks: Part II*, Springer-Verlag, 1989, pp. 150–153; MR
      90b:01039.
[41] L. Lewin, *Polylogarithms and Associated Functions*, North-Holland, 1981, pp. 38–45, 106,
      166, 190; MR 83b:33019.

1.8 Khintchine–Lévy Constants

Let x be a real number. Expand x (uniquely) as a regular continued fraction:

$$x = q_0 + \frac{1|}{|q_1} + \frac{1|}{|q_2} + \frac{1|}{|q_3} + \cdots,$$

where q_0 is an integer and $q_1, q_2, q_3, \ldots$ are positive integers. Unlike a decimal expansion, the properties of a regular continued fraction do not depend on the choice of base.
Hence, to number theorists, terms of a continued fraction are more "natural" to look at
than decimal digits.

What can be said about the average behavior of q_k, where $k > 0$ is arbitrary? Consider, for example, the geometric mean

$$M(n, x) = (q_1 q_2 q_3 \cdots q_n)^{\frac{1}{n}}$$

in the limit as $n \to \infty$. One would expect this limiting value to depend on x in some
possibly complicated way. Since any sequence of qs determines a unique x, there
exist xs for which the qs obey any conceivable condition. To attempt to compute
$\lim_{n\to\infty} M(n, x)$ would thus seem to be impossibly difficult.

Here occurs one of the most astonishing facts in mathematics. Khintchine [1–4] proved that

$$\lim_{n \to \infty} M(n, x) = \prod_{k=1}^{\infty} \left(1 + \frac{1}{k(k+2)}\right)^{\frac{\ln(k)}{\ln(2)}} = K = e^{0.9878490568\ldots} = 2.6854520010\ldots,$$

a *constant*, for almost all real numbers x. This means that the set of exceptions x to Khintchine's result (e.g., all rationals, quadratic irrationals, and more) is of Lebesgue measure zero. We can be probabilistically certain that a truly randomly selected x will obey Khintchine's law. This is a profound statement about the nature of real numbers. Another proof, drawing upon ergodic theory and due to Ryll-Nardzewski [5], is found in Kac [6].

The infinite product representation of K converges very slowly. Fast numerical procedures for computing K appear in [7–13]. Among several different representations of K are [8, 11, 13, 14]

$$\ln(2)\ln(K) = -\sum_{i=2}^{\infty} \ln\left(1 - \frac{1}{i}\right) \ln\left(1 + \frac{1}{i}\right) = \sum_{j=2}^{\infty} \frac{(-1)^j (2 - 2^j)}{j} \zeta'(j),$$

$$\ln(2)\ln(K) = \sum_{k=1}^{\infty} \frac{\zeta(2k) - 1}{k}\left(1 - \frac{1}{2} + \frac{1}{3} - + \cdots + \frac{1}{2k - 1}\right),$$

$$\ln(2)\ln(K) = -\int_0^1 \frac{1}{x(1 + x)} \ln\left(\frac{\sin(\pi x)}{\pi x}\right) dx$$

$$= \frac{\pi^2}{12} + \frac{\ln(2)^2}{2} + \int_0^{\pi} \frac{\ln|\theta \cot(\theta)|}{\theta} d\theta,$$

where $\zeta(x)$ denotes the Riemann zeta function [1.6] and $\zeta'(x)$ is its derivative.

Many questions arise. Is K irrational? What well-known irrational numbers are among the meager exceptions to Khintchine's result? Lehmer [7, 15] observed that e is an exception; whether $\sqrt[3]{2}$, π, and K itself (!) are likewise remains unsolved.

Related ideas include the asymptotic behavior of the coprime positive integers P_n and Q_n, where P_n/Q_n is the nth partial convergent of x. That is, P_n/Q_n is the value of the finite regular continued fraction expansion of x up through q_n. Lévy [16, 17] determined that

$$\lim_{n \to \infty} Q_n^{\frac{1}{n}} = e^{\frac{\pi^2}{12\ln(2)}} = e^{1.1865691104\ldots} = 3.2758229187\ldots = \lim_{n \to \infty} \left(\frac{P_n}{x}\right)^{\frac{1}{n}}$$

for almost all real x. Philipp [18, 19] provided improvements to error bounds associated with both Khintchine and Lévy limits. A different perspective is given by [20–22]:

$$-\lim_{n \to \infty} \frac{1}{n} \log_{10}\left|x - \frac{P_n}{Q_n}\right| = \frac{\pi^2}{6\ln(2)\ln(10)} = 1.0306408341\ldots,$$

which indicates that the information in a typical continued fraction term is approximately 1.03 decimal digits (valid for almost all real x). Equivalently, the metric entropy of the continued fraction map $x \mapsto \{1/x\}$ is [23, 24]

$$\lim_{n \to \infty} \frac{Q_{n+1}^2}{Q_n^2} = e^{\frac{\pi^2}{6 \ln(2)}} = 10.7310157948\ldots = (0.0931878229\ldots)^{-1},$$

where $\{x\}$ denotes the fractional part of x. That is, an additional term reduces the uncertainty in x by a factor of 10.73. The corresponding entropy for the shift map $x \mapsto \{10x\}$ is 10.

Corless [13, 25] pointed out the interesting contrasting formulas

$$\ln(K) = \int_0^1 \frac{\ln \lfloor \frac{1}{x} \rfloor}{\ln(2)(1+x)} dx, \quad \frac{\pi^2}{12 \ln(2)} = \int_0^1 \frac{\ln\left(\frac{1}{x}\right)}{\ln(2)(1+x)} dx,$$

where $\lfloor x \rfloor$ is the largest integer $\leq x$.

Let us return to the original question: What can be said about the average behavior of the kth partial denominator q_k, $k > 0$? We have examined the situation for only one type of mean value, the geometric mean. A generalization [26] of mean value is

$$M(s, n, x) = \left(\frac{1}{n} \sum_{k=1}^{n} q_k^s \right)^{\frac{1}{s}},$$

which reduces to the harmonic mean, geometric mean, arithmetic mean, and root mean square, respectively, when $s = -1$, 0, 1, and 2. Thus the well-known means fit into a continuous hierarchy of mean values. It is known [3, 27] that, if $s \geq 1$, then $\lim_{n \to \infty} M(s, n, x) = \infty$ for almost all real x. What can be said about the value of $M(s, n, x)$ for $s < 1$, $s \neq 0$? The analog of Khintchine's formula here is

$$\lim_{n \to \infty} M(s, n, x) = \left[\frac{1}{\ln(2)} \sum_{k=1}^{\infty} k^s \ln\left(1 + \frac{1}{k(k+2)}\right) \right]^{\frac{1}{s}} = K_s$$

for almost all real x. It is known [13, 28] that $K_{-1} = 1.7454056624\ldots$, $K_{-2} = 1.4503403284\ldots$, $K_{-3} = 1.3135070786\ldots$, and clearly $K_s = 1 + O(1/s)$ as $s \to -\infty$.

Closely related topics are discussed in [2.17], [2.18], and [2.19].

1.8.1 Alternative Representations

There are alternative ways of representing real numbers, akin to regular continued fractions, that have associated Khintchine–Lévy constants. For example, every real number $0 < x < 1$ can be uniquely expressed in the form

$$x = \frac{1}{a_1 + 1} + \sum_{n=2}^{\infty} \left(\prod_{k=1}^{n-1} \frac{1}{a_k(a_k + 1)} \right) \frac{1}{a_n + 1}$$

$$= \frac{1}{b_1} + \sum_{n=2}^{\infty} \left(\prod_{k=1}^{n-1} \frac{1}{b_k(b_k + 1)} \right) \frac{(-1)^{n-1}}{b_n},$$

where $a_1, a_2, a_3, \ldots$ and $b_1, b_2, b_3, \ldots$ are positive integers. These are called the **Lüroth**
and **alternating Lüroth representations** of x, respectively. The limiting constants are
the same whether we use as or bs, and [29–31]

$$\lim_{n \to \infty} (a_1 a_2 a_3 \cdots a_n)^{\frac{1}{n}} = \prod_{k=1}^{\infty} k^{\frac{1}{k(k+1)}} = e^{0.7885305659\ldots} = 2.2001610580 \ldots = U,$$

$$\lim_{n \to \infty} \left| x - \frac{P_n}{Q_n} \right|^{\frac{1}{n}} = \prod_{k=1}^{\infty} [k(k+1)]^{\frac{-1}{k(k+1)}} = e^{-2.0462774528\ldots} = V,$$

where P_n/Q_n is the nth partial sum. A variation of this [32],

$$\lim_{n \to \infty} ((a_1 + 1)(a_2 + 1) \cdots (a_n + 1))^{\frac{1}{n}} = \prod_{k=1}^{\infty} (k+1)^{\frac{1}{k(k+1)}} = e^{1.2577468869\ldots} = W,$$

also appears in [2.9]. Of course, $UVW = 1$ and

$$\ln(U) = -\sum_{i=2}^{\infty} (-1)^i \zeta'(i), \quad \ln(V) = 2\sum_{j=1}^{\infty} \zeta'(2j), \quad \ln(W) = -\sum_{k=2}^{\infty} \zeta'(k).$$

A second example [22] is the **Bolyai–Rényi representation** of $0 < x < 1$,

$$x = -1 + \sqrt{a_1 + \sqrt{a_2 + \sqrt{a_3 + \cdots}}},$$

where each $a_k \in \{0, 1, 2\}$. Whereas an exact expression $\pi^2/(6\ln(2)) = 2.373138\ldots$
arises for the entropy of continued fractions, only a numerical result $1.056313\ldots$ exists
for the entropy of radical expansions [33].

A third example [34–41] is the **nearest integer continued fraction** of $-1/2 < x < 1/2$,

$$x = \frac{1|}{|c_1} + \frac{1|}{|c_2} + \frac{1|}{|c_3} + \cdots,$$

which is generated according to

$$c_1 = \left\lfloor \frac{1}{x} + \frac{1}{2} \right\rfloor, \quad x_1 = \frac{1}{x} - c_1, \quad c_2 = \left\lfloor \frac{1}{x_1} + \frac{1}{2} \right\rfloor, \quad x_2 = \frac{1}{x_1} - c_2, \ldots.$$

Some of the cs may be negative. The formulas for the Khintchine–Lévy constants in
this case are

$$\lim_{n \to \infty} |c_1 c_2 \cdots c_n|^{\frac{1}{n}} = \left(\frac{5\varphi + 3}{5\varphi + 2} \right)^{\frac{\ln(2)}{\ln(\varphi)}} \prod_{k=3}^{\infty} \left(\frac{8(k-1)\varphi + (2k-3)^2 + 4}{8(k-1)\varphi + (2k-3)^2} \right)^{\frac{\ln(k)}{\ln(\phi)}}$$

$$= e^{1.6964441175\ldots} = 5.4545172445 \ldots,$$

$$\lim_{n \to \infty} Q_n^{\frac{1}{n}} = e^{\frac{\pi^2}{12 \ln(\varphi)}} = e^{1.7091579853\ldots} = 5.5243079702 \ldots,$$

Table 1.2. *Nonexplicit Constants Recursively Derived from K*

$y = 2.3038421962\ldots$	q_n is the largest possible integer: $\prod\limits_{k=0}^{n} q_k < K^{n+1}$
$y = 3.3038421963\ldots$	q_n is the smallest possible integer: $\prod\limits_{k=0}^{n} q_k > K^{n+1}$
$y = 2.2247514809\ldots$	$\prod\limits_{k=0}^{n} q_k$ is just less than K^{n+1} when n is even, and $\prod\limits_{k=0}^{n} q_k$ is just greater than K^{n+1} when n is odd
$y = 3.4493588902\ldots$	$\prod\limits_{k=0}^{n} q_k$ is just greater than K^{n+1} when n is even, and $\prod\limits_{k=0}^{n} q_k$ is just less than K^{n+1} when n is odd

where P_n/Q_n is the nth partial convergent and φ is the Golden mean [1.2]. Such expansions are also called **centered continued fractions** [42].

1.8.2 Derived Constants

Although we know exceptions x (which all belong to a set of measure zero) to Khintchine's law, we do not know a single explicit y that provably satisfies it. This is remarkable because one would expect y to be easy to find, being so much more plentiful than x. The requirement that y be "explicit" is the difficult part. It means, in particular, that the partial denominators q_n in the regular continued fraction for y should not depend on knowing K to arbitrary precision. Robinson [43] described four nonexplicit constants that are recursively derived from K in a simple manner (see Table 1.2). Bailey, Borwein & Crandall [13] gave other, more sophisticated constructions in which at least the listing $q_0, q_1, q_2, \ldots$ is explicit (although the constant y still is not).

1.8.3 Complex Analog

Schmidt [44–46] introduced what appears to be the most natural approach for generalizing continued fraction theory to the complex field. For example [47–50], the complex analog of Lévy's constant is $\exp(G/\pi)$, where G is Catalan's constant [1.7]. Does Khintchine's constant possess a complex analog?

[1] A. Khintchine, Metrische Kettenbruchprobleme, *Compositio Math.* 1 (1935) 361–382.
[2] A. Khintchine, Zur metrischen Kettenbruchprobleme, *Compositio Math.* 3 (1936) 276–285.
[3] A. Khintchine, *Continued Fractions*, Univ. of Chicago Press, 3rd ed., 1961; MR 28 #5038.
[4] A. M. Rockett and P. Szüsz, *Continued Fractions*, World Scientific, 1992; MR 93m:11060.
[5] C. Ryll-Nardzewski, On the ergodic theorems. II: Ergodic theory of continued fractions, *Studia Math.* 12 (1951) 74–79; MR 13,757b.
[6] M. Kac, *Statistical Independence in Probability, Analysis and Number Theory*, Math. Assoc. Amer., 1959; MR 22 #996.

[7]   D. H. Lehmer, Note on an absolute constant of Khintchine, *Amer. Math. Monthly* 46 (1939) 148–152.

[8]   D. Shanks and J. W. Wrench, Khintchine's constant, *Amer. Math. Monthly* 66 (1959) 276–279; MR 21 #1950.

[9]   J. W. Wrench, Further evaluation of Khintchine's constant, *Math. Comp.* 14 (1960) 370–371; MR 30 #693.

[10] J. W. Wrench and D. Shanks, Questions concerning Khintchine's constant and the efficient computation of regular continued fractions, *Math. Comp.* 20 (1966) 444–448.

[11] I. Vardi, *Computational Recreations in Mathematica*, Addison-Wesley, 1991; MR 93e:00002.

[12] P. Flajolet and I. Vardi, Zeta function expansions of classical constants, unpublished note (1996).

[13] D. H. Bailey, J. M. Borwein, and R. E. Crandall, On the Khintchine constant, *Math. Comp.* 66 (1997) 417–431; CECM preprint 95:036; MR 97c:11119.

[14] V. S. Adamchik and H. M. Srivastava, Some series of the zeta and related functions, *Analysis* 18 (1998) 131–144; MR 99d:11096.

[15] P. Shiu, Computations of continued fractions without input values, *Math. Comp.* 64 (1995) 1307–1317; MR 87h:11127.

[16] P. Lévy, Sur les lois probabilité dont dépendent les quotients complets et incomplets d'une fraction continue, *Bull. Soc. Math. France* 57 (1929) 178–194; also in *Oeuvres*, v. 6, ed. D. Dugué, Gauthier-Villars, 1980, pp. 266–282.

[17] P. Lévy, Sur le développement en fraction continue d'un nombre choisi au hasard, *Compositio Math.* 3 (1936) 286–303; also in *Oeuvres*, v. 6, ed. D. Dugué, Gauthier-Villars, 1980, pp. 285–302.

[18] W. Philipp, Some metrical theorems in number theory, *Pacific J. Math.* 20 (1967) 109–127; MR 34 #5755.

[19] W. Philipp, Some metrical theorems in number theory. II, *Duke Math. J.* 37 (1970) 447–458; MR 42 #7620.

[20] G. Lochs, Vergleich der Genauigkeit von Dezimalbruch und Kettenbruch, *Abh. Math. Sem. Univ. Hamburg* 27 (1964) 142–144; MR 29 #57.

[21] C. Kraaikamp, A new class of continued fraction expansions, *Acta Arith.* 57 (1991) 1–39; MR 92a:11090.

[22] W. Bosma, K. Dajani, and C. Kraaikamp, Entropy and counting correct digits, Univ. of Nijmegen Math. Report 9925 (1999).

[23] V. A. Rohlin, Exact endomorphisms of a Lebesgue space (in Russian), *Izv. Akad. Nauk SSSR Ser. Mat.* 25 (1961) 499–530; MR 26 #1423.

[24] P. Flajolet, B. Vallée, and I. Vardi, Continued fractions from Euclid to the present day, École Polytechnique preprint (2000).

[25] R. M. Corless, Continued fractions and chaos, *Amer. Math. Monthly* 99 (1992) 203–215; also in *Organic Mathematics*, Proc. 1995 Burnaby workshop, ed. J. Borwein, P. Borwein, L. Jörgenson, and R. Corless, Amer. Math. Soc., 1997; MR 94g:58135.

[26] E. F. Beckenbach and R. Bellman, *Inequalities*, Springer-Verlag, 1965; MR 33 #236.

[27] D. E. Knuth, *The Art of Computer Programming*, v. 2, *Seminumerical Algorithms*, 2nd ed., Addison-Wesley, 1981, pp. 361–362, 604–606; MR 44 #3531.

[28] H. Riesel, On the metric theory of nearest integer continued fractions, *BIT* 27 (1987) 248–263; errata 28 (1988) 188; MR 88k:11048 and MR 89f:11114; Zbl. 617.10036 and Zbl. 644.10036.

[29] A. David and S. Dvorak, The estimations of the limit of the geometric means of Lüroth's digits, *Acta Fac. Rerum Natur. Univ. Comenian. Math.* 35 (1979) 95–107; MR 82c:10062.

[30] S. Kalpazidou, Khintchine's constant for Lüroth representation, *J. Number Theory* 29 (1988) 196–205; MR 89f:11105.

[31] S. Kalpazidou, A. Knopfmacher, and J. Knopfmacher, Metric properties of alternating Lüroth series, *Portugal. Math.* 48 (1991) 319–325; MR 92h:11068.

[32] H. Jager and C. de Vroedt, Lüroth series and their ergodic properties, *Proc. Konink. Nederl. Akad. Wetensch. Ser. A* 72 (1969) 31–42; *Indag. Math.* 31 (1969) 31–42; MR 39 #157.

[33] O. Jenkinson and M. Pollicott, Ergodic properties of the Bolyai-Rényi expansion, *Indag. Math.* 11 (2000) 399–418.

[34] G. J. Rieger, Über die mittlere Schrittanzahl bei Divisionsalgorithmen, *Math. Nachr.* 82 (1978) 157–180; MR 58 #533.

[35] G. J. Rieger, Ein Gauss-Kusmin-Levy-Satz für Kettenbrüche nach nächsten Ganzen, *Manuscripta Math.* 24 (1978) 437–448; MR 58 #27875.

[36] G. J. Rieger, Mischung und Ergodizität bei Kettenbrüchen nach nächsten Ganzen, *J. Reine Angew. Math.* 310 (1979) 171–181; MR 81c:10066.

[37] A. M. Rockett, The metrical theory of continued fractions to the nearer integer, *Acta Arith.* 38 (1980/81) 97–103; MR 82d:10074.

[38] S. Kalpazidou, Some asymptotic results on digits of the nearest integer continued fraction, *J. Number Theory* 22 (1986) 271–279; MR 87i:11101.

[39] L. Degeratu, Some metrical results for the nearest integer continued fraction, *Politehn. Univ. Bucharest Sci. Bull. Ser. A* 57/58 (1995/96) 61–67; MR 99e:11107.

[40] V. S. Adamchik, Evaluation of the nearest integer analog of Khintchine's constant, unpublished note (2001).

[41] J. Bourdon, On the Khintchine constant for centred continued fraction expansions, unpublished note (2001).

[42] P. Flajolet and B. Vallée, Continued fractions, comparison algorithms, and fine structure constants, *Constructive, Experimental, and Nonlinear Analysis*, Proc. 1999 Limoges conf., ed. M. Théra, Amer. Math. Soc., 2000, pp. 53–82; INRIA preprint RR4072; MR 2001h:11161.

[43] H. P. Robinson and E. Potter, *Mathematical Constants*, UCRL-20418 (1971), Univ. of Calif. at Berkeley; available through the National Technical Information Service, Springfield VA 22151.

[44] A. L. Schmidt, Diophantine approximation of complex numbers, *Acta Math.* 134 (1975) 1–85; MR 54 #10160.

[45] A. L. Schmidt, Ergodic theory for complex continued fractions, *Monatsh. Math.* 93 (1982) 39–62; MR 83g:10036.

[46] A. L. Schmidt, Ergodic theory of complex continued fractions, *Number Theory with an Emphasis on the Markoff Spectrum*, Proc. 1991 Provo conf., ed. A. D. Pollington and W. Moran, Dekker, 1993, pp. 215–226; MR 95f:11055.

[47] H. Nakada, On ergodic theory of A. Schmidt's complex continued fractions over Gaussian field, *Monatsh. Math.* 105 (1988) 131–150; MR 89f:11113.

[48] H. Nakada, On metrical theory of diophantine approximation over imaginary quadratic field, *Acta Arith.* 51 (1988) 393–403; MR 89m:11070.

[49] H. Nakada, The metrical theory of complex continued fractions, *Acta Arith.* 56 (1990) 279–289; MR 92e:11081.

[50] H. Nakada, Dynamics of complex continued fractions and geodesics over H^3, *Dynamical Systems and Chaos*, v. 1, Proc. 1994 Tokyo conf., ed. N. Aoki, K. Shiraiwa, and Y. Takahashi, World Scientific, 1995, pp. 192–199; MR 99c:11103.

1.9 Feigenbaum–Coullet–Tresser Constants

Let $f(x) = ax(1 - x)$, where a is constant. The interval $[0, 1]$ is mapped into itself by f for each value of $a \in [0, 4]$. This family of functions, parametrized by a, is known as the family of **logistic maps** [1–8].

What are the 1-cycles (i.e., fixed points) of f? Solving $x = f(x)$, we obtain

$$x = 0 \quad \text{(which attracts for } a < 1 \text{ and repels for } a > 1)$$

and

$$x = \frac{a - 1}{a} \quad \text{(which attracts for } 1 < a < 3 \text{ and repels for } a > 3\text{)}.$$

What are the 2-cycles of f? That is, what are the fixed points of the iterate f^2 that are not fixed points of f? Solving $x = f^2(x)$, $x \neq f(x)$, we obtain the 2-cycle

$$x = \frac{a + 1 \pm \sqrt{a^2 - 2a - 3}}{2a} \quad \text{(which attracts for } 3 < a < 1 + \sqrt{6}$$
$$\text{and repels for } a > 1 + \sqrt{6}\text{)}.$$

For $a > 1 + \sqrt{6} = 3.4495\ldots$, an attracting 4-cycle emerges. We can obtain the 4-cycle by numerically solving $x = f^4(x)$, $x \neq f^2(x)$. It can be shown that the 4-cycle attracts for $3.4495\ldots < a < 3.5441\ldots$ and repels for $a > 3.5441\ldots$.

For $a > 3.5441$, an attracting 8-cycle emerges. We can obtain the 8-cycle by numerically solving $x = f^8(x)$, $x \neq f^4(x)$. It can be shown that the 8-cycle attracts for $3.5441\ldots < a < 3.5644\ldots$ and repels for $a > 3.5644\ldots$.

For how long does the sequence of period-doubling bifurcations continue? It is interesting that this behavior stops far short of 4. Letting

$$a_0 = 1, \quad a_1 = 3, \quad a_2 = 3.4495\ldots, \quad a_3 = 3.5441\ldots, \quad a_4 = 3.5644\ldots,$$

etc. denote the sequence of **bifurcation points** of f, it can be proved that

$$a_\infty = \lim_{n \to \infty} a_n = 3.5699\ldots < 4.$$

This limiting point marks the separation between the "periodic regime" and the "chaotic regime" for this family of quadratic functions. Much research has been aimed at developing a theory of chaos and applying it to the study of physical, chemical, and biological systems. We will focus on only a small aspect of the theory: two "universal" constants associated with the exponential accumulation described earlier. The bifurcation diagram in Figure 1.5 is helpful for defining the following additional symbols. The sequence of **superstable points** of f is

$$\tilde{a}_1 = 1 + \sqrt{5} = 3.2360\ldots, \quad \tilde{a}_2 = 3.4985\ldots, \quad \tilde{a}_3 = 3.5546\ldots, \quad \tilde{a}_4 = 3.5666\ldots,$$

where $\tilde{a}_n$ is the least parameter value at which a 2^n-cycle contains the critical element $1/2$. Call this cycle $\tilde{C}(n)$. The sequence of **superstable widths** of f is

$$\tilde{w}_1 = (\sqrt{5} - 1)/4 = 0.3090\ldots, \quad \tilde{w}_2 = 0.1164\ldots, \quad \tilde{w}_3 = 0.0459\ldots,$$

where $\tilde{w}_n$ is the distance between $1/2$ and the element $f^{2^{n-1}}(1/2) \in \tilde{C}(n)$ nearest to $1/2$. Also, the sequence of **bifurcation widths** of f is

$$w_1 = \sqrt{2}(\sqrt{6} - 1)/5 = 0.4099\ldots, \quad w_2 = 0.1603\ldots, \quad w_3 = 0.0636\ldots,$$

where w_n is the corresponding cycle distance at a_{n+1}. The superstable variants $\tilde{a}_n$ and $\tilde{w}_n$ are numerically easier to compute than a_n and w_n. Define the two **Feigenbaum–**

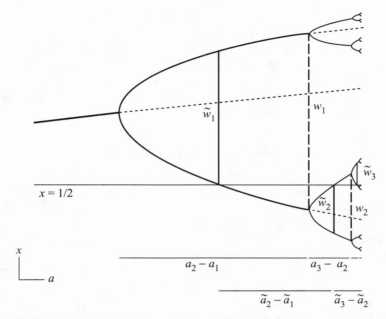

Figure 1.5. Horizontal and vertical characteristics of the bifurcation are quantified by a_n and w_n.

Coullet–Tresser constants to be [9–17]

$$\delta = \lim_{n\to\infty} \frac{a_n - a_{n-1}}{a_{n+1} - a_n} = \lim_{n\to\infty} \frac{\tilde{a}_n - \tilde{a}_{n-1}}{\tilde{a}_{n+1} - \tilde{a}_n} = 4.6692016091\ldots$$

and

$$\alpha = \lim_{n\to\infty} \frac{w_n}{w_{n+1}} = \lim_{n\to\infty} \frac{\tilde{w}_n}{\tilde{w}_{n+1}} = 2.5029078750\ldots = (0.3995352805\ldots)^{-1}.$$

As indicated here, the tildes can be included or excluded without change to the limiting ratios δ and α.

What qualifies these constants to be called "universal"? If we replace the logistic maps f by, for example, $g(x) = b\sin(\pi x)$, $0 \le b \le 1$, then interestingly the same constants δ and α occur. Both functions f and g have quadratic maximum points; we extend this condition to obtain generalized Feigenbaum constants [1.9.1]. We mention a two-dimensional example [1.9.2] as well. Rigorous proofs of universality for the one-dimensional, quadratic maximum case were first given by Lanford [18–22] and Campanino & Epstein [23–28]; the former apparently was the first computer-assisted proof of its kind in mathematics.

Does there exist a simpler definition of the Feigenbaum constants? One would like to see a more classical characterization in terms of a limit or an integral that would not require quite so much explanation. The closest thing to this involves a certain functional equation [1.9.3], which in fact appears to provide the most practical algorithm for calculating the constants to high precision [29–37]. We also mention maps on a circle [1.9.4] and a different form of chaos.

The numbers $3.5441\ldots$ and $3.5644\ldots$ mentioned previously are known to be algebraic of degrees 12 and 240, as discussed in [38, 39].

Salamin [40] has speculated that the (unitless) fine structure constant $(137.0359\ldots)^{-1}$ from quantum electrodynamics will, in a better theory than we have today, be related to a Feigenbaum-like constant.

1.9.1 Generalized Feigenbaum Constants

Consider the functions f and g defined earlier. Consider also the function $h(x) = 1 - c|x|^r$ defined on the interval $[-1, 1]$, where $1 < c < 2$ and $r > 1$ are constants. Each function is unimodal, concave, symmetric, and analytic everywhere with the possible exception of h at $x = 0$. Further, each second derivative, evaluated at the maximum point, is strictly negative if $r = 2$. That is, f, g, and h have quadratic maximum points.

In contrast, the order of the maximum of h is cubic if $r = 3$, quartic if $r = 4$, etc. This is an important distinction with regard to the values of the Feigenbaum constants.

Many authors have used the word "universal" to describe δ and α, and this is appropriate if quadratic maximums are all one is concerned about. Vary r, however, and different values of δ and α emerge. Numerical evidence indicates that δ increases with r, and α decreases to a limiting value of 1 [36, 41] (see Table 1.3). In fact, we have [42–48]

$$\lim_{r \to \infty} \delta(r) = 29.576303\ldots, \quad \lim_{r \to \infty} \alpha(r)^{-r} = 0.0333810598\ldots.$$

At the other extreme [15, 31], $\lim_{r \to 1^+} \delta(r) = 2$ whereas $\lim_{r \to 1^+} \alpha(r) = \infty$.

A somewhat different generalization involves period triplings rather than period doublings [1, 16, 29, 30, 49–51]. For the logistic map f, when $3.8284\ldots \le a \le 3.8540\ldots$, a cascade of trifurcations to 3^n-cycles at parameter values $\hat{a}_n$ occur with Feigenbaum constants:

$$\hat{\delta} = \lim_{n \to \infty} \frac{\hat{a}_n - \hat{a}_{n-1}}{\hat{a}_{n+1} - \hat{a}_n} = 55.247\ldots, \quad \hat{\alpha} = \lim_{n \to \infty} \frac{\hat{w}_n}{\hat{w}_{n+1}} = 9.27738\ldots.$$

Three-cycles are of special interest since they guarantee the existence of chaos [2]. We do not know precisely the minimum value of a for which f has points that are not asymptotically periodic. The first 6-cycle appears [2] at $3.6265\ldots$, and the first odd-cycle appears [1] at $3.6786\ldots$.

The constants $55.247\ldots$ and $9.27738\ldots$ have not been computed to the same precision as the original Feigenbaum constants. Existing theory [27, 28] seems to apply

Table 1.3. *Feigenbaum Constants as Functions of Order r*

r	3	4	5	6
$\delta(r)$	$5.9679687038\ldots$	$7.2846862171\ldots$	$8.3494991320\ldots$	$9.2962468327\ldots$
$\alpha(r)$	$1.9276909638\ldots$	$1.6903029714\ldots$	$1.5557712501\ldots$	$1.4677424503\ldots$

only to period doublings. Our knowledge of period triplings is evidently based more on numerical heuristics than on mathematical rigor at present.

Incidently, the bifurcation points of h, when $r = 2$, are

$$c_2 = \tfrac{5}{4} = 1.25, \quad c_3 = 1.3680\ldots, \quad c_4 = 1.3940\ldots, \quad \ldots, \quad c_\infty = 1.4011\ldots$$

and are related to a_n via the transformation $c_n = a_n(a_n - 2)/4$. The limit point $c_\infty = 1.4011551890\ldots$ is due to Myrberg[52] but is not universal in any sense. Similarly, we can find the successive superstable width ratios of h, when $r = 2$:

$$\alpha_1 = 3.2185\ldots, \quad \alpha_2 = 2.6265\ldots, \quad \alpha_3 = 2.5281\ldots, \quad \ldots \alpha_\infty = \alpha = 2.5029\ldots,$$

in terms of symbols defined earlier: $\alpha_n = \tilde{w}_n(\tilde{a}_{n+1} - 2)\tilde{w}_{n+1}^{-1}(\tilde{a}_n - 2)^{-1}$. Both sequences $\{c_n\}$ and $\{\alpha_n\}$ are needed in [1.9.3].

1.9.2 Quadratic Planar Maps

The quadratic area-preserving (conservative) **Hénon map** [53, 54]

$$\begin{pmatrix} x_{n+1} \\ y_{n+1} \end{pmatrix} = \begin{pmatrix} 1 - ax_n^2 + y_n \\ x_n \end{pmatrix}$$

also leads to a cascade of period doublings, but with Feigenbaum constants $\alpha = 4.0180767046\ldots$, $\beta = 16.3638968792\ldots$ (scaling for two directions), and $\delta = 8.7210972\ldots$ that are larger than those for the one-dimensional case. These are characteristic for a certain subclass of the class of two-dimensional maps with quadratic maxima [50, 55, 56]. There is a different subclass, however, for which the *original* Feigenbaum constant $\delta = 4.6692016091\ldots$ appears: the area-contracting (dissipative) Hénon maps [49, 57, 58]

$$\begin{pmatrix} x_{n+1} \\ y_{n+1} \end{pmatrix} = \begin{pmatrix} 1 - ax_n^2 + y_n \\ bx_n \end{pmatrix}$$

(where the additional parameter b satisfies $|b| < 1$). It appears in higher dimensions too. The extent of the universality of δ is therefore larger than one may have expected!

Like period-tripling constants discussed in [1.9.1], the quantities $4.01808\ldots$, $16.36389\ldots$, and $8.72109\ldots$ have not been computed to the same precision as the original Feigenbaum constants. For two-dimensional conservative maps, Eckmann, Koch & Wittwer [59, 60] proved that these are indeed universal. For N-dimensional dissipative maps, Collet, Eckmann & Koch [61, 62] sketched a proof that the constant $4.66920\ldots$ is likewise universal.

1.9.3 Cvitanovic–Feigenbaum Functional Equation

Let D be an open, connected set in the complex plane containing the interval $[0, 1]$. Let X be the real Banach space of functions F satisfying $F(0) = 0$ that are complex-analytic on D, continuous on the closure of D, and real on $[0, 1]$, equipped with the supremum norm.

Fix a real number $r > 1$. Let Ω_r be the set of functions $f : [-1, 1] \to (-1, 1]$ of the form $f(x) = 1 + F(|x|^r)$, $F \in X$, with $F'(y) < 0$ for all $y \in [0, 1]$. In words, Ω_r is the set of even, folding self-maps f of the interval $[-1, 1]$ that can be written as power series in $|x|^r$ and satisfy $-1 < f^2(0) < f(0) = 1$. Define also $\Omega_{r,0}$ to be the subset of Ω_r subject to the additional constraint $f^2(0) < 0 < f^4(0) < -f^2(0) < f^3(0) < 1$.

By using the correspondence between f and F, the sets $\Omega_{r,0}$ and Ω_r are naturally identified with nested, open subsets of X. Hence $\Omega_{r,0}$ and Ω_r are Banach manifolds, both based on X. We can thus perform differential calculus on what is called the **period-doubling operator** $T_r : \Omega_{r,0} \to \Omega_r$, obtaining a linear operator $L_r : X \to X$ that best fits T_r in the vicinity of a certain function φ. This will be done shortly and is necessary to rigorously formulate the Feigenbaum constants [15, 27, 63].

Consider the function h defined earlier. Let us make its dependence on the parameter c explicit and write h_c from now on. Clearly $h_c \in \Omega_r$. Recall the sequences $\{c_n\}$ and $\{\alpha_n\}$ defined at the conclusion of [1.9.1] for $r = 2$; analogous sequences can be defined for arbitrary $r > 1$. We are interested in the "universality" of iterates of h_c as the parameter c increases to c_∞ and as the middle portion of the graph is magnified without bound. The remarkable limit

$$\lim_{n \to \infty} (-\alpha_n)^n \cdot h_{c_n}^{2^n} \left(\frac{x}{\alpha_n^n} \right) = \varphi(x)$$

exists [64–67] and satisfies the **Cvitanovic–Feigenbaum functional equation**

$$\varphi(x) = \varphi(1)^{-1} \cdot \varphi(\varphi(\varphi(1) \cdot x)) = T_r[\varphi](x)$$

with $\varphi \in \Omega_{r,0}$. See Figure 1.6 for a nice geometric interpretation. Moreover, the solution φ has been proven to be unique if r is an even integer [68–71]. Extending this uniqueness

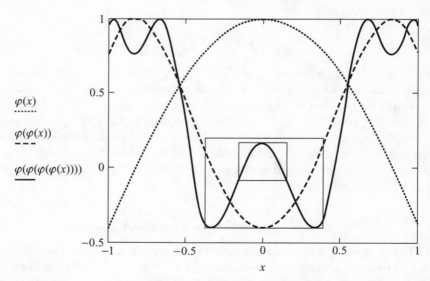

$\varphi(x)$

$\varphi(\varphi(x))$

$\varphi(\varphi(\varphi(\varphi(x))))$

Figure 1.6. Self-similarity of iterates of φ are illustrated inside diminishing rectangular windows: The condition $\varphi(1) < 0$ reverses orientation.

result to arbitrary $r > 1$ is an unsolved challenge [72]. As a consequence, for each r, we have $\alpha(r) = -\varphi(1)^{-1}$.

Consider now the local linearization (Fréchet derivative) of T_r at the fixed point φ:

$$L_r[\psi](x) = \varphi(1)^{-1} \cdot \left\{ \varphi'(\varphi(\varphi(1) \cdot x)) \cdot \psi(\varphi(1) \cdot x) + \psi(\varphi(\varphi(1) \cdot x)) \right.$$
$$\left. + \psi(1) \cdot [\varphi'(x) \cdot x - \varphi(x)] \right\}.$$

Then, for each r, $\delta(r)$ is the largest eigenvalue associated with L_r and is, in fact, the only eigenvalue that lies outside the unit disk. This is the basis for accurate estimates of $\delta(r)$. Fortunately, only the first two of the three terms in $L_r[\psi](x)$ are needed for computations [27, 36]. Alternatively, $\delta(r) = \lim_{n \to \infty} \sigma_{n+1}/\sigma_n$, where [45–47]

$$\sigma_n = \frac{1}{\xi(1)^n} \sum_{k=1}^{2^n-1} \xi^k(0) \cdot \left(\prod_{j=0}^{k-1} \xi'(\xi^j(0)) \right)^{-1}$$

and $\xi(x) = \left| \varphi(x^{1/r}) \right|^r$ for $0 \leq x \leq 1$. This formula is attractive, but unfortunately it is not numerically feasible for high-precision results. More formulas for δ appear in [73–75].

For period tripling [1.9.1], the analog of the Cvitanovic–Feigenbaum equation [29]

$$\varphi(x) = \varphi(1)^{-1} \cdot \varphi(\varphi(\varphi(\varphi(1) \cdot x)))$$

gives an estimate of $\hat{\alpha}$, and a linearization of the right-hand side gives $\hat{\delta}$. For planar maps, a matrix analog applies. Other functional equations will appear shortly.

1.9.4 Golden and Silver Circle Maps

We briefly mention a different example [76–79]:

$$\theta_{n+1} = k_a(\theta_n) = \theta_n + a - \frac{1}{2\pi} \sin(2\pi\theta_n),$$

which can be thought of as a homeomorphic mapping of a circle of circumference 1 onto itself. For any such circle map l, the limit

$$\rho(l) = \lim_{n \to \infty} \frac{l^n(\theta) - \theta}{n}$$

exists and is independent of θ. The quantity $\rho(l)$ is called the **winding** or **rotation number** of l. Our interest here is not in period doubling but rather quasiperiodicity: The subject offers an alternative transition into chaos and is rooted in the tension created under conditions when ρ is irrational.

Let $f_1 = f_2 = 1$, $f_3 = 2, \ldots$ denote the Fibonacci numbers [1.2], and define sequences $\{a_n\}$ and $\{w_n\}$ by [80, 81]

$$k_{a_n}^{f_n}(0) = f_{n-1}, \quad w_n = k_{a_n}^{f_{n-1}}(0) - f_{n-2}.$$

It can be proved that $\rho(k_{a_\infty}) = (1 - \sqrt{5})/2$; hence the family of circle maps k_{a_n} is **golden** and the corresponding Feigenbaum constants are $\alpha = 1.2885745539\ldots$ and $\delta = 2.8336106558\ldots$. Moreover, for all golden circle maps with a single cubic point of inflection, the constants α and δ are universal. If we replace the Fibonacci numbers by Pell numbers [1.1], then $\rho(k_{a_\infty}) = \sqrt{2} - 1$; hence the family of circle maps k_{a_n} is **silver** with $\alpha = 1.5868266790\ldots$ and $\delta = 6.7992251609\ldots$. Similar universality holds for cubic silver circle maps; other irrational winding numbers have been studied too [30]. If, instead, we examine golden circle maps with a single r^{th}-order inflection point, then functions $\alpha(r)$ and $\delta(r)$ emerge, satisfying [47, 80, 82–86]

$$\lim_{r\to\infty} \alpha(r) = 1, \qquad \lim_{r\to\infty} \alpha(r)^r = 3.63600703\ldots,$$

$$\alpha\left(\tfrac{1}{r}\right) = \alpha(r)^r \text{ for all } r > 0, \qquad \lim_{r\to\infty} \delta(r) = 4.121326\ldots.$$

It is conjectured, but not yet proven, that $\delta(1/r) = \delta(r)$ for all r.

As with interval maps, certain functional equations provide the numerical key to precisely computing $\alpha(r)$ and $\delta(r)$ associated with circle maps [81]:

$$\varphi(\theta) = \varphi(1)^{-1} \cdot \varphi(\varphi(\varphi(1)^2 \cdot \theta))$$

for the golden case and

$$\varphi(\theta) = \varphi(1)^{-1} \cdot \varphi(\varphi(1) \cdot \varphi(\varphi(\varphi(1)^2 \cdot \theta)))$$

for the silver case.

McCarthy [87] compared the two famous functional equations

$$\varphi(x) \cdot \varphi(y) = \varphi(x + y), \quad \varphi(\varphi(y)) = s^{-1}\varphi(s\,y).$$

In the former, multiplication is simply a form of addition; in the latter, self-composition is just a rescaling. He invoked the appropriate phrase "twentieth-century exponential function" for a solution of the latter. Research in this area will, however, continue for many more years.

[1] R. M. May, Simple mathematical models with very complicated dynamics, *Nature* 261 (1976) 459–467.

[2] T. Y. Li and J. A. Yorke, Period three implies chaos, *Amer. Math. Monthly* 82 (1975) 985–992; MR 52 #5898.

[3] D. Singer, Stable orbits and bifurcations of maps on the interval, *SIAM J. Appl. Math.* 35 (1978) 260–271; MR 58 #13206.

[4] R. L. Devaney, *An Introduction to Chaotic Dynamical Systems*, 2nd ed., Addison-Wesley, 1989; MR 91a:58114.

[5] M. Martelli, *Discrete Dynamical Systems and Chaos*, Longman, 1992; MR 97i:58104.

[6] H. G. Schuster, *Deterministic Chaos: An Introduction*, 3rd ed., VCH Verlagsgesellschaft mbH, 1995; MR 97c:58103.

[7] R. A. Holmgren, *A First Course in Discrete Dynamical Systems*, 2nd ed., Springer-Verlag, 1996; MR 97f:58052.

[8] R. L. Kraft, Chaos, Cantor sets, and hyperbolicity for the logistic maps, *Amer. Math. Monthly* 106 (1999) 400–408; MR 2000f:37042.

[9] M. J. Feigenbaum, Quantitative universality for a class of nonlinear transformations, *J. Stat. Phys.* 19 (1978) 25–52; MR 58 #18601.

[10] M. J. Feigenbaum, The universal metric properties of nonlinear transformations, *J. Stat. Phys.* 21 (1979) 669–706; MR 82e:58072.

[11] M. J. Feigenbaum, Universal behavior in nonlinear systems, *Los Alamos Sci.* 1 (1980) 4–27; MR 82h:58031.

[12] C. Tresser and P. Coullet, Itérations d'endomorphismes et groupe de renormalisation, *C. R. Acad. Sci. Paris Sér. A-B* 287 (1978) A577–A580; MR 80b:58043.

[13] C. Tresser and P. Coullet, Itérations d'endomorphismes et groupe de renormalisation, *J. de Physique Colloque* C5, n. 8, t. 39 (1978) C5-25–C5-27.

[14] P. Collet and J.-P. Eckmann, Properties of continuous maps of the interval to itself, *Mathematical Problems in Theoretical Physics*, ed. K. Osterwalder, Lect. Notes in Physics 116, Springer-Verlag, 1979, pp. 331–339; MR 82b:58051.

[15] P. Collet, J.-P. Eckmann, and O. E. Lanford, Universal properties of maps on an interval, *Commun. Math. Phys.* 76 (1980) 211–254; MR 83d:58036.

[16] P. Collet and J.-P. Eckmann, *Iterated Maps on the Interval as Dynamical Systems*, Birkhaüser, 1980; MR 82j:58078.

[17] P. Cvitanovic, *Universality in Chaos*, Adam Hilger, 1984; MR 91e:58124.

[18] O. E. Lanford, Remarks on the accumulation of period-doubling bifurcations, *Mathematical Problems in Theoretical Physics*, ed. K. Osterwalder, Lect. Notes in Physics 116, Springer-Verlag, 1979, pp. 340–342; MR 82b:58052.

[19] O. E. Lanford, Smooth transformations of intervals, *Séminaire Bourbaki 1980/81*, n. 563, Lect. Notes in Math. 901, Springer-Verlag, 1981, pp. 36–54; MR 83k:58066.

[20] O. E. Lanford, A computer-assisted proof of the Feigenbaum conjectures, *Bull. Amer. Math. Soc.* 6 (1982) 427–434; MR 83g:58051.

[21] O. E. Lanford, Computer-assisted proofs in analysis, *Physica A* 124 (1984) 465–470; MR 86a:00013.

[22] O. E. Lanford, A shorter proof of the existence of the Feigenbaum fixed point, *Commun. Math. Phys.* 96 (1984) 521–538; MR 86c:58121.

[23] M. Campanino and H. Epstein, On the existence of Feigenbaum's fixed point, *Commun. Math. Phys.* 79 (1981) 261–302; MR 82j:58099.

[24] M. Campanino, H. Epstein, and D. Ruelle, On Feigenbaum's functional equation $g \circ g(\lambda x) + \lambda g(x) = 0$, *Topology* 21 (1982) 125–129; MR 83g:58039.

[25] J.-P. Eckmann and P. Wittwer, A complete proof of the Feigenbaum conjectures, *J. Stat. Phys.* 46 (1987) 455–475; MR 89b:58131.

[26] H. Koch, A. Schenkel, and P. Wittwer, Computer-assisted proofs in analysis and programming in logic: A case study, *SIAM Rev.* 38 (1996) 565–604; Université de Genève physics preprint 94–394; MR 97k:39001.

[27] E. B. Vul, Ya. G. Sinai, and K. M. Khanin, Feigenbaum universality and thermodynamic formalism (in Russian), *Uspekhi Mat. Nauk*, v. 39 (1984) n. 3, 3–37; Engl. transl. in *Russian Math. Surveys*, v. 39 (1984) n. 3, 1–40; MR 86g:58106.

[28] D. Rand, Universality and renormalisation, *New Directions in Dynamical Systems*, ed. T. Bedford and J. Swift, Lect. Notes 127, London Math. Soc., 1988, pp. 1–56; MR 89j:58082.

[29] R. Delbourgo and B. G. Kenny, Universality relations, *Phys. Rev. A* 33 (1986) 3292–3302.

[30] R. Delbourgo, Relations between universal scaling constants in dissipative maps, *Nonlinear Dynamics and Chaos*, Proc. Fourth Physics Summer School, ed. R. L. Dewar and B. I. Henry, World Scientific, 1992, pp. 231–256; MR 93c:58121.

[31] J. P. van der Weele, H. W. Capel, and R. Kluiving, Period doubling in maps with a maximum of order z, *Physica A* 145 (1987) 425–460; MR 89f:58109.

[32] J. W. Stephenson and Y. Wang, Numerical solution of Feigenbaum's equation, *Appl. Math. Notes* 15 (1990) 68–78; MR 92c:58085.

[33] J. W. Stephenson and Y. Wang, Relationships between the solutions of Feigenbaum's equations, *Appl. Math. Lett.* 4 (1991) 37–39; MR 92g:39003.

[34] J. W. Stephenson and Y. Wang, Relationships between eigenfunctions associated with solutions of Feigenbaum's equation, *Appl. Math. Lett.* 4 (1991) 53–56; MR 92g:39004.

[35] K. M. Briggs, How to calculate the Feigenbaum constants on your PC, *Austral. Math. Soc. Gazette* 16 (1989) 89–92; also in *Feigenbaum Scaling in Discrete Dynamical Systems*, Ph.D. thesis, Univ. of Melbourne, 1997.

[36] K. M. Briggs, A precise calculation of the Feigenbaum constants, *Math. Comp.* 57 (1991) 435–439; MR 91j:11117.

[37] D. J. Broadhurst, Feigenbaum constants to 1018 decimal places, unpublished note (1999).

[38] D. H. Bailey, Multiprecision translation and execution of Fortran programs, *ACM Trans. Math. Software* 19 (1993) 288–319.

[39] D. H. Bailey and D. J. Broadhurst, Parallel integer relation detection: Techniques and applications, *Math. Comp.* 70 (2001) 1719–1736; math.NA/9905048; MR 2002b:11174.

[40] E. Salamin, Fine structure constant, unpublished note (2000).

[41] A. P. Kuznetsov, S. P. Kuznetsov, and I. R. Sataev, A variety of period-doubling universality classes in multi-parameter analysis of transition to chaos, *Physica D* 109 (1997) 91–112; MR 98k:58159.

[42] J.-P. Eckmann and P. Wittwer, *Computer Methods and Borel Summability Applied to Feigenbaum's Equation*, Lect. Notes in Physics 227, Springer-Verlag, 1985; MR 86m:58129.

[43] J.-P. Eckmann and H. Epstein, Bounds on the unstable eigenvalue for period doubling, *Commun. Math. Phys.* 128 (1990) 427–435; MR 91a:582134.

[44] J. Groeneveld, On constructing complete solution classes of the Cvitanovic-Feigenbaum equation, *Physica A* 138 (1986) 137–166; MR 88k:58079.

[45] J. B. McGuire and C. J. Thompson, Asymptotic properties of sequences of iterates of nonlinear transformations, *J. Stat. Phys.* 27 (1982) 183–200; MR 84h:58123.

[46] C. J. Thompson and J. B. McGuire, Asymptotic and essentially singular solutions of the Feigenbaum equation, *J. Stat. Phys.* 51 (1988) 991–1007; MR 90c:58134.

[47] K. M. Briggs, T. W. Dixon, and G. Szekeres, Analytic solutions of the Cvitanovic-Feigenbaum and Feigenbaum-Kadanoff-Shenker equations, *Int. J. Bifurcat. Chaos Appl. Sci. Eng.* 8 (1998) 347–357; MR 99h:58054.

[48] H. Thunberg, Feigenbaum numbers for certain flat-top families, *Experim. Math.* 3 (1994) 51–57; MR 96f:58085.

[49] B. Derrida, A. Gervois, and Y. Pomeau, Universal metric properties of bifurcations of endomorphisms, *J. Phys. A* 12 (1979) 269–296; MR 80k:58078.

[50] B. Derrida and Y. Pomeau, Feigenbaum's ratios of two-dimensional area preserving maps, *Phys. Lett. A* 80 (1980) 217–219; MR 81m:58051.

[51] A. I. Golberg, Ya. G. Sinai, and K. M. Khanin, Universal properties of sequences of period-tripling bifurcations (in Russian), *Uspekhi Mat. Nauk*, v. 38 (1983) n. 1, 159–160; Engl. transl. in *Russian Math. Surveys*, v. 38 (1983) n. 1, 187–188; MR 84i:58085.

[52] P. J. Myrberg, Iteration der reellen Polynome zweiten Grades. III, *Annales Acad. Sci. Fenn. A*, v. 336 (1963) n. 3, 1–18; MR 27 #1552.

[53] M. Hénon, A two-dimensional mapping with a strange attractor, *Commun. Math. Phys.* 50 (1976) 69–77; MR 54 #10917.

[54] K. M. Briggs, G. R. W. Quispel, and C. J. Thompson, Feigenvalues for Mandelsets, *J. Phys. A* 24 (1991) 3363–3368; MR 92h:58167.

[55] P. Collet, J.-P. Eckmann, and H. Koch, On universality for area-preserving maps of the plane, *Physica D* 3 (1981) 457–467; MR 83b:58055.

[56] J. M. Greene, R. S. MacKay, F. Vivaldi, and M. J. Feigenbaum, Universal behaviour in families of area-preserving maps, *Physica D* 3 (1981) 468–486; MR 82m:58041.

[57] J.-P. Eckmann, Roads to turbulence in dissipative dynamical systems, *Rev. Mod. Phys.* 53 (1981) 643–654; MR 82j:58079.

[58] J. M. T. Thompson and H. B. Stewart, *Nonlinear Dynamics and Chaos*, Wiley, 1986; MR 87m:58098.

[59] J.-P. Eckmann, H. Koch, and P. Wittwer, Existence of a fixed point of the doubling transformation for area-preserving maps of the plane, *Phys. Rev. A* 26 (1982) 720–722.

[60] J.-P. Eckmann, H. Koch, and P. Wittwer, *A Computer-Assisted Proof of Universality for Area-Preserving Maps*, Amer. Math. Soc., 1984; MR 85e:58119.

[61] P. Collet, J.-P. Eckmann, and H. Koch, Period doubling bifurcations for families of maps on $\mathbb{R}^n$, *J. Stat. Phys.* 25 (1981) 1–14; MR 82i:58052.

[62] O. E. Lanford, Period doubling in one and several dimensions, *Physica D* 7 (1983) 124–125.

[63] Y. Jiang, T. Morita, and D. Sullivan, Expanding direction of the period doubling operator, *Commun. Math. Phys.* 144 (1992) 509–520; MR 93c:58169.

[64] H. Epstein, New proofs of the existence of the Feigenbaum functions, *Commun. Math. Phys.* 106 (1986) 395–426; MR 88i:58124.

[65] J.-P. Eckmann and H. Epstein, Fixed points of composition operators, *Proc. 1986 International Congress on Mathematical Physics*, ed. M. Mebkhout and R. Seneor, World Scientific, 1987, pp. 517–530; MR 89d:58080.

[66] H. Epstein, Fixed points of composition operators, *Nonlinear Evolution and Chaotic Phenomena*, ed. G. Gallavotti and P. F. Zweifel, Plenum Press, 1988, pp. 71–100; MR 92f:58003.

[67] H. Epstein, Fixed points of composition operators. II, *Nonlinearity* 2 (1989) 305–310; MR 90j:58086.

[68] D. Sullivan, Bounds, quadratic differentials, and renormalization conjectures, *Mathematics into the Twenty-first Century*, ed. F. Browder, Amer. Math. Soc., 1992, pp. 417–466; MR 93k:58194.

[69] W. de Melo and S. van Strien, *One-Dimensional Dynamics*, Springer-Verlag, 1993; MR 95a:58035.

[70] C. T. McMullen, *Complex Dynamics and Renormalization*, Princeton Univ. Press, 1994; MR 96b:58097.

[71] M. Lyubich, The quadratic family as a qualitatively solvable model of chaos, *Notices Amer. Math. Soc.* 47 (2000) 1042–1052; MR 2001g:37063.

[72] Y. Jiang, Renormalization on one-dimensional folding maps, *Dynamical Systems and Chaos*, v. 1, Proc. 1994 Hachioji conf., ed. N. Aoki, K. Shiraiwa, and Y. Takahashi, World Scientific, 1995, pp. 116–125; MR 98g:58045.

[73] F. Christiansen, P. Cvitanovic, and H. H. Rugh, The spectrum of the period-doubling operator in terms of cycles, *J. Phys. A* 23 (1990) L713–L717; MR 91d:58136.

[74] R. Artuso, E. Aurell, and P. Cvitanovic, Recycling of strange sets. II: Applications. *Nonlinearity* 3 (1990) 361–386; MR 92c:58105.

[75] M. Pollicott, A note on the Artuso-Aurell-Cvitanovic approach to the Feigenbaum tangent operator, *J. Stat. Phys.* 62 (1991) 257–267; MR 92d:58166.

[76] S. J. Shenker, Scaling behavior in a map of a circle onto itself: Empirical results, *Physica D* 5 (1982) 405–411; MR 84f:58066.

[77] M. J. Feigenbaum, L. P. Kadanoff, and S. J. Shenker, Quasiperiodicity in dissipative systems: A renormalization group analysis, *Physica D* 5 (1982) 370–386; MR 84f:58101.

[78] S. Östlund, D. Rand, J. Sethna, and E. Siggia, Universal properties of the transition from quasiperiodicity to chaos in dissipative systems, *Physica D* 8 (1983) 303–342; MR 85d:58066.

[79] O. E. Lanford, Functional equations for circle homeomorphisms with golden ratio rotation number, *J. Stat. Phys.* 34 (1984) 57–73; MR 86a:58064.

[80] T. W. Dixon, B. G. Kenny, and K. M. Briggs, On the universality of singular circle maps, *Phys. Lett. A* 231 (1997) 359–366.

[81] T. W. Dixon, T. Gherghetta, and B. G. Kenny, Universality in the quasiperiodic route to chaos, *Chaos* 6 (1996) 32–42; also in *Chaos and Nonlinear Dynamics*, ed. R. C. Hilborn and N. B. Tufillaro, Amer. Assoc. Physics Teachers, 1999, pp 90–100; MR 97a:58162.

[82] L. Jonker and D. A. Rand, Universal properties of maps of the circle with ε-singularities, *Commun. Math. Phys.* 90 (1983) 273–292; MR 85j:58103.

[83] A. Arneodo and M. Holschneider, Fractal dimensions and homeomorphic conjugacies, *J. Stat. Phys.* 50 (1988) 995–1020; MR 90a:58092.

[84] B. Hu, A. Valinia, and O. Piro, Universality and asymptotic limits of the scaling exponents in circle maps, *Phys. Lett. A* 144 (1990) 7–10; MR 90k:58131.

[85] R. Delbourgo and B. G. Kenny, Relations between universal scaling constants for the circle map near the golden mean, *J. Math. Phys.* 32 (1991) 1045–1051; MR 92e:58109.

[86] T. W. Dixon and B. G. Kenny, Transition to criticality in circle maps at the golden mean, *J. Math. Phys.* 39 (1998) 5952–5963; MR 99h:58169.

[87] P. J. McCarthy, Ultrafunctions, projective function geometry, and polynomial functional equations, *Proc. London Math. Soc.* 53 (1986) 321–339; MR 88c:39009.

1.10 Madelung's Constant

Consider the square lattice in the plane with unit charges located at integer lattice points $(i, j) \neq (0, 0)$ and of sign $(-1)^{i+j}$. The electrostatic potential at the origin due to the charge at (i, j) is $(-1)^{i+j}/\sqrt{i^2 + j^2}$. The total electrostatic potential at the origin due to all charges is hence [1]

$$M_2 = \sum_{i,j=-\infty}^{\infty}{}' \frac{(-1)^{i+j}}{\sqrt{i^2 + j^2}},$$

where the prime indicates that we omit $(0, 0)$ from the summation.

How is this infinite lattice sum to be interpreted? This is a delicate issue since the subseries with $i = j$ is divergent, so the alternating character of the full series needs to be carefully exploited [2–7]. We may, nonetheless, work with either expanding circles or with expanding squares and still obtain the same convergent sum [8–15]:

$$M_2 = 4(\sqrt{2} - 1)\zeta\left(\frac{1}{2}\right)\beta\left(\frac{1}{2}\right) = -1.6155426267\ldots,$$

where $\zeta(x)$ is Riemann's zeta function [1.6] and $\beta(x)$ is Dirichlet's beta function [1.7]. The sum M_2 is called Madelung's constant for a two-dimensional NaCl crystal. Rewriting lattice sums in terms of well-known functions as such is essential because convergence rates otherwise are extraordinarily slow.

The three-dimensional analog

$$M_3 = \sum_{i,j,k=-\infty}^{\infty}{}' \frac{(-1)^{i+j+k}}{\sqrt{i^2 + j^2 + k^2}}$$

is trickier because, surprisingly, the expanding-spheres method for summation leads to divergence! This remarkable fact was first noticed by Emersleben [16]. Using expanding cubes instead, we obtain the Benson–Mackenzie formula [17, 18]

$$M_3 = -12\pi \sum_{m,n=1}^{\infty} \operatorname{sech}\left(\frac{\pi}{2}\sqrt{(2m-1)^2 + (2n-1)^2}\right)^2 = -1.7475645946\ldots,$$

which is rapidly convergent. Of many possible reformulations, there is a formula due to Hautot [19]

$$M_3 = \frac{\pi}{2} - \frac{9}{2}\ln(2) + 12 \sum_{m,n=1}^{\infty} (-1)^m \frac{\operatorname{csch}\left(\pi\sqrt{m^2 + n^2}\right)}{\sqrt{m^2 + n^2}},$$

that is not quite as fast but is formally consistent with other lattice sums we discuss later. The quantity M_3 is called Madelung's constant for a three-dimensional NaCl crystal or, more simply, **Madelung's constant**. Note that, in their splendid survey, Glasser &

Zucker[20] called $\pm 2M_3$ the same, so caution should be exercised when reviewing the literature. Other representations of M_3 appear in [21–23].

The four-, six-, and eight-dimensional analogs can also be found [24]:

$$M_4 = \sum_{i,j,k,l=-\infty}^{\infty}{}' \frac{(-1)^{i+j+k+l}}{\sqrt{i^2 + j^2 + k^2 + l^2}} = -8\left(5 - 3\sqrt{2}\right) \zeta\left(\frac{1}{2}\right) \zeta\left(-\frac{1}{2}\right)$$
$$= -1.8393990840\ldots,$$

$$M_6 = \frac{3}{\pi^2}\left[4\left(\sqrt{2} - 1\right)\zeta\left(\frac{1}{2}\right)\beta\left(\frac{5}{2}\right) - \left(4\sqrt{2} - 1\right)\zeta\left(\frac{5}{2}\right)\beta\left(\frac{1}{2}\right)\right]$$
$$= -1.9655570390\ldots,$$

$$M_8 = \frac{15}{4\pi^3}\left(8\sqrt{2} - 1\right)\zeta\left(\frac{1}{2}\right)\zeta\left(\frac{7}{2}\right) = -2.0524668272\ldots.$$

A general result due to Borwein & Borwein[4] shows that the n-dimensional analog of Madelung's constant is convergent for any $n \geq 1$. Of course, $M_1 = -2\ln(2)$. Rapidly convergent series expressions for $M_5 = -1.9093378156\ldots$ or $M_7 = -2.0124059897\ldots$ seem elusive [25]. It is known, however, that for all n,

$$M_n = \frac{1}{\sqrt{\pi}} \int_0^{\infty} \left\{\left(\sum_{k=-\infty}^{\infty} (-1)^k e^{-k^2 t}\right)^n - 1\right\} \frac{dt}{\sqrt{t}},$$

from which high-precision numerical computations are possible [26, 27]. Using this integral, it can be proved [28] that $M_n \sim -\sqrt{4\ln(n)/\pi}$ as $n \to \infty$.

There are many possible variations on these lattice sums. One could, for example, remove the square root in the denominator and obtain [15, 20]

$$N_1 = \sum_{i=-\infty}^{\infty}{}' \frac{(-1)^i}{i^2} = -\frac{\pi^2}{6}, \quad N_2 = \sum_{i,j=-\infty}^{\infty}{}' \frac{(-1)^{i+j}}{i^2 + j^2} = -\pi\ln(2),$$

$$N_3 = \sum_{i,j,k=-\infty}^{\infty}{}' \frac{(-1)^{i+j+k}}{i^2 + j^2 + k^2}$$
$$= \frac{\pi^2}{3} - \pi\ln(2) - \frac{\pi}{\sqrt{2}}\ln\left(2(\sqrt{2} + 1)\right) + 8\pi \sum_{m,n=1}^{\infty} (-1)^n \frac{\operatorname{csch}\left(\pi\sqrt{m^2 + 2n^2}\right)}{\sqrt{m^2 + 2n^2}}$$
$$= -2.5193561520\ldots,$$

$$N_4 = \sum_{i,j,k,l=-\infty}^{\infty}{}' \frac{(-1)^{i+j+k+l}}{i^2 + j^2 + k^2 + l^2} = -4\ln(2),$$

with asymptotics $N_n \sim -\ln(n)$ determined similarly. One could alternatively perform the summation over a different lattice; for example, a regular hexagonal lattice in the plane rather than the square lattice $[2, 7]$, with basis vectors $(1, 0)$ and $(1/2, \sqrt{3}/2)$. This yields the expression

$$H_2 = \frac{4}{3} \sum_{i,j=-\infty}^{\infty}{}' \frac{\sin((i+1)\theta)\sin((j+1)\theta) - \sin(i\theta)\sin((j-1)\theta)}{\sqrt{i^2 + ij + j^2}},$$

where $\theta = 2\pi/3$, which may be rewritten as

$$H_2 = -3\left(\sqrt{3} - 1\right)\varsigma\left(\frac{1}{2}\right)$$
$$\times \left(1 - \frac{1}{\sqrt{2}} + \frac{1}{\sqrt{4}} - \frac{1}{\sqrt{5}} + \frac{1}{\sqrt{7}} - \frac{1}{\sqrt{8}} + \frac{1}{\sqrt{10}} - \frac{1}{\sqrt{11}} + - \cdots\right)$$
$$= 1.5422197217\ldots.$$

This is Madelung's constant for the planar hexagonal lattice; the three-dimensional analog H_3 of this perhaps has a chemical significance akin to M_3. If we remove the square root in the denominator as well, then

$$K_2 = \frac{4}{3} \sum_{i,j=-\infty}^{\infty}{}' \frac{\sin((i+1)\theta)\sin((j+1)\theta) - \sin(i\theta)\sin((j-1)\theta)}{i^2 + ij + j^2} = \sqrt{3}\pi \ln(3).$$

A lattice sum generalization of the Euler–Mascheroni constant [1.5] appears in [1.10.1]. This, by the way, has no connection with different extensions due to Stieltjes [2.21] or to Masser and Gramain [7.2].

Forrester & Glasser [29] discovered that

$$\sum_{i,j,k=-\infty}^{\infty} \frac{(-1)^{i+j+k}}{\sqrt{\left(i - \frac{1}{6}\right)^2 + \left(j - \frac{1}{6}\right)^2 + \left(k - \frac{1}{6}\right)^2}} = \sqrt{3},$$

which may be as close to an exact evaluation of M_3 as possible (in the sense that no such formula is known at any point closer to the origin). Some variations involving trigonometric functions were explored in [30, 31]. There are many more relevant summations available than we can possibly give here [20, 32].

1.10.1 Lattice Sums and Euler's Constant

For any integer $p \geq 2$, define

$$\Delta(n, p) = \sum_{i_1,i_2,\ldots,i_p=-n}^{n}{}' \frac{1}{\sqrt{i_1^2 + i_2^2 + \cdots + i_p^2}} - \int_{x_1,x_2,\ldots,x_p=-n-\frac{1}{2}}^{n+\frac{1}{2}} \frac{dx_1 dx_2 \cdots dx_p}{\sqrt{x_1^2 + x_2^2 + \cdots + x_p^2}}.$$

The integral converges in spite of the singularity at the origin. In two dimensions, we have [33]

$$\Delta(n,2) = \sum_{i,j=-n}^{n}{}' \frac{1}{\sqrt{i^2+j^2}} - 4\ln\left(\frac{\sqrt{2}+1}{\sqrt{2}-1}\right)\left(n+\frac{1}{2}\right)$$

$$\rightarrow 4\zeta\left(\frac{1}{2}\right)\beta\left(\frac{1}{2}\right)$$

$$= \left(\sqrt{2}+1\right)M_2 = -3.9002649200\ldots = \delta_2$$

as $n \rightarrow \infty$. It is interesting that if we define a function

$$f(z) = \sum_{i,j=-\infty}^{\infty}{}' \frac{1}{(i^2+j^2)^z}, \quad \text{Re}(z) > 1,$$

then f can be analytically continued to a function F over the whole complex plane via the formula $F(z) = 4\zeta(z)\beta(z)$ with just one singularity, a simple pole, at $z = 1$. So although the lattice sum $f(1/2) = \infty$, we have $\delta_2 = F(1/2) = -3.90026\ldots$; that is, the integral "plays no role" in the final answer.

In the same way, by starting with the function

$$g(z) = \sum_{i,j,k=-\infty}^{\infty}{}' \frac{1}{(i^2+j^2+k^2)^z}, \quad \text{Re}(z) > \frac{3}{2},$$

g can be analytically continued to a function G that is analytic everywhere except for a simple pole at $z = 3/2$. Unlike the two-dimensional case, however, we here have [33]

$$\Delta(n,3) = \sum_{i,j,k=-n}^{n}{}' \frac{1}{\sqrt{i^2+j^2+k^2}} - 12\left(-\frac{\pi}{6} + \ln\left(\frac{\sqrt{3}+1}{\sqrt{3}-1}\right)\right)\left(n+\frac{1}{2}\right)^2$$

$$\rightarrow G\left(\frac{1}{2}\right) + \frac{\pi}{6}$$

$$= -2.3136987039\ldots = \delta_3$$

as $n \rightarrow \infty$; that is, here the integral *does* play a role and a "correction term" $\pi/6$ is needed. A fast expression for evaluating $G(1/2)$ is [20, 34]

$$G\left(\frac{1}{2}\right) = \frac{7\pi}{6} - \frac{19}{2}\ln(2) + 4\sum_{m,n=1}^{\infty} [3 + 3(-1)^m + (-1)^{m+n}] \frac{\text{csch}\left(\pi\sqrt{m^2+n^2}\right)}{\sqrt{m^2+n^2}}$$

$$= -2.8372974794\ldots,$$

which bears some similarity to Hautot's formula for M_3.

Now define, for any integer $p \geq 1$,

$$\gamma_p = \lim_{n\rightarrow\infty}\left(\sum_{i_1,i_2,\ldots,i_p=1}^{n} \frac{1}{\sqrt{i_1^2+i_2^2+\cdots+i_p^2}} - \int_{x_1,x_2,\ldots,x_p=1} \frac{dx_1dx_2\cdots dx_p}{\sqrt{x_1^2+x_2^2+\cdots+x_p^2}}\right).$$

Everyone knows that $\gamma_1 = \gamma$ is the Euler–Mascheroni constant [1.5], but comparatively few people know that [35–37]

$$\gamma_2 = \frac{1}{4}\left\{\delta_2 + 2\ln\left(\frac{\sqrt{2}+1}{\sqrt{2}-1}\right) - 4\gamma_1\right\} = -0.6709083078\ldots,$$

$$\gamma_3 = \frac{1}{8}\left\{\delta_3 + 3\left[-\frac{\pi}{6} + \ln\left(\frac{\sqrt{3}+1}{\sqrt{3}-1}\right)\right] + 12\gamma_2 - 6\gamma_1\right\} = 0.5817480456\ldots.$$

No one has computed the value of γ_p for any $p \geq 4$.

[1] E. Madelung, Das elektrische Feld in Systemen von regelmässig angeordneten Punktladun-
     gen, *Phys. Z.* 19 (1918) 524–533.
[2] D. Borwein, J. M. Borwein, and K. F. Taylor, Convergence of lattice sums and Madelung's
     constant, *J. Math. Phys.* 26 (1985) 2999–3009; MR 86m:82047.
[3] K. F. Taylor, On Madelung's constant, *J. Comput. Chem.* 8 (1987) 291–295; MR 88h:82066.
[4] D. Borwein and J. M. Borwein, A note on alternating series in several dimensions, *Amer.
     Math. Monthly* 93 (1986) 531–539; MR 87j:40008.
[5] J. P. Buhler and R. E. Crandall, On the convergence problem for lattice sums, *J. Phys. A* 23
     (1990) 2523–2528; MR 91h:82008.
[6] J. Buhler and S. Wagon, Secrets of the Madelung constant, *Mathematica Educ. Res.* 5
     (1996) 49–55.
[7] D. Borwein, J. M. Borwein, and C. Pinner, Convergence of Madelung-like lattice sums,
     Trans. Amer. Math. Soc. 350 (1998) 3131–3167; CECM preprint 95:040; MR 98k:11135.
[8] G. H. Hardy and E. M. Wright, *An Introduction to the Theory of Numbers*, 5th ed., Oxford
     Univ. Press, 1985, pp. 256–257; MR 81i:10002.
[9] M. L. Glasser, The evaluation of lattice sums. I: Analytic procedures, *J. Math. Phys.* 14
     (1973) 409–413; comments by A. Hautot, 15 (1974) 268; MR 47 #5328 and MR 55 #741b.
[10] M. L. Glasser, The evaluation of lattice sums. II: Number-theoretic approach, *J. Math.
     Phys.* 14 (1973) 701–703; erratum 15 (1974) 520; MR 48 #8409 and MR 49 #6849.
[11] I. J. Zucker, A note on lattice sums in two dimensions, *J. Math. Phys.* 15 (1974) 187; MR
     55 #741a.
[12] I. J. Zucker and M. M. Robertson, Exact values for some two-dimensional lattice sums,
     J. Phys. A 8 (1975) 874–881; MR 54 #9515.
[13] I. J. Zucker and M. M. Robertson, Some properties of Dirichlet L-series, *J. Phys. A* 9 (1976)
     1207–1214; MR 54 #253.
[14] I. J. Zucker and M. M. Robertson, A systematic approach to the evaluation of
     $\sum_{(m,n\neq0,0)}(am^2 + bmn + cn^2)^{-s}$, *J. Phys. A* 9 (1976) 1215–1225; MR 54 #244.
[15] J. M. Borwein and P. B. Borwein, *Pi and the AGM: A Study in Analytic Number Theory
     and Computational Complexity*, Wiley, 1987, pp. 288–305; MR 99h:11147.
[16] O. Emersleben, Über die Konvergenz der Reihen Epsteinscher Zetafunktionen, *Math.
     Nachr.* 4 (1951) 468–480.
[17] G. C. Benson, A simple formula for evaluating the Madelung constant of a NaCl-type
     crystal, *Canad. J. Phys.* 34 (1956) 888–890.
[18] J. K. Mackenzie, A simple formula for evaluating the Madelung constant of an NaCl-type
     crystal, *Canad. J. Phys.* 35 (1957) 500–501.
[19] A. Hautot, A new method for the evaluation of slowly convergent series, *J. Math. Phys* 15
     (1974) 1722–1727; MR 53 #9575.
[20] M. L. Glasser and I. J. Zucker, Lattice sums, *Theoretical Chemistry: Advances and Per-
     spectives*, v. 5, ed. H. Eyring and D. Henderson, Academic Press, 1980, pp. 67–139.
[21] R. E. Crandall and J. P. Buhler, Elementary function expansions for Madelung constants,
     J. Phys. A 20 (1987) 5497–5510; MR 88m:82034.
[22] R. E. Crandall, New representations for the Madelung constant, *Experim. Math.* 8 (1999)
     367–379; MR 2000m:11125.

[23] R. E. Crandall, Fast evaluation for a certain class of lattice sums, Perfectly Scientific Inc. preprint (2000).

[24] I. J. Zucker, Exact results for some lattice sums in 2, 4, 6 and 8 dimensions, *J. Phys. A* 7 (1974) 1568–1575; MR 53 #11258.

[25] M. L. Glasser, Evaluation of lattice sums. IV: A five-dimensional sum, *J. Math. Phys.* 16 (1975) 1237–1238; MR 55 #7228.

[26] H. Essén and A. Nordmark, Some results on the electrostatic energy of ionic crystals, *Canad. J. Chem.* 74 (1996) 885–891.

[27] J. Keane, Computations of M_n and N_n for $n \leq 64$, unpublished note (1997).

[28] P. Flajolet, A problem in asymptotics, unpublished note (2001).

[29] P. J. Forrester and M. L. Glasser, Some new lattice sums including an exact result for the electrostatic potential within the NaCl lattice, *J. Phys. A* 15 (1982) 911–914; MR 83d:82047.

[30] J. Boersma and P. J. De Doelder, On alternating multiple series, *SIAM Rev.* 35 (1993) 497–500.

[31] D. Borwein and J. M. Borwein, On some trigonometric and exponential lattice sums, *J. Math. Anal. Appl.* 188 (1994) 209–218; MR 95i:11089.

[32] Q. C. Johnson and D. H. Templeton, Madelung constants for several structures, *J. Chem. Phys.* 34 (1961) 2004–2007.

[33] D. Borwein, J. M. Borwein, and R. Shail, Analysis of certain lattice sums, *J. Math. Anal. Appl.* 143 (1989) 126–137; MR 90j:82038.

[34] I. J. Zucker, Functional equations for poly-dimensional zeta functions and the evaluation of Madelung constants, *J. Phys. A* 9 (1976) 499–505; MR 54 #6800.

[35] V. V. Kukhtin and O. V. Shramko, Lattice sums within the Euler-Maclaurin approach, *Phys. Lett. A* 156 (1991) 257–259; MR 92d:82101.

[36] V. V. Kukhtin and O. V. Shramko, A new evaluation of the energy of Wigner BCC and FCC crystals, *J. Phys. A* 26 (1993) L963–L965.

[37] V. V. Kukhtin and O. V. Shramko, Analogues of the Euler constant for two- and three-dimensional spaces (in Ukrainian), *Dopovidi Akad. Nauk Ukrain.* (1993) n. 8, 42-43; MR 94m:11152.

1.11 Chaitin's Constant

Here is a brief discussion of algorithmic information theory [1–4]. Our perspective is number-theoretic and our treatment is informal: We will not attempt, for example, to define "computer" (Turing machine) here.

A **diophantine equation** involves a polynomial $p(x_1, x_2, \ldots, x_n)$ with integer co-efficients. Hilbert's tenth problem asked for a general algorithm that could ascertain whether $p(x_1, x_2, \ldots, x_n) = 0$ has positive integer solutions $x_1, x_2, \ldots, x_n$, given arbitrary p. The work of Matiyasevic, Davis, Putnam, and Robinson [5] culminated in a proof that no such algorithm can exist. In fact, one can find a **universal diophantine equation** $P(N, x_1, x_2, \ldots, x_n) = 0$ such that, by varying the parameter N, the corresponding set D_N of solutions x can be any recursively enumerable set of positive integers. Equivalently, any set of positive integers x that could *possibly* be the output of a deterministic computer program *must* be D_N for some N. The existence of P is connected to Gödel's incompleteness theorem in mathematical logic and Turing's negative solution of the halting problem in computability theory.

Now, define a real number A in terms of its binary expansion $0.A_1 A_2 A_3 \ldots$ as follows:

$$A_N = \begin{cases} 1 & \text{if } D_N \neq \emptyset, \\ 0 & \text{if } D_N = \emptyset. \end{cases}$$

There is no algorithm for deciding, given arbitrary N, whether $A_N = 1$ or 0, so A is an uncomputable real number. Is it possible to say more about A?

There is an interesting interplay between computability and randomness. We say that a real number z is **random** if the first N bits of z cannot be compressed into a program shorter than N bits. It follows that the successive bits of z cannot be distinguished from the result of independent tosses of a fair coin. The thought that randomness might occur in number theory staggers the imagination. No *computable* real number z is random [6, 7]. It turns out that A is not random either! We must look a little harder to find unpredictability in arithmetic.

An **exponential diophantine equation** involves a polynomial $q(x_1, x_2, \ldots, x_n)$ with integer coefficients as before, with the added freedom that there may be certain positive integers c and $1 \leq i < j \leq n$ for which $x_j = c^{x_i}$, and there may be certain $1 \leq i \leq j < k \leq n$ for which $x_k = x_i^{x_j}$. That is, exponents are allowed to be variables as well. Starting with the work of Jones and Matiyasevic, Chaitin [6, 7] found an exponential diophantine equation $Q(N, x_1, x_2, \ldots, x_n) = 0$ with the following remarkable property. Let E_N denote the set of positive integer solutions x of $Q = 0$ for each N. Define a real number Ω in terms of $0.\Omega_1\Omega_2\Omega_3 \ldots$ as follows:

$$\Omega_N = \begin{cases} 1 & \text{if } E_N \text{ is infinite,} \\ 0 & \text{if } E_N \text{ is finite.} \end{cases}$$

Then Ω is not merely uncomputable, but it is random too! So although the equation $P = 0$ gave us uncomputable A, the equation $Q = 0$ gives us random Ω; this provides our first glimpse of genuine uncertainity in mathematics [8–10].

Chaitin explicitly wrote down his equation $Q = 0$, which has 17000 variables and requires 200 pages for printing. The corresponding constant Ω is what we call **Chaitin's constant**. Other choices of the expression Q are possible and thus other random Ω exist. The basis for Chaitin's choice of Q is akin to Gödel numbering - Chaitin's modified LISP implementations make this very concrete - but the details are too elaborate to explain here.

Chaitin's constant is the halting probability of a certain self-delimiting universal computer. A different machine will, as before, usually give a different constant. So whereas Turing's fundamental result is that the halting *problem* is unsolvable, Chaitin's result is that the halting *probability* is random. We have a striking formula [2–4]:

$$\Omega = \sum_{\pi} 2^{-|\pi|},$$

the infinite sum being over all self-delimiting programs π that cause Chaitin's universal computer to eventually halt. Here $|\pi|$ denotes the length of π (thinking of programs as strings of bits).

It turns out that the first several bits of Chaitin's original Ω are known and all are ones thus far. This observation gives rise to some interesting philosophical developments. Assume that ZFC (Zermelo–Fraenkel set theory, coupled with the Axiom of Choice) is arithmetically sound. That is, assume any theorem of arithmetic proved by ZFC is true. Under this condition, there is an explicit finite bound on the number of bits of Ω that

ZFC can determine. Solovay [11, 12] dramatically constructed a worst-case machine U for which ZFC cannot calculate any bits of $\Omega(U)$ at all! Further, ZFC cannot predict more than the initial block of ones for any Chaitin constant Ω; although the kth bit may be a zero in truth, this fact is unprovable in ZFC. As Calude [13] wrote, "As soon as you get a 0, it's all over". Solovay's Ω starts with a zero; hence it is unknowable. More recently, a procedure for computing the first 64 bits of such an Ω was implemented [14] via the construction of a non-Solovay machine V that satisfies $\Omega(V) = \Omega(U)$ but is more manageable than U.

It is also known that the set of computably enumerable, random reals coincides with the set of all halting probabilities Ω of Chaitin universal computers [15–17]. Is it possible to define a "simpler" random Ω whose description would not be so complicated as to strain credibility? The latter theorem states that all such numbers have a Diophantine representation $Q = 0$; whether we can significantly reduce the size of the equation remains an open question.

[1] G. J. Chaitin, *Algorithmic Information Theory*, Cambridge Univ. Press, 1987; MR 89g:68022.

[2] C. S. Calude, *Information and Randomness*, Springer-Verlag, 1994; MR 96d:68103.

[3] G. J. Chaitin, *The Limits of Mathematics*, Springer-Verlag, 1997; MR 98m:68056.

[4] G. J. Chaitin, *The Unknowable*, Springer-Verlag, 1999; MR 2000h:68071.

[5] M. Davis, *Computability and Unsolvability*, Dover, 1973; MR 23 #A1525 (Appendix 2, "Hilbert's tenth problem is unsolvable," appeared originally in *Amer. Math. Monthly* 80 (1973) 233–269; MR 47 #6465).

[6] G. J. Chaitin, Randomness and Gödel's theorem, *Mondes en Développement,* Proc. 1985 Brussels Symp. on Laws of Nature and Human Conduct, n. 54–55 (1986) 125–128; also *Information, Randomness and Incompleteness: Papers on Algorithmic Information Theory*, World Scientific, 1987, pp. 66–69; MR 89f:01089.

[7] G. J. Chaitin, Incompleteness theorems for random reals, *Adv. Appl. Math.* 8 (1987) 119–146; MR 88h:68038.

[8] G. J. Chaitin, Randomness and mathematical proof, *Sci. Amer.*, v. 232 (1975) n. 5, 47–52.

[9] C. H. Bennett, On random and hard-to-describe numbers: Chaitin's Ω, quoted by M. Gardner, *Fractal Music, Hypercards and More . . .*, W. H. Freeman, 1992; MR 92m:00005 (appeared originally in *Sci. Amer.*, v. 241 (1979) n. 5, 20–34).

[10] G. J. Chaitin, Randomness in arithmetic, *Sci. Amer.*, v. 259 (1988) n. 1, 80–85.

[11] R. M. Solovay, A version of Ω for which ZFC cannot predict a single bit, *Finite Versus Infinite: Contributions to an Eternal Dilemma*, ed. C. S. Calude and G. Paun, Springer-Verlag, 2000, pp. 323–334; CDMTCS report 104.

[12] C. S. Calude and G. J. Chaitin, Randomness everywhere, *Nature* 400 (1999) 319–320.

[13] C. S. Calude, Chaitin Ω numbers, Solovay machines and Gödel incompleteness, *Theoret. Comput. Sci.* 284 (2002) 269–277; CDMTCS report 114.

[14] C. S. Calude, M. J. Dinneen, and C.-K. Shu, Computing a glimpse of randomness, *Experim. Math.*, to appear; CDMTCS report 167; nlin.CD/0112022.

[15] C. S. Calude, P. H. Hertling, B. Khoussainov, and Y. Wang, Recursively enumerable reals and Chaitin Ω numbers, *Theoret. Comput. Sci.* 255 (2002) 125–149; also in *Proc. 1998 Symp. on Theoretical Aspects of Computer Science (STACS)*, Paris, ed. M. Morvan, C. Meinel, and D. Krob, Lect. Notes in Comp. Sci. 1373, Springer-Verlag, 1998, pp. 596–606; CDMTCS report 59; MR 99h:68089 and MR 2002f:68065.

[16] A. Kucera and T. A. Slaman, Randomness and recursive enumerability, *SIAM J. Comput.* 31 (2001) 199–211.

[17] C. S. Calude, A characterization of c.e. random reals, *Theoret. Comput. Sci.* 271 (2002) 3–14; CDMTCS report 95.

2

Constants Associated with Number Theory

2.1 Hardy–Littlewood Constants

The sequence of prime numbers $2, 3, 5, 7, 11, 13, 17, \ldots$ has fascinated mathematicians for centuries. Consider, for example, the counting function

$$P_n = \sum_{p \leq n} 1 = \text{the number of primes} \leq n,$$

where the sum is over all primes p. We write $P_n(p) = P_n$, and the motivation behind this unusual notation will become clear momentarily. It was not until 1896 that Hadamard and de la Vallée Poussin (building upon the work of many) proved what is known as the **Prime Number Theorem**:

$$P_n(p) \sim \frac{n}{\ln(n)}$$

as $n \to \infty$. For every problem that has been solved in prime number theory, however, there are several that remain unsolved. Two of the most famous problems are the following:

Goldbach's Conjecture. *Every even number > 2 can be expressed as a sum of two primes.*

Twin Prime Conjecture. *There are infinitely many primes p such that $p + 2$ is also prime.*

The latter can be rewritten in the following way:

If $P_n(p, p + 2)$ is the number of twin primes with the lesser of the two $\leq n$, then $\lim_{n \to \infty} P_n(p, p + 2) = \infty$.

Striking theoretical progress has been achieved toward proving these conjectures, but insurmountable gaps remain. We focus on certain heuristic formulas, developed by Hardy & Littlewood [1]. These formulas attempt to answer the following question: Putting aside the existence issue, what is the distribution of primes satisfying various

84

additional constraints? In essence, one desires asymptotic distributional formulas analogous to that in the Prime Number Theorem.

Extended Twin Prime Conjecture [2–6].

$$P_n(p, p+2) \sim 2C_{\text{twin}} \frac{n}{\ln(n)^2},$$

where $C_{\text{twin}} = \prod_{p>2} \frac{p(p-2)}{(p-1)^2} = 0.6601618158\ldots = \frac{1}{2}(1.3203236316\ldots).$

Conjectures involving two different kinds of prime triples [2].

$$P_n(p, p+2, p+6) \sim P_n(p, p+4, p+6) \sim D \frac{n}{\ln(n)^3},$$

where $D = \frac{9}{2} \prod_{p>3} \frac{p^2(p-3)}{(p-1)^3} = 2.8582485957\ldots.$

Conjectures involving two different kinds of prime quadruples [2].

$$P_n(p, p+2, p+6, p+8) \sim \frac{1}{2} P_n(p, p+4, p+6, p+10) \sim E \frac{n}{\ln(n)^4},$$

where $E = \frac{27}{2} \prod_{p>3} \frac{p^3(p-4)}{(p-1)^4} = 4.1511808632\ldots.$

Conjecture involving primes of the form m^2+1 [3, 4, 7–9]. *If Q_n is defined to be the number of primes $p \le n$ satisfying $p = m^2 + 1$ for some integer m, then*

$$Q_n \sim 2C_{\text{quad}} \frac{\sqrt{n}}{\ln(n)},$$

where $C_{\text{quad}} = \frac{1}{2} \prod_{p>2} \left(1 - \frac{(-1)^{\frac{p-1}{2}}}{p-1} \right) = 0.6864067314\ldots = \frac{1}{2}(1.3728134628\ldots).$

Extended Goldbach Conjecture [3, 4, 10, 11]. *If R_n is defined to be the number of representations of an even integer n as a sum of two primes (order counts), then*

$$R_n \sim 2C_{\text{twin}} \cdot \prod_{\substack{p>2 \\ p|n}} \frac{p-1}{p-2} \cdot \frac{n}{\ln(n)^2},$$

where the product is over all primes p dividing n.

It is intriguing that both the Extended Twin Prime Conjecture and the Extended Goldbach Conjecture involve the same constant C_{twin}. It is often said that the Goldbach conjecture is "conjugate" to the Twin Prime conjecture [12]. We talk about recent progress in estimating Q_n [2.1.1] and in estimating R_n [2.1.2]. Shah & Wilson [13] extensively tested the asymptotic formula for R_n; thus C_{twin} is sometimes called the Shah–Wilson constant [14]. A formula for computing C_{twin} is given in [2.4].

The Hardy–Littlewood constants discussed here all involve infinite products over primes. Other such products occur in our essays on the Landau–Ramanujan constant [2.3], Artin's constant [2.4], the Hafner–Sarnak–McCurley constant [2.5], Bateman–Grosswald constants [2.6.1], Euler totient constants [2.7], and Pell–Stevenhagen constants [2.8].

Riesel [2] discussed prime constellations, which generalize prime triples and quadruples, and demonstrated how one computes the corresponding Hardy–Littlewood constants. He emphasized the remarkable fact that, although we do not know the sequence of primes in its entirety, we can compute Hardy–Littlewood constants to *any decimal accuracy* due to a certain transformation in terms of Riemann's zeta function $\zeta(x)$ [1.6].

There is a cubic analog [2.1.3] of the conjecture for prime values taken by the preceding quadratic polynomial. Incidently, if we perturb the product $2C_{\text{quad}}$ only slightly, we obtain a closed-form expression:

$$\prod_{p>2}\left(1 - \frac{(-1)^{\frac{p-1}{2}}}{p}\right) = \frac{4}{\pi} = \frac{1}{\beta(1)},$$

where $\beta(x)$ is Dirichlet's beta function [1.7].

Mertens' well-known formula gives [2.2]

$$\lim_{n\to\infty} \frac{1}{\ln(n)} \prod_{2<p<n} \frac{p}{p-1} = \frac{1}{2}e^{\gamma} = 0.8905362089\ldots,$$

where γ is the Euler–Mascheroni constant [1.5]. Here is a less famous result [15–17]:

$$\lim_{n\to\infty} \frac{1}{\ln(n)^2} \prod_{2<p<n} \frac{p}{p-2} = \frac{1}{4C_{\text{twin}}}e^{2\gamma} = 1.2013035599\ldots = \frac{1}{0.8324290656\ldots}.$$

Here also is an extension of $C_{\text{twin}} = C_2$ introduced by Hardy & Littlewood [16–20]:

$$C_n = \prod_{p>n}\left(\frac{p}{p-1}\right)^{n-1} \frac{p-n}{p-1} = \prod_{p>n}\left(1 - \frac{1}{p}\right)^{-n}\left(1 - \frac{n}{p}\right),$$

for which $C_3 = 0.6351663546\ldots = 2D/9$, $C_4 = 0.3074948787\ldots = 2E/27$, $C_5 = 0.4098748850\ldots$, $C_6 = 0.1866142973\ldots$, and $C_7 = 0.3694375103\ldots$.

In a study of Waring's problem, Bateman & Stemmler [21–24] examined the conjecture

$$P_n(p, p^2 + p + 1) \sim H\frac{n}{\ln(n)^2},$$

where

$$H = \frac{1}{2}\prod_p \left(1 - \frac{1}{p}\right)^{-2}\left(1 - \frac{2+\chi(p)}{p}\right) = 1.5217315350\ldots = 2 \cdot 0.7608657675\ldots$$

and $\chi(p) = -1, 0, 1$ accordingly as $p \equiv -1, 0, 1 \bmod 3$, respectively. See also [25–28].

We give two problems vaguely related to Goldbach's conjecture. Let $f(n)$ denote the number of representations of n as the sum of one or more *consecutive* primes.

For example, $f(41) = 3$ since $41 = 11 + 13 + 17 = 2 + 3 + 5 + 7 + 11 + 13$. Moser [29] proved that

$$\lim_{N \to \infty} \frac{1}{N} \sum_{n=1}^{N} f(n) = \ln(2) = 0.6931471805 \dots.$$

Let $g(n)$ denote the number of integers not exceeding n that can be represented as a sum of a prime and a power of 2. Romani [30] numerically investigated the ratio $g(n)/n$ and concluded that the asymptotic density of such integers is $0.434 \dots$.

2.1.1 Primes Represented by Quadratics

We defined Q_n earlier. Let $\tilde{Q}_n$ be the number of positive integers $k \leq n$ having ≤ 2 prime factors and satisfying $k = m^2 + 1$ for some integer m. Hardy & Littlewood's conjecture regarding the limiting behavior of Q_n remains unproven; some supporting numerical work appeared long ago [31, 32]. Iwaniec, however, recently demonstrated the asymptotic inequality [4, 33]

$$\tilde{Q}_n > \frac{1}{77} \cdot 2C_{\text{quad}} \cdot \frac{\sqrt{n}}{\ln(n)} = 0.0178 \dots \cdot \frac{\sqrt{n}}{\ln(n)},$$

which shows that there are infinitely many **almost primes** of the required form. His results extend to any irreducible quadratic polynomial $am^2 + bm + c$ with $a > 0$ and c odd. A good upper bound on Q_n does not seem to be known.

Shanks [32] mentioned a formula

$$C_{\text{quad}} = \frac{3}{4G} \frac{\zeta(6)}{\zeta(3)} \prod_{p \equiv 1 \bmod 4} \left(1 + \frac{2}{p^3 - 1} \right) \left(1 - \frac{2}{p(p-1)^2} \right),$$

where $G = \beta(2)$ is Catalan's constant [1.7]. He added that more rapid convergence may be obtained by multiplying through by the identity

$$1 = \frac{17}{16} \frac{\zeta(8)}{\zeta(4)\beta(4)} \prod_{p \equiv 1 \bmod 4} \left(1 + \frac{2}{p^4 - 1} \right).$$

2.1.2 Goldbach's Conjecture

Some progress has been made recently in proving Goldbach's conjecture, that is, in turning someone's guess into a theorem. Here are both binary and ternary versions:

Conjecture G. *Every even integer > 2 can be expressed as a sum of two primes.*

Conjecture G′. *Every odd integer > 5 can be expressed as a sum of three primes.*

Note that if G is true, then G′ is true. Here are the corresponding asymptotic versions:

Conjecture AG. *There exists N so large that every even integer $> N$ can be expressed as a sum of two primes.*

Conjecture AG′. *There exists N' so large that every odd integer $> N'$ can be expressed as a sum of three primes.*

The circle method of Hardy & Littlewood [1] led Vinogradov [34] to prove that AG' is true; moreover, he showed that

$$S_n \sim \prod_p \left(1 + \frac{1}{(p-1)^3}\right) \cdot \prod_{\substack{p>2 \\ p\mid n}} \left(1 - \frac{1}{p^2 - 3p + 3}\right) \cdot \frac{n^2}{2\ln(n)^3},$$

where S_n is the number of representations of the large odd integer n as a sum of three primes. Observe that this is not a conjecture, but a theorem. Further, Borodzkin [35] showed that **Vinogradov's number** N' could be taken to be $3^{3^{15}} \approx 10^{7000000}$ and Chen & Wang [36, 37] improved this to 10^{7194}. It is not possible with today's technology to check all odd integers up to this threshold and hence deduce G'. But by *assuming* the truth of a generalized Riemann hypothesis, the number N' was reduced to 10^{20} by Zinoviev [38], and Saouter [39] and Deshouillers et al. [40] successfully diminished N' to 5. Therefore G' is true, subject to the truth of a generalized Riemann hypothesis.

We do not have any analogous conditional proof for AG or for G. Here are two known weakenings of these:

Theorem (Ramaré [41, 42]). *Every even integer can be expressed as a sum of six or fewer primes (in other words, **Schnirelmann's number** is ≤ 6).*

Theorem (Chen [11, 12, 43, 44]). *Every sufficiently large even integer can be expressed as a sum of a prime and a positive integer having ≤ 2 prime factors.*

In fact, Chen proved the asymptotic inequality

$$\tilde{R}_n > 0.67 \cdot \prod_{p>2} \left(1 - \frac{1}{(p-1)^2}\right) \cdot \prod_{\substack{p>2 \\ p\mid n}} \frac{p-1}{p-2} \cdot \frac{n}{\ln(n)^2},$$

where $\tilde{R}_n$ is the number of corresponding representations. Chen also proved that there are infinitely many primes p such that $p + 2$ is an almost prime, a weakening of the twin prime conjecture, and the same coefficient 0.67 appears.

Here are additional details on these results. Kaniecki [45] proved that every odd integer can be expressed as a sum of at most five primes, under the condition that the Riemann hypothesis is true. With a large amount of computation, this will eventually be improved to at most four primes. By way of contrast, Ramaré's result that every even integer is a sum of at most six primes is unconditional (not dependent on the Riemann hypothesis).

Vinogradov's result may be rewritten as

$$\liminf_{n\to\infty} \frac{\ln(n)^3}{n^2} S_n = \frac{1}{2} \prod_p \left(1 + \frac{1}{(p-1)^3}\right) \cdot \prod_{p>2} \left(1 - \frac{1}{p^2 - 3p + 3}\right) = C_{\text{twin}}$$
$$= 0.6601618158\ldots,$$

$$\limsup_{n\to\infty} \frac{\ln(n)^3}{n^2} S_n = \frac{1}{2} \prod_p \left(1 + \frac{1}{(p-1)^3}\right) = 1.1504807723\ldots.$$

That is, although $S(n)$ is asymptotically misbehaved, its growth remains within the same order of magnitude. This cannot be said for Chen's result:

$$\liminf_{n\to\infty} \frac{\ln(n)^2}{n} \tilde{R}_n > 0.67 \cdot C_{\text{twin}} = 0.44,$$

$$\limsup_{n\to\infty} \frac{\ln(n)}{n} \tilde{R}_n > 0.67 \cdot \frac{1}{2} e^{\gamma} = 0.59.$$

Note that the limit superior bound grows at a logarithmic factor faster than the limit inferior bound. We have made use of Mertens' formulas in obtaining these expressions.

Chen's coefficient 0.67 for the Goldbach conjecture [43] was replaced by 0.81 in [46] and by 2 in [11]. His inequality for the twin prime conjecture can likewise be improved; the sharpenings in this case include 1.42 in [47], 1.94 in [48], 2.03 in [49], and 2.1 in [50].

Chen [51], building upon [52–54], proved the upper bound

$$R_n \leq 7.8342 \cdot \prod_{p>2} \left(1 - \frac{1}{(p-1)^2}\right) \cdot \prod_{\substack{p>2 \\ p|n}} \frac{p-1}{p-2} \cdot \frac{n}{\ln(n)^2}.$$

Pan [55] gave a simpler proof but a weaker result with coefficient 7.9880. Improvements on the corresponding coefficient 7.8342 for twin primes include 7.8156 in [56], 7.5555 in [57], 7.5294 in [58], 7 in [59], 6.9075 in [47], 6.8354 in [50], and 6.8325 in [60]. (A claimed upper bound of 6.26, mentioned in [3] and in the review of [50], was incorrect.)

Most of the sharpenings for twin primes are based on [59], which does *not* apply to the Goldbach conjecture for complicated reasons.

There is also a sense in which the set of possible counterexamples to Goldbach's conjecture must be small [61–66]. The number $\varepsilon(n)$ of positive even integers $\leq n$ that are *not* sums of two primes provably satisfies $\varepsilon(n) = o\left(n^{0.914}\right)$ as $n \to \infty$. Of course, we expect $\varepsilon(n) = 1$ for all $n \geq 2$. See also [67–69].

2.1.3 Primes Represented by Cubics

Hardy & Littlewood [1] conjectured that there exist infinitely many primes of the form $m^3 + k$, where the fixed integer k is not a cube. Further, if T_n is defined to be the number of primes $p \leq n$ satisfying $p = m^3 + 2$ for some integer m, then

$$\lim_{n\to\infty} \frac{\ln(n)}{\sqrt[3]{n}} T_n = A = \prod_{p \equiv 1 \bmod 6} \frac{p - \alpha(p)}{p - 1} = 1.2985395575\ldots,$$

where

$$\alpha(p) = \begin{cases} 3 & \text{if 2 is a cubic residue mod } p \text{ (i.e., if } x^3 \equiv 2 \bmod p \text{ is solvable)}, \\ 0 & \text{otherwise.} \end{cases}$$

Likewise, if U_n is defined to be the number of primes $p \leq n$ satisfying $p = m^3 + 3$ for some integer m, then

$$\lim_{n\to\infty} \frac{\ln(n)}{\sqrt[3]{n}} U_n = B = \prod_{p\equiv 1 \bmod 6} \frac{p - \beta(p)}{p - 1} = 1.3905439387\ldots,$$

where

$$\beta(p) = \begin{cases} 3 & \text{if 3 is a cubic residue mod } p \text{ (i.e., if } x^3 \equiv 3 \bmod p \text{ is solvable)}, \\ 0 & \text{otherwise.} \end{cases}$$

The constants A and B are known as **Bateman's constants** and were first computed to high precision by Shanks & Lal [3, 22, 70, 71].

Here is an example involving a quartic [72]. If V_n is defined to be the number of primes $p \leq n$ satisfying $p = m^4 + 1$ for some integer m, then

$$\lim_{n\to\infty} \frac{\ln(n)}{\sqrt[4]{n}} V_n = 4I = 2.6789638796\ldots,$$

where

$$I = \frac{\pi^2}{16\ln(1 + \sqrt{2})} \prod_{p\equiv 1 \bmod 8} \left(1 - \frac{4}{p}\right)\left(\frac{p+1}{p-1}\right)^2 = 0.6697409699\ldots.$$

It seems appropriate to call this **Shanks' constant**. Similar estimates for primes of the form $m^5 + 2$ or $m^5 + 3$ evidently do not appear in the literature.

The Bateman–Horn conjecture [3, 21, 73] extends this theory to polynomials of arbitrary degree. It also applies in circumstances when several such polynomials must simultaneously be prime. For example [74–77], if F_n is defined to be the number of prime pairs of the form $(m - 1)^2 + 1$ and $(m + 1)^2 + 1$ with the lesser of the two $\leq n$, then

$$\lim_{n\to\infty} \frac{\ln(n)^2}{\sqrt{n}} F_n = 4J = 1.9504911124\ldots,$$

where

$$J = \frac{\pi^2}{8} \prod_{p\equiv 1 \bmod 4} \left(1 - \frac{4}{p}\right)\left(\frac{p+1}{p-1}\right)^2 = 0.4876227781\ldots.$$

Note that F_n is also the number of Gaussian twin primes $(m - 1 + i, m + 1 + i)$ situated on the line $x + i$ in the complex plane; hence J might be called the **Gaussian twin prime constant**. (These are *not* all Gaussian twin primes in the plane: On the line $x + 2i$, consider $m = 179984$.)

As another example, if G_n is defined to be the number of prime pairs of the form $(m - 1)^4 + 1$ and $(m + 1)^4 + 1$ with the lesser of the two $\leq n$, then

$$\lim_{n\to\infty} \frac{\ln(n)^2}{\sqrt[4]{n}} G_n = 16K = 12.6753318106\ldots,$$

where

$$K = 2I^2 \prod_{p \equiv 1 \bmod 8} \frac{p(p-8)}{(p-4)^2} = 0.7922082381\ldots.$$

The latter is known as **Lal's constant**. Sebah [77] computed this and many of the constants in this essay.

[1] G. H. Hardy and J. E. Littlewood, Some problems of 'Partitio Numerorum.' III: On the expression of a number as a sum of primes, *Acta Math.* 44 (1923) 1–70; also in *Collected Papers of G. H. Hardy*, v. 1, Oxford Univ. Press, 1966, pp. 561–630.

[2] H. Riesel, *Prime Numbers and Computer Methods for Factorization*, Birkhäuser, 1985; MR 95h:11142.

[3] P. Ribenboim, *The New Book of Prime Number Records*, Springer-Verlag, 1996, pp. 259–265, 291–299, 403–411; MR 96k:11112.

[4] R. K. Guy, *Unsolved Problems in Number Theory*, 2nd ed., Springer-Verlag, 1994, sect. A1, A8, C1; MR 96e:11002.

[5] G. H. Hardy and E. M. Wright, *An Introduction to the Theory of Numbers*, 5th ed., Oxford Univ. Press, 1985, pp. 371–373; MR 81i:10002.

[6] S. W. Golomb, The twin prime constant, *Amer. Math. Monthly* 67 (1960) 767–769.

[7] D. Shanks, On the conjecture of Hardy & Littlewood concerning the number of primes of the form $n^2 + a$, *Math. Comp.* 14 (1960) 321–332; MR 22 #10960.

[8] D. Shanks, Supplementary data and remarks concerning a Hardy-Littlewood conjecture, *Math. Comp.* 17 (1963) 188–193; MR 28 #3013.

[9] D. Shanks, Polylogarithms, Dirichlet series, and certain constants, *Math. Comp.* 18 (1964) 322–324; MR 30 #5460.

[10] W. Ellison and F. Ellison, *Prime Numbers*, Wiley, 1985, p. 333; MR 87a:11082.

[11] M. B. Nathanson, *Additive Number Theory: The Classical Bases*, Springer-Verlag, 1996, pp. 151–298; MR 97e:11004.

[12] H. Halberstam and H.-E. Richert, *Sieve Methods*, Academic Press, 1974, pp. 116–117; MR 54 #12689.

[13] N. M. Shah and B. M. Wilson, On an empirical formula connected with Goldbach's theorem, *Proc. Cambridge Philos. Soc.* 19 (1919) 238–244.

[14] F. Le Lionnais, *Les Nombres Remarquables*, Hermann, 1983.

[15] B. Rosser, The nth prime is greater than $n \log(n)$, *Proc. London Math. Soc.* 45 (1938) 21–44.

[16] J. W. Wrench, Evaluation of Artin's constant and the twin prime constant, *Math. Comp.* 15 (1961) 396–398; MR 23 #A1619.

[17] A. Fletcher, J. C. P. Miller, L. Rosenhead, and L. J. Comrie, *An Index of Mathematical Tables*, 2nd ed., v. 1, Addison-Wesley, 1962; MR 26 #365a-b.

[18] H. P. Robinson and E. Potter, *Mathematical Constants*, UCRL-20418 (1971), Univ. of Calif. at Berkeley; available through the National Technical Information Service, Springfield VA 22151.

[19] R. Harley, Some estimates due to Richard Brent applied to the "high jumpers" problem, unpublished note (1994).

[20] G. Niklasch and P. Moree, Some number-theoretical constants: Products of rational functions over primes, unpublished note (2000).

[21] P. T. Bateman and R. A. Horn, A heuristic asymptotic formula concerning the distribution of prime numbers, *Math. Comp.* 16 (1962) 363–367; MR 26 #6139.

[22] P. T. Bateman and R. A. Horn, Primes represented by irreducible polynomials in one variable, *Theory of Numbers*, ed. A. L. Whiteman, Proc. Symp. Pure Math. 8, Amer. Math. Soc., 1965, pp. 119–132; MR 31 #1234.

[23] D. Shanks and J. W. Wrench, The calculation of certain Dirichlet series, *Math. Comp.* 17 (1963) 136–154; corrigenda 17 (1963) 488 and 22 (1968) 699; MR 28 #3012 and MR 37 #2414.

[24] P. T. Bateman and R. M. Stemmler, Waring's problem for algebraic number fields and primes of the form $(p^r - 1)/(p^d - 1)$, *Illinois J. Math.* 6 (1962) 142–156; MR 25 #2059.

[25] E. Grosswald, Arithmetic progressions that consist only of primes, *J. Number Theory* 14 (1982) 9–31; MR 83k:10081.

[26] N. Kurokawa, Special values of Euler products and Hardy-Littlewood constants, *Proc. Japan Acad. Ser. A. Math. Sci.* 62 (1986) 25–28; MR 87j:11127.

[27] E. Bogomolny and P. Leboeuf, Statistical properties of the zeros of zeta functions - beyond the Riemann case, *Nonlinearity* 7 (1994) 1155–1167; MR 95k:11108.

[28] R. Gross and J. H. Smith, A generalization of a conjecture of Hardy and Littlewood to algebraic number fields, *Rocky Mount. J. Math.* 30 (2000) 195–215; MR 2001g:11175.

[29] L. Moser, Notes on number theory. III: On the sum of consecutive primes, *Canad. Math. Bull.* 6 (1963) 159–161; MR 28 #75.

[30] F. Romani, Computations concerning primes and powers of two, *Calcolo* 20 (1983) 319–336: MR 86c:11082.

[31] A. E. Western, Note on the number of primes of the form $n^2 + 1$, *Cambridge Philos. Soc.* 21 (1922) 108–109.

[32] D. Shanks, A sieve method for factoring numbers of the form $n^2 + 1$, *Math. Comp.* 13 (1959) 78–86.

[33] H. Iwaniec, Almost-primes represented by quadratic polynomials, *Invent. Math.* 47 (1978) 171–188; MR 58 #5553.

[34] I. M. Vinogradov, Representation of an odd number as a sum of three primes (in Russian), *Dokl. Akad. Nauk SSSR* 15 (1937) 169–172; Engl. trans. in *Goldbach Conjecture*, ed. Y. Wang, World Scientific, 1984.

[35] K. G. Borozdkin, On the problem of I. M. Vinogradov's constant (in Russian), *Proc. Third All-Union Math. Conf.*, v. 1, Moscow, Izdat. Akad. Nauk SSSR, 1956, p. 3; MR 34 #5784.

[36] J. R. Chen and T. Z. Wang, On the odd Goldbach problem (in Chinese), *Acta Math. Sinica* 32 (1989) 702–718; addendum 34 (1991) 143–144; MR 91e:11108 and MR 92g:11101.

[37] J. R. Chen and T. Z. Wang, The Goldbach problem for odd numbers (in Chinese), *Acta Math. Sinica* 39 (1996) 169–174; MR 97k:11138.

[38] D. Zinoviev, On Vinogradov's constant in Goldbach's ternary problem, *J. Number Theory* 65 (1997) 334–358; MR 98f:11107.

[39] Y. Saouter, Checking the odd Goldbach conjecture up to 10^{20}, *Math. Comp.* 67 (1998) 863–866; MR 98g:11115.

[40] J.-M. Deshouillers, G. Effinger, H. te Riele, and D. Zinoviev, A complete Vinogradov 3-primes theorem under the Riemann hypothesis, *Elec. Res. Announce. Amer. Math. Soc.* 3 (1997) 99–104; MR 98g:11112.

[41] O. Ramaré and R. Rumely, Primes in arithmetic progressions, *Math. Comp.* 65 (1996) 397–425; MR 97a:11144.

[42] O. Ramaré, On Schnirelmann's constant, *Annali Scuola Norm. Sup. Pisa Cl. Sci.* 22 (1995) 645–706; MR 97a:11167.

[43] J. R. Chen, On the representation of a large even integer as the sum of a prime and the product of at most two primes, *Sci. Sinica* 16 (1973) 157–176; MR 55 #7959.

[44] P. M. Ross, On Chen's theorem that each large even number has the form $p_1 + p_2$ or $p_1 + p_2 p_3$, *J. London Math. Soc.* 10 (1975) 500–506; MR 52 #10646.

[45] L. Kaniecki, On Snirelman's constant under the Riemann hypothesis, *Acta Arith.* 72 (1995) 361–374; MR 96i:11112.

[46] J. R. Chen, On the representation of a large even integer as the sum of a prime and the product of at most two primes. II, *Sci. Sinica* 21 (1978) 421–430; MR 80e:10037.

[47] É. Fouvry and F. Grupp, On the switching principle in sieve theory, *J. Reine Angew. Math.* 370 (1986) 101–126; MR 87j:11092.

[48] J. H. Kan, On the sequence $p + h$, *Arch. Math. (Basel)* 56 (1991) 454–464; MR 92d:11110.

[49] H. Q. Liu, On the prime twins problem, *Sci. China Ser. A* 33 (1990) 281–298; MR 91i:11125.

[50] J. Wu, Sur la suite des nombres premiers jumeaux, *Acta Arith.* 55 (1990) 365–394; MR 91j:11074.

[51] J. R. Chen, On the Goldbach's problem and the sieve methods, *Sci. Sinica* 21 (1978) 701–739; MR 80b:10069.

[52] A. Selberg, On elementary methods in primenumber-theory and their limitations, *Den 11ᵗᵉ Skandinaviske Matematikerkongress,* Proc. 1949 Trondheim conf., Johan Grundt Tanums Forlag, 1952, pp. 13–22; MR 14,726k.

[53] C. D. Pan, A new application of the Ju. V. Linnik large sieve method (in Chinese), *Acta Math. Sinica* 14 (1964) 597–606; Engl. transl. in *Chinese Math. - Acta* 5 (1964) 642–652; MR 30 #3871.

[54] E. Bombieri and H. Davenport, Small differences between prime numbers, *Proc. Royal Soc. Ser. A* 293 (1966) 1–18; MR 33 #7314.

[55] C. B. Pan, On the upper bound of the number of ways to represent an even integer as a sum of two primes, *Sci. Sinica* 23 (1980) 1368–1377; MR 82j:10078.

[56] D. H. Wu, An improvement of J. R. Chen's theorem (in Chinese), *Shanghai Keji Daxue Xuebao* (1987) n. 1, 94–99; MR 88g:11072.

[57] É. Fouvry and H. Iwaniec, Primes in arithmetic progressions, *Acta Arith.* 42 (1983) 197–218; MR 84k:10035.

[58] É. Fouvry, Autour du théorème de Bombieri-Vinogradov, *Acta Math.* 152 (1984) 219–244; MR 85m:11052.

[59] E. Bombieri, J. B. Friedlander, and H. Iwaniec, Primes in arithmetic progressions to large moduli, *Acta Math.* 156 (1986) 203–251; MR 88b:11058.

[60] J. K. Haugland, *Application of Sieve Methods to Prime Numbers*, Ph.D. thesis, Oxford Univ., 1999.

[61] H. L. Montgomery and R. C. Vaughan, The exceptional set in Goldbach's problem, *Acta Arith.* 27 (1975) 353–370; MR 51 #10263.

[62] J. R. Chen and C. D. Pan, The exceptional set of Goldbach numbers. I, *Sci. Sinica* 23 (1980) 416–430; MR 82f:10060.

[63] J. R. Chen, The exceptional set of Goldbach numbers. II, *Sci. Sinica Ser. A* 26 (1983) 714–731; MR 85m:11059.

[64] J. R. Chen and J. M. Liu, The exceptional set of Goldbach numbers. III, *Chinese Quart. J. Math.* 4 (1989) 1–15; MR 90k:11129.

[65] H. Li, The exceptional set of Goldbach numbers, *Quart. J. Math.* 50 (1999) 471–482; MR 2001a:11172.

[66] H. Li, The exceptional set of Goldbach numbers. II, *Acta Arith.* 92 (2000) 71–88; MR 2001c:11110.

[67] J.-M. Deshouillers, A. Granville, W. Narkiewicz, and C. Pomerance, An upper bound in Goldbach's problem, *Math. Comp.* 61 (1993) 209–213; MR 94b:11101.

[68] T. Oliveira e Silva, Goldbach conjecture verification, unpublished note (2001).

[69] J. Richstein, Verifying Goldbach's conjecture up to $4 \cdot 10^{14}$, *Math. Comp.* 70 (2001) 1745–1749; MR 2002c:11131.

[70] D. Shanks and M. Lal, Bateman's constants reconsidered and the distribution of cubic residues, *Math. Comp.* 26 (1972) 265–285; MR 46 #1734.

[71] D. Shanks, Calculation and applications of Epstein zeta functions, *Math. Comp.* 29 (1975) 271–287; corrigenda 29 (1975) 1167 and 30 (1976) 900; MR 53 #13114a-c.

[72] D. Shanks, On numbers of the form $n^4 + 1$, *Math. Comp.* 15 (1961) 186–189; corrigenda 16 (1962) 513; MR 22 #10941.

[73] D. Shanks, *Solved and Unsolved Problems in Number Theory*, 2ⁿᵈ ed., Chelsea, 1978; MR 86j:11001.

[74] D. Shanks, A note on Gaussian twin primes, *Math. Comp.* 14 (1960) 201–203; MR 22 #2586.

[75] M. Lal, Primes of the form $n^4 + 1$, *Math. Comp.* 21 (1967) 245–247; MR 36 #5059.

[76] D. Shanks, Lal's constant and generalizations, *Math. Comp.* 21 (1967) 705–707; MR 36 #6363.

[77] X. Gourdon and P. Sebah, Some constants from number theory (Numbers, Constants and Computation).

2.2 Meissel–Mertens Constants

All of the infinite series discussed here and in [2.14] involve reciprocals of the prime numbers 2, 3, 5, 7, 11, 13, 17, ... The sum of the reciprocals of all primes is divergent and, in fact [1–6],

$$\lim_{n\to\infty} \left(\sum_{p\le n} \frac{1}{p} - \ln(\ln(n)) \right) = M = \gamma + \sum_{p} \left[\ln\left(1 - \frac{1}{p}\right) + \frac{1}{p} \right] = 0.2614972128\ldots,$$

where both sums are over all primes p and where γ is Euler's constant [1.5]. According to [7,8], the definition of M was confirmed to be valid by Meissel in 1866 and independently by Mertens in 1874. The quantity M is sometimes called Kronecker's constant [9] or the prime reciprocal constant [10]. A rapidly convergent series for M is [11–13]

$$M = \gamma + \sum_{k=2}^{\infty} \frac{\mu(k)}{k} \ln(\zeta(k)),$$

where $\zeta(k)$ is the Riemann zeta function [1.6] and $\mu(k)$ is the Möbius mu function

$$\mu(k) = \begin{cases} 1 & \text{if } k = 1, \\ (-1)^r & \text{if } k \text{ is a product of } r \text{ distinct primes,} \\ 0 & \text{if } k \text{ is divisible by a square } > 1. \end{cases}$$

If $\omega(n)$ denotes the number of *distinct* prime factors of an arbitrary integer n, then interestingly the average value of $\omega(1), \omega(2), \ldots, \omega(n)$:

$$E_n(\omega) = \frac{1}{n} \sum_{k=1}^{n} \omega(k)$$

can be expressed asymptotically via the formula [2, 9, 14–16]

$$\lim_{n\to\infty} (E_n(\omega) - \ln(\ln(n))) = M.$$

A somewhat larger average value for the *total* number, $\Omega(n)$, of prime factors of n (repeated factors counted) is as follows:

$$M' = \lim_{n\to\infty} (E_n(\Omega) - \ln(\ln(n))) = M + \sum_{p} \frac{1}{p(p-1)}$$

$$= \gamma + \sum_{p} \left[\ln\left(1 - \frac{1}{p}\right) + \frac{1}{p-1} \right] = \gamma + \sum_{k=2}^{\infty} \frac{\varphi(k)}{k} \ln(\zeta(k))$$

$$= 1.0346538818\ldots,$$

where $\varphi(k)$ is the Euler totient function [2.7]. A related limit [1, 17] is

$$\lim_{n\to\infty} \left(\sum_{p\le n} \frac{\ln(p)}{p} - \ln(n) \right) = -M'' = -\gamma - \sum_{p} \frac{\ln(p)}{p(p-1)} = -1.3325822757\ldots,$$

and a fast way to compute M'' uses the series [18]

$$M'' = \gamma + \sum_{k=2}^{\infty} \mu(k) \frac{\zeta'(k)}{\zeta(k)}.$$

Dirichlet's famous theorem states that if a and b are coprime positive integers then there exist infinitely many prime numbers of the form $a + bl$. What can be said about the sum of the reciprocals of all such primes? The limit

$$m_{a,b} = \lim_{n \to \infty} \left(\sum_{\substack{p \le n \\ p \equiv a \bmod b}} \frac{1}{p} - \frac{1}{\varphi(b)} \ln(\ln(n)) \right)$$

can be shown to exist and is finite for each a and b. For example [19–23],

$$m_{1,4} = \ln\left(\frac{\sqrt{\pi}}{4K} \right) + \frac{\gamma}{2} + \sum_{p \equiv 1 \bmod 4} \left[\ln\left(1 - \frac{1}{p} \right) + \frac{1}{p} \right] = -0.2867420562\ldots,$$

$$m_{3,4} = \ln\left(\frac{2K}{\sqrt{\pi}} \right) + \frac{\gamma}{2} + \sum_{p \equiv 3 \bmod 4} \left[\ln\left(1 - \frac{1}{p} \right) + \frac{1}{p} \right] = 0.0482392690\ldots,$$

where K is the Landau–Ramanujan constant [2.3]. Of course, $m_{1,4} + m_{3,4} + 1/2 = M$.

The sum of the squared reciprocals of primes is

$$N = \sum_p \frac{1}{p^2} = \sum_{k=1}^{\infty} \frac{\mu(k)}{k} \ln(\zeta(2k)) = 0.4522474200\ldots,$$

which is connected to the variance of $\omega(1), \omega(2), \ldots, \omega(n)$:

$$\text{Var}_n(\omega) = E_n(\omega^2) - E_n(\omega)^2$$

via the formula [9, 14]

$$\lim_{n \to \infty} (\text{Var}_n(\omega) - \ln(\ln(n))) = M - N - \pi^2/6 = -1.8356842740\ldots.$$

Likewise,

$$N' = \sum_p \frac{1}{(p-1)^2} = 1.3750649947\ldots$$

appears in the following:

$$\lim_{n \to \infty} (\text{Var}_n(\Omega) - \ln(\ln(n))) = M' + N' - \pi^2/6 = 0.7647848097\ldots.$$

See [15, 24] for detailed accounts of evaluating N and N' and [25–27] for the asymptotic probability distributions of ω and Ω.

Given a positive integer n, let $D_n = \max\{d : d^2|n\}$. Define S to be the set of n such that D_n is prime, and define $\tilde{S}$ to be the set of $n \in S$ such that $D_n^3 \nmid n$. The asymptotic densities of S and $\tilde{S}$ are, respectively [28–30],

$$\frac{6}{\pi^2} \sum_p \frac{1}{p^2} = 0.2749334633\ldots, \qquad \frac{6}{\pi^2} \sum_p \frac{1}{p(p+1)} = 0.2007557220\ldots.$$

In words, S is the set of integers, each of whose prime factors are simple with exactly one exception; in $\tilde{S}$, the exception must be a prime squared. See related discussions of square-free sets [2.5] and square-full sets [2.6].

Bach [12] estimated the computational complexity of calculating M, as well as Artin's constant C_{Artin} [2.4] and the twin prime constant C_{twin} [2.1].

The alternating series

$$\sum_{k=1}^{\infty}(-1)^k\frac{1}{p_k} = -0.2696063519\ldots,$$

where $p_1 = 2$, $p_2 = 3$, $p_3 = 5,\ldots$, is clearly convergent [31]. This is perhaps not so interesting as the two non-alternating series [32–35]

$$\sum_{k=2}^{\infty}\varepsilon_k\frac{1}{p_k} = 0.3349813253\ldots, \quad \sum_{k=1}^{\infty}\varepsilon'_k\frac{1}{p_k} = 0.6419448385\ldots,$$

where

$$\varepsilon_k = \begin{cases} -1 & \text{if } p_k \equiv 1 \bmod 4, \\ 1 & \text{if } p_k \equiv 3 \bmod 4, \end{cases} \quad \varepsilon'_k = \begin{cases} -1 & \text{if } p_k \equiv 1 \bmod 3, \\ 1 & \text{if } p_k \equiv 2 \bmod 3, \\ 0 & \text{if } p_k \equiv 0 \bmod 3. \end{cases}$$

Of course, the following is also convergent [36]:

$$\sum_{k=2}^{\infty}\varepsilon_k\frac{1}{p_k^2} = 0.0946198928\ldots.$$

Erdös [37, 38] wondered if the same is true for the series $\sum_{k=1}^{\infty}(-1)^k k/p_k$.

Merrifield [39] and Lienard [40] tabulated values of the series $\sum_p p^{-n}$ for $2 \leq n \leq 167$, as well as M and $\gamma - M = 0.3157184521\ldots$.

2.2.1 Quadratic Residues

Let $f(p)$ denote the smallest positive quadratic nonresidue modulo p, where p is prime. The average value of $f(p)$ is [41, 42]

$$\lim_{n\to\infty}\frac{\displaystyle\sum_{p\leq n} f(p)}{\displaystyle\sum_{p\leq n} 1} = \lim_{n\to\infty}\frac{\ln(n)}{n}\sum_{p\leq n} f(p) = \sum_{k=1}^{\infty}\frac{p_k}{2^k} = 3.6746439660\ldots.$$

More generally, if m is odd, let $f(m)$ denote the least positive integer k for which the Jacobi symbol $(k/m) < 1$, where m is nonsquare, and $f(m) = 0$ if m is square. (If $(k/m) = -1$, for example, then k is a quadratic nonresidue modulo m.) The average value of $f(m)$ is [41, 43, 44]

$$\lim_{n\to\infty}\frac{2}{n}\sum_{\substack{m\leq n \\ m \text{ odd}}} f(m) = 1 + \sum_{j=2}^{\infty}\frac{p_j+1}{2^{j-1}}\prod_{i=1}^{j-1}\left(1 - \frac{1}{p_i}\right) = 3.1477551485\ldots.$$

[1] J. B. Rosser and L. Schoenfeld, Approximate formulas for some functions of prime numbers, *Illinois J. Math.* 6 (1962) 64–94; MR 25 #1139.

[2] G. H. Hardy and E. M. Wright, *An Introduction to the Theory of Numbers*, 5ᵗʰ ed., Oxford Univ. Press, 1985, pp. 351–358; MR 81i:10002.

[3] A. E. Ingham, *The Distribution of Prime Numbers*, Cambridge Univ. Press, 1932; MR 91f:11064.

[4] H. M. Terrill and L. Sweeny, Two constants connected with the theory of prime numbers, *J. Franklin Inst.* 239 (1945) 242–243; MR 6,169a.

[5] D. H. Greene and D. E. Knuth, *Mathematics for the Analysis of Algorithms*, 3ʳᵈ ed., Birkhäuser, 1990, pp. 60–63; MR 92c:68067.

[6] G. Tenenbaum, *Introduction to Analytic and Probabilistic Number Theory*, Cambridge Univ. Press, 1995, pp. 14–18; MR 97e:11005b.

[7] P. Lindqvist and J. Peetre, On a number theoretic sum considered by Meissel – A historical observation, *Nieuw Arch. Wisk.* 15 (1997) 175–179; MR 99b:11141.

[8] P. Lindqvist and J. Peetre, On the remainder in a series of Mertens, *Expos. Math.* 15 (1997) 467–478; MR 98i:11110.

[9] M. R. Schroeder, *Number Theory in Science and Communication: With Applications in Cryptography, Physics, Digital Information, Computing and Self-Similarity*, 2ⁿᵈ ed., Springer-Verlag, 1986; MR 99c:11165.

[10] E. Bach and J. Shallit, *Algorithmic Number Theory*, v. 1. *Efficient Algorithms*, MIT Press, 1996, pp. 233–237, 263; MR 97e:11157.

[11] P. Flajolet and I. Vardi, Zeta function expansions of classical constants, unpublished note (1996).

[12] E. Bach, The complexity of number-theoretic constants, *Inform. Process. Lett.* 62 (1997) 145–152; MR 98g:11148.

[13] X. Gourdon and P. Sebah, Some constants from number theory (Numbers, Constants and Computation).

[14] P. Diaconis, F. Mosteller and H. Onishi, Second-order terms for the variances and covariances of the number of prime factors – including the square free case, *J. Number Theory* 9 (1977) 187–202; MR 55 #7953.

[15] H. Cohen, High precision computation of Hardy-Littlewood constants, unpublished note (1999).

[16] R. L. Duncan, A class of arithmetical functions, *Amer. Math. Monthly* 69 (1962) 34–36.

[17] H. L. Montgomery, *Topics in Multiplicative Number Theory*, Lect. Notes in Math. 227, Springer-Verlag, 1971, p. 43; MR 49 #2616.

[18] T. Jameson, Asymptotics of $\sum_{n \leq x} \mu(n)^2 / \varphi(n)$, unpublished note (1999).

[19] S. Uchiyama, On some products involving primes, *Proc. Amer. Math. Soc.* 28 (1971) 629–630; MR 43 #3227.

[20] K. S. Williams, Mertens' theorem for arithmetic progressions, *J. Number Theory* 6 (1974) 353–359; MR 51 #392.

[21] E. Grosswald, Some number theoretical products, *Rev. Colombiana Mat.* 21 (1987) 231–242; MR 90e:11129.

[22] E. A. Vasil'kovskaja, Mertens' formula for an arithmetic progression (in Russian), *Voprosy Mat. Sbornik Naucn. Trudy Taskent. Gos. Univ.* (1977) n. 548, 14–17, 139–140; MR 58 #27848.

[23] G. Niklasch and P. Moree, Generalized Meissel-Mertens constants, unpublished note (2000).

[24] J. W. L. Glaisher, On the sums of the inverse powers of the prime numbers, *Quart. J. Pure Appl. Math.* 25 (1891) 347–362.

[25] P. Erdös and M. Kac, The Gaussian law of errors in the theory of additive number theoretic functions, *Amer. J. Math.* 62 (1940) 738–742; MR 2,42c.

[26] D. E. Knuth and L. Trabb Pardo, Analysis of a simple factorization algorithm, *Theoret. Comput. Sci.* 3 (1976) 321–348; also in *Selected Papers on Analysis of Algorithms*, CSLI, 2000, pp. 303–339; MR 58 #16485.

[27] S. Guiasu, On the distribution of the number of distinct prime factors, *J. Inst. Math. Comp. Sci. (Math. Ser.)* 4 (1991) 171–179; MR 92j:11106.

[28] A. Rényi, On the density of certain sequences of integers, *Acad. Serbe Sci. Publ. Inst. Math.* 8 (1955) 157–162; also in *Selected Papers*, v. 1, Akadémiai Kiadó, 1976, pp. 506–512; MR 17,944f.

[29] E. Cohen, Arithmetical notes. VIII: An asymptotic formula of Rényi, *Proc. Amer. Math. Soc.* 13 (1962) 536–539; MR 25 #2049.

[30] E. Cohen, Some asymptotic formulas in the theory of numbers, *Trans. Amer. Math. Soc.* 112 (1964) 214–227; MR 29 #3458.

[31] H. P. Robinson and E. Potter, *Mathematical Constants*, UCRL-20418 (1971), Univ. of Calif. at Berkeley; available through the National Technical Information Service, Springfield VA 22151.

[32] L. Euler, De summa seriei ex numeris primis formatae $1/3 - 1/5 + 1/7 + 1/11 - 1/13 - \cdots$ ubi numeri primi formae $4n - 1$ habent signum positivum formae autem $4n + 1$ signum negativum, 1775, *Opera Omnia Ser. I*, v. 4, Lipsiae, 1911, pp. 146–162.

[33] J. W. L. Glaisher, On the series $1/3 - 1/5 + 1/7 + 1/11 - 1/13 - \cdots$, *Quart. J. Pure Appl. Math.* 25 (1891) 375–383.

[34] A. Weil, *Number Theory: An Approach Through History from Hammurapi to Legendre*, Birkhäuser, 1984, pp. 266–267; MR 85c:01004.

[35] J. W. L. Glaisher, On the series $1/2 + 1/5 - 1/7 + 1/11 - 1/13 + \cdots$, *Quart. J. Pure Appl. Math.* 25 (1891) 48–65.

[36] J. W. L. Glaisher, On the series $1/3^2 - 1/5^2 + 1/7^2 + 1/11^2 - 1/13^2 - \cdots$, *Quart. J. Pure Appl. Math.* 26 (1893) 33–47.

[37] P. Erdös, Some of my new and almost new problems and results in combinatorial number theory, *Number Theory: Diophantine, Computational and Algebraic Aspects*, Proc. 1996 Elger conf., ed. K. Györy, A. Pethö, and V. T. Sós, Gruyter, 1998, pp. 169–180; MR 2000a:11001.

[38] R. K. Guy, *Unsolved Problems in Number Theory*, 2nd ed., Springer-Verlag, 1994, sect. E7; MR 96e:11002.

[39] C. W. Merrifield, The sums of the series of the reciprocals of the prime numbers and of their powers, *Proc. Royal Soc. London* 33 (1881) 4–10.

[40] R. Lienard, *Tables fondamentales à 50 décimales des sommes S_n, u_n, Σ_n*, Paris, 1948; MR 10,149i.

[41] P. Ribenboim, *The New Book of Prime Number Records*, 3rd ed., Springer-Verlag, 1996, p. 142; MR 96k:11112.

[42] P. Erdös, Remarks on number theory. I, *Mat. Lapok* 12 (1961) 10–17; MR 26 #2410.

[43] R. Baillie and S. S. Wagstaff, Lucas pseudoprimes, *Math. Comp.* 35 (1980) 1391–1417; MR 81j:10005.

[44] N. J. A. Sloane, On-Line Encyclopedia of Integer Sequences, A053760 and A053761.

2.3 Landau–Ramanujan Constant

Let $B(x)$ denote the number of positive integers not exceeding x that can be expressed as a sum of two integer squares. Clearly $B(x) \to \infty$ as $x \to \infty$, but the rate at which it does so is quite fascinating!

Landau [1–3] and Ramanujan [4, 5] independently proved that the following limit exists:

$$\lim_{x \to \infty} \frac{\sqrt{\ln(x)}}{x} B(x) = K,$$

where K is the remarkable constant

$$K = \frac{1}{\sqrt{2}} \prod_{p \equiv 3 \bmod 4} \left(1 - \frac{1}{p^2}\right)^{-\frac{1}{2}} = \frac{\pi}{4} \prod_{p \equiv 1 \bmod 4} \left(1 - \frac{1}{p^2}\right)^{\frac{1}{2}}$$

and the two products are restricted to primes p. An empirical confirmation of this limit is found in [6]. Shanks [7, 8] discovered a rapidly convergent expression for K:

$$K = \frac{1}{\sqrt{2}} \prod_{k=1}^{\infty} \left[\left(1 - \frac{1}{2^{2^k}}\right) \frac{\zeta(2^k)}{\beta(2^k)} \right]^{\frac{1}{2^{k+1}}} = 0.7642236535\ldots,$$

where $\zeta(x)$ is the Riemann zeta function [1.6] and $\beta(x)$ is the Dirichlet beta function [1.7]. A stronger conclusion, due to Landau, is that

$$\lim_{x \to \infty} \frac{\ln(x)^{\frac{3}{2}}}{Kx} \left(B(x) - \frac{Kx}{\sqrt{\ln(x)}} \right) = C,$$

where C is given by [7, 9–12]

$$C = \frac{1}{2} + \frac{\ln(2)}{4} - \frac{\gamma}{4} - \frac{\beta'(1)}{4\beta(1)} + \frac{1}{4} \frac{d}{ds} \ln \left(\prod_{p \equiv 3 \bmod 4} \left(1 - \frac{1}{p^{2s}}\right) \right)\Bigg|_{s=1}$$

$$= \frac{1}{2} \left(1 - \ln\left(\frac{\pi e^{\gamma}}{2L}\right)\right) - \frac{1}{4} \sum_{k=1}^{\infty} \left(\frac{\zeta'(2^k)}{\zeta(2^k)} - \frac{\beta'(2^k)}{\beta(2^k)} + \frac{\ln(2)}{2^{2^k} - 1} \right)$$

$$= 0.5819486593\ldots,$$

γ is Euler's constant [1.5], and $L = 2.6220575542\ldots$ is Gauss' lemniscate constant [6.1]. These formulas were the basis for several recent high-precision computations by Flajolet & Vardi, Zimmermann, Adamchik, Golden & Gosper, MacLeod, and Hare.

2.3.1 Variations

Here are some variations. Define K_n to be the analog of K when counting positive integers of the form $a^2 + nb^2$. Clearly $K = K_1$. Define C_n likewise. It can be proved that [10, 13–16]

$$K_2 = \frac{1}{\sqrt[4]{2}} \prod_{p \equiv 5 \text{ or } 7 \bmod 8} \left(1 - \frac{1}{p^2}\right)^{-\frac{1}{2}} = 0.8728875581\ldots,$$

$$K_3 = \frac{1}{\sqrt{2\sqrt{3}}} \prod_{p \equiv 2 \bmod 3} \left(1 - \frac{1}{p^2}\right)^{-\frac{1}{2}} = 0.6389094054\ldots,$$

$$K_4 = \tfrac{3}{4}K = 0.5731677401\ldots, \quad C_4 = C = 0.5819486593\ldots.$$

Moree & te Riele [17] recently computed $C_3 = 0.5767761224\ldots$, but no one has yet found the value of C_n for $n = 2$ or $n > 4$. In the case $n = 3$, counting positive integers of the form $a^2 + 3b^2$ is equivalent to counting those of the form $a^2 + ab + b^2$.

Define instead $K_{l,m}$ to be the analog of K when counting positive integers simultaneously of the form $a^2 + b^2$ and $lc + m$, where l and m are coprime. Here, $K_{l,m}$ is simply a rational multiple of K depending on l only [18, 19].

Here are more variations. Let $B_{\text{sqfr}}(x)$ be the number of positive square-free integers not exceeding x that can be expressed as a sum of two squares. Also, let $B_{\text{copr}}(x)$ be the number of positive integers not exceeding x that can be expressed as a sum of two coprime squares. It can be proved that [20–22]

$$\lim_{x \to \infty} \frac{\sqrt{\ln(x)}}{x} B_{\text{sqfr}}(x) = \frac{6K}{\pi^2} = 0.4645922709\ldots,$$

$$\lim_{x \to \infty} \frac{\sqrt{\ln(x)}}{x} B_{\text{copr}}(x) = \frac{3}{8K} = 0.4906940504\ldots.$$

A conclusion from the first limit is that being square-free and being a sum of two squares are asymptotically independent properties. Of course, the two squares must be coprime; otherwise the sum could not be square-free.

Dividing the first expression by the second expression, we obtain that the asymptotic relative density of the first set as a subset of the second set is [22]

$$\lim_{x \to \infty} \frac{B_{\text{sqfr}}(x)}{B_{\text{copr}}(x)} = \frac{16K^2}{\pi^2} = \prod_{p \equiv 1 \bmod 4} \left(1 - \frac{1}{p^2}\right) = 0.9468064072\ldots.$$

This is a large density! On the one hand, if we randomly select two coprime integers, square them, and then add them, the sum is very likely to be square-free. On the other hand, there are infinitely many counterexamples: Consider, for example, the primitive Pythagorean triples [5.2].

Let $B_j(x)$ be the number of positive integers up to x, all of whose prime factors are congruent to j modulo 4, where $j = 1$ or 3. It can be shown that [20, 21, 23, 24]

$$\lim_{x \to \infty} \frac{\sqrt{\ln(x)}}{x} B_1(x) = \frac{1}{4K} = 0.3271293669\ldots,$$

$$\lim_{x \to \infty} \frac{\sqrt{\ln(x)}}{x} B_3(x) = \frac{2K}{\pi} = 0.4865198884\ldots.$$

It is interesting that these are not equal! This is a manifestation of the **Chebyshev effect** described by Rubenstein & Sarnak [25]. See [2.8] for a related discussion.

We mention two limits discovered by Uchiyama [26]:

$$\lim_{x \to \infty} \sqrt{\ln(x)} \prod_{\substack{p \leq x \\ p \equiv 1 \bmod 4}} \left(1 - \frac{1}{p}\right) = \frac{4}{\sqrt{\pi}} \exp\left(-\frac{\gamma}{2}\right) K = 1.2923041571\ldots,$$

$$\lim_{x \to \infty} \sqrt{\ln(x)} \prod_{\substack{p \leq x \\ p \equiv 3 \bmod 4}} \left(1 - \frac{1}{p}\right) = \frac{\sqrt{\pi}}{2} \exp\left(-\frac{\gamma}{2}\right) \frac{1}{K} = 0.8689277682\ldots,$$

which when multiplied together give Mertens' famous theorem [2.2]. Extensions of these results appear in [27–29]. As corollaries, we have

$$\lim_{x \to \infty} \frac{1}{\sqrt{\ln(x)}} \prod_{\substack{p \le x \\ p \equiv 1 \bmod 4}} \left(1 + \frac{1}{p}\right) = \frac{4}{\pi^{\frac{3}{2}}} \exp\left(\frac{\gamma}{2}\right) K = 0.7326498193\ldots,$$

$$\lim_{x \to \infty} \frac{1}{\sqrt{\ln(x)}} \prod_{\substack{p \le x \\ p \equiv 3 \bmod 4}} \left(1 + \frac{1}{p}\right) = \frac{1}{\sqrt{\pi}} \exp\left(\frac{\gamma}{2}\right) \frac{1}{K} = 0.9852475810\ldots.$$

Here are formulas that complement the expression for $16K/\pi^2$ earlier:

$$\prod_{p \equiv 3 \bmod 4} \left(1 - \frac{1}{p^2}\right) = \frac{1}{2K^2} = 0.8561089817\ldots,$$

$$\prod_{p \equiv 1 \bmod 4} \left(1 + \frac{1}{p^2}\right) = \frac{192K^2G}{\pi^4} = 1.0544399448\ldots,$$

$$\prod_{p \equiv 3 \bmod 4} \left(1 + \frac{1}{p^2}\right) = \frac{\pi^2}{16K^2G} = 1.1530805616\ldots,$$

where $G = \beta(2)$ denotes Catalan's constant [1.7]. A similar expression emerges when dealing with the following situation. Let $\hat{B}(x)$ be the number of positive square-free integers that belong to the sequence $n^2 + 1$ with $1 \le n \le x$. Then [30, 31]

$$\lim_{x \to \infty} \frac{\hat{B}(x)}{x} = \prod_{p \equiv 1 \bmod 4} \left(1 - \frac{2}{p^2}\right) = 0.8948412245\ldots.$$

Vast generalizations of this result are described in [32–34].

Let $\tilde{B}(x)$ denote the number of positive integers n not exceeding x for which n^2 *cannot* be expressed as a sum of two *distinct nonzero* squares. Shanks [35, 36] called these **non-hypotenuse numbers**, proved that

$$\tilde{K} = \lim_{x \to \infty} \frac{\sqrt{\ln(x)}}{x} \tilde{B}(x) = \frac{4K}{\pi} = 0.9730397768\ldots,$$

$$\lim_{x \to \infty} \frac{\ln(x)^{\frac{3}{2}}}{\tilde{K}x} \left(\tilde{B}(x) - \frac{\tilde{K}x}{\sqrt{\ln(x)}}\right) = C + \frac{1}{2} \ln\left(\frac{\pi e^\gamma}{2L^2}\right) = 0.7047534517\ldots,$$

and also mentioned that a third-order term is known to be positive (but did not compute this).

Let $A(x)$ denote the number of *primes* not exceeding x that can be expressed as a sum of two squares. Since odd primes of the form $a^2 + b^2$ are precisely those that are 1 modulo 4, we have

$$\lim_{x \to \infty} \frac{\ln(x)}{x} A(x) = \frac{1}{2}.$$

Define $U(x)$ to be the number of primes not exceeding x that can be expressed in the form $a^2 + b^4$. Friedlander & Iwaniec [37, 38] proved that

$$\lim_{x \to \infty} \frac{\ln(x)}{x^{\frac{3}{4}}} U(x) = \frac{4L}{3\pi} = 1.1128357889 \ldots.$$

By coincidence, the constant L appeared in the second-order approximation of $B(x)$ as well. Drawing inspiration from this achievement, Heath-Brown [39] recently proved an analogous result for primes of the form $a^3 + 2b^3$.

Let $V(x)$ be the number of positive integers not exceeding x that can be expressed in the form $a^2 + b^4$. It turns out that for almost all integers, the required representation is unique; hence a formula in [38] is applicable and

$$\lim_{x \to \infty} x^{-\frac{3}{4}} V(x) = \frac{L}{3} = 0.8740191847 \ldots.$$

The corresponding asymptotics for positive integers of the form $a^3 + 2b^3$ would be good to see. Related material appears in [40, 41].

Let $Q(x)$ be the number of positive integers not exceeding x that can be expressed as a sum of three squares. Landau [1] proved that $Q(x)/x \to 5/6$ as $x \to \infty$. The error term $\Delta(x) = Q(x) - 5x/6$ is not well behaved asymptotically [42–44], in the sense that

$$0 = \liminf_{x \to \infty} \Delta(x) < \limsup_{x \to \infty} \Delta(x) = \frac{1}{3 \ln(2)}.$$

The average value of $\Delta(x)$ can be precisely quantified in terms of a periodic, continuous, nowhere-differentiable function. More about such formulation is found in [2.16]. The asymptotics for counts of x of the form $a^3 + b^3 + c^3$ or $a^4 + b^4 + c^4 + d^4$ remain open [45].

[1] E. Landau, Über die Einteilung der positiven ganzen Zahlen in vier Klassen nach der Min-destzahl der zu ihrer additiven Zusammensetzung erforderlichen Quadrate, *Archiv Math. Phys.* 13 (1908) 305–312; also in *Collected Works*, v. 4, ed. L. Mirsky, I. J. Schoenberg, W. Schwarz, and H. Wefelscheid, Thales Verlag, 1985, pp. 59–66.

[2] G. H. Hardy, *Ramanujan: Twelve Lectures on Subjects Suggested by His Life and Work*, Chelsea, 1940, pp. 60–63; MR 21 #4881.

[3] W. J. LeVeque, *Topics in Number Theory, II*, Addison-Wesley, 1956, pp. 257–263; MR 18,283d.

[4] B. C. Berndt, *Ramanujan's Notebooks: Part IV*, Springer-Verlag, 1994, pp. 52, 60–66; MR 95e:11028.

[5] P. Moree and J. Cazaran, On a claim of Ramanujan in his first letter to Hardy, *Expos. Math* 17 (1999) 289–312; MR 2001c:11103.

[6] P. Shiu, Counting sums of two squares: The Meissel-Lehmer method, *Math. Comp.* 47 (1986) 351–360; MR 87h:11127.

[7] D. Shanks, The second-order term in the asymptotic expansion of $B(x)$, *Math. Comp.* 18 (1964) 75–86; MR 28 #2391.

[8] P. Flajolet and I. Vardi, Zeta function expansions of classical constants, unpublished note (1996).

[9] G. K. Stanley, Two assertions made by Ramanujan, *J. London Math. Soc.* 3 (1928) 232–237; corrigenda 4 (1929) 32.

[10] W. Heupel, Die Verteilung der ganzen Zahlen, die durch quadratische Formen dargestellt werden, *Arch. Math. (Basel)* 19 (1968) 162–166; MR 37 #2686.

[11] A. MacLeod, The Landau-Ramanujan second-order constant, unpublished note (1996).

[12] P. Moree, Chebyshev's bias for composite numbers with restricted prime divisors, *Math. Comp.*, to appear; math.NT/0112100.

[13] R. D. James, The distribution of integers represented by quadratic forms, *Amer. J. Math.* 60 (1938) 737–744.

[14] G. Pall, The distribution of integers represented by binary quadratic forms, *Bull. Amer. Math. Soc.* 49 (1943) 447–449; MR 4,240g.

[15] D. Shanks and L. P. Schmid, Variations on a theorem of Landau. Part I, *Math. Comp.* 20 (1966) 551–569; MR 35 #1564.

[16] K. S. Williams, Note on integers representable by binary quadratic forms, *Canad. Math. Bull.* 18 (1975) 123–125; MR 52 #269.

[17] P. Moree and H. J. J. te Riele, The hexagonal versus the square lattice, *Math. Comp.*, to appear; math.NT/0204332.

[18] K. Prachar, Über Zahlen der Form $a^2 + b^2$ in einer arithmetischen Progression, *Math. Nachr.* 10 (1953) 51–54; MR 15,289b.

[19] H. Iwaniec, The half dimensional sieve, *Acta Arith.* 29 (1976) 69–95; MR 54 #261.

[20] P. Moree, Variations on the Landau-Ramanujan problem, unpublished note (2000).

[21] G. J. Rieger, Über die Anzahl der als Summe von zwei Quadraten darstellbaren und in einer primen Restklasse gelegenen Zahlen unterhalb einer positiven Schranke. II, *J. Reine Angew. Math.* 217 (1965) 200–216; MR 30 #4734.

[22] W. Bosma and P. Stevenhagen, Density computations for real quadratic units, *Math. Comp.* 65 (1996) 1327–1337; MR 96j:11171.

[23] P. Stevenhagen, A density conjecture for the negative Pell equation, *Computational Algebra and Number Theory*, Proc. 1992 Sydney conf., ed. W. Bosma and A. van der Poorten, Kluwer, 1995, pp. 187–200; MR 96g:11137.

[24] G. Tenenbaum, *Introduction to Analytic and Probabilistic Number Theory*, Cambridge Univ. Press, 1995, p. 265; MR 97e:11005b.

[25] M. Rubinstein and P. Sarnak, Chebyshev's bias, *Experim. Math.* 3 (1994) 173–197; MR 96d:11099.

[26] S. Uchiyama, On some products involving primes, *Proc. Amer. Math. Soc.* 28 (1971) 629–630; MR 43 #3227.

[27] K. S. Williams, Mertens' theorem for arithmetic progressions, *J. Number Theory* 6 (1974) 353–359; MR 51 #392.

[28] E. Grosswald, Some number theoretical products, *Rev. Colombiana Mat.* 21 (1987) 231–242; MR 90e:11129.

[29] E. A. Vasil'kovskaja, Mertens' formula for an arithmetic progression (in Russian), *Voprosy Mat. Sbornik Naucn. Trudy Taskent. Gos. Univ.* (1977) n. 548, 14–17, 139–140; MR 58 #27848.

[30] P. Moree, Square-free polynomial values, unpublished note (2000).

[31] P. Sebah, Approximation of an infinite product, unpublished note (2000).

[32] P. Erdös, Arithmetical properties of polynomials, *J. London Math. Soc.* 28 (1953) 416–425; MR 15,104f.

[33] C. Hooley, On the power free values of polynomials, *Mathematika* 14 (1967) 21–26; MR 35 #5405.

[34] A. Granville, ABC allows us to count squarefrees, *Int. Math. Res. Notices* (1998) 991–1009; MR 99j:11104.

[35] D. Shanks, Non-hypotenuse numbers, *Fibonacci Quart.* 13 (1975) 319–321; MR 52 #8062.

[36] N. J. A. Sloane, On-Line Encyclopedia of Integer Sequences, A001481, A004144, A009003, and A022544.

[37] J. Friedlander and H. Iwaniec, Using a parity-sensitive sieve to count prime values of a polynomial, *Proc. Nat. Acad. Sci. USA* 94 (1997) 1054–1058; MR 98b:11097.

[38] J. Friedlander and H. Iwaniec, The polynomial $X^2 + Y^4$ captures its primes, *Annals of Math.* 148 (1998) 945–1040; MR 2000c:11150a.

[39] D. R. Heath-Brown, Primes represented by $x^3 + 2y^3$, *Acta Math.* 186 (2001) 1–84; MR 2002b:11122.
[40] P. Erdös and K. Mahler, On the number of integers which can be represented by a binary form, *J. London Math. Soc.* 13 (1938) 134–139.
[41] R. K. Guy, *Unsolved Problems in Number Theory*, 2nd ed., Springer-Verlag, 1994, sect. D4; MR 96e:11002.
[42] M. C. Chakrabarti, On the limit points of a function connected with the three-square problem, *Bull. Calcutta Math. Soc.* 32 (1940) 1–6; MR 3,162i.
[43] P. Shiu, Counting sums of three squares, *Bull. London Math. Soc.* 20 (1988) 203–208; MR 89c:11054.
[44] A. H. Osbaldestin and P. Shiu, A correlated digital sum problem associated with sums of three squares, *Bull. London Math. Soc.* 21 (1989) 369–374; MR 90f:11023.
[45] J.-M. Deshouillers, F. Hennecart, and B. Landreau, Do sums of 4 biquadrates have a positive density?, *Proc. 1998 Algorithmic Number Theory Sympos. (ANTS-III)*, Portland, ed. J. P. Buhler, Lect. Notes in Comp. Sci. 1423, Springer-Verlag, 1998, pp. 196–203; MR 2000k:11051.

2.4 Artin's Constant

Fermat's Little Theorem says that if p is a prime and n is an integer not divisible by p, then $n^{p-1} - 1$ is divisible by p.

Consider now the set of all positive integers e such that $n^e - 1$ is divisible by p. If $e = p - 1$ is the smallest such positive integer, then n is called a **primitive root modulo** p.

For example, 6 is a primitive root mod 11 since none of the remainders of $6^1, 6^2, 6^3, \ldots, 6^9$ upon division by 11 are equal to 1; thus $e = 10 = 11 - 1$. However, 6 is not a primitive root mod 19 since $6^9 - 1$ is divisible by 19 and $e = 9 < 19 - 1$.

Here is an alternative, more algebraic phrasing. The set $Z_p = \{0, 1, 2, \ldots, p - 1\}$ with addition and multiplication mod p forms a field. Further, the subset $U_p = \{1, 2, \ldots, p - 1\}$ with multiplication mod p forms a cyclic group. Hence we see that the integer n (more precisely, its residue class mod p) is a primitive root mod p if and only if n is a generator of the group U_p.

Here is another interpretation. Let $p > 5$ be a prime. The decimal expansion of the fraction $1/p$ has maximal period $(= p - 1)$ if and only if 10 is a primitive root modulo p. Primes satisfying this condition are also known as **long primes** [1–4].

Artin [5] conjectured in 1927 that if $n \neq -1, 0, 1$ is not an integer square, then the set $S(n)$ of all primes for which n is a primitive root must be infinite. Some remarkable progress toward proving this conjecture is indicated in [6–9]. For example, it is known that at least one of the sets $S(2)$, $S(3)$, or $S(5)$ is infinite.

Suppose additionally that n is not an rth integer power for any $r > 1$. Let n' denote the square-free part of n, equivalently, the divisor of n that is the outcome after all factors of the form d^2 have been eliminated. Artin further conjectured that the density of the set $S(n)$, relative to the primes, exists and equals

$$C_{\text{Artin}} = \prod_p \left(1 - \frac{1}{p(p-1)}\right) = 0.3739558136\ldots$$

independently of the choice of n, if $n' \not\equiv 1 \bmod 4$. A proof of this incredible conjecture is still unknown. For other cases, a rational correction factor is needed – see [2.4.2] – but

Artin's constant remains the central feature of such formulas. Hooley [10, 11] proved that such formulas are valid, subject to the truth of a generalized Riemann hypothesis.

A rapidly convergent expression for Artin's constant is as follows [12–18]. Define **Lucas' sequence** as

$$l_0 = 2, \qquad l_1 = 1, \qquad l_n = l_{n-1} + l_{n-2} \quad \text{for } n \geq 2$$

and observe that $l_n = \varphi^n + (1 - \varphi)^n$, where φ is the Golden mean [1.2]. Then

$$C_{\text{Artin}} = \prod_{n \geq 2} \zeta(n)^{-\frac{1}{n} \sum_{k|n} l_k \cdot \mu\left(\frac{n}{k}\right)}$$

$$= \zeta(2)^{-1} \zeta(3)^{-1} \zeta(4)^{-1} \zeta(5)^{-2} \zeta(6)^{-2} \zeta(7)^{-4} \zeta(8)^{-5} \zeta(9)^{-8} \cdots,$$

where $\zeta(n)$ is Riemann's zeta function [1.6] and $\mu(n)$ is Möbius' mu function [2.2]. For comparison's sake, here is the analogous expression for the twin prime constant [2.1]:

$$C_{\text{twin}} = \prod_{n \geq 2} \left[\left(1 - \frac{1}{2^n}\right) \zeta(n) \right]^{-\frac{1}{n} \sum_{k|n} 2^k \cdot \mu\left(\frac{n}{k}\right)}$$

$$= \left(\frac{3\zeta(2)}{4}\right)^{-1} \left(\frac{7\zeta(3)}{8}\right)^{-2} \left(\frac{15\zeta(4)}{16}\right)^{-3} \left(\frac{31\zeta(5)}{32}\right)^{-6} \left(\frac{63\zeta(6)}{64}\right)^{-9} \left(\frac{127\zeta(7)}{128}\right)^{-18} \cdots.$$

We briefly examine two k-dimensional generalizations of Artin's constant, omitting technical details. First, let $S(n_1, n_2, \ldots, n_k)$ denote the set of all primes p for which the integers $n_1, n_2, \ldots, n_k$ are simultaneously primitive roots mod p. Matthews [19, 20] deduced the analog of C_{Artin} corresponding to the density of $S(n_1, n_2, \ldots, n_k)$, relative to the primes [21]:

$$C_{\text{Matthews},k} = \prod_p \left(1 - \frac{p^k - (p-1)^k}{p^k(p-1)}\right) = \begin{cases} 0.1473494003\ldots & \text{if } k = 2, \\ 0.0608216553\ldots & \text{if } k = 3, \\ 0.0261074464\ldots & \text{if } k = 4, \end{cases}$$

which is valid up to a rational correction factor. Second, let N denote the subgroup of the cyclic group U_p generated by the set $\{n_1, n_2, \ldots, n_k\} \subseteq U_p$, and define $\tilde{S}(n_1, n_2, \ldots, n_k)$ to be the set of all primes p for which $N = U_p$. Pappalardi [22, 23] obtained the analog of C_{Artin} corresponding to the density of $\tilde{S}(n_1, n_2, \ldots, n_k)$, relative to the primes [17]:

$$C_{\text{Pappalardi},k} = \prod_p \left(1 - \frac{1}{p^k(p-1)}\right) = \begin{cases} 0.6975013584\ldots & \text{if } k = 2, \\ 0.8565404448\ldots & \text{if } k = 3, \\ 0.9312651841\ldots & \text{if } k = 4, \end{cases}$$

which again is valid up to a rational correction factor. Niklasch & Moree [17] computed $C_{\text{Pappalardi},k}$ and many of the constants in this essay.

In the context of quadratic number fields [24, 25], a suitably extended Artin's conjecture involves $C_{\text{Pappalardi},2}$ as well as the constant

$$\frac{8C_{\text{twin}}}{\pi^2} = \prod_{p > 2} \left(1 - \frac{2}{p(p-1)}\right) = 0.5351070126\ldots.$$

A generalization to arbitrary algebraic number fields seems to be an open problem. See [26–28] for a curious variation of C_{Artin} involving Fibonacci primitive roots, and see [29] likewise for pseudoprimes and Carmichael numbers.

We describe an unsolved problem. Define, for any odd prime p, $g(p)$ to be the least positive integer that is a primitive root mod p, and define $G(p)$ to be the least prime that is a primitive root mod p. What are the expected values of $g(p)$ and $G(p)$? Murata [21,30] argued heuristically that $g(p)$ is never very far from

$$1 + C_{\text{Murata}} = 1 + \prod_p \left(1 + \frac{1}{(p-1)^2}\right) = 3.8264199970\ldots$$

for almost all p. This estimate turns out to be too low. Empirical data [21,31,32] suggest that $\text{E}(g(p)) = 4.9264\ldots$ and $\text{E}(G(p)) = 5.9087\ldots$. There is a complicated infinite series for $\text{E}(g(p))$ involving Matthews' constants [21], but it is perhaps computationally infeasible. See [2.7] for another occurrence of C_{Murata}.

2.4.1 Relatives

Here are some related constants from various parts of number theory. Let nonzero integers a and b be multiplicatively independent in the sense that $a^m b^n \neq 1$ except when $m = n = 0$. Let $T(a, b)$ denote the set of all primes p for which $p | (a^k - b)$ for some nonnegative integer k. Assuming a generalized Riemann hypothesis, Stephens [33] proved that the density of $T(a, b)$ relative to the primes is

$$\prod_p \left(1 - \frac{p}{p^3 - 1}\right) = 0.5759599688\ldots$$

up to a rational correction factor. Moree & Stevenhagen [34] extended Stephens' work and offered adjustments to the correction factors. They further proved unconditionally that the density of $T(a, b)$ must be positive. A rapidly convergent expression for Stephens' constant is given in [16,17].

The Feller–Tornier constant [35–37]

$$\frac{1}{2} + \frac{1}{2} \prod_p \left(1 - \frac{2}{p^2}\right) = \frac{1}{2} + \frac{3}{\pi^2} \prod_p \left(1 - \frac{1}{p^2 - 1}\right) = 0.6613170494\ldots$$

is the density of integers that have an even number of powers of primes in their canonical factorization. By *power*, we mean a power higher than the first. Thus $2 \cdot 3^2 \cdot 5^3$ has two powers of primes in it and contributes to the density, whereas $3 \cdot 7 \cdot 19 \cdot 31^2$ has one power of a prime in it and does not contribute to the density.

Consider the set of integer vectors (x_0, x_1, x_2, x_3) satisfying the equation $x_0^3 = x_1 x_2 x_3$ and the constraints $0 < x_j \leq X$ for $1 \leq j \leq 3$ and $\gcd(x_1, x_2, x_3) = 1$. What are the asymptotics of the cardinality, $N(X)$, of this set as $X \to \infty$? Heath-Brown & Moroz [38] proved that

$$\lim_{X \to \infty} \frac{2880 N(X)}{X \ln(X)^6} = \prod_p \left(1 - \frac{1}{p^7}\right) \left(1 + \frac{7}{p} + \frac{1}{p^2}\right) = 0.0013176411\ldots.$$

Counting problems such as these for arbitrary cubic surfaces are very difficult.

Given a positive integer n, let $D_n^2 = n/n'$, the largest square divisor of n. Define Σ to be the set of n such that D_n and n' are coprime. Then Σ has asymptotic density [37]

$$\chi = \prod_p \left(1 - \frac{1}{p^2(p+1)}\right) = 0.8815138397\ldots.$$

Interestingly, the constant χ appears in the following as well.

If d is the fundamental discriminant of an imaginary quadratic field ($d < 0$) and $h(d)$ is the associated class number, then the ratio $2\pi h(d)/\sqrt{-d}$ is equal to χ on average [39, 40]. This constant plays a role for real quadratic fields too ($d > 0$). In connection with indefinite binary quadratic forms, Sarnak [41] obtained that the average value of $h(d)$, taken over the thin subset of discriminants $0 < d < D$ of the form $c^2 - 4$, is asymptotically

$$\frac{5\pi^2}{48} \prod_p \left(1 - \frac{1}{p^2} - \frac{2}{p^3}\right) \cdot \frac{\sqrt{D}}{\ln(D)} = 0.7439711933\ldots \cdot \frac{\sqrt{D}}{\ln(D)}$$

as $D \to \infty$. The analogous constants for $0 < d < D$ of the form $c^{2\nu} - 4$, $\nu \geq 2$, do not appear to possess similar formulation.

The $2k^{\text{th}}$ moment (over the critical line) of the Riemann zeta function

$$m_{2k}(T) = \frac{1}{T} \int_0^T |\zeta(1/2 + it)|^{2k} dt$$

is known to satisfy $m_2(T) \sim \ln(T)$ and $m_4(T) \sim (1/(2\pi^2))\ln(T)^4$ as $T \to \infty$. It is conjectured that $m_{2k}(T) \sim \gamma_k \ln(T)^{k^2}$ and further that [42–44]

$$\frac{9!}{42}\gamma_6 = \prod_p \left(1 - \frac{1}{p}\right)^4 \left(1 + \frac{4}{p} + \frac{1}{p^2}\right),$$

$$\frac{16!}{24024}\gamma_8 = \prod_p \left(1 - \frac{1}{p}\right)^9 \left(1 + \frac{9}{p} + \frac{9}{p^2} + \frac{1}{p^3}\right).$$

This analysis can be extended to Dirichlet L-functions. Understanding the behavior of moments such as these could have numerous benefits for number theory.

2.4.2 Correction Factors

We have assumed that $n \neq -1, 0, 1$ is not an rth power for any $r > 1$ and that n' is the square-free part of n. If $n' \equiv 1 \bmod 4$, then the density of the set $S(n)$ relative to the primes is conjectured to be [8, 10, 14, 45, 46]

$$\left(1 - \mu(|n'|) \prod_{q|n'} \frac{1}{q^2 - q - 1}\right) \cdot C_{\text{Artin}},$$

where the product is restricted to primes q. For example, if $n' = u$ is prime, then this formula simplifies to

$$\left(1 + \frac{1}{u^2 - u - 1}\right) \cdot C_{\text{Artin}}.$$

If instead $n' = uv$, where $u \equiv 1 \bmod 4$ and $v \equiv 1 \bmod 4$ are both primes, then the formula instead simplifies to

$$\left(1 - \frac{1}{u^2 - u - 1} \frac{1}{v^2 - v - 1}\right) \cdot C_{\text{Artin}}.$$

If n is an rth power, a slightly more elaborate formula applies.

[1]　D. H. Lehmer, A note on primitive roots, *Scripta Math.* 26 (1961) 117–119; MR 26 #7128.
[2]　D. Shanks, *Solved and Unsolved Problems in Number Theory*, 2nd ed., Chelsea, 1978, pp. 80–83, 222–225; MR 86j:11001.
[3]　J. H. Conway and R. K. Guy, *The Book of Numbers*, Springer-Verlag, 1996, pp. 157–163, 166–171; MR 98g:00004.
[4]　N. J. A. Sloane, On-Line Encyclopedia of Integer Sequences, A001122, A001913, A006883, A019334–A019421.
[5]　E. Artin, *Collected Papers*, ed. S. Lang and J. T. Tate, Springer-Verlag, 1965, pp. viii–ix.
[6]　M. Ram Murty, Artin's conjecture for primitive roots, *Math. Intellig.* 10 (1988) 59–67; MR 89k:11085.
[7]　K. Ireland and M. Rosen, *A Classical Introduction to Modern Number Theory*, 2nd ed., Springer-Verlag, 1990, pp. v, 39–47; MR 92e:11001.
[8]　P. Ribenboim, *The New Book of Prime Number Records*, Springer-Verlag, 1996, pp. 22–25, 379–386; MR 96k:11112.
[9]　R. K. Guy, *Unsolved Problems in Number Theory*, 2nd ed., Springer-Verlag, 1994, sect. F9; MR 96e:11002.
[10]　C. Hooley, On Artin's conjecture, *J. Reine Angew. Math.* 225 (1967) 209–220; MR 34 #7445.
[11]　C. Hooley, *Applications of Sieve Methods to the Theory of Numbers*, Cambridge Univ. Press, 1976; MR 53 #7976.
[12]　J. W. Wrench, Evaluation of Artin's constant and the twin prime constant, *Math. Comp.* 15 (1961) 396–398; MR 23 #A1619.
[13]　P. Flajolet and I. Vardi, Zeta function expansions of classical constants, unpublished note (1996).
[14]　E. Bach, The complexity of number-theoretic constants, *Inform. Process. Lett.* 62 (1997) 145–152; MR 98g:11148.
[15]　H. Cohen, High precision computation of Hardy-Littlewood constants, unpublished note (1999).
[16]　P. Moree, Approximation of singular series and automata, *Manuscripta Math.* 101 (2000) 385–399; MR 2001f:11204.
[17]　G. Niklasch and P. Moree, Some number-theoretical constants: Products of rational functions over primes, unpublished note (2000).
[18]　X. Gourdon and P. Sebah, Some constants from number theory (Numbers, Constants and Computation).
[19]　K. R. Matthews, A generalisation of Artin's conjecture for primitive roots, *Acta Arith.* 29 (1976) 113–146; MR 53 #313.
[20]　R. N. Buttsworth, An inclusion-exclusion transform, *Ars Combin.* 15 (1983) 279–300; MR 85k:05007.

[21] P. D. T. A. Elliott and L. Murata, On the average of the least primitive root modulo p, *J. London Math. Soc.* 56 (1997) 435–454 (computations by A. Paszkiewicz); MR 98m:11094.

[22] F. Pappalardi, On the r-rank Artin conjecture, *Math. Comp.* 66 (1997) 853–868; MR 97f:11082.

[23] L. Cangelmi and F. Pappalardi, On the r-rank Artin conjecture. II, *J. Number Theory* 75 (1999) 120–132; MR 2000i:11149.

[24] H. Roskam, A quadratic analogue of Artin's conjecture on primitive roots, *J. Number Theory* 81 (2000) 93–109; errata 85 (2000) 108; MR 2000k:11128.

[25] H. Roskam, Artin's primitive root conjecture for quadratic fields, *J. Théorie Nombres Bordeaux*, to appear; report MI-2000–22, Univ. of Leiden.

[26] D. Shanks, Fibonacci primitive roots, *Fibonacci Quart.* 10 (1972) 163–168, 181; MR 45 #6747.

[27] H. W. Lenstra, Jr., On Artin's conjecture and Euclid's algorithm in global fields, *Invent. Math.* 42 (1977) 201–224; MR 58 #576.

[28] J. W. Sander, On Fibonacci primitive roots, *Fibonacci Quart.* 28 (1990) 79–80; MR 91b:11094.

[29] S. S. Wagstaff, Pseudoprimes and a generalization of Artin's conjecture, *Acta Arith.* 41 (1982) 141–150; MR 83m:10004.

[30] L. Murata, On the magnitude of the least prime primitive root, *J. Number Theory* 37 (1991) 47–66; MR 91j:11082.

[31] T. Oliveira e Silva, Least primitive root of prime numbers, unpublished note (2001).

[32] A. Paszkiewicz and A. Schinzel, On the least prime primitive root modulo a prime, *Math. Comp.* 71 (2002) 1307–1321.

[33] P. J. Stephens, Prime divisors of second-order linear recurrences. I, *J. Number Theory* 8 (1976) 313–332; MR 54 #5142.

[34] P. Moree and P. Stevenhagen, A two-variable Artin conjecture, *J. Number Theory* 85 (2000) 291–304; MR 2001k:11188.

[35] W. Feller and E. Tornier, Mengentheoretische Untersuchungen von Eigenschaften der Zahlenreihe, *Math. Annalen* 107 (1933) 188–232.

[36] I. J. Schoenberg, On asymptotic distributions of arithmetical functions, *Trans. Amer. Math. Soc.* 39 (1936) 315–330.

[37] E. Cohen, Some asymptotic formulas in the theory of numbers, *Trans. Amer. Math. Soc.* 112 (1964) 214–227; MR 29 #3458.

[38] D. R. Heath-Brown and B. Z. Moroz, The density of rational points on the cubic surface $X_0^3 = X_1 X_2 X_3$, *Math. Proc. Cambridge Philos. Soc.* 125 (1999) 385–395; MR 2000f:11080.

[39] R. Ayoub, *An Introduction to the Analytic Theory of Numbers*, Amer. Math. Soc., 1963, pp. 320–322; MR 28 #3954.

[40] H. Cohen, *A Course in Computational Algebraic Number Theory*, Springer-Verlag, 1993, pp. 290–293; MR 94i:11105.

[41] P. C. Sarnak, Class numbers of indefinite binary quadratic forms. II, *J. Number Theory* 21 (1985) 333–346; MR 87h:11027.

[42] J. B. Conrey and A. Ghosh, A conjecture for the sixth power moment of the Riemann zeta-function, *Int. Math. Res. Notices* (1998) 775–780; MR 99h:11096.

[43] J. B. Conrey and S. M. Gonek, High moments of the Riemann zeta-function, *Duke Math. J.* 107 (2001) 577–604; MR 2002b:11112.

[44] J. B. Conrey, L-functions and random matrices, *Mathematics Unlimited – 2001 and Beyond*, ed. B. Engquist and W. Schmid, Springer-Verlag, 2001, pp. 331–352; MR 2002g: 11134.

[45] D. H. Lehmer and E. Lehmer, Heuristics, anyone?, *Studies in Mathematical Analysis and Related Topics*, ed. G. Szegö, C. Loewner, S. Bergman, M. M. Schiffer, J. Neyman, D. Gilbarg, and H. Solomon, Stanford Univ. Press, 1962, pp. 202–210; MR 26 #2409.

[46] A. E. Western and J. C. P. Miller, *Tables of Indices and Primitive Roots*, Royal Soc. Math. Tables, v. 9, Cambridge Univ. Press, 1968, pp. xxxvii–xlii; MR 39 #7792.

2.5 Hafner–Sarnak–McCurley Constant

We start with a well-known theorem [1]. The probability that two randomly chosen integers are coprime is $6/\pi^2 = 0.6079271018\ldots$ (in the limit over large intervals). What happens if we replace the integers by integer square matrices? Given two randomly chosen integer $n \times n$ matrices, what is the probability, $\Delta(n)$, that the two corresponding determinants are coprime?

Hafner, Sarnak & McCurley [2] showed that

$$\Delta(n) = \prod_p \left[1 - \left(1 - \prod_{k=1}^{n} \left(1 - p^{-k} \right) \right)^2 \right]$$

for each n, where the outermost product is restricted to primes p. It can be proved that

$$\Delta(1) = \frac{6}{\pi^2} > \Delta(2) > \Delta(3) > \ldots > \Delta(n-1) > \Delta(n) > \ldots,$$

and Vardi [3,4] computed the limiting value

$$\lim_{n \to \infty} \Delta(n) = \prod_p \left[1 - \left(1 - \prod_{k=1}^{\infty} \left(1 - p^{-k} \right) \right)^2 \right] = 0.3532363719\ldots.$$

2.5.1 Carefree Couples

It is also well known that $6/\pi^2$ is the probability that a randomly chosen integer x is square-free [1], meaning x is divisible by no square exceeding 1. Schroeder [5] asked the following question: Are the properties of being square-free and coprime statistically independent? The answer is no: There appears to be a positive correlation between the two properties. More precisely, define two randomly chosen integers x and y to be **carefree** [5,6] if x and y are coprime and x is square-free. The probability that x and y are carefree is somewhat larger than $36/\pi^4 = 0.3695\ldots$ and is exactly equal to

$$P = \frac{6}{\pi^2} \prod_p \left(1 - \frac{1}{p(p+1)} \right) = 0.4282495056\ldots.$$

Moree [7] proved that Schroeder's formula is correct. Further, he defined x and y to be **strongly carefree** when x and y are coprime, and x and y are both square-free. The probability in this case is [8]

$$Q = \frac{6}{\pi^2} \prod_p \left(1 - \frac{2}{p(p+1)} \right) = \frac{36}{\pi^4} \prod_p \left(1 - \frac{1}{(p+1)^2} \right) = 0.2867474284\ldots.$$

Define finally x and y to be **weakly carefree** when x and y are coprime, and x or y is square-free. As a corollary, the probability here is $2P - Q = 0.5697515829\ldots$, using the fact that $P(A \cup B) = P(A) + P(B) - P(A \cap B)$. Do there exist matrix analogs of these joint probabilities?

The constants P and Q appear elsewhere in number theory [7]. Let $D_n = \max\{d : d^2 | n\}$. Define

$$\kappa(n) = \frac{n}{D_n^2}, \quad \text{the \textbf{square-free part} of } n,$$

$$K(n) = \prod_{p|n} p, \quad \text{the \textbf{square-free kernel} of } n;$$

then [9–11]

$$\lim_{N\to\infty} \frac{1}{N^2} \sum_{n=1}^{N} \kappa(n) = \frac{\pi^2}{30} = 0.3289\ldots, \quad \lim_{N\to\infty} \frac{1}{N^2} \sum_{n=1}^{N} K(n) = \frac{\pi^2 P}{12} = 0.3522\ldots$$

(see [2.10] for the average of D_n instead). Let $\omega(n)$ be the number of distinct prime factors of n, as in [2.2]; then [11–13]

$$\lim_{N\to\infty} \frac{1}{N \ln(N)} \sum_{n=1}^{N} 2^{\omega(n)} = \frac{6}{\pi^2} = 0.6079\ldots,$$

$$\lim_{N\to\infty} \frac{1}{N \ln(N)^2} \sum_{n=1}^{N} 3^{\omega(n)} = \frac{Q}{2} = 0.1433\ldots.$$

If $\omega(n)$ is replaced by $\Omega(n)$, the total number of prime factors of n, then alternatively [11, 14, 15]

$$\lim_{N\to\infty} \frac{1}{N \ln(N)^2} \sum_{n=1}^{N} 2^{\Omega(n)} = \frac{1}{8 \ln(2) C_{\text{twin}}} = 0.2731707223\ldots,$$

where C_{twin} is the twin prime constant [2.1], which seems to be unrelated to P and Q.

We conclude with a generalization. The probability that k randomly chosen integers are coprime is $1/\zeta(k)$, as suggested in [1.6]. The probability that they are *pairwise* coprime is known to be [5, 7]

$$\prod_{p} \left(1 - \frac{1}{p}\right)^{k-1} \left(1 + \frac{k-1}{p}\right)$$

for $2 \leq k \leq 3$, but a proof for $k > 3$ has not yet been found. The expression naturally reduces to $6/\pi^2$ if $k = 2$. More surprisingly, if $k = 3$, it reduces to Q.

[1] G. H. Hardy and E. M. Wright, *An Introduction to the Theory of Numbers*, 5th ed., Oxford Univ. Press, 1985, p. 269; MR 81i:10002.

[2] J. L. Hafner, P. Sarnak, and K. McCurley, Relatively prime values of polynomials, *A Tribute to Emil Grosswald: Number Theory and Related Analysis*, ed. M. Knopp and M. Sheingorn, Contemp. Math. 143, Amer. Math. Soc., 1993, pp. 437–443; MR 93m:11094.

[3] I. Vardi, *Computational Recreations in Mathematica*, Addison-Wesley, 1991, p. 174; MR 93e:00002.

[4] P. Flajolet and I. Vardi, Zeta function expansions of classical constants, unpublished note (1996).

[5] M. R. Schroeder, *Number Theory in Science and Communication: With Applications in Cryptography, Physics, Digital Information, Computing and Self-Similarity*, 2nd ed., Springer-Verlag, 1986, pp. 25, 48–51, 54; MR 99c:11165.

[6] M. R. Schroeder, Square-free and coprime, unpublished note (1998).

[7] P. Moree, Counting carefree couples, unpublished note (1999).

[8] G. Niklasch and P. Moree, Some number-theoretical constants: Products of rational functions over primes, unpublished note (2000).

[9] E. Cohen, Arithmetical functions associated with the unitary divisors of an integer, *Math. Z.* 74 (1960) 66–80; MR 22 #3707.

[10] E. Cohen, Some asymptotic formulas in the theory of numbers, *Trans. Amer. Math. Soc.* 112 (1964) 214–227; MR 29 #3458.

[11] G. Tenenbaum, *Introduction to Analytic and Probabilistic Number Theory*, Cambridge Univ. Press, 1995, pp. 53–54; MR 97e:11005b.

[12] A. Selberg, Note on a paper by L. G. Sathe, *J. Indian Math. Soc.* 18 (1954) 83–87; MR 16,676a.

[13] H. Delange, Sur des formules de Atle Selberg, *Acta Arith.* 19 (1971) 105–146 (errata insert); MR 44 #6623.

[14] E. Grosswald, The average order of an arithmetic function, *Duke Math. J.* 23 (1956) 41–44; MR 17,588f.

[15] P. Bateman, Proof of a conjecture of Grosswald, *Duke Math. J.* 25 (1957) 67–72; MR 19,1040a.

2.6 Niven's Constant

Let m be a positive integer with prime factorization $p_1^{a_1} p_2^{a_2} p_3^{a_3} \cdots p_k^{a_k}$. We assume that each exponent $a_i \geq 1$ and each prime $p_i \neq p_j$ for all $i \neq j$. Define two functions

$$h(m) = \begin{cases} 1 & \text{if } m = 1, \\ \min\{a_1, \ldots, a_k\} & \text{if } m > 1, \end{cases} \quad H(m) = \begin{cases} 1 & \text{if } m = 1, \\ \max\{a_1, \ldots, a_k\} & \text{if } m > 1, \end{cases}$$

that is, the smallest and largest exponents for m. Niven [1, 2] proved that

$$\lim_{n \to \infty} \frac{1}{n} \sum_{m=1}^{n} h(m) = 1$$

and, moreover,

$$\lim_{n \to \infty} \frac{\left(\displaystyle\sum_{m=1}^{n} h(m) \right) - n}{\sqrt{n}} = \frac{\zeta(\frac{3}{2})}{\zeta(3)} = 2.1732543125 \ldots,$$

where $\zeta(x)$ denotes Riemann's zeta function [1.6]. He also proved that

$$\lim_{n \to \infty} \frac{1}{n} \sum_{m=1}^{n} H(m) = C$$

and we call C **Niven's constant**:

$$C = 1 + \sum_{k=2}^{\infty} \left(1 - \frac{1}{\zeta(k)} \right) = 1.7052111401 \ldots.$$

Subsequent authors discovered the following extended results [3, 4]:

$$\sum_{m=1}^{n} h(m) = n + c_{02}n^{\frac{1}{2}} + (c_{12} + c_{03})n^{\frac{1}{3}} + (c_{13} + c_{04})n^{\frac{1}{4}} + (c_{23} + c_{14} + c_{05})n^{\frac{1}{5}} + O(n^{\frac{1}{6}}),$$

$$\sum_{m=1}^{n} \frac{1}{h(m)} = n - \frac{c_{02}}{2}n^{\frac{1}{2}} - \frac{3c_{12} + c_{03}}{6}n^{\frac{1}{3}} - \frac{2c_{13} + c_{04}}{12}n^{\frac{1}{4}}$$
$$- \frac{10c_{23} + 5c_{14} + 3c_{05}}{60}n^{\frac{1}{5}} + O(n^{\frac{1}{6}}),$$

where the coefficients c_{ij} are given in [2.6.1]; additionally, we have

$$\lim_{n\to\infty} \frac{1}{n}\sum_{m=1}^{n} \frac{1}{H(m)} = \sum_{k=2}^{\infty} \frac{1}{k(k-1)\zeta(k)} = 0.7669444905\ldots.$$

Averages for H are not as well understood asymptotically as averages for h.

The constant $c_{02} = \zeta(3/2)/\zeta(3)$ also occurs when estimating the asymptotic growth of the number of square-full integers [2.6.1], as does $c_{12} = \zeta(2/3)/\zeta(2) = -1.4879506635\ldots$. In contrast, the constant $6/\pi^2$ arises in connection with the square-free integers [2.5].

A generalization of Niven's theorem to the setting of a free abelian normed semigroup appears in [5].

Here is a problem that gives expressions similar to C. First, observe that [6, 7]

$$\sum_{l=2}^{\infty}\sum_{n=2}^{\infty} \frac{1}{n^l} = \sum_{l=2}^{\infty}(\zeta(l) - 1) = 1, \quad \sum_{p}\sum_{n=2}^{\infty} \frac{1}{n^p} = \sum_{p}(\zeta(p) - 1) = 0.8928945714\ldots,$$

where the sum over p is restricted to primes. Both series involve reciprocal nontrivial integer powers with duplication, for example, $2^4 = 4^2$ and $4^3 = 8^2$. Now, let $S = \{4, 8, 9, 16, 25, 27, 32, 36, 49, 64, 81, \ldots\}$ be the set of nontrivial integer powers *without* duplication. It follows that [8]

$$\sum_{s\in S} \frac{1}{s} = -\sum_{k=2}^{\infty} \mu(k)(\zeta(k) - 1) = 0.8744643684\ldots,$$

where $\mu(k)$ is Möbius' mu function [2.2]; we also have [8, 9]

$$\sum_{s\in S} \frac{1}{s-1} = 1, \quad \sum_{s\in S} \frac{1}{s+1} = \frac{\pi^2}{3} - \frac{5}{2}.$$

Given an arbitrary integer $c \notin S$, what can be said about $\sum_{s\in S}(s-c)^{-1}$? (By Mihailescu's recent proof of Catalan's conjecture, the only two integers in S that differ by 1 are 8 and 9.) See other expressions in [5.1].

2.6.1 Square-Full and Cube-Full Integers

Let $k \geq 2$ be an integer. A positive integer m is k-**full** (or **powerful of type** k) if $m = 1$ or if, for any prime number p, $p|m$ implies $p^k|m$.

Let $N_k(x)$ denote the number of k-full integers not exceeding x. For the case $k = 2$, Erdös & Szekeres [10] showed that

$$N_2(x) = \frac{\zeta(\frac{3}{2})}{\zeta(3)} x^{\frac{1}{2}} + O\left(x^{\frac{1}{3}}\right)$$

and Bateman & Grosswald [11–13] proved the more accurate result

$$N_2(x) = \frac{\zeta(\frac{3}{2})}{\zeta(3)} x^{\frac{1}{2}} + \frac{\zeta(\frac{2}{3})}{\zeta(2)} x^{\frac{1}{3}} + o\left(x^{\frac{1}{6}}\right).$$

This is essentially as sharp an error estimate as possible without additional knowledge concerning the unsolved Riemann hypothesis. A number of researchers have studied this problem. The current best-known error term [14, 15], assuming Riemann's hypothesis, is $O(x^{1/7+\varepsilon})$ for any $\varepsilon > 0$, and several authors conjecture that $1/7$ can be replaced by $1/10$.

For the case $k = 3$, Bateman & Grosswald [12] and Krätzel [16, 17] demonstrated unconditionally that

$$N_3(x) = c_{03}x^{\frac{1}{3}} + c_{13}x^{\frac{1}{4}} + c_{23}x^{\frac{1}{5}} + o\left(x^{\frac{1}{8}}\right).$$

By assuming Riemann's hypothesis, the error term [15] can be improved to $O(x^{97/804+\varepsilon})$. Formulas for the coefficients c_{ij} include [3, 12, 18–20]

$$c_{0j} = \prod_p \left(1 + \sum_{m=j+1}^{2j-1} p^{-\frac{m}{j}}\right) = \begin{cases} 4.6592661225\ldots & \text{if } j = 3, \\ 9.6694754843\ldots & \text{if } j = 4, \\ 19.4455760839\ldots & \text{if } j = 5, \end{cases}$$

$$c_{1j} = \zeta\left(\frac{j}{j+1}\right) \prod_p \left(1 + \sum_{m=j+2}^{2j-1} p^{-\frac{m}{j+1}} - \sum_{m=2j+2}^{3j} p^{-\frac{m}{j+1}}\right)$$
$$= \begin{cases} -5.8726188208\ldots & \text{if } j = 3, \\ -16.9787814834\ldots & \text{if } j = 4, \end{cases}$$

$$c_{23} = \zeta\left(\tfrac{3}{5}\right) \zeta\left(\tfrac{4}{5}\right) \prod_p \left(1 - p^{-\frac{8}{5}} - p^{-\frac{9}{5}} - p^{-\frac{10}{5}} + p^{-\frac{13}{5}} + p^{-\frac{14}{5}}\right) = 1.6824415102\ldots,$$

where all products are restricted to primes p. The decimal approximations for the **Bateman–Grosswald constants** listed here are due to Niklasch & Moree [21] and Sebah [22]. Higher-order coefficients appear in the expansions of $N_k(x)$ for $k \geq 4$.

We observe that the Erdös–Szekeres paper [10] also plays a crucial role in the asymptotics of abelian group enumeration [5.1]. The books by Ivić [23] and Krätzel [24] provide detailed analyses and background. See also [5.4] for discussion of the smallest and largest prime factors of m.

[1] I. Niven, Averages of exponents in factoring integers, *Proc. Amer. Math. Soc.* 22 (1969) 356–360; MR 39 #2713.

[2] F. Le Lionnais, *Les Nombres Remarquables*, Hermann, 1983.

[3] D. Suryanarayana and R. Sitaramachandrarao, On the maximum and minimum exponents in factoring integers, *Arch. Math. (Basel)* 28 (1977) 261–269; MR 55 #10368.

[4]   H. Z. Cao, The asymptotic formulas related to exponents in factoring integers, *Math. Balkanica* 5 (1991) 105–108; MR 93e:11107.

[5]   S. Porubský, On exponents in arithmetical semigroups, *Monatsh. Math.* 84 (1977) 49–53; MR 56 #15591.

[6]   G. Pólya and G. Szegö, *Problems and Theorems in Analysis*, v. 2, Springer-Verlag, 1976, ex. 262.1; MR 81e:00002.

[7]   G. Salamin and D. Wilson, Sum of reciprocal powers, unpublished note (1999).

[8]   V. F. Lev and P. Pleasants, Sum of reciprocal powers, unpublished note (2002).

[9]   J. D. Shallit and K. Zikan, A theorem of Goldbach, *Amer. Math. Monthly* 93 (1986) 402–403.

[10] P. Erdös and G. Szekeres, Über die Anzahl der Abelschen Gruppen gegebener Ordnung und über ein verwandtes zahlentheoretisches Problem, *Acta Sci. Math. (Szeged)* 7 (1934–35) 95–102.

[11] P. T. Bateman, Squarefull integers, *Amer. Math. Monthly* 61 (1954) 477–479.

[12] P. T. Bateman and E. Grosswald, On a theorem of Erdös and Szekeres, *Illinois J. Math.* 2 (1958) 88–98; MR 20 #2305.

[13] E. Cohen, On the distribution of certain sequences of integers, *Amer. Math. Monthly* 70 (1963) 516–521; MR 26 #6105.

[14] X. Cao, On the distribution of square-full integers, *Period. Math. Hungar.* 34 (1998) 169–175; MR 99a:11104.

[15] J. Wu, On the distribution of square-full and cube-full integers, *Monatsh. Math.* 126 (1998) 353–367; MR 2000a:11125.

[16] E. Krätzel, Zahlen k^{ter} art, *Amer. Math. J.* 94 (1972) 209–328; MR 45 #5093.

[17] E. Krätzel, Zweifache Exponentialsummen und dreidimensionale Gitterpunktprobleme, *Elementary and Analytic Theory of Numbers*, Proc. 1982 Warsaw conf., ed. H. Iwaniec, Banach Center Publ., 1985, pp. 337–369; MR 87m:11091.

[18] A. Ivić and P. Shiu, The distribution of powerful numbers, *Illinois J. Math.* 26 (1982) 576–690; MR 84a:10047.

[19] P. Shiu, The distribution of cube-full numbers, *Glasgow Math. J.* 33 (1991) 287–295; MR 92g:11091.

[20] P. Shiu, Cube-full numbers in short intervals, *Math. Proc. Cambridge Philos. Soc.* 112 (1992) 1–5; MR 93d:11097.

[21] G. Niklasch and P. Moree, Some number-theoretical constants: Products of rational functions over primes, unpublished note (2000).

[22] P. Sebah, Evaluating certain prime products, unpublished note (2001).

[23] A. Ivić, *The Riemann Zeta-Function*, Wiley, 1985, pp. 33–34, 407–413, 438–439; MR 87d:11062.

[24] E. Krätzel, *Lattice Points*, Kluwer, 1988, pp. 276–293; MR 90e:11144.

2.7 Euler Totient Constants

When n is a positive integer, Euler's totient function, $\varphi(n)$, is defined to be the number of positive integers not greater than n and relatively prime to n. For example, if p and q are distinct primes and r and s are positive integers, then

$$\varphi(p^r) = p^{r-1}(p - 1),$$

$$\varphi(p^r q^s) = p^{r-1}q^{s-1}(p - 1)(q - 1).$$

In the language of group theory, $\varphi(n)$ is the number of generators in a cyclic group of order n. Landau [1–4] showed that

$$\limsup_{n \to \infty} \frac{\varphi(n)}{n} = 1$$

but

$$\liminf_{n \to \infty} \frac{\varphi(n) \ln(\ln(n))}{n} = e^{-\gamma} = 0.5614594835\ldots,$$

where γ is the Euler–Mascheroni constant [1.5].

The average behavior of $\varphi(n)$ over all positive integers has been of interest to many authors. Walfisz [5, 6], building on the work of Dirichlet and Mertens [2], proved that

$$\sum_{n=1}^{N} \varphi(n) = \frac{3N^2}{\pi^2} + O\left(N \ln(N)^{\frac{2}{3}} \ln(\ln(N))^{\frac{4}{3}}\right)$$

as $N \to \infty$, which is the sharpest such asymptotic formula known. (A claim in [7] that the exponent 4/3 could be replaced by $1 + \varepsilon$, for any $\varepsilon > 0$, is incorrect [8].) It is also known [9, 10] that the error term is not $o(N \ln(\ln(\ln(N))))$.

Interesting constants emerge if we consider instead the series of reciprocals of $\varphi(n)$. Landau [11–13] proved that

$$\sum_{n=1}^{N} \frac{1}{\varphi(n)} = A \cdot (\ln(N) + B) + O\left(\frac{\ln(N)}{N}\right),$$

where

$$A = \frac{\zeta(2)\zeta(3)}{\zeta(6)} = \frac{315}{2\pi^4}\zeta(3) = 1.9435964368\ldots,$$

$$B = \gamma - \sum_{p} \frac{\ln(p)}{p^2 - p + 1} = \gamma - 0.6083817178\ldots = \frac{-0.0605742294\ldots}{A},$$

and $\zeta(x)$ is Riemann's zeta function [1.6]. Sums and products over p are restricted to primes. The sum within B has inspired several accurate computations by Jameson [14], Moree [15] and Sebah [16]. Landau's error term $O(\ln(N)/N)$ was improved to $O(\ln(N)^{2/3}/N)$ by Sitaramachandra Rao [17, 18].

Define $K(x)$ to be the number of all positive integers n that satisfy $\varphi(n) \leq x$. It is known [19–22] that the following distributional result is true:

$$K(x) = Ax + O\left(x \exp\left(-c\sqrt{\ln(x)\ln(\ln(x))}\right)\right)$$

for any $0 < c < 1/\sqrt{2}$. Other relevant formulas are [18, 23, 24]

$$\sum_{n=1}^{N} \frac{\varphi(n)}{n} = \frac{6N}{\pi^2} + O\left(\ln(N)^{\frac{2}{3}} \ln(\ln(N))^{\frac{4}{3}}\right),$$

$$\sum_{n=1}^{N} \frac{n}{\varphi(n)} = AN - \frac{1}{2}\ln(N) - \frac{1}{2}C + O\left(\ln(N)^{\frac{2}{3}}\right),$$

$$\sum_{n=1}^{N} \frac{1}{n\varphi(n)} = D - \frac{A}{N} + O\left(\frac{\ln(N)}{N^2}\right),$$

where

$$C = \ln(2\pi) + \gamma + \sum_p \frac{\ln(p)}{p(p-1)} = \ln(2\pi) + 1.3325822757\ldots = 3.1704593421\ldots,$$

which occurred in [2.2], and

$$D = \frac{\pi^2}{6} \prod_p \left(1 + \frac{1}{p^2(p-1)}\right) = 2.2038565964\ldots,$$

which came from a sharpening by Moree [24] of estimates in [25]. See [26] for numerical evaluations of such prime products. The constant A occurs in [27, 28] as the asymptotic mean of a certain prime divisor function and elsewhere too [29]. The constant D also occurs in a certain Hardy–Littlewood conjecture proved by Chowla [30].

We note the following alternative representation of A:

$$A = \prod_p \frac{1 - p^{-6}}{(1 - p^{-2})(1 - p^{-3})} = \prod_p \left(1 + \frac{1}{p(p-1)}\right),$$

which bears a striking resemblance to Artin's constant [2.4]. The only distinction is that an addition is replaced by a subtraction. Curiously, Artin's constant and Murata's constant [2.4] arise explicitly in the following asymptotic results [31, 32]:

$$\lim_{N\to\infty} \frac{\ln(N)}{N} \sum_{p \leq N} \frac{\varphi(p-1)}{p-1} = C_{\text{Artin}} = 0.3739558136\ldots,$$

$$\lim_{N\to\infty} \frac{\ln(N)}{N} \sum_{p \leq N} \frac{p-1}{\varphi(p-1)} = C_{\text{Murata}} = 2.8264199970\ldots.$$

Let $L(x)$ denote the number of all positive integers n not exceeding x for which n and $\varphi(n)$ are relatively prime. Erdös [33, 34] proved that

$$\lim_{n\to\infty} \frac{L(n)\ln(\ln(\ln(n)))}{n} = e^{-\gamma},$$

another interesting occurrence of the Euler–Mascheroni constant.

[1] E. Landau, Über den Verlauf der zahlentheoretischen Funktion $\varphi(x)$, *Archiv Math. Phys.* 5 (1903) 86–91; also in *Collected Works*, v. 1, ed. L. Mirsky, I. J. Schoenberg, W. Schwarz, and H. Wefelscheid, Thales Verlag, 1983, pp. 378–383.
[2] G. H. Hardy and E. M. Wright, *An Introduction to the Theory of Numbers*, 5th ed., Oxford Univ. Press, 1985, pp. 267–268, 272; MR 81i:10002.
[3] N. J. A. Sloane, On-Line Encyclopedia of Integer Sequences, A000010 and A002088.
[4] M. Hausman, Generalization of a theorem of Landau, *Pacific J. Math.* 84 (1979) 91–95; MR 81d:10005.
[5] A. Walfisz, Über die Wirksamkeit einiger Abschätzungen trigonometrischer Summen, *Acta Arith.* 4 (1958) 108–180; MR 21 #2623.
[6] A. Walfisz, *Weylsche Exponentialsummen in der neueren Zahlentheorie*, Mathematische Forschungsberichte, XV, VEB Deutscher Verlag der Wissenschaften, 1963; MR 36 #3737.
[7] A. I. Saltykov, On Euler's function (in Russian), *Vestnik Moskov. Univ. Ser. I Mat. Mekh.* (1960) n. 6, 34–50; MR 23 #A2395.

[8] U. Balakrishnan and Y.-F. S. Pétermann, Errata to: "The Dirichlet series of $\zeta(s)\zeta^\alpha(s + 1)f(s + 1)$: On an error term associated with its coefficients," *Acta Arith.* 87 (1999) 287–289; MR 99m:11105.

[9] S. S. Pillai and S. D. Chowla, On the error terms in some asymptotic formulae in the theory of numbers, *J. London Math. Soc.* 5 (1930) 95–101.

[10] S. Chowla, Contributions to the analytic theory of numbers, *Math. Z.* 35 (1932) 279–299.

[11] E. Landau, Über die zahlentheoretische Function $\varphi(n)$ und ihre Beziehung zum Goldbachschen Satz, *Nachr. Königlichen Ges. Wiss. Göttingen, Math.-Phys. Klasse* (1900) 177–186; also in *Collected Works*, v. 1, ed. L. Mirsky, I. J. Schoenberg, W. Schwarz, and H. Wefelscheid, Thales Verlag, 1983, pp. 106–115.

[12] J.-M. DeKoninck and A. Ivić, *Topics in Arithmetic Functions: Asymptotic Formulae for Sums of Reciprocals of Arithmetical Functions and Related Fields*, North-Holland, 1980, pp. 1–3; MR 82a:10047.

[13] H. Halberstam and H.-E. Richert, *Sieve Methods*, Academic Press, 1974, pp. 110–111; MR 54 #12689.

[14] T. Jameson, Asymptotics of $\sum_{n\le x} 1/\varphi(n)$, unpublished note (1999).

[15] P. Moree, Expressing B as $\gamma - \sum_{k\ge 2} e_k \zeta'(k)/\zeta(k)$, unpublished note (2000).

[16] X. Gourdon and P. Sebah, Some constants from number theory (Numbers, Constants and Computation).

[17] R. Sitaramachandrarao, On an error term of Landau, *Indian J. Pure Appl. Math.* 13 (1982) 882–885; MR 84b:10069.

[18] R. Sitaramachandrarao, On an error term of Landau. II, *Rocky Mount. J. Math.* 15 (1985) 579–588; MR 87g:11116.

[19] P. Erdös, Some remarks on Euler's φ-function and some related problems, *Bull. Amer. Math. Soc.* 51 (1945) 540–544; MR 7,49f.

[20] R. E. Dressler, A density which counts multiplicity, *Pacific J. Math.* 34 (1970) 371–378; MR 42 #5940.

[21] P. T. Bateman, The distribution of values of the Euler function, *Acta Arith.* 21 (1972) 329–345; MR 46 #1730.

[22] M. Balazard and A. Smati, Elementary proof of a theorem of Bateman, *Analytic Number Theory*, Proc. 1989 Allerton Park conf., ed. B. C. Berndt, H. G. Diamond, H. Halberstam, and A. Hildebrand, Birkhäuser, 1990, pp. 41–46; MR 92a:11104.

[23] W. G. Nowak, On an error term involving the totient function, *Indian J. Pure Appl. Math.* 20 (1989) 537–542; MR 90g:11135.

[24] P. Moree, On the error terms in Stephens' work, unpublished note (2000).

[25] P. J. Stephens, Prime divisors of second-order linear recurrences. I, *J. Number Theory* 8 (1976) 313–332; MR 54 #5142.

[26] G. Niklasch and P. Moree, Some number-theoretical constants: Products of rational functions over primes, unpublished note (2000).

[27] J. Knopfmacher, A prime-divisor function, *Proc. Amer. Math. Soc.* 40 (1973) 373–377; MR 48 #6036.

[28] J. Knopfmacher, Arithmetical properties of finite rings and algebras, and analytic number theory. VI, *J. Reine Angew. Math.* 277 (1975) 45–62; MR 52 #3088.

[29] D. S. Mitrinovic, J. Sándor, and B. Crstici, *Handbook of Number Theory*, Kluwer, 1996, pp. 9–37, 49–51, 332; MR 97f:11001.

[30] S. Chowla, The representation of a number as a sum of four squares and a prime, *Acta Arith.* 1 (1935) 115–122.

[31] P. Moree, On some sums connected with primitive roots, preprint MPI 98-42, Max-Planck-Institut für Mathematik.

[32] P. Moree, On primes in arithmetic progression having a prescribed primitive root, *J. Number Theory* 78 (1999) 85–98; MR 2001i:11118.

[33] P. Erdös, Some asymptotic formulas in number theory, *J. Indian Math. Soc.* 12 (1948) 75–78; MR 10,594d.

[34] I. Z. Ruzsa, Erdös and the integers, *J. Number Theory* 79 (1999) 115–163; MR 2002e:11002.

2.8 Pell–Stevenhagen Constants

If an integer $d > 1$ is not a square, then the **Pell equation**

$$x^2 - dy^2 = 1$$

has a solution in integers (in fact, infinitely many). This fact was known long ago [1–5]. We are here concerned with a more difficult question. What can be said about the set D of integers $d > 1$ for which the **negative Pell equation**

$$x^2 - dy^2 = -1$$

has a solution in integers? Only recently has progress been made in answering this.

First, define the **Pell constant**

$$P = 1 - \prod_{\substack{j \geq 1 \\ j \text{ odd}}} \left(1 - \frac{1}{2^j}\right) = 0.5805775582\ldots,$$

which is needed in the following. The constant P is provably irrational [6] but only conjectured to be transcendental. Define also a function

$$\psi(p) = \frac{2 + \left(1 + 2^{1-v_p}\right)p}{2(p+1)},$$

where v_p is the number of factors of 2 occurring in $p - 1$.

For any set S of positive integers, let $f_S(n)$ denote the number of elements in S not exceeding n. Stevenhagen [6–8] developed several conjectures regarding the distribution of D. He hypothesized that the counting function $f_D(n)$ satisfies the following [7]:

$$\lim_{n \to \infty} \frac{\sqrt{\ln(n)}}{n} f_D(n) = \frac{3P}{2\pi} \prod_{p \equiv 1 \bmod 4} \left(1 + \frac{\psi(p)}{p^2 - 1}\right) \left(1 - \frac{1}{p^2}\right)^{\frac{1}{2}} = 0.28136\ldots,$$

where the product is restricted to primes p.

Let U be the set of positive integers not divisible by 4, and let V be the set of positive integers not divisible by any prime congruent to 3 module 4. Clearly D is a subset of $U \cap V$, and $U \cap V$ is the set of positive integers that can be written as a sum of two coprime squares. By the conjectured limit mentioned here and by a coprimality result given in [2.3.1] due to Rieger [9], the density of D inside $U \cap V$ is [7]

$$\lim_{n \to \infty} \frac{f_D(n)}{f_{U \cap V}(n)} = P \prod_{p \equiv 1 \bmod 4} \left(1 + \frac{\psi(p)}{p^2 - 1}\right) \left(1 - \frac{1}{p^2}\right) = 0.57339\ldots.$$

Here is another conjecture. Let W be the set of square-free integers, that is, integers that are divisible by no square exceeding 1. Stevenhagen [6] hypothesized that

$$\lim_{n \to \infty} \frac{\sqrt{\ln(n)}}{n} f_{D \cap W}(n) = \frac{6}{\pi^2} PK = 0.2697318462\ldots,$$

where K is the Landau–Ramanujan constant [2.3]. Clearly $V \cap W$ is the set of positive square-free integers that can be written as a sum of two (coprime) squares. By the second conjectured limit and by a square-free result given in [2.3.1] due to Moree [10], the density of $D \cap W$ inside $V \cap W$ is [8]

$$\lim_{n \to \infty} \frac{f_{D \cap W}(n)}{f_{V \cap W}(n)} = P = 0.5805775582\ldots.$$

A fascinating connection to continued fractions is as follows [7]: An integer $d > 1$ is in D if and only if $\sqrt{d}$ is irrational and has a regular continued fraction expansion with *odd* period length.

A constant Q similar to P here appears in [5.14]; however, exponents in Q are not constrained to be odd integers.

[1] T. Nagell, *Introduction to Number Theory*, Chelsea, 1981, pp. 195–204; MR 30 #4714.
[2] K. Ireland and M. Rosen, *A Classical Introduction to Modern Number Theory*, 2nd ed., Springer-Verlag, 1990, pp. 276–278; MR 92e:11001.
[3] K. H. Rosen, *Elementary Number Theory and Its Applications*, Addison-Wesley, 1985, pp. 401–409; MR 93i:11002.
[4] D. A. Buell, *Binary Quadratic Forms: Classical Theory and Modern Computations*, Springer-Verlag, 1989, pp. 31–34; MR 92b:11021.
[5] M. R. Schroeder, *Number Theory in Science and Communication: With Applications in Cryptography, Physics, Digital Information, Computing and Self-Similarity*, 2nd ed., Springer-Verlag, 1986, pp. 98–99; MR 99c:11165.
[6] P. Stevenhagen, The number of real quadratic fields having units of negative norm, *Experim. Math.* 2 (1993) 121–136; MR 94k:11120.
[7] P. Stevenhagen, A density conjecture for the negative Pell equation, *Computational Algebra and Number Theory*, Proc. 1992 Sydney conf., ed. W. Bosma and A. van der Poorten, Kluwer, 1995, pp. 187–200; MR 96g:11137.
[8] W. Bosma and P. Stevenhagen, Density computations for real quadratic units, *Math. Comp.* 65 (1996) 1327–1337; MR 96j:11171.
[9] G. J. Rieger, Über die Anzahl der als Summe von zwei Quadraten darstellbaren und in einer primen Restklasse gelegenen Zahlen unterhalb einer positiven Schranke. II, *J. Reine Angew. Math.* 217 (1965) 200–216; MR 30 #4734.
[10] P. Moree, Variations on the Landau-Ramanujan problem, unpublished note (2000).

2.9 Alladi–Grinstead Constant

Let n be a positive integer. The well-known formula

$$n! = 1 \cdot 2 \cdot 3 \cdot 4 \cdots (n-1) \cdot n$$

is only one of many available ways to decompose $n!$ as a product of n positive integer factors. Let us agree to disallow 1 as a factor and to further restrict each of the n factors to be a prime power:

$$p_k^{b_k}, \text{ each } p_k \text{ is prime and } b_k \geq 1, \ k = 1, 2, \ldots, n.$$

(Thus the previously stated natural decomposition of $n!$ is inadmissible.) Let us also write the factors in nondecreasing order from left to right. If $n = 9$, for example, all of the admissible decompositions are

$$
\begin{aligned}
9! &= 2 \cdot 2 \cdot 2 \cdot 2 \cdot 2 \cdot 2^2 \cdot 5 \cdot 7 \cdot 3^4 \\
&= 2 \cdot 2 \cdot 2 \cdot 2 \cdot 3 \cdot 5 \cdot 7 \cdot 2^3 \cdot 3^3 \\
&= 2 \cdot 2 \cdot 2 \cdot 2 \cdot 5 \cdot 7 \cdot 2^3 \cdot 3^2 \cdot 3^2 \\
&= 2 \cdot 2 \cdot 2 \cdot 3 \cdot 2^2 \cdot 2^2 \cdot 5 \cdot 7 \cdot 3^3 \\
&= 2 \cdot 2 \cdot 2 \cdot 2^2 \cdot 2^2 \cdot 5 \cdot 7 \cdot 3^2 \cdot 3^2 \\
&= 2 \cdot 2 \cdot 2 \cdot 3 \cdot 3 \cdot 5 \cdot 7 \cdot 3^2 \cdot 2^4 \\
&= 2 \cdot 2 \cdot 3 \cdot 3 \cdot 2^2 \cdot 5 \cdot 7 \cdot 2^3 \cdot 3^2 \\
&= 2 \cdot 2 \cdot 3 \cdot 3 \cdot 3 \cdot 3 \cdot 5 \cdot 7 \cdot 2^5 \\
&= 2 \cdot 3 \cdot 3 \cdot 2^2 \cdot 2^2 \cdot 2^2 \cdot 5 \cdot 7 \cdot 3^2 \\
&= 2 \cdot 3 \cdot 3 \cdot 3 \cdot 3 \cdot 2^2 \cdot 5 \cdot 7 \cdot 2^4 \\
&= 2 \cdot 3 \cdot 3 \cdot 3 \cdot 3 \cdot 5 \cdot 7 \cdot 2^3 \cdot 2^3 \\
&= 3 \cdot 3 \cdot 3 \cdot 3 \cdot 2^2 \cdot 2^2 \cdot 5 \cdot 7 \cdot 2^3.
\end{aligned}
$$

Note that eleven of the leftmost factors are 2 and one is 3. The maximum leftmost factor, considering all admissible decompositions of 9! into 9 prime powers, is therefore 3. We define

$$
\alpha(9) = \frac{\ln(3)}{\ln(9)}.
$$

In the same way, for arbitrary n, one determines the maximum leftmost factor p^b over all admissible decompositions of $n!$ into n prime powers and defines

$$
\alpha(n) = \frac{\ln(p^b)}{\ln(n)}.
$$

Clearly $\alpha(n) < 1$ for each n. What can be said about $\alpha(n)$ for large n?

Alladi & Grinstead [1, 2] determined that the limit of $\alpha(n)$ as $n \to \infty$ exists and

$$
\lim_{n \to \infty} \alpha(n) = e^{c-1} = 0.8093940205\ldots,
$$

where

$$
c = -\sum_{k=2}^{\infty} \frac{1}{k} \ln\left(1 - \frac{1}{k}\right) = \sum_{j=2}^{\infty} \frac{\zeta(j) - 1}{j - 1} = 0.7885305659\ldots
$$
$$
= -\ln(0.4545121805\ldots)
$$

and $\zeta(x)$ is Riemann's zeta function [1.6].

How strongly does Alladi & Grinstead's result depend on decomposing $n!$ and not some other function $f(n)$? It is assumed that f provides sufficiently many small and varied prime factors for each n. See [3] for a related unsolved problem.

Let $d(m)$ denote the number of positive integer divisors of m. What can be said about $d(n!)$? Erdös et al. [4] proved that

$$\lim_{n\to\infty} \frac{\ln(\ln(n!))^2}{\ln(n!)} \ln(d(n!)) = C,$$

where

$$C = \sum_{k=2}^{\infty} \frac{1}{k(k-1)} \ln(k) = -\sum_{j=2}^{\infty} \zeta'(j) = 1.2577468869\ldots$$

as mentioned in [1.8]. The similarity between c and C is quite interesting.

Here are four related infinite products [5, 6]:

$$\prod_{n\geq 2}\left(1+\frac{1}{n}\right)^{\frac{1}{n}} = 1.7587436279\ldots, \quad \prod_{n\geq 2}\left(1-\frac{1}{n}\right)^{\frac{1}{n}} = 0.4545121805\ldots,$$

$$\prod_{p}\left(1+\frac{1}{p}\right)^{\frac{1}{p}} = 1.4681911223\ldots, \quad \prod_{p}\left(1-\frac{1}{p}\right)^{\frac{1}{p}} = 0.5598656169\ldots,$$

the latter two of which are restricted to primes p. The second product is e^{-c}, and the fourth appears in [7, 8]. A related problem, regarding the asymptotics of the smallest and largest prime factors of n, is discussed in [5.4].

[1] K. Alladi and C. Grinstead, On the decomposition of $n!$ into prime powers, *J. Number Theory* 9 (1977) 452–458; MR 56 #11934.
[2] R. K. Guy, *Unsolved Problems in Number Theory*, 2nd ed., Springer-Verlag, 1994, sect. B22; MR 96e:11002.
[3] R. K. Guy and J. L. Selfridge, Factoring factorial n, *Amer. Math. Monthly* 105 (1998) 766–767.
[4] P. Erdös, S. W. Graham, A. Ivić, and C. Pomerance, On the number of divisors of $n!$, *Analytic Number Theory*, Proc. 1995 Allerton Park conf., v. 1, ed. B. C. Berndt, H. G. Diamond, and A. J. Hildebrand, Birkhäuser, 1996, pp. 337–355; MR 97d:11142.
[5] P. Sebah, Evaluating $\prod_{n\geq 2}(1\pm 1/n)^{1/n}$, unpublished note (2000).
[6] M. Deleglise, Computing $\prod_{p}(1\pm 1/p)^{1/p}$, unpublished note (1999).
[7] P. Erdös, Remarks on two problems of the Matematikai Lapok (in Hungarian), *Mat. Lapok* 7 (1956) 10–17; MR 20 #4534.
[8] I. Z. Ruzsa, Erdös and the integers, *J. Number Theory* 79 (1999) 115–163; MR 2002e:11002.

2.10 Sierpinski's Constant

In his 1908 dissertation, Sierpinski [1] studied certain series involving the function $r(n)$, defined to be the number of representations of the positive integer n as a sum of two squares, counting order and sign. For example, $r(1) = 4$, $r(p) = 0$ for primes $p \equiv 3 \bmod 4$, and $r(q) = 8$ for primes $q \equiv 1 \bmod 4$.

Certain results about $r(n)$ are not difficult to see; for example [2–4],

$$\sum_{k=1}^{n} r(k) = \pi n + O\left(n^{\frac{1}{2}}\right)$$

as $n \to \infty$. More details on this estimate are in [2.10.1]. Sierpinski's series include [1, 5, 6]

$$\sum_{k=1}^{n} \frac{r(k)}{k} = \pi \left(\ln(n) + S \right) + O \left(n^{-\frac{1}{2}} \right),$$

$$\sum_{k=1}^{n} r(k^2) = \frac{4}{\pi} \left(\ln(n) + \hat{S} \right) n + O \left(n^{\frac{2}{3}} \right),$$

$$\sum_{k=1}^{n} r(k)^2 = 4 \left(\ln(n) + \tilde{S} \right) n + O \left(n^{\frac{3}{4}} \ln(n) \right),$$

where the constants $\hat{S}$ and $\tilde{S}$ are defined in terms of S as

$$\hat{S} = \gamma + S + \frac{12}{\pi^2} \zeta'(2) + \frac{\ln(2)}{3} - \frac{1}{\pi}, \quad \tilde{S} = 2S + \frac{12}{\pi^2} \zeta'(2) + \frac{\ln(2)}{3} - 1,$$

where γ is the Euler–Mascheroni constant [1.5] and $\zeta(x)$ is Riemann's zeta function [1.6]. See [2.15] and [2.18] for other occurrences of $\zeta'(2)$.

The constant S, which we call **Sierpinski's constant**, thus plays a role in the summation of all three series. It can be defined as

$$S = \gamma + \frac{\beta'(1)}{\beta(1)} = \ln \left(\frac{\pi^2 e^{2\gamma}}{2L^2} \right) = \ln \left(\frac{4\pi^3 e^{2\gamma}}{\Gamma \left(\frac{1}{4} \right)^4} \right) = \frac{2.5849817595\ldots}{\pi},$$

where $\beta(x)$ is Dirichlet's beta function [1.7], $L = 2.6220575542\ldots$ is Gauss' lemniscate constant [6.1], and $\Gamma(x)$ is the Euler gamma function [1.5.4]. It also appears in our essays on the Landau–Ramanujan constant [2.3] and the Masser–Gramain constant [7.2]. Sierpinski, in fact, defined S as a limit:

$$S = \frac{1}{\pi} \lim_{z \to 1} \left(F(z) - \frac{\pi}{z-1} \right),$$

and the function $F(z) = 4\zeta(z)\beta(z)$ is central to our discussion of lattice sums [1.10.1]. Other formulas for S include a definite integral representation:

$$S = 2\gamma + \frac{4}{\pi} \int_{0}^{\infty} \frac{e^{-x} \ln(x)}{1 + e^{-2x}} dx.$$

Clearly this is a meeting place for many ideas, all coming together at once.

2.10.1 Circle and Divisor Problems

More precisely [7–12], the sum of the first n values of r provably satisfies

$$\sum_{k=1}^{n} r(k) = \pi n + O \left(n^{\frac{23}{73}} \ln(n)^{\frac{315}{146}} \right),$$

and it is conjectured that

$$\sum_{k=1}^{n} r(k) = \pi n + O\left(n^{\frac{1}{4}+\varepsilon}\right)$$

for all $\varepsilon > 0$. The problem of estimating the error term is known as the **circle problem** since this is the same as counting the number of integer ordered pairs falling within the disk of radius $\sqrt{n}$ centered at the origin.

Here is a related problem, known as the **divisor problem**, mentioned briefly in [1.5]. If $d(n)$ is the number of distinct divisors of n, then

$$\sum_{k=1}^{n} d(k) = n\ln(n) + (2\gamma - 1)n + O\left(n^{\frac{23}{73}} \ln(n)^{\frac{461}{146}}\right)$$

is the best-known estimate of the sum of the first n values of d. Again, the conjectured exponent is $1/4 + \varepsilon$, but this remains unproven. The analog of Sierpinski's third series, for example, is [13–15]

$$\sum_{k=1}^{n} d(k)^2 = \left(A\ln(n)^3 + B\ln(n)^2 + C\ln(n) + D\right)n + O\left(n^{\frac{1}{2}+\varepsilon}\right),$$

where

$$A = \frac{1}{\pi^2}, \quad B = \frac{12\gamma - 3}{\pi^2} - \frac{36}{\pi^4}\zeta'(2),$$

and the constants C and D have more complicated expressions. The analog of Sierpinski's first series is [16]

$$\sum_{k=1}^{n} \frac{d(k)}{k} = \frac{1}{2}\ln(n)^2 + 2\gamma \ln(n) + (\gamma^2 - 2\gamma_1) + O(n^{-\frac{1}{2}}),$$

where $\gamma_1 = -0.0728158454\ldots$ is the first Stieltjes constant [2.21].

In a variation of $d(n)$, we might restrict attention to divisors of n that are square-free [17]. Likewise, for $r(n)$, we might count only representations $n = u^2 + v^2$ for which u, v are coprime, or examine differences rather than sums. Here is another variation: Define $r_m(n)$ to be the number of representations $n = |u|^m + |v|^m$, where u, v are arbitrary integers. It is known that, if $m \geq 3$, then [12, 18, 19]

$$\sum_{k=1}^{n} r_m(k) = \frac{2\Gamma\left(\frac{1}{m}\right)^2}{m\Gamma\left(\frac{2}{m}\right)} n^{\frac{2}{m}} + O\left(n^{\frac{1}{m}\left(1-\frac{1}{m}\right)}\right)$$

and, further, the error term may be replaced by

$$2^{3-\frac{1}{m}} \pi^{-1-\frac{1}{m}} m^{\frac{1}{m}} \Gamma\left(1+\frac{1}{m}\right) \cdot \sum_{k=1}^{\infty} k^{-1-\frac{1}{m}} \sin\left(2\pi k n^{\frac{1}{m}} - \frac{\pi}{2m}\right) \cdot n^{\frac{1}{m}\left(1-\frac{1}{m}\right)}$$

$$+ O\left(n^{\frac{46}{73m}} \ln(n)^{\frac{315}{146}}\right).$$

A full asymptotic analysis of such circle or divisor sums will be exceedingly difficult and cannot be expected soon.

In a related 1908 paper, Sierpinski [20–22] discovered the following fact. Let $D_n = \max\{d : d^2 | n\}$; that is, D_n^2 is the largest square divisor of n. Then

$$\frac{1}{n} \sum_{k=1}^{n} D_n = \frac{3}{\pi^2} \ln(n) + \frac{9\gamma}{\pi^2} - \frac{36}{\pi^4} \zeta'(2) + o(1)$$

as $n \to \infty$. By way of contrast, the average square-free part of n appears in [2.5].

[1]   W. Sierpinski, On the summation of the series $\sum_{n>a}^{n \leq b} \tau(n) f(n)$, where $\tau(n)$ denotes the number of decompositions of n into a sum of two integer squares (in Polish), *Prace Matematyczno-Fizyczne* 18 (1908) 1–59; French transl. in *Oeuvres Choisies*, t. 1, Editions Scientifiques de Pologne, 1974, pp. 109–154; MR 54 #2405.

[2]   G. H. Hardy and E. M. Wright, *An Introduction to the Theory of Numbers*, 5th ed., Oxford Univ. Press, 1985, pp. 241–243, 256–258, 270–271; MR 81i:10002.

[3]   D. Shanks, *Solved and Unsolved Problems in Number Theory*, 2nd ed., Chelsea, 1978, pp. 162–165; MR 86j:11001.

[4]   E. C. Titchmarsh, *The Theory of the Riemann Zeta Function*, Oxford Univ. Press, 1951, pp. 262–275; MR 88c:11049.

[5]   A. Schinzel, Waclaw Sierpinski's papers on the theory of numbers, *Acta Arith.* 21 (1972) 7–13; MR 46 #9b.

[6]   S. Plouffe, Sierpinski constant (Plouffe's Tables).

[7]   E. Grosswald, *Representations of Integers as Sums of Squares*, Springer-Verlag, 1985, pp. 20–21; MR 87g:11002.

[8]   H. Iwaniec and C. J. Mozzochi, On the divisor and circle problems, *J. Number Theory* 29 (1988) 60–93; MR 89g:11091.

[9]   M. N. Huxley, Exponential sums and lattice points. II, *Proc. London Math. Soc.* 66 (1993) 279–301; corrigenda 68 (1994) 264; MR 94b:11100 and MR 95d:11134.

[10] R. K. Guy, *Unsolved Problems in Number Theory*, 2nd ed., Springer-Verlag, 1994, sect. F1; MR 96e:11002.

[11] A. Ivić, *The Riemann Zeta-Function*, Wiley, 1985, pp. 35–36, 93–94, 351–384; MR 87d:11062.

[12] E. Krätzel, *Lattice Points*, Kluwer, 1988, pp. 140–142, 228–230; MR 90e:11144.

[13] S. Ramanujan, Some formulae in the analytic theory of numbers, *Messenger of Math.* 45 (1916) 81–84; also in *Collected Papers*, ed. G. H. Hardy, P. V. Seshu Aiyar, and B. M. Wilson, Cambridge Univ. Press, 1927, pp. 133–135, 339–340.

[14] B. M. Wilson, Proofs of some formulae enunciated by Ramanujan, *Proc. London Math. Soc.* 21 (1922) 235–255.

[15] D. Suryanarayana and R. Sitaramachandra Rao, On an asymptotic formula of Ramanujan, *Math. Scand.* 32 (1973) 258–264; MR 49 #2611.

[16] S. A. Amitsur, Some results on arithmetic functions, *J. Math. Soc. Japan* 11 (1959) 275–290; MR 26 #67.

[17] R. C. Baker, The square-free divisor problem, *Quart. J. Math* 45 (1994) 269–277; part II, *Quart. J. Math* 47 (1996) 133–146; MR 95h:11098 and MR 97f:11080.

[18] W. G. Nowak, On sums and differences of two relative prime cubes, *Analysis* 15 (1995) 325–341; part II, *Tatra Mount. Math. Publ.* 11 (1997) 23–34; MR 96m:11085 and MR 98j:11073.

[19] M. Kühleitner, On sums of two k^{th} powers: An asymptotic formula for the mean square of the error term, *Acta Arith.* 92 (2000) 263–276; MR 2001a:11164.

[20] W. Sierpinski, On the average values of several numerical functions (in Polish), *Sprawozdania Towarzystwo Naukowe Warszawskie* 1 (1908) 215–226.

[21] S. M. Lee, On the sum of the largest k^{th} divisors, *Kyungpook Math. J.* 15 (1975) 105–108; MR 51 #5528.

[22] K. Greger, Square divisors and square-free numbers, *Math. Mag.* 51 (1978) 211–219; MR 58 #21916.

2.11 Abundant Numbers Density Constant

If n is a positive integer, let $\sigma(n)$ denote the sum of all positive divisors of n. Then n is said to be **perfect** if $\sigma(n) = 2n$, **deficient** if $\sigma(n) < 2n$, and **abundant** if $\sigma(n) > 2n$.

The smallest examples of perfect numbers are 6 and 28. If the Mersenne number $2^{m+1} - 1$ is prime, then $2^m(2^{m+1} - 1)$ is perfect. Here are two famous unanswered questions [1]. Do there exist infinitely many even perfect numbers? Does there exist an odd perfect number? (According to [2], a counterexample cannot be less than 10^{300}.)

For positive real x, define the density function

$$A(x) = \lim_{n \to \infty} \frac{|\{n : \sigma(n) \geq x\,n\}|}{n}.$$

Behrend [3, 4], Davenport [5], and Chowla [6] independently proved that $A(x)$ exists and is continuous for all x. Erdös [7, 8] gave a proof requiring only elementary considerations. Clearly $A(x) = 1$ for $x \leq 1$, and $A(x) \to 0$ as $x \to \infty$. Refining Behrend's technique, Wall [9, 10] obtained the following bounds on the **abundant numbers density constant**:

$$0.2441 < A(2) < 0.2909,$$

and Deléglise [11] improved this to

$$|A(2) - 0.2477| < 0.0003.$$

Further, it can be demonstrated [12] that $A(x)$ is differentiable everywhere except on a set of Lebesgue measure zero, and

$$\int\limits_0^\infty x^{s-1} A(x)\,dx = \frac{1}{s} \prod_p \left[\left(1 - \frac{1}{p}\right)^{-s+1} \sum_{k=0}^\infty \frac{1}{p^k} \left(1 - \frac{1}{p^{k+1}}\right)^s \right]$$

for complex s satisfying $\text{Re}(s) > 1$. The product is over all primes p. An inversion of this identity (Mellin transform) is theoretically possible but not yet numerically feasible [11].

As an aside, define an **exponential divisor** d of $n = p_1^{a_1} \cdots p_r^{a_r}$ to be a divisor of the form $d = p_1^{b_1} \cdots p_r^{b_r}$, where $b_j | a_j$ for each j. Let $\sigma^{(e)}(n)$ denote the sum of all exponential divisors of n, with the convention $\sigma^{(e)}(1) = 1$. Then [13–16]

$$\lim_{N \to \infty} \frac{1}{N^2} \sum_{n=1}^N \sigma(n) = \frac{\pi^2}{12}, \quad \lim_{N \to \infty} \frac{1}{N^2} \sum_{n=1}^N \sigma^{(e)}(n) = B,$$

where

$$B = \frac{1}{2} \prod_p \left[1 + \frac{1}{p(p^2 - 1)} - \frac{1}{p^2 - 1} + \left(1 - \frac{1}{p}\right) \sum_{k=2}^\infty \frac{p^k}{p^{2k} - 1} \right]$$

$$= 0.5682854937\ldots.$$

A study of the corresponding density function $A^{(e)}(x)$ was begun in [17].

[1] K. Ireland and M. Rosen, *A Classical Introduction to Modern Number Theory*, 2nd ed., Springer-Verlag, 1990; MR 92e:11001.

[2] R. K. Guy, *Unsolved Problems in Number Theory*, 2nd ed., Springer-Verlag, 1994, sect. B1, B2; MR 96e:11002.

[3] F. Behrend, Über numeri abundantes, *Sitzungsber. Preuss. Akad. Wiss.* (1932) 322–328.

[4] F. Behrend, Über numeri abundantes. II, *Sitzungsber. Preuss. Akad. Wiss.* (1933) 280–293.

[5] H. Davenport, Über numeri abundantes, *Sitzungsber. Preuss. Akad. Wiss.* (1933) 830–837.

[6] S. Chowla, On abundant numbers, *J. Indian Math. Soc.* 1 (1934) 41–44.

[7] P. Erdös, On the density of the abundant numbers, *J. London Math. Soc.* 9 (1934) 278–282.

[8] P. D. T. A. Elliott, *Probabilistic Number Theory*. I: *Mean-Value Theorems*, Springer-Verlag, 1979, pp. 3–4, 187–189, 203–213; MR 82h:10002a.

[9] C. R. Wall, Density bounds for the sum of divisors function, *The Theory of Arithmetic Functions*, Proc. 1971 Kalamazoo conf., ed. A. A. Gioia and D. L. Goldsmith, Lect. Notes in Math. 251, Springer-Verlag, 1971, pp. 283–287; MR 49 #10650.

[10] C. R. Wall, P. L. Crews, and D. B. Johnson, Density bounds for the sum of divisors function, *Math. Comp.* 26 (1972) 773–777; errata 31 (1977) 616; MR 48 #6042 and MR 55 #286.

[11] M. Deléglise, Bounds for the density of abundant integers, *Experim. Math.* 7 (1998) 137–143; MR 2000a:11137.

[12] J. Martinet, J. M. Deshouillers, and H. Cohen, La fonction somme des diviseurs, *Séminaire de Théorie des Nombres, 1972-1973*, exp. 11, Centre Nat. Recherche Sci., Talence, 1973; MR 52 #13607.

[13] M. V. Subbarao, On some arithmetic convolutions, *The Theory of Arithmetic Functions*, Proc. 1971 Kalamazoo conf., ed. A. A. Gioia and D. L. Goldsmith, Lect. Notes in Math. 251, Springer-Verlag, 1972, pp. 247–271; MR 49 #2510.

[14] J. Fabrykowski and M. V. Subbarao, The maximal order and the average order of multiplicative function $\sigma^{(e)}(n)$, *Théorie des nombres*, Proc. 1987 Québec conf., ed. J.-M. De Koninck and C. Levesque, Gruyter, 1989, pp. 201–206; MR 90m:11012.

[15] J. Wu, Problème de diviseurs exponentiels et entiers exponentiellement sans facteur carré, *J. Théorie Nombres Bordeaux* 7 (1995) 133–141; MR 98e:11108.

[16] A. Smati and J. Wu, On the exponential divisor function, *Publ. Inst. Math. (Beograd)*, v. 61 (1997) n. 75, 21–32; MR 98k:11127.

[17] P. Hagis, Some results concerning exponential divisors, *Int. J. Math. Math. Sci.* 11 (1988) 343–349; MR 90d:11011.

2.12 Linnik's Constant

We first discuss prime values of a specific sequence. Dirichlet's theorem states that any arithmetic progression $\{an + b : n \geq 0\}$, for which $a \geq 1$ and $b \geq 1$ are coprime, must contain infinitely many primes. This raises a natural question: How large is the first such prime $p(a, b)$?

Define $p(a)$ to be the maximum of $p(a, b)$ over all b satisfying $1 \leq b < a$, $\gcd(a, b) = 1$ and let

$$K = \sup_{a \geq 2} \frac{\ln(p(a))}{\ln(a)}, \quad L = \lim_{a \to \infty} \frac{\ln(p(a))}{\ln(a)}.$$

That is, K is the infimum of κ satisfying $p(a) < a^\kappa$ for all $a \geq 2$, and L is the infimum of λ satisfying $p(a) < a^\lambda$ for all sufficiently large a. Much research [1, 2] has been devoted to evaluating K and L, as well as to determining other forms of upper and lower bounds on $p(a, b)$.

Clearly $K > 1.82$ (witness the case $p(5) = 19$). Schinzel & Sierpinski [3] and Kanold [4, 5] conjectured that $K \leq 2$. If true, this would imply that there exists a prime somewhere in the following list:

$$b, a + b, 2a + b, \ldots, (a - 1)a + b$$

if $\gcd(a, b) = 1$. Such a statement is beyond the reach of present-day mathematics. Schinzel & Sierpinski that confessed they did not know what the fate of their hypothesis (among several) might be. Ribenboim [2] wondered if such hypotheses might be undecidable within the framework of Peano axiomatic arithmetic.

Linnik [6, 7] proved that L exists and is finite. Clearly $L \leq K$. If we assume a generalized Riemann hypothesis, it is known that [8–10]

$$p(a) = O(\varphi(a)^2 \ln(a)^2),$$

which would imply that $L \leq 2$. Here $\varphi(x)$ denotes the Euler totient function [2.7]. The search for an unconditional upper bound for **Linnik's constant** L has occupied many researchers [11–13]. A culmination of this work is Heath-Brown's proof [14] that $L \leq 5.5$.

Partial evidence for $L \leq 2$ includes the following. For any fixed positive integers b and k, Bombieri, Friedlander & Iwaniec [15] proved that

$$p(a, b) < \frac{a^2}{\ln(a)^k}$$

for every a outside a set of density zero, as observed by Granville [16, 17]. We may therefore infer $L \leq 2$ for *almost all* integers a.

Chowla [18] believed that $L = 1$. Subsequent authors [19–23] conjectured that

$$p(a) = O(\varphi(a) \ln(a)^2),$$

which would imply that $L = 1$. An earlier theorem of Elliott & Halberstam [24] provides partial support for this new estimate.

We now turn attention to prime solutions of a specific equation. Liu & Tsang [25–28], among others, investigated existence issues of prime solutions p, q, r of the linear equation $ap + bq + cr = d$, where a, b, c are nonzero integers and where it is further assumed that $a + b + c - d$ is even and that $\gcd(a, b, c)$, $\gcd(d, a, b)$, $\gcd(d, a, c)$, $\gcd(d, b, c)$ are each 1. (Note that, if we were to allow $c = 0$, then the case $a = b = 1$ would be equivalent to Goldbach's conjecture and the case $a = 1, b = -1, d = 2$ would be equivalent to the twin prime conjecture.)

There are two cases, depending on whether a, b, c are all positive or not. We discuss only one case here: Suppose a, b, c are not all of the same sign. Then there exists a constant μ with the property that the equation $ap + bq + cr = d$ must have a solution in primes p, q, r satisfying

$$\max(p, q, r) \leq 3|d| + (\max(3, |a|, |b|, |c|))^\mu .$$

This result is a generalization of Linnik's original theorem.

The infimum M of all such μ is known as **Baker's constant** [29] and it can be proved that $L \leq M$. The best-known upper bound [30, 31] for M is 45 (unconditional) and 4 (assuming a generalized Riemann hypothesis). Liu & Tsang, like Chowla, conjectured that $M = 1$.

[1] R. K. Guy, *Unsolved Problems in Number Theory*, 2nd ed., Springer-Verlag, 1994, sect. A4; MR 96e:11002.

[2] P. Ribenboim, *The New Book of Prime Number Records*, Springer-Verlag, 1996, pp. 277–284, 397–400; MR 96k:11112.

[3] A. Schinzel and W. Sierpinski, Sur certaines hypothèses concernant les nombres premiers, *Acta Arith.* 4 (1958) 185–208; erratum 5 (1959) 259; MR 21 #4936.

[4] H.-J. Kanold, Elementare Betrachtungen zur Primzahltheorie, *Arch. Math.* 14 (1963) 147–151; MR 27 #89.

[5] H.-J. Kanold, Über Primzahlen in arithmetischen Folgen, *Math. Annalen* 156 (1964) 393–395; 157 (1965) 358–362; MR 30 #70 and MR 37 #5168.

[6] U. V. Linnik, On the least prime in an arithmetic progression. I: The basic theorem, *Mat. Sbornik* 15 (1944) 139–178; MR 6,260b.

[7] U. V. Linnik, On the least prime in an arithmetic progression. II: The Deuring-Heilbronn phenomenon, *Mat. Sbornik* 15 (1944) 347–368; MR 6,260c.

[8] E. C. Titchmarsh, A divisor problem, *Rend. Circ. Mat. Palmero* 54 (1930) 414–429.

[9] Y. Wang, S.-K. Hsieh, and K.-J. Yu, Two results on the distribution of prime numbers (in Chinese), *J. China Univ. Sci. Technol.* 1 (1965) 32–38; MR 34 #7482.

[10] C. Hooley, The distribution of sequences in arithmetic progressions, *International Congress of Mathematicians*, v. 1, Proc. 1974 Vancouver conf., ed. R. D. James, Canad. Math. Congress, 1975, pp. 357–364; MR 58 #16560.

[11] M. Jutila, On Linnik's constant, *Math. Scand.* 41 (1977) 45–62; MR 57 #16230.

[12] S. Graham, On Linnik's constant, *Acta Arith.* 39 (1981) 163–179; MR 83d:10050.

[13] J. R. Chen and J. M. Liu, On the least prime in an arithmetical progression and theorems concerning the zeros of Dirichlet's L-functions. V, *International Symposium in Memory of Hua Loo Keng*, v. 1, Proc. 1988 Beijing conf., ed. S. Gong, Q. K. Lu, Y. Wang, and L. Yang, Springer-Verlag, 1991, pp. 19–42; MR 92m:11093.

[14] D. R. Heath-Brown, Zero-free regions for Dirichlet L-functons and the least prime in an arithmetic progression, *Proc. London Math. Soc.* 64 (1992) 265–338; MR 93a:11075.

[15] E. Bombieri, J. B. Friedlander, and H. Iwaniec, Primes in arithmetic progressions to large moduli. III, *J. Amer. Math. Soc.* 2 (1989) 215–224; MR 89m:11087.

[16] A. Granville, Least primes in arithmetic progressions, *Théorie des nombres*, Proc. 1987 Québec conf., ed. J. M. De Koninck and C. Levesque, Gruyter, 1989, pp. 306–321; MR 91c:11052.

[17] A. Granville, Some conjectures in analytic number theory and their connection with Fermat's last theorem, *Analytic Number Theory*, Proc. 1989 Allerton Park conf., ed. B. C. Berndt, H. G. Diamond, H. Halberstam, and A. Hildebrand, Birkhäuser, 1990, pp. 311–326; MR 92a:11031.

[18] S. Chowla, On the least prime in an arithmetical progression, *J. Indian Math. Soc.* 1 (1934) 1–3.

[19] D. R. Heath-Brown, Almost-primes in arithmetic progressions and short intervals, *Math. Proc. Cambridge Philos. Soc.* 83 (1978) 357–375; MR 58 #10789.

[20] S. S. Wagstaff, Greatest of the least primes in arithmetic progressions having a given modulus, *Math. Comp.* 33 (1979) 1073–1080; MR 81e:10038.

[21] C. Pomerance, A note on the least prime in an arithmetic progression, *J. Number Theory* 12 (1980) 218–223; MR 81m:10081.

[22] K. S. McCurley, The least r-free number in an arithmetic progression, *Trans. Amer. Math. Soc.* 293 (1986) 467–475; MR 87b:11016.

[23] A. Granville and C. Pomerance, On the least prime in certain arithmetic progressions, *J. London Math. Soc.* 41 (1990) 193–200; MR 91i:11119.

[24] P. D. T. A. Elliott and H. Halberstam, The least prime in an arithmetic progression, *Studies in Pure Mathematics*, ed. L. Mirsky, Academic Press, 1971, pp. 59–61; MR 42 #7609.

[25] M. C. Liu and K. M. Tsang, Small prime solutions of linear equations, *Théorie des nombres*, Proc. 1987 Québec conf., ed. J. M. De Koninck and C. Levesque, Gruyter, 1989, pp. 595–624; MR 90i:11112.

[26] K. K. Choi, M. C. Liu, and K. M. Tsang, Small prime solutions of linear equations. II, *Proc. Amalfi Conf. on Analytic Number Theory*, Maiori, 1989, ed. E. Bombieri. A. Perelli, S. Salerno, and U. Zannier, Univ. Salerno, 1992, pp. 1–16; MR 94i:11080.

[27] K. K. Choi, M. C. Liu, and K. M. Tsang, Conditional bounds for small prime solutions of linear equations, *Manuscripta Math.* 74 (1992) 321–340; MR 93a:11084.

[28] M. C. Liu and K. M. Tsang, Recent progress on a problem of A. Baker, *Séminaire de Théorie des Nombres, Paris, 1991–92*, ed. S. David, Birkhäuser, 1993, pp. 121–133; MR 95h:11107.

[29] A. Baker, On some diophantine inequalities involving primes, *J. Reine Angew. Math.* 228 (1967) 166–181; MR 36 #111.

[30] K. K. Choi, A numerical bound for Baker's constant – Some explicit estimates for small prime solutions of linear equations, *Bull. Hong Kong Math. Soc.* 1 (1997) 1–19; MR 98k:11137.

[31] M. C. Liu and T. Wang, A numerical bound for small prime solutions of some ternary linear equations, *Acta Arith.* 86 (1998) 343–383; MR 99m:11115.

2.13 Mills' Constant

Mills [1] demonstrated the surprising existence of a positive constant C such that the expression $\left\lfloor C^{3^N} \right\rfloor$ yields only prime numbers for all positive integers N. (Recall that $\lfloor x \rfloor$ denotes the largest integer not exceeding x.) The proof is based on a difficult theorem in prime number theory due to Hoheisel [2] and refined by Ingham [3]: If $p < p'$ are consecutive primes, then given $\varepsilon > 0$,

$$p' - p < p^{(5/8)+\varepsilon}$$

for sufficiently large p. This inequality is used to define the following recursive sequence. Let $q_0 = 2$ and q_{n+1} be the least prime exceeding q_n^3 for each $n \geq 0$. For example [4,5], $q_1 = 11$, $q_2 = 1361$, and $q_3 = 2521008887$. The Hoheisel–Ingham theorem implies that

$$q_n^3 < q_{n+1} < q_{n+1} + 1 < q_n^3 + q_n^{(15/8)+3\varepsilon} + 1 < (q_n + 1)^3$$

for large n; hence

$$q_n^{3^{-n}} < q_{n+1}^{3^{-(n+1)}} < (q_{n+1} + 1)^{3^{-(n+1)}} < (q_n + 1)^{3^{-n}}.$$

We deduce that $C = \lim_{n \to \infty} q_n^{3^{-n}}$ exists, which yields the desired prime-representing result. For the particular sequence selected here [4, 6, 7], it is easily computed that $C = 1.3063778838\ldots$.

A different choice of starting value q_0 or variation in the exponent 3 will provide a different value of C. There are infinitely many such quantities C; that is, Mills' constant $1.3063778838\ldots$ is not the unique value of C to give only prime numbers. A generalization of Mills' theorem (to arbitrary sequences of positive integers obeying a growth restriction) is an exercise in [8].

Another constant, $c = 1.9287800\ldots$, appears in Wright [9] as part of an alternative prime-representing function:

$$\left\lfloor 2^{2^{2^{\cdot^{\cdot^{\cdot^{2^c}}}}}} \right\rfloor,$$

the iterated exponential with N 2s and c at the top. Unlike Mills' example, this example does not require a deep theorem to work. All that is needed is the fact that $p' < 2p$, which is known as Bertrand's postulate.

Several authors [6, 7, 10] wisely pointed out that formulas like that of Mills are not very useful. One would need to know C correctly to many places to compute only a few primes. To make matters worse, there does not seem to be any way of estimating C *except* via the primes $q_1, q_2, q_3, \ldots$ (i.e., the reasoning becomes circular). The only manner in which Mills' formula could be useful is if an *exact* value for C were to somehow become available, which no one has conjectured might ever happen.

Nevertheless, the sheer existence of C is striking. It is not known whether C must necessarily be irrational. A similar constant, $1.6222705028\ldots$, due to Odlyzko & Wilf, arises in [2.30]. See [11] for a related problem concerning expressions of the form $\lfloor C^N \rfloor$.

Huxley [12], among others, succeeded in replacing the exponent 5/8 by 7/12. Recent work in sharpening the Hoheisel–Ingham theorem includes [13–16]. The best result known to date is

$$p' - p = O(p^{0.525}).$$

Assuming the Riemann hypothesis to be true, Cramér [17, 18] proved that

$$p' - p = O(\sqrt{p}\ln(p)),$$

which would be a dramatic improvement if the unproved assertion someday falls to analysis. He subsequently conjectured that [19]

$$p' - p = O(\ln(p)^2)$$

and, moreover,

$$\limsup_{p\to\infty} \frac{p' - p}{\ln(p)^2} = 1.$$

Granville [20, 21], building upon the work of Maier [22], revised this conjecture as follows:

$$\limsup_{p\to\infty} \frac{p' - p}{\ln(p)^2} \geq 2e^{-\gamma} = 1.122\ldots,$$

where γ is Euler's constant [1.5]. It has been known for a long time [23] that

$$\limsup_{p\to\infty} \frac{p' - p}{\ln(p)} = \infty;$$

thus Cramér's bound $\ln(p)^2$ cannot be replaced by $\ln(p)$. However, we have [24–26]

$$\liminf_{p \to \infty} \frac{p' - p}{\ln(p)} \leq 0.248.$$

Is further improvement possible? If the twin prime conjecture is true [2.1], then the limit infimum is clearly 0.

[1]   W. H. Mills, A prime-representing function, *Bull. Amer. Math. Soc.* 53 (1947) 604; MR 8,567d.

[2]   G. Hoheisel, Primzahlprobleme in der Analysis, *Sitzungsber. Preuss. Akad. Wiss.* (1930) 580–588.

[3]   A. E. Ingham, On the difference between consecutive primes, *Quart. J. Math.* 8 (1937) 255–266.

[4]   C. K. Caldwell, Mills' theorem – A generalization (Prime Pages).

[5]   N. J. A. Sloane, On-Line Encyclopedia of Integer Sequences, A051254 and A016104.

[6]   P. Ribenboim, *The New Book of Prime Number Records*, Springer-Verlag, 1996, pp. 186–187, 252–257; MR 96k:11112.

[7]   R. L. Graham, D. E. Knuth, and O. Patashnik, *Concrete Mathematics*, 2nd ed., Addison-Wesley, 1994, pp. 109, 150, and 523; MR 97d:68003.

[8]   W. Ellison and F. Ellison, *Prime Numbers*, Wiley, 1985, pp. 22, 31–32; MR 87a:11082.

[9]   E. M. Wright, A prime-representing function, *Amer. Math. Monthly* 58 (1951) 616–618; MR 13,321e.

[10]   G. H. Hardy and E. M. Wright, *An Introduction to the Theory of Numbers*, 5th ed., Oxford Univ. Press, 1985, pp. 344–345, 414; MR 81i:10002.

[11]   R. C. Baker and G. Harman, Primes of the form $\lfloor c^p \rfloor$, *Math. Z.* 221 (1996) 73–81; MR 96k:11115.

[12]   M. N. Huxley, On the difference between consecutive primes, *Invent. Math.* 15 (1972) 164–170; MR 45 #1856.

[13]   C. J. Mozzochi, On the difference between consecutive primes, *J. Number Theory* 24 (1986) 181–187; MR 88b:11057.

[14]   S. T. Lou and Q. Yao, The number of primes in a short interval, *Hardy-Ramanujan J.* 16 (1993) 21–43; MR 94b:11089.

[15]   R. C. Baker and G. Harman, The difference between consecutive primes, *Proc. London Math. Soc.* 72 (1996) 261–280; MR 96k:11111.

[16]   R. C. Baker, G. Harman, and J. Pintz, The difference between consecutive primes. II, *Proc. London Math. Soc.* 83 (2001) 532–562; MR 2002f:11125.

[17]   H. Cramér, Some theorems concerning prime numbers, *Ark. Mat. Astron. Fysik*, v. 15 (1920) n. 5, 1–32; also in *Collected Works*, v. 1, ed. A. Martin-Löf, Springer-Verlag, 1994, pp. 138–170.

[18]   A. Ivić, *The Riemann Zeta-Function*, Wiley, 1985, pp. 321–330, 349–350; MR 87d:11062.

[19]   H. Cramér, On the order of magnitude of the differences between consecutive prime numbers, *Acta Arith.* 2 (1936) 23–46; also in *Collected Works*, v. 2, ed. A. Martin-Löf, Springer-Verlag, 1994, pp. 871–894.

[20]   A. Granville, Unexpected irregularities in the distribution of prime numbers, *International Congress of Mathematicians*, v. 1, Proc. 1994 Zürich conf., ed. S. D. Chatterji, Birkhäuser, 1995, pp. 388–399; MR 97d:11139.

[21]   A. Granville, Harald Cramér and the distribution of prime numbers, *Scand. Actuar. J.* (1995) n. 1, 12–28; MR 96g:01002.

[22]   H. Maier, Primes in short intervals, *Michigan Math. J.* 32 (1985) 221–225; MR 86i:11049.

[23]   E. Westzynthius, Über die Verteilung der Zahlen die zu den n ersten Primzahlen teilerfremd sind, *Comment. Phys. Math. Soc. Sci. Fenn.*, v. 5 (1931) n. 25, 1–37.

[24]   E. Bombieri and H. Davenport, Small differences between prime numbers, *Proc. Royal Soc. Ser. A* 293 (1966) 1–18; MR 33 #7314.

[25] M. N. Huxley, Small differences between consecutive primes. II, *Mathematika* 24 (1977) 142–152; MR 57 #5925.

[26] H. Maier, Small differences between prime numbers, *Michigan Math. J.* 35 (1988) 323–344; MR 90e:11126.

2.14 Brun's Constant

Brun's constant is defined to be the sum of the reciprocals of all twin primes [1,2]:

$$B_2 = \left(\frac{1}{3} + \frac{1}{5}\right) + \left(\frac{1}{5} + \frac{1}{7}\right) + \left(\frac{1}{11} + \frac{1}{13}\right) + \left(\frac{1}{17} + \frac{1}{19}\right) + \left(\frac{1}{29} + \frac{1}{31}\right) + \cdots.$$

Note that the prime 5 is taken twice (some authors do not do this). If this series were divergent, then a proof of the twin prime conjecture [2.1] would follow immediately. Brun proved, however, that the series is convergent and thus B_2 is finite [3–8]. His result demonstrates the scarcity of twin primes relative to all primes (whose reciprocal sum is divergent [2.2]), but it does not shed any light on whether the number of twin primes is finite or infinite.

Selmer [9], Fröberg [10], Bohman [11], Shanks & Wrench [12], Brent [13,14], Nicely [15–18], Sebah [19], and others successively improved numerical estimates of B_2. The most recent calculations give

$$B_2 = 1.9021605831\ldots$$

using large datasets of twin primes and assuming the truth of the extended twin prime conjecture [2.1]. Let us elaborate on the latter issue. Under Hardy & Littlewood's hypothesis, the raw summation of twin prime reciprocals converges very slowly:

$$\sum_{\substack{\text{twin} \\ p \leq n}} \frac{1}{p} - B_2 = O\left(\frac{1}{\ln(n)}\right),$$

but the following extrapolation helps to accelerate the process [10,12,15]:

$$\left(\sum_{\substack{\text{twin} \\ p \leq n}} \frac{1}{p} + \frac{4C_{\text{twin}}}{\ln(n)}\right) - B_2 = O\left(\frac{1}{\sqrt{n}\ln(n)}\right),$$

where $C_{\text{twin}} = 0.6601618158\ldots$ is the twin prime constant. Higher order extrapolations exist but do not present practical advantages as yet. In the midst of his computations, Nicely [15] uncovered the infamous Intel Pentium error.

We discuss three relevant variations. Let A_3 denote the reciprocal sum of prime 3-tuples of the form $(p, p+2, p+6)$, A_3' the reciprocal sum of prime 3-tuples of the form $(p, p+4, p+6)$, and A_4 the reciprocal sum of prime 4-tuples of the form $(p, p+2, p+6, p+8)$. Nicely [2,20] calculated

$$A_3 = 1.0978510391\ldots, \quad A_3' = 0.8371132125\ldots, \quad A_4 = 0.8705883800\ldots.$$

Define B_h, where $h \geq 2$ is an even integer, to be the reciprocal sum of primes separated by h, and define $\tilde{B}_h$ to be the reciprocal sum of *consecutive* primes separated by h. Segal proved that B_h is finite for all h [5, 21, 22]; thus $\tilde{B}_h$ is finite as well. Clearly $B_2 = \tilde{B}_2$ and

$$B_4 = \left(\frac{1}{3} + \frac{1}{7}\right) + \left(\frac{1}{7} + \frac{1}{11}\right) + \left(\frac{1}{13} + \frac{1}{17}\right) + \left(\frac{1}{19} + \frac{1}{23}\right) + \cdots = \tilde{B}_4 + \frac{10}{21},$$

but highly precise computations of B_h or $\tilde{B}_h$, $h \geq 4$, have not yet been performed. Wolf [23] speculated that, for $h \geq 6$,

$$\tilde{B}_h = \frac{4C_{\text{twin}}}{h} \prod_{\substack{p|h \\ p>2}} \frac{p-1}{p-2}$$

on the basis of a small dataset. Even if his conjecture is eventually shown to be false, it should inspire more attempts to relate such generalized Brun's constants to other constants found in number theory.

[1] H. Riesel, *Prime Numbers and Computer Methods for Factorization*, Birkhäuser, 1985, pp. 64–65; MR 95h:11142.

[2] P. Ribenboim, *The New Book of Prime Number Records*, 3rd ed., Springer-Verlag, 1996, pp. 261, 509–510; MR 96k:11112.

[3] V. Brun, La série $1/5 + 1/7 + 1/11 + 1/13 + 1/17 + 1/19 + 1/29 + 1/31 + 1/41 + 1/43 + 1/59 + 1/61 + \cdots$ où les dénominateurs sont "nombres premiers jumeaux" est convergente ou finie, *Bull. Sci. Math.* 43 (1919) 100–104, 124–128.

[4] H. Rademacher, *Lectures on Elementary Number Theory*, Blaisdell, 1964, pp. 137–144; MR 58 #10677.

[5] H. Halberstam and H.-E. Richert, *Sieve Methods*, Academic Press, 1974, pp. 50–52, 91–92, 116–117; MR 54 #12689.

[6] W. J. LeVeque, *Fundamentals of Number Theory*, Addison-Wesley, 1977, pp. 173–177; MR 58 #465.

[7] M. B. Nathanson, *Additive Number Theory: The Classical Bases*, Springer-Verlag, 1996, pp. 167–174; MR 97e:11004.

[8] K. D. Boklan, Fugitive pieces: Elementary results for twin primes, unpublished note (2000).

[9] E. S. Selmer, A special summation method in the theory of prime numbers and its application to "Brun's sum" (in Norwegian), *Norsk. Mat. Tidsskr.* 24 (1942) 74–81; MR 8,316g.

[10] C.-E. Fröberg, On the sum of inverses of primes and twin primes, *Nordisk Tidskr. Informat. (BIT)* 1 (1961) 15–20.

[11] J. Bohman, Some computational results regarding the prime numbers below 2,000,000,000, *Nordisk Tidskr. Informat. (BIT)* 13 (1973) 242–244; errata 14 (1974) 127; MR 48 #217.

[12] D. Shanks and J. W. Wrench, Brun's constant, *Math. Comp.* 28 (1974) 293–299; corrigenda 28 (1974) 1183; MR 50 #4510.

[13] R. P. Brent, Irregularities in the distribution of primes and twin primes, *Math. Comp.* 29 (1975) 43–56, correction 30 (1976) 198; MR 51 #5522 and 53 #302.

[14] R. P. Brent, Tables concerning irregularities in the distribution of primes and twin primes up to 10^{11}, *Math. Comp.* 29 (1975) 331; 30 (1976) 379.

[15] T. R. Nicely, Enumeration to 10^{14} of the twin primes and Brun's constant, *Virginia J. Sci.* 46 (1995) 195–204; MR 97e:11014.

[16] R. P. Brent, Review of T. R. Nicely's paper, *Math. Comp.* 66 (1997) 924–925.

[17] T. R. Nicely, Enumeration to $1.6 \cdot 10^{15}$ of the twin primes and Brun's constant, unpublished note (1999).

[18] T. R. Nicely, A new error analysis for Brun's constant, *Virginia J. Sci.* 52 (2001) 45–55.

[19] P. Sebah, Counting twin primes and estimating Brun's constant up to 10^{16} (Numbers, Constants and Computation).
[20] T. R. Nicely, Enumeration to $1.6 \cdot 10^{15}$ of the prime quadruplets, unpublished note (1999).
[21] B. Segal, Generalization of a theorem of Brun's (in Russian), *C. R. Acad. Sci. URSS A* (1930) 501–507.
[22] W. Narkiewicz, *Number Theory*, World Scientific, 1983, pp. 144–153; MR 85j:11002.
[23] M. Wolf, Generalized Brun's constants, unpublished note (1997).

2.15 Glaisher–Kinkelin Constant

Stirling's formula [1]

$$\lim_{n \to \infty} \frac{n!}{e^{-n} n^{n+\frac{1}{2}}} = \sqrt{2\pi}$$

provides a well-known estimate for large factorials. If we replace $n! = \Gamma(n+1)$ by different expressions, for example,

$$K(n+1) = \prod_{m=1}^{n} m^m \text{ or } G(n+1) = \frac{(n!)^n}{K(n+1)} = \prod_{m=1}^{n-1} m!$$

then the approximation takes different forms. Kinkelin [2], Jeffery [3], and Glaisher [4–6] demonstrated that

$$\lim_{n \to \infty} \frac{K(n+1)}{e^{-\frac{1}{4}n^2} n^{\frac{1}{2}n^2 + \frac{1}{2}n + \frac{1}{12}}} = A \text{ and } \lim_{n \to \infty} \frac{G(n+1)}{e^{-\frac{3}{4}n^2} (2\pi)^{\frac{1}{2}n} n^{\frac{1}{2}n^2 - \frac{1}{12}}} = \frac{e^{\frac{1}{12}}}{A}.$$

The constant A, which plays the same role in these approximations as $\sqrt{2\pi}$ plays in Stirling's formula, has the following closed-form expression:

$$A = \exp\left(\frac{1}{12} - \zeta'(-1) \right) = \exp\left(\frac{-\zeta'(2)}{2\pi^2} + \frac{\ln(2\pi) + \gamma}{12} \right) = 1.2824271291\ldots,$$

where $\zeta'(x)$ is the derivative of the Riemann zeta function [1.6] and γ is the Euler–Mascheroni constant [1.5]. See [2.10] and [2.18] for other occurrences of $\zeta'(2)$.

Many beautiful formulas involving A exist, including two infinite products [6]:

$$1^{\frac{1}{1}} \cdot 2^{\frac{1}{4}} \cdot 3^{\frac{1}{9}} \cdot 4^{\frac{1}{16}} \cdot 5^{\frac{1}{25}} \cdots = \left(\frac{A^{12}}{2\pi e^{\gamma}} \right)^{\frac{\pi^2}{6}},$$

$$1^{\frac{1}{1}} \cdot 3^{\frac{1}{9}} \cdot 5^{\frac{1}{25}} \cdot 7^{\frac{1}{49}} \cdot 9^{\frac{1}{81}} \cdots = \left(\frac{A^{36}}{2^4 \pi^3 e^{3\gamma}} \right)^{\frac{\pi^2}{24}},$$

and two definite integrals [4, 7]:

$$\int_0^{\infty} \frac{x \ln(x)}{e^{2\pi x} - 1} dx = \frac{1}{24} - \frac{1}{2} \ln(A),$$

$$\int_0^{1/2} \ln(\Gamma(x+1)) dx = -\frac{1}{2} - \frac{7}{24} \ln(2) + \frac{1}{4} \ln(\pi) + \frac{3}{2} \ln(A).$$

More formulas are found in [8–12].

A generalization of the latter integral,

$$\int_0^x \ln(\Gamma(t+1))dt = \frac{1}{2}\ln(2\pi)x - \frac{1}{2}x(x+1) + x\ln(\Gamma(x+1)) - \ln(G(x+1)),$$

was obtained by Alexeiewsky [13], Hölder [14], and Barnes [15–17] using an analytic extension of $G(n+1)$. Just as the gamma function extends the factorial function $\Gamma(n+1)$ to the complex z-plane, the **Barnes G-function**

$$G(z+1) = (2\pi)^{\frac{1}{2}z} e^{-\frac{1}{2}z(z+1)-\frac{\gamma}{2}z^2} \prod_{n=1}^{\infty} \left(1+\frac{z}{n}\right)^n e^{-z+\frac{1}{2n}z^2}$$

extends $G(n+1)$. Just as the gamma function assumes a special value at $z = 1/2$:

$$\Gamma\left(\frac{1}{2}\right) = \left(-\frac{1}{2}\right)! = \sqrt{\pi},$$

the Barnes function satisfies

$$G\left(\frac{1}{2}\right) = 2^{\frac{1}{24}} e^{\frac{1}{8}} \pi^{-\frac{1}{4}} A^{-\frac{3}{2}}.$$

A similar, natural extension of Kinkelin's function via $K(z+1) = \Gamma(z+1)^z / G(z+1)$ has been comparatively neglected by researchers in favor of G. Here is a sample application. Define

$$D(x) = \lim_{n\to\infty} \prod_{k=1}^{2n+1} \left(1+\frac{x}{k}\right)^{(-1)^{k+1}k} = \exp(x) \cdot \lim_{n\to\infty} \prod_{k=1}^{2n} \left(1+\frac{x}{k}\right)^{(-1)^{k+1}k}.$$

Melzak [18] proved that $D(2) = \pi e/2$. Borwein & Dykshoorn [19] extended this result to

$$D(x) = \left(\frac{\Gamma(\frac{x}{2}+\frac{1}{2})}{\Gamma(\frac{x}{2})}\right)^x \left(\frac{K(\frac{x}{2})K(\frac{1}{2})}{K(\frac{x}{2}+\frac{1}{2})}\right)^2 \exp(-\frac{x}{2}).$$

where $x > 0$. As a special case, $D(1) = A^6/(2^{\frac{1}{6}}\pi^{\frac{1}{2}})$.

Apart from infrequent whispers [20–27], the Glaisher–Kinkelin constant seemed largely forgotten until recently. Vignéras [28], Voros [29], Sarnak [30], Vardi [31], and others revived interest in the Barnes G-function because of its connection to certain spectral functions in mathematical physics and differential geometry. There is also a connection with random matrix theory and the spacing of zeta function zeros [32–34]. See [2.15.3] and [5.22] as well. Thus generalizations of the formulas here for $\Gamma(1/2)$ and $G(1/2)$ possess a significance unanticipated by their original discoverers.

2.15.1 Generalized Glaisher Constants

Bendersky [35, 36] studied the product $1^{1^k} \cdot 2^{2^k} \cdot 3^{3^k} \cdot 4^{4^k} \cdots n^{n^k}$, which is $n!$ for $k = 0$ and $K(n+1)$ for $k = 1$. More precisely, he examined the logarithm of the product and determined the value of the limit

$$\ln(A_k) = \lim_{n \to \infty} \left(\sum_{m=1}^{n} m^k \ln(m) - p_k(n) \right),$$

where

$$p_k(n) = \left(\frac{n^{k+1}}{k+1} + \frac{n^k}{2} + \frac{B_{k+1}}{k+1} \right) \ln(n) - \frac{n^{k+1}}{(k+1)^2}$$

$$+ k! \sum_{j=1}^{k-1} \frac{B_{j+1}}{(j+1)!} \frac{n^{k-j}}{(k-j)!} \left(\ln(n) + \sum_{i=1}^{j} \frac{1}{k-i+1} \right)$$

and B_n is the nth Bernoulli number [1.6.1]. Clearly $A_0 = \sqrt{2\pi}$ and $A_1 = A$. Choudhury [37] and Adamchik [38] obtained the following exact expression for all $k \geq 0$:

$$A_k = \exp \left(\frac{B_{k+1}}{k+1} \sum_{j=1}^{k} \frac{1}{j} - \zeta'(-k) \right) = \begin{cases} 1.0309167521\ldots & \text{if } k = 2, \\ 0.9795555269\ldots & \text{if } k = 3, \\ 0.9920479745\ldots & \text{if } k = 4, \\ 1.0096803872\ldots & \text{if } k = 5. \end{cases}$$

Zeta derivatives at negative integers can be transformed: If $n > 0$, then [12, 39]

$$\zeta'(-2n) = (-1)^n \frac{(2n)!}{2(2\pi)^{2n}} \zeta(2n + 1),$$

$$\zeta'(-2n + 1) = \frac{1}{2n} \left[(-1)^{n+1} \frac{2(2n)!}{(2\pi)^{2n}} \zeta'(2n) + \left(\sum_{j=1}^{2n-1} \frac{1}{j} - \ln(2\pi) - \gamma \right) B_{2n} \right].$$

It follows that $\ln(A_2) = \zeta(3)/(4\pi^2)$ and $\ln(A_3) = 3\zeta'(4)/(4\pi^4) - (\ln(2\pi) + \gamma)/120$.

2.15.2 Multiple Barnes Functions

Barnes [40] defined a sequence of functions $\{G_n(z)\}$ on the complex plane satisfying

$$G_0(z) = z, \qquad G_n(1) = 1, \qquad G_{n+1}(z + 1) = \frac{G_{n+1}(z)}{G_n(z)} \quad \text{for } n \geq 0.$$

The sequence is unique, by an argument akin to the Bohr–Mollerup theorem [41], if it is further assumed that

$$(-1)^n \frac{d^{n+1}}{dx^{n+1}} \ln(G_n(x)) \geq 0 \quad \text{for } x > 0.$$

Clearly $G_1(z) = 1/\Gamma(z)$ and $G_2(z) = G(z)$. Properties of $\{G_n(z)\}$ are given in [31, 42, 43]. Of special interest are the values of $G_n(1/2)$. Adamchik [42] determined the simplest known formula for these:

$$\ln \left(G_n \left(\tfrac{1}{2} \right) \right) = \frac{1}{(n-1)!} \left[-\frac{\ln(\pi)}{2^n} \prod_{k=2}^{n} (2k - 3) + \sum_{m=1}^{n} \left(\ln(2) \frac{B_{m+1}}{m+1} + (2^{m+1} - 1)\zeta'(-m) \right) \frac{q_{m,n}}{2^m} \right],$$

where $q_{m,n}$ is the coefficient of x^m in the expansion of the polynomial $2^{1-n} \prod_{j=1}^{n-1}(2x + 2j - 1)$. We may hence write

$$\ln\left(G_3\left(\frac{1}{2}\right)\right) = \frac{1}{8} + \frac{1}{24}\ln(2) - \frac{3}{16}\ln(\pi) - \frac{3}{2}\ln(A_1) - \frac{7}{8}\ln(A_2),$$

$$\ln\left(G_4\left(\frac{1}{2}\right)\right) = \frac{265}{2304} + \frac{229}{5760}\ln(2) - \frac{5}{32}\ln(\pi) - \frac{23}{16}\ln(A_1)$$
$$- \frac{21}{16}\ln(A_2) - \frac{5}{16}\ln(A_3)$$

in terms of the generalized Glaisher constants A_k.

2.15.3 GUE Hypothesis

Assume that the Riemann hypothesis [1.6.2] is true. Let

$$\gamma_1 = 14.1347251417\ldots \leq \gamma_2 = 21.0220396387\ldots$$
$$\leq \gamma_3 = 25.0108575801\ldots \leq \gamma_4 \leq \gamma_5 \leq \cdots$$

denote the imaginary parts of the nontrivial zeros of $\zeta(z)$ in the upper half-plane. If $N(T)$ denotes the number of such zeros with imaginary part $< T$, then the Riemann–von Mongoldt formula [44] gives

$$N(T) = \frac{T}{2\pi}\ln\left(\frac{T}{2\pi e}\right) + O(\ln(T))$$

as $T \to \infty$, and hence

$$\gamma_n \sim \frac{2\pi n}{\ln(n)}$$

as $n \to \infty$. The mean spacing between γ_n and γ_{n+1} tends to zero as $n \to \infty$, so it is useful to renormalize (or "unfold") the consecutive differences to be

$$\delta_n = \frac{\gamma_{n+1} - \gamma_n}{2\pi}\ln\left(\frac{\gamma_n}{2\pi}\right),$$

and thus δ_n has mean value 1.

What can be said about the probability distribution of δ_n? That is, what density function $p(s)$ satisfies

$$\lim_{N\to\infty}\frac{1}{N}|\{n : 1 \leq n \leq N, \ \alpha \leq \delta_n \leq \beta\}| = \int_\alpha^\beta p(s)ds$$

for all $0 < \alpha < \beta$?

Here is a fascinating conjectured answer. A random Hermitian $N \times N$ matrix X is said to belong to the **Gaussian unitary ensemble** (GUE) if its (real) diagonal elements x_{jj} and (complex) upper triangular elements $x_{jk} = u_{jk} + iv_{jk}$ are independently chosen from zero-mean Gaussian distributions with $\text{Var}(x_{jj}) = 2$ for $1 \leq j \leq N$ and

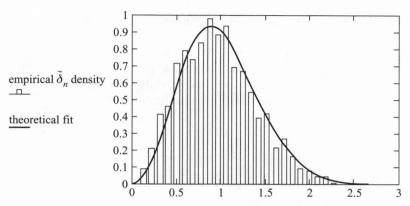

Figure 2.1. In a small simulation, the eigenvalues of fifty 120×120 random GUE matrices were generated. The resulting histogram plot of $\tilde{\delta}_n$ compares well against $p(s)$.

$\mathrm{Var}(u_{jk}) = \mathrm{Var}(v_{jk}) = 1$ for $1 \le j < k \le N$. Let $\lambda_1 \le \lambda_2 \le \lambda_3 \le \ldots \le \lambda_N$ denote the (real) eigenvalues of X and consider the normalized spacings

$$\tilde{\delta}_n = \frac{\lambda_{n+1} - \lambda_n}{4\pi} \sqrt{8N - \lambda_n^2}, \quad n \approx \frac{N}{2}.$$

With this choice of scaling, $\tilde{\delta}_n$ has mean value 1. The probability density of $\tilde{\delta}_n$, in the limit as $N \to \infty$, tends to what is called the **Gaudin density** $p(s)$. Inspired by some theoretical work by Montgomery [45], Odlyzko [46–50] experimentally determined that the distributions for δ_n and $\tilde{\delta}_n$ are very close. The **GUE hypothesis** (or **Montgomery–Odlyzko law**) is the astonishing conjecture that the two distributions are identical. See Figure 2.1.

Furthermore, there are extensive results concerning the function $p(s)$. Define

$$E(s) = \exp \left(\int_0^{\pi s} \frac{\sigma(t)}{t} dt \right),$$

where $\sigma(t)$ satisfies the Painlevé V differential equation (in "sigma form")

$$(t \cdot \sigma'')^2 + 4(t \cdot \sigma' - \sigma)[t \cdot \sigma' - \sigma + (\sigma')^2] = 0$$

with boundary conditions

$$\sigma(t) \sim -\frac{t}{\pi} - \left(\frac{t}{\pi}\right)^2 \text{ as } t \to 0^+, \quad \sigma(t) \sim -\left(\frac{t}{2}\right)^2 - \frac{1}{4} \text{ as } t \to \infty;$$

then $p(s) = d^2 E / ds^2$.

The Painlevé representation [51–56] above allows straightforward numerical calculation of $p(s)$, although historically a Fredholm determinant representation [49, 57, 58] for $E(s)$ came earlier. (Incidently, Painlevé II arises in our discussion of the longest increasing subsequence problem [5.20], and Painlevé III arises in connection with the Ising model [5.22].)

Using $p(s)$, one could compute the median, mode, and variance of $\tilde{\delta}_n$, as well as higher moments.

Here is an interesting problem having to do with the tail of the Gaudin distribution [59, 60]. The function $E(s)$ can be interpreted as the probability that the interval $[0, s]$ contains no (scaled) eigenvalues. If the specific interval $[0, s]$ is replaced by an arbitrary interval of length s, then the probability remains the same. We know that [49, 61]

$$E(s) \sim 1 - s + \frac{\pi^2 s^4}{360} \text{ as } s \to 0^+, \quad E(s) \sim C \cdot (\pi s)^{-\frac{1}{4}} \exp\left(-\frac{1}{8}(\pi s)^2\right) \text{ as } s \to \infty,$$

where C is a constant. Dyson [49, 62] nonrigorously identified

$$C = 2^{\frac{1}{3}} e^{3\zeta'(-1)} = 2^{\frac{1}{4}} e^{2B}$$

using a result of Widom [63], where

$$B = \frac{1}{24} \ln(2) + \frac{3}{2} \zeta'(-1) = -0.2192505830\ldots.$$

This, in turn, is related to Glaisher's constant A via the formula [22]

$$e^{2B} = 2^{\frac{1}{12}} e^{\frac{1}{4}} A^{-3}.$$

It is curious that a complete asymptotic expansion for $E(s)$ is now known [60, 64–66], all rigorously obtained except for the factor C! Similar phenomena were reported in [67–70] in connection with certain associated problems.

There is another way of looking at the GUE hypothesis. Let us return to the normalized differences δ_n of consecutive zeta function zeros and define

$$\Delta_{nk} = \sum_{j=0}^{k} \delta_{n+j}.$$

Earlier, k was constrained to be 0. If now $k \geq 0$ is allowed to vary, what is the "distribution" of Δ_{nk}? Montgomery [45] conjectured that the following simple formula is true:

$$\lim_{N \to \infty} \frac{1}{N} |\{(n, k) : 1 \leq n \leq N, \ k \geq 0, \ \alpha \leq \Delta_{nk} \leq \beta\}| = \int_{\alpha}^{\beta} \left[1 - \left(\frac{\sin(\pi r)}{\pi r}\right)^2\right] dr.$$

In other words, $1 - (\sin(\pi r)/(\pi r))^2$ is the **pair correlation function** of zeros of the zeta function, as predicted by Montgomery's partial results. Incredibly, it has been proved that GUE eigenvalues possess the same pair correlation function. Odlyzko [46–49] again has accumulated extensive numerical evidence supporting this conjecture. The implications of the pair correlation conjecture for prime number theory were explored in [71]. Hejhal [72] studied a three-dimensional analog, known as the triple correlation conjecture; higher level correlations were examined in [73].

Careful readers will note the restriction $n \approx N/2$ in the preceding definition of $\tilde{\delta}_n$. In our small simulation, we took only the middle third of the eigenvalues, sampling what is known as the "bulk" of the spectrum. If we sampled instead the "edges" of the spectrum, a different density emerges [69, 70]. The sine kernel in the Fredholm determinant for the "bulk" is replaced by the Airy kernel for the "edges."

Rudnick & Sarnak [73, 74] and Katz & Sarnak [75, 76] generalized the GUE hypothesis to a wider, more abstract setting. They gave proofs in certain important special cases, but not in the original case discussed here.

There is interest in the limit superior and limit inferior of δ_n, which are conjectured to be ∞ and 0, respectively [77–80].

A huge amount of research has been conducted in the area of random matrices (with no symmetry assumed) and the related subject of random polynomials. We mention only one sample result. Let $q(x)$ be a random polynomial, with real coefficients independently chosen from a standard Gaussian distribution. Let z_n denote the expected number of real zeros of $q(x)$. Kac [81, 82] proved that

$$\lim_{n \to \infty} \frac{z_n}{\ln(n)} = \frac{2}{\pi},$$

and it is known that [82–88]

$$\lim_{n \to \infty} z_n - \frac{2}{\pi} \ln(n) = c,$$

where

$$c = \frac{2}{\pi} \left[\ln(2) + \int_0^\infty \left(\sqrt{x^{-2} - 4e^{-2x}(1 - e^{-2x})^{-2}} - (x+1)^{-1} \right) dx \right]$$

$$= 0.6257358072\ldots.$$

More terms of the asymptotic expansion are known; see [82, 87] for an overview.

[1] A. E. Taylor and R. Mann, *Advanced Calculus*, 2nd ed., Wiley, 1972, pp. 740–745; MR 83m:26001.

[2] J. Kinkelin, Über eine mit der Gammafunction verwandte Transcendente und deren Anwendung auf die Integralrechnung, *J. Reine Angew. Math.* 57 (1860) 122–158.

[3] H. M. Jeffery, On the expansion of powers of the trigonometrical ratios in terms of series of ascending powers of the variable, *Quart. J. Pure Appl. Math.* 5 (1862) 91–108.

[4] J. W. L. Glaisher, On the product $1^1 \cdot 2^2 \cdot 3^3 \cdots n^n$, *Messenger of Math.* 7 (1878) 43–47.

[5] J. W. L. Glaisher, On certain numerical products in which the exponents depend upon the numbers, *Messenger of Math.* 23 (1893) 145–175.

[6] J. W. L. Glaisher, On the constant which occurs in the formula for $1^1 \cdot 2^2 \cdot 3^3 \cdots n^n$, *Messenger of Math.* 24 (1894) 1–16.

[7] G. Almkvist, Asymptotic formulas and generalized Dedekind sums, *Experim. Math.* 7 (1998) 343–359; MR 2000d:11126.

[8] R. W. Gosper, $\int_{n/4}^{m/6} \ln(\Gamma(z)) dz$, *Special Functions, q-Series and Related Topics*, ed. M. Ismail, D. Masson, and M. Rahman, Fields Inst. Commun., v. 14, Amer. Math. Soc., 1997, pp. 71–76; MR 98m:33004.

[9] J. Choi and H. M. Srivastava, Sums associated with the zeta function, *J. Math. Anal. Appl.* 206 (1997) 103–120; MR 97i:11092.

[10] J. Choi and C. Nash, Integral representations of the Kinkelin's constant A, *Math. Japon.* 45 (1997) 223–230; MR 98j:33002.

[11] J. Choi, H. M. Srivastava, and N.-Y. Zhang, Integrals involving a function associated with the Euler-Maclaurin summation formula, *Appl. Math. Comput.* 93 (1998) 101–116; MR 99h:33004.

[12] J. Choi and H. M. Srivastava, Certain classes of series associated with the zeta function and multiple gamma functions, *J. Comput. Appl. Math.* 118 (2000) 87–109; MR 2001f:11147.

[13] W. Alexeiewsky, Über eine Classe von Functionen, die der Gammafunction analog sind, *Berichte über die Verhandlungen der Königlich Sächsischen Gesellschaft der Wissenschaften zu Leipzig, Math.-Phys. Klasse* 46 (1894) 268–275.

[14] O. Hölder, Über eine transcendente Function, *Nachrichten von der Königlichen Gesellschaft der Wissenschaften und der Georg Augusts Universität zu Göttingen* (1886) 514–522.

[15] E. W. Barnes, The theory of the G-function, *Quart. J. Pure Appl. Math.* 31 (1900) 264–314.

[16] E. W. Barnes, The genesis of the double gamma functions, *Proc. London Math. Soc.* 31 (1899) 358–381.

[17] E. W. Barnes, The theory of the double gamma function, *Philos. Trans. Royal Soc. London Ser. A* 196 (1901) 265–388.

[18] Z. A. Melzak, Infinite products for πe and π/e, *Amer. Math. Monthly* 68 (1961) 39–41; MR 23 #A252.

[19] P. Borwein and W. Dykshoorn, An interesting infinite product, *J. Math. Anal. Appl.* 179 (1993) 203–207; MR 94j:11131.

[20] E. T. Whittaker and G. N. Watson, *A Course of Modern Analysis*, 4th ed., Cambridge Univ. Press, 1963, p. 264; MR 97k:01072.

[21] F. W. J. Olver, *Asymptotics and Special Functions*, Academic Press, 1974, pp. 285–292; MR 97i:41001.

[22] B. M. McCoy and T. T. Wu, *The Two-Dimensional Ising Model*, Harvard Univ. Press, 1973, Appendix B.

[23] D. H. Greene and D. E. Knuth, *Mathematics for the Analysis of Algorithms*, Birkhäuser, 1981, pp. 99–100; MR 92c:68067.

[24] G. H. Norton, On the asymptotic analysis of the Euclidean algorithm, *J. Symbolic Comput.* 10 (1990) 53–58; MR 91k:11088.

[25] T. Shintani, A proof of the classical Kronecker limit formula, *Tokyo J. Math.* 3 (1980) 191–199; MR 82f:10038.

[26] R. A MacLeod, Fractional part sums and divisor functions, *J. Number Theory* 14 (1982) 185–227; MR 83m:10080.

[27] B. C. Berndt, *Ramanujan's Notebooks: Part I*, Springer-Verlag, 1985, pp. 273–288; MR 86c:01062.

[28] M.-F. Vignéras, L'équation fonctionnelle de la fonction zêta de Selberg du groupe modulaire $PSL(2, Z)$, *Astérisque* 61 (1979) 235–249; MR 81f:10040.

[29] A. Voros, Spectral functions, special functions and the Selberg zeta function, *Commun. Math. Phys.* 110 (1987) 439–465; MR 89b:58173.

[30] P. Sarnak, Determinants of Laplacians, *Commun. Math. Phys.* 110 (1987) 113–120; MR 89e:58116.

[31] I. Vardi, Determinants of Laplacians and multiple gamma functions, *SIAM J. Math. Anal.* 19 (1988) 493–507; MR 89g:33004.

[32] J. P. Keating and N. C. Snaith, Random matrix theory and $\zeta(1/2 + it)$, *Commun. Math. Phys.* 214 (2000) 57–89; MR 2002c:11107.

[33] J. P. Keating and N. C. Snaith, Random matrix theory and L-functions at $s = 1/2$, *Commun. Math. Phys.* 214 (2000) 91–110; MR 2002c:11108.

[34] P. J. Forrester, *Log-Gases and Random Matrices*, unpublished manuscript (2000).

[35] L. Bendersky, Sur la fonction gamma généralisée, *Acta Math.* 61 (1933) 263–322.

[36] H. T. Davis, *The Summation of Series*, Principia Press of Trinity Univ., 1962, pp. 85–91; MR 25 #5305

[37] B. K. Choudhury, The Riemann zeta-function and its derivatives, *Proc. Royal Soc. London A* 450 (1995) 477–499; MR 97e:11095.

[38] V. S. Adamchik, Polygamma functions of negative order, *J. Comput. Appl. Math.* 100 (1999) 191–199; MR 99j:33001.

[39] J. Miller and V. S. Adamchik, Derivatives of the Hurwitz zeta function for rational arguments, *J. Comput. Appl. Math.* 100 (1998) 201–206; MR 2000g:11085.

[40] E. W. Barnes, On the theory of the multiple gamma function, *Trans. Cambridge Philos. Soc.* 19 (1904) 374–425.

[41] J. B. Conway, *Functions of One Complex Variable*, 2nd ed., Springer-Verlag, 1978; MR 80c:30003.

[42] V. S. Adamchik, On the Barnes function, *Proc. 2001 Int. Symp. Symbolic and Algebraic Computation (ISSAC)*, ed. B. Mourrain, Univ. of Western Ontario, ACM, 2001, pp. 15–20.

[43] J. Choi, H. M. Srivastava, and V. S. Adamchik, Multiple gamma and related functions, *Appl. Math. Comput.*, to appear.

[44] A. Ivić, *The Riemann Zeta-Function*, Wiley, 1985, pp. 17–21, 251–252; MR 87d:11062.

[45] H. L. Montgomery, The pair correlation of zeros of the zeta function, *Analytic Number Theory*, ed. H. G. Diamond, Proc. Symp. Pure Math. 24, Amer. Math. Soc., 1973, pp. 181–193; MR 49 #2590.

[46] A. M. Odlyzko, On the distribution of spacings between zeros of the zeta function, *Math. Comp.* 48 (1987) 273–308; MR 88d:11082.

[47] A. M. Odlyzko, The 10^{20th} zero of the Riemann zeta function and 175 million of its neighbors, unpublished manuscript (1992).

[48] A. M. Odlyzko, The 10^{22nd} zero of the Riemann zeta function, *Dynamical, Spectral, and Arithmetic Zeta Functions*, Proc. 1999 San Antonio conf., ed. M. L. Lapidus and M. van Frankenhuysen, Amer. Math. Soc., 2001, pp. 139–144.

[49] M. L. Mehta, *Random Matrices*, Academic Press, 1991; MR 92f:82002.

[50] B. Cipra, A prime case of chaos, *What's Happening in the Mathematical Sciences*, v. 4, Amer. Math. Soc., 1998–1999.

[51] M. Jimbo, T. Miwa, Y. Mori, and M. Sato, Density matrix of an impenetrable Bose gas and the fifth Painlevé transcendent, *Physica D* 1 (1980) 80–158; MR 84k:82037.

[52] A. R. Its, A. G. Izergin, V. E. Korepin, and N. A. Slavnov, Differential equations for quantum correlation functions, *Int. J. Mod. Phys. B* 4 (1990) 1003–1037; MR 91k:82009.

[53] M. L. Mehta, A nonlinear differential equation and a Fredholm determinant, *J. Physique I* 2 (1992) 1721–1729; MR 93i:58163.

[54] M. L. Mehta, Painlevé transcendents in the theory of random matrices, *An Introduction to Methods of Complex Analysis and Geometry for Classical Mechanics and Non-Linear Waves*, Proc. Third Workshop on Astronomy and Astrophysics, ed. D. Benest and C. Froeschlé, Frontières, 1994, pp. 197–208; MR 96k:82007.

[55] C. A. Tracy and H. Widom, Introduction to random matrices, *Geometric and Quantum Aspects of Integrable Systems*, Proc. 1992 Scheveningen conf., ed. G. F. Helminck, Lect. Notes in Physics 424, Springer-Verlag, 1993, pp. 103–130; hep-th/9210073; MR 95a:82050.

[56] C. A. Tracy and H. Widom, Universality of the distribution functions of random matrix theory, *Integrable Systems: From Classical to Quantum*, Proc. 1999 Montréal conf., ed. J. Harnad, G. Sabidussi, and P. Winternitz, Amer. Math. Soc, 2000, pp. 251–264; math-ph/9909001; MR 2002f:15036.

[57] M. Gaudin, Sur la loi limite de l'éspacement des valeurs propres d'une matrice aléatorie, *Nucl. Phys.* 25 (1961) 447–458; also in C. E. Porter, *Statistical Theories of Spectra: Fluctuations*, Academic Press, 1965.

[58] M. L. Mehta and M. Gaudin, On the density of eigenvalues of a random matrix, *Nucl. Phys.* 18 (1960) 420–427; MR 22 #3741.

[59] E. L. Basor, C. A. Tracy, and H. Widom, Asymptotics of level-spacing distributions for random matrices, *Phys. Rev. Lett.* 69 (1992) 5–8, 2880; MR 93g:82004a-b.

[60] C. A. Tracy and H. Widom, Asymptotics of a class of Fredholm determinants, *Spectral Problems in Geometry and Arithmetic*, Proc. 1997 Iowa City conf., Amer. Math. Soc., 1999, pp. 167–174; solv-int/9801008; MR 2000e:47077.

[61] J. des Cloizeaux and M. L. Mehta, Asymptotic behavior of spacing distributions for the eigenvalues of random matrices, *J. Math. Phys.* 14 (1973) 1648–1650; MR 48 #6500.

[62] F. J. Dyson, Fredholm determinants and inverse scattering problems, *Commun. Math. Phys.* 47 (1976) 171–183; MR 53 #9993.

[63] H. Widom, The strong Szegö limit theorem for circular arcs, *Indiana Univ. Math. J.* 21 (1971) 277–283; MR 44 #5693.

[64]   H. Widom, The asymptotics of a continuous analogue of orthogonal polynomials, *J. Approx. Theory* 77 (1994) 51–64; MR 95f:42041.

[65]   H. Widom, Asymptotics for the Fredholm determinant of the sine kernel on a union of intervals, *Commun. Math. Phys.* 171 (1995) 159–180; MR 96i:47050.

[66]   P. A. Deift, A. R. Its, and X. Zhou, A Riemann-Hilbert approach to asymptotic problems arising in the theory of random matrix models, and also in the theory of integrable statistical mechanics, *Annals of Math.* 146 (1997) 149–235; MR 98k:47097.

[67]   P. J. Forrester and A. M. Odlyzko, A nonlinear equation and its application to nearest neighbor spacings for zeros of the zeta function and eigenvalues of random matrices, *Organic Mathematics*, Proc. 1995 Burnaby workshop, ed. J. Borwein, P. Borwein, L. Jörgenson, and R. Corless, Amer. Math. Soc., 1995, pp. 239–251; MR 99c:11107.

[68]   P. J. Forrester and A. M. Odlyzko, Gaussian unitary ensemble eigenvalues and Riemann zeta function zeros: A non-linear equation for a new statistic, *Phys. Rev. E* 54 (1996) R4493–R4495; MR 98a:82054.

[69]   C. A. Tracy and H. Widom, Level-spacing distributions and the Airy kernel, *Phys. Lett. B* 305 (1993) 115–118; hep-th/9210074; MR 94f:82046.

[70]   C. A. Tracy and H. Widom, Level-spacing distributions and the Airy kernel, *Commun. Math. Phys.* 159 (1994) 151–174; hep-th/9211141; MR 95e:82003.

[71]   D. A. Goldston and H. L. Montgomery, Pair correlation of zeros and primes in short intervals, *Analytic Number Theory and Diophantine Problems*, Proc. 1984 Stillwater conf., ed. A. C. Adolphson, J. B. Conrey, A. Ghosh, and R. I. Yager, Birkhäuser, 1987, pp. 183–203; MR 90h:11084.

[72]   D. A. Hejhal, On the triple correlation of zeros of the zeta function, *Int. Math. Res. Notices* (1994) n. 7, 293–302; MR 96d:11093.

[73]   Z. Rudnick and P. Sarnak, The *n*-level correlations of zeros of the zeta function, *C. R. Acad. Sci. Paris Ser. I Math.* 319 (1994) 1027–1032; MR 96b:11124.

[74]   Z. Rudnick and P. Sarnak, Zeros of principal L-functions and random matrix theory, *Duke Math. J.* 81 (1996) 269–322; MR 97f:11074.

[75]   N. M. Katz and P. Sarnak, *Random Matrices, Frobenius Eigenvalues, and Monodromy*, Amer. Math. Soc., 1999; MR 2000b:11070.

[76]   N. M. Katz and P. Sarnak, Zeroes of zeta functions and symmetry, *Bull. Amer. Math. Soc.* 36 (1999) 1–26; MR 2000f:11114.

[77]   H. L. Montgomery and A. M. Odlyzko, Gaps between zeros of the zeta function, *Topics in Classical Number Theory*, v. II, Proc. 1981 Budapest conf., Colloq. Math. Soc. János Bolyai 34, North-Holland, 1984, pp. 1079–1106; MR 86e:11072.

[78]   J. B. Conrey, A. Ghosh, and S. M. Gonek, A note on gaps between zeros of the zeta function, *Bull. London Math. Soc.* 16 (1984) 421–424; MR 86i:11048.

[79]   J. B. Conrey, A. Ghosh, D. Goldston, S. M. Gonek, and D. R. Heath-Brown, On the distribution of gaps between zeros of the zeta function, *Quart. J. Math.* 36 (1985) 43–51; MR 86j:11083.

[80]   J. B. Conrey, A. Ghosh, and S. M. Gonek, Large gaps between zeros of the zeta function, *Mathematika* 33 (1986) 212–238; MR 88g:11057.

[81]   A. T. Bharucha-Reid and M. Sambandham, *Random Polynomials*, Academic Press, 1986, pp. 11–14, 90–91; MR 87m:60118.

[82]   K. Farahmand, *Topics in Random Polynomials*, Longman, 1998, pp. 34–35, 59–71; MR 2000d:60092.

[83]   B. R. Jamrom, The average number of real roots of a random algebraic polynomial (in Russian), *Vestnik Leningrad. Univ.* (1971) n. 19, 152–156; MR 45 #7791.

[84]   B. R. Jamrom, The average number of real zeros of random polynomials (in Russian), *Dokl. Akad. Nauk SSSR* 206 (1972) 1059–1060; Engl. transl. in *Soviet Math. Dokl.* 13 (1972) 1381–1383; MR 47 #2666.

[85]   Y. J. Wang, Bounds on the average number of real roots of a random algebraic equation, *Chinese Annals Math. Ser. A* 4 (1983) 601–605; Engl. summary in *Chinese Annals Math. Ser. B* 4 (1983) 527; MR 85c:60081.

[86] Z. M. Yu, Bounds on the average number of real roots for a class of random algebraic equations, *J. Math. Res. Expos.* 2 (1982) 81–85; MR 84h:60081.

[87] J. E. Wilkins, An asymptotic expansion for the expected number of real zeros of a random polynomial, *Proc. Amer. Math. Soc.* 103 (1988) 1249–1258; MR 90f:60105.

[88] A. Edelman and E. Kostlan, How many zeros of a random polynomial are real?, *Bull. Amer. Math. Soc.* 32 (1995) 1–37; erratum 33 (1996) 325; MR 95m:60082.

2.16 Stolarsky–Harborth Constant

Given a positive integer k, let $b(k)$ denote the number of ones in the binary expansion of k. Glaisher [1–6] showed that the number of odd binomial coefficients of the form $\binom{k}{j}$, $0 \leq j \leq k$, is $2^{b(k)}$. As a consequence, the number of odd elements in the first n rows of Pascal's triangle is

$$f(n) = \sum_{k=0}^{n-1} 2^{b(k)}$$

and satisfies the recurrence

$$f(0) = 0, \quad f(1) = 1, \quad f(n) = \begin{cases} 3f(m) & \text{if } n = 2m \\ 2f(m) + f(m+1) & \text{if } n = 2m+1 \end{cases} \quad \text{for } n \geq 2.$$

The question is: Can a simple approximation for $f(n)$ be found? The answer is yes. Let $\theta = \ln(3)/\ln(2) = 1.5849625007\ldots$, the fractal dimension [7,8] of Pascal's triangle modulo 2. It turns out that n^θ is a reasonable approximation for $f(n)$. It also turns out that $f(n)$ is not well behaved asymptotically. Stolarsky [9] and Harborth [10] determined that

$$0.812556 < \lambda = \liminf_{n\to\infty} \frac{f(n)}{n^\theta} < 0.812557 < \limsup_{n\to\infty} \frac{f(n)}{n^\theta} = 1,$$

and we call $\lambda = 0.8125565590\ldots$ the **Stolarsky–Harborth constant**.

Here is a generalization. Let p be a prime and $f_p(n)$ be the number of elements in the first n rows of Pascal's triangle that are not divisible by p. Define

$$\theta_p = \frac{\ln\left(\frac{p(p+1)}{2}\right)}{\ln(p)}$$

and note that $\lim_{n\to\infty} \theta_p = 2$. Of course, $f_2(n) = f(n)$ and $\theta_2 = \theta$. It is known that [11–14]

$$\lambda_p = \liminf_{n\to\infty} \frac{f_p(n)}{n^{\theta_p}} < \limsup_{n\to\infty} \frac{f_p(n)}{n^{\theta_p}} = 1,$$

$$\lambda_3 = \left(\tfrac{3}{2}\right)^{1-\theta_3} = 0.7742\ldots, \quad \lim_{p\to\infty} \lambda_p = \tfrac{1}{2}$$

and further conjectured that

$$\lambda_5 = \left(\tfrac{3}{2}\right)^{1-\theta_5} = 0.7582\ldots, \quad \lambda_7 = \left(\tfrac{3}{2}\right)^{1-\theta_7} = 0.7491\ldots,$$

$$\lambda_{11} = \tfrac{59}{44}\left(\tfrac{22}{31}\right)^{\theta_{11}} = 0.7364\ldots.$$

Curiously, no such exact formula for $\lambda_2 = \lambda$ has been found. A broader generalization involves multinomial coefficients [15–17].

2.16.1 Digital Sums

The expression $f_2(n)$ is an **exponential sum of digital sums**. Another example is

$$m_p(n) = \sum_{k=0}^{n-1}(-1)^{b(p\,k)},$$

which, in the case $p = 3$, quantifies an empirical observation that multiples of 3 prefer to have an even number of 1-digits. We will first discuss, however, a **power sum of digital sums**:

$$s_q(n) = \sum_{k=0}^{n-1} b(k)^q$$

and set $q = 1$ for the sake of concreteness.

Trollope [18] and Delange [19], building upon [20–26], proved that

$$s_1(n) = \frac{1}{2\ln(2)}n\ln(n) + n\,S\left(\frac{\ln(n)}{\ln(2)}\right)$$

exactly, where $S(x)$ is a certain continuous nowhere-differentiable function of period 1,

$$-0.2075\ldots = \frac{\ln(3)}{2\ln(2)} - 1 = \inf_x S(x) < \sup_x S(x) = 0,$$

and the Fourier coefficients of $S(x)$ are all known. See Figure 2.2. The mean value of $S(x)$ is [19, 27]

$$\int_0^1 S(x)dx = \frac{1}{2\ln(2)}\left(\ln(2\pi) - 1\right) - \frac{3}{4} = -0.1455\ldots.$$

Extensions of this remarkable result to arbitrary q appear in [28–36].

Let $\omega = \theta/2$ and $\varepsilon(n) = (-1)^{b(3n-1)}$ if n is odd, 0 otherwise. Newman [37–39] proved that $m_3(n) > 0$ always and is $O(n^\omega)$. Coquet [40] strengthened this to

$$m_3(n) = n^\omega M\left(\frac{\ln(n)}{2\ln(2)}\right) + \frac{1}{3}\varepsilon(n),$$

where $M(x)$ is a continuous nowhere-differentiable function of period 1,

$$1.1547\ldots = \frac{2\sqrt{3}}{3} = \inf_x M(x) < \sup_x M(x) = \frac{55}{3}\left(\frac{3}{65}\right)^\omega = 1.6019\ldots$$

and, again, the Fourier coefficients of $M(x)$ are all known. The mean value [27] of $M(x)$ is $1.4092203477\ldots$ but has a complicated integral expression. Extensions of this result to $p = 5$ and 17 appear in [41–43]. The pattern in $\{(-1)^{b(k)}\}$ follows the well-known Prouhet–Thue–Morse sequence [6.8], and associated sums of subsequences of the form $\{(-1)^{b(pk+r)}\}$ are discussed in [44–46].

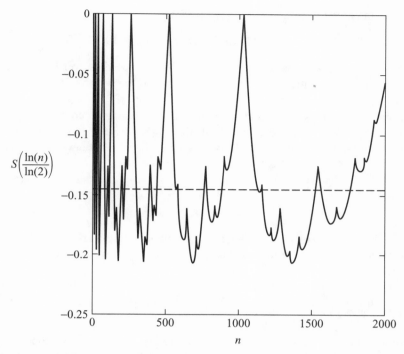

Figure 2.2. The Trollope–Delange function is pictured, as well as its mean value.

We return to binomial coefficients. Stein [47] proved that

$$f_2(n) = n^\theta \, F\left(\frac{\ln(n)}{\ln(2)}\right),$$

where $F(x)$ is a continuous function of period 1; by way of contrast, $F(x)$ is differentiable almost everywhere, but is nowhere monotonic [48]. This fact, however, does not appear to give any insight concerning an exact formula for $\lambda_2 = \inf_x F(x)$. The Fourier coefficients of $F(x)$ are all known, and the mean value [27] of $F(x)$ is $0.8636049963\ldots$. Again, the underlying integral is complicated.

This material plays a role in the analysis of algorithms, for example, in approximating the register function for binary trees [49], and in studying mergesort [50], maxima finding [51], and other divide-and-conquer recurrences [52, 53].

2.16.2 Ulam 1-Additive Sequences

There is an unexpected connection between digital sums and **Ulam 1-additive sequences** [54]. Let $u < v$ be positive integers. The 1-additive sequence with base u, v is the infinite sequence $(u, v) = a_1, a_2, a_3, \ldots$ with $a_1 = u, a_2 = v$ and a_n is the least integer exceeding a_{n-1} and possessing a unique representation $a_n = a_i + a_j, i < j,$

$n \geq 3$. Ulam's archetypal sequence

$$(1, 2) = 1, 2, 3, 4, 6, 8, 11, 13, 16, 18, 26, 28, 36, 38, 47, 48, 53, \ldots$$

remains a mystery. No pattern in its successive differences has ever been observed. Ulam conjectured that the density of $(1, 2)$, relative to the positive integers, is 0. No one has yet found a proof of this.

Substantially more is known about the cases $(2, v)$, where v is odd, and $(4, v)$, where v additionally is congruent to 1 modulo 4. Cassaigne & Finch [55] proved that the successive differences of the Ulam 1-additive sequence $(4, v)$ are eventually periodic and that the density of $(4, v)$ is

$$d(v) = \frac{1}{2(v+1)} \sum_{k=0}^{(v-1)/2} 2^{-b(k)}.$$

It can be shown that $d(v) \to 0$ as $v \to \infty$. The techniques giving rise to the Stolarsky–Harborth constant λ can be modified to give the following more precise asymptotic estimate of the density:

$$\frac{1}{4} = \liminf_{\substack{v \to \infty \\ v \equiv 1 \bmod 4}} \left(\frac{v}{2}\right)^{2-\theta} d(v) < 0.272190 < \limsup_{\substack{v \to \infty \\ v \equiv 1 \bmod 4}} \left(\frac{v}{2}\right)^{2-\theta} d(v) < 0.272191.$$

A certain family of ternary quadratic recurrences and its periodicity properties play a crucial role in the proof in [55]. It is natural to ask how far this circle of ideas and techniques can be extended.

2.16.3 Alternating Bit Sets

If n is a positive integer satisfying $2^{k-1} \leq n < 2^k$, clearly the binary expansion of n has k bits. Define an **alternating bit set** in n to be a subset of the k bit positions of n with the following properties [6, 56–58]:

- The bits of n that lie in these positions are alternatively 1s and 0s.
- The leftmost (most significant) of these is a 1.
- The rightmost (least significant) of these is a 0.

Let $c(n)$ be the cardinality of all alternating bit sets of n. For example, $c(26) = 8$ since 26 is 11010 in binary and hence all alternating bit sets of 26 are

$$\{\}, \{5, 3\}, \{5, 1\}, \{4, 3\}, \{4, 1\}, \{2, 1\}, \{5, 3, 2, 1\}, \text{ and } \{4, 3, 2, 1\}.$$

Although $c(n)$ is not a digital sum like $b(n)$, it has similarly interesting combinatorial properties: $c(n)$ is the number of ways of writing n as a sum of powers of 2, with each power used at most twice. It satisfies the recurrence

$$c(0) = 1, \qquad c(n) = \begin{cases} c(m) + c(m-1) & \text{if } n = 2m \\ c(m) & \text{if } n = 2m+1 \end{cases} \quad \text{for } n \geq 1.$$

It is also linked to the Fibonacci sequence in subtle ways and one can prove that [57]

$$0.9588 < \limsup_{n \to \infty} \frac{c(n)}{n^{\ln(\varphi)/\ln(2)}} < 1.1709,$$

where φ is the Golden mean [1.2]. What is the exact value of this limit supremum? Is there a reason to doubt that its exact value is 1?

[1] J. W. L. Glaisher, On the residue of a binomial-theorem coefficient with respect to a prime modulus, *Quart. J. Math.* 30 (1899) 150–156.

[2] N. J. Fine, Binomial coefficients modulo a prime, *Amer. Math. Monthly* 54 (1947) 589–592; MR 9,331b.

[3] L. Carlitz, The number of binomial coefficients divisible by a fixed power of a prime, *Rend. Circ. Mat. Palermo* 16 (1967) 299–320; MR 40 #2554.

[4] D. Singmaster, Notes on binomial coefficients III – Any integer divides almost all binomial coefficients, *J. London Math. Soc.* 8 (1974) 555–560; MR 53 #153.

[5] A. Granville, The arithmetic properties of binomial coefficients, *Organic Mathematics*, Proc. 1995 Burnaby workshop, ed. J. Borwein, P. Borwein, L. Jörgenson, and R. Corless, Amer. Math. Soc., 1997, pp. 253–276; MR 99h:11016.

[6] N. J. A. Sloane, On-Line Encyclopedia of Integer Sequences, A000120, A000788, A001316, A002487, A002858, A003670, A005599, A006046, A006047, A006048, and A006844.

[7] S. Wolfram, Geometry of binomial coefficients, *Amer. Math. Monthly* 91 (1984) 566–571; MR 86d:05007.

[8] D. Flath and R. Peele, Hausdorff dimension in Pascal's triangle, *Applications of Fibonacci Numbers*, v. 5, Proc. 1992 St. Andrews conf., ed. G. E. Bergum, A. N. Philippou, and A. F. Horadam, Kluwer, 1993, pp. 229–244; MR 95a:11068.

[9] K. B. Stolarsky, Power and exponential sums of digital sums related to binomial coefficient parity, *SIAM J. Appl. Math.* 32 (1977) 717–730; MR 55 #12621.

[10] H. Harborth, Number of odd binomial coefficients, *Proc. Amer. Math. Soc.* 62 (1977) 19–22; MR 55 #2725.

[11] A. H. Stein, Binomial coefficients not divisible by a prime, *Number Theory: New York Seminar 1985-1988*, ed. D. V. Chudnovsky, G. V. Chudnovsky, H. Cohn, and M. B. Nathanson, Lect. Notes in Math. 1383, Springer-Verlag, 1989, pp. 170–177; MR 91c:11012.

[12] Z. M. Franco, Distribution of binomial coefficients modulo p, *Number Theory: Diophantine, Computational and Algebraic Aspects*, Proc. 1996 Elger conf., ed. K. Györy, A. Pethö, and V. T. Sós, Gruyter, 1998, pp. 199–209; MR 99d:11017.

[13] Z. M. Franco, Distribution of binomial coefficients modulo three, *Fibonacci Quart.* 36 (1998) 272–274.

[14] B. Wilson, Asymptotic behavior of Pascal's triangle modulo a prime, *Acta Arith.* 83 (1998) 105–116; MR 98k:11012.

[15] N. A. Volodin, Number of multinomial coefficients not divisible by a prime, *Fibonacci Quart.* 32 (1994) 402–406; MR 95j:11017.

[16] N. A. Volodin, Multinomial coefficients modulo a prime, *Proc. Amer. Math. Soc.* 127 (1999) 349–353; MR 99c:11019.

[17] Y.-G. Chen and C. Ji, The number of multinomial coefficients not divided by a prime, *Acta Sci. Math. (Szeged)* 64 (1998) 37–48; MR 99j:11020.

[18] J. R. Trollope, An explicit expression for binary digital sums, *Math. Mag.* 41 (1968) 21–25; MR 38 #2084.

[19] H. Delange, Sur la fonction sommatoire de la fonction "somme des chiffres," *Enseign. Math.* 21 (1975) 31–47; MR 52 #319.

[20] L. E. Bush, An asymptotic formula for the average sum of the digits of integers, *Amer. Math. Monthly* 47 (1940) 154–156; MR 1 #199.

[21] R. Bellman and H. N. Shapiro, On a problem in additive number theory, *Annals of Math.* 49 (1948) 333–340; MR 9 #414.

[22] L. Mirsky, A theorem on representations of integers in the scale of r, *Scripta Math.* 15 (1949) 11–12; MR 11 #83.

[23] M. P. Drazin and J. S. Griffith, On the decimal representation of integers, *Proc. Cambridge Philos. Soc.* 48 (1952) 555–565; MR 14 #253.

[24] P.-H. Cheo and S.-C. Yien, A problem on the k-adic representation of positive integers (in Chinese), *Acta Math. Sinica* 5 (1955) 433–438; MR 17,828b.

[25] G. F. Clements and B. Lindström, A sequence of (± 1) determinants with large values, *Proc. Amer. Math. Soc.* 16 (1965) 548–550; MR 31 #2259.

[26] M. D. McIlroy, The number of 1's in binary integers: Bounds and extremal properties, *SIAM J. Comput.* 3 (1974) 255–261; MR 55 #9628.

[27] P. Flajolet, P. Grabner, P. Kirschenhofer, H. Prodinger, and R.F. Tichy, Mellin transforms and asymptotics: Digital sums, *Theoret. Comput. Sci.* 123 (1994) 291–314; MR 94m:11090.

[28] J. Coquet, Power sums of digital sums, *J. Number Theory* 22 (1986) 161–176; MR 87d:11070.

[29] P. Kirschenhofer, On the variance of the sum of digits function, *Number-Theoretic Analysis: Vienna 1988-89*, ed. E. Hlawka and R. F. Tichy, Lect. Notes in Math. 1452, Springer-Verlag, 1990, pp. 112–116; MR 92f:11103.

[30] P. J. Grabner, P. Kirschenhofer, H. Prodinger, and R. Tichy, On the moments of the sum-of-digits function, *Applications of Fibonacci Numbers*, v. 5, Proc. 1992 St. Andrews conf., ed. G. E. Bergum, A. N. Philippou, and A. F. Horadam, Kluwer, 1993, pp. 263–271; MR 95d:11123.

[31] C. Cooper and R. E. Kennedy, A generalization of a result by Trollope on digital sums, *J. Inst. Math. Comput. Sci. Math. Ser.* 12 (1999) 17–22; MR 2000e:11008.

[32] J.-P. Allouche and J. Shallit, Sums of digits and the Hurwitz zeta function, *Analytic Number Theory*, Proc. 1988 Tokyo conf., ed. K. Nagasaka and É. Fouvry, Lect. Notes in Math. 1434, Springer-Verlag, 1990, pp. 19–30; MR 91i:11111.

[33] A. H. Osbaldestin, Digital sum problems, *Fractals in the Fundamental and Applied Sciences*, ed. H.-O. Peitgen, J. M. Henriques, and L. F. Penedo, North-Holland, 1991, pp. 307–328; MR 93g:58102.

[34] T. Okada, T. Sekiguchi, and Y. Shiota, Applications of binomial measures to power sums of digital sums, *J. Number Theory* 52 (1995) 256–266; MR 96d:11084.

[35] J. M. Dumont and A. Thomas, Digital sum problems and substitutions on a finite alphabet, *J. Number Theory* 39 (1991) 351–366; MR 92m:11074.

[36] G. Tenenbaum, Sur la non-dérivabilité de fonctions périodiques associées à certaines formules sommatoires, *The Mathematics of Paul Erdös*, v. 1, ed. R. L. Graham and J. Nesetril, Springer-Verlag, 1997, pp. 117–128; MR 97k:11010.

[37] D. J. Newman, On the number of binary digits in a multiple of three, *Proc. Amer. Math. Soc.* 21 (1969) 719–721; MR 39 #5466.

[38] D. J. Newman and M. Slater, Binary digit distribution over naturally defined sequences, *Trans. Amer. Math. Soc.* 213 (1975) 71–78; MR 52 #5607.

[39] J.-M. Dumont, Discrépance des progressions arithmétiques dans la suite de Morse, *C. R. Acad. Sci. Paris Sér. I Math.* 297 (1983) 145–148; MR 85f:11058.

[40] J. Coquet, A summation formula related to the binary digits, *Invent. Math.* 73 (1983) 107–115; MR 85c:11012.

[41] P. J. Grabner, A note on the parity of the sum-of-digits function, *Séminaire Lotharingien de Combinatoire*, Proc. 1993 Gerolfingen session, ed. R. König and V. Strehl, Univ. Louis Pasteur, 1993, pp. 35–42; MR 95k:11125.

[42] P. J. Grabner, Completely q-multiplicative functions: The Mellin transform approach, *Acta Arith.* 65 (1993) 85–96; MR 94k:11111.

[43] P. J. Grabner, T. Herendi, and R. F. Tichy, Fractal digital sums and codes, *Appl. Algebra Engin. Commun. Comput.* 8 (1997) 33–39; MR 99c:11150.

[44] S. Goldstein, K. A. Kelly, and E. R. Speer, The fractal structure of rarefied sums of the Thue-Morse sequence, *J. Number Theory* 42 (1992) 1–19; MR 93m:11020.

[45] M. Drmota and M. Skalba, Sign-changes of the Thue-Morse fractal function and Dirichlet L-series, *Manuscripta Math.* 86 (1995) 519–541; MR 96b:11027.
[46] M. Drmota and M. Skalba, Rarified sums of the Thue-Morse sequence, *Trans. Amer. Math. Soc.* 352 (2000) 609–642; MR 2000c:11038.
[47] A. H. Stein, Exponential sums of sum-of-digit functions, *Illinois J. Math.* 30 (1986) 660–675; MR 89a:11014.
[48] G. Larcher, On the number of odd binomial coefficients, *Acta Math. Hungar.* 71 (1996) 183–203; MR 97e:11026.
[49] P. Flajolet, J.-C. Raoult, and J. Vuillemin, The number of registers required for evaluating arithmetic expressions, *Theoret. Comput. Sci.* 9 (1979) 99–125; MR 80e:68101.
[50] P. Flajolet and M. Golin, Mellin transforms and asymptotics: The mergesort recurrence, *Acta Inform.* 31 (1994) 673–696; MR 95h:68035.
[51] P. Flajolet and M. Golin, Exact asymptotics of divide-and-conquer recurrences, *Proc. 1993 Int. Colloq. on Automata, Languages and Programming (ICALP)*, Lund, ed. A. Lingas, R. Karlsson, and S. Carlsson, Lect. Notes in Comp. Sci. 700, Springer-Verlag, 1993, pp. 137–149.
[52] R. Sedgewick and P. Flajolet, *Introduction to the Analysis of Algorithms*, Addison-Wesley, 1996, pp. 62–70.
[53] P. Flajolet and R. Sedgewick, *Analytic Combinatorics*, unpublished manuscript (2001), ch. 7.
[54] R. K. Guy, *Unsolved Problems in Number Theory*, 2nd ed., Springer-Verlag, 1994, sect. C4; MR 96e:11002.
[55] J. Cassaigne and S. R. Finch, A class of 1-additive sequences and quadratic recurrences, *Experim. Math.* 4 (1995) 49–60; MR 96g:11007.
[56] B. Reznick, Some binary partition functions, *Analytic Number Theory*, Proc. 1989 Allerton Park conf., ed. B. C. Berndt, H. G. Diamond, H. Halberstam, and A. Hildebrand, Birkhäuser, 1990, pp. 451–477; MR 91k:11092.
[57] N. J. Calkin and H. S. Wilf, Binary partitions of integers and Stern-Brocot-like trees, unpublished note (1998).
[58] N. J. Calkin and H. S. Wilf, Recounting the rationals, *Amer. Math. Monthly* 107 (2000) 360–363; MR 2001d:11024.

2.17 Gauss–Kuzmin–Wirsing Constant

Let x_0 be a random number drawn uniformly from the interval $(0, 1)$. Write x_0 (uniquely) as a regular continued fraction

$$x_0 = 0 + \frac{1|}{|a_1|} + \frac{1|}{|a_2|} + \frac{1|}{|a_3|} + \cdots,$$

where each a_k is a positive integer, and define for all $n > 0$,

$$x_n = 0 + \frac{1|}{|a_{n+1}|} + \frac{1|}{|a_{n+2}|} + \frac{1|}{|a_{n+3}|} + \cdots.$$

For each n, x_n is also a number in $(0, 1)$ since $x_n = \{1/x_{n-1}\}$, where $\{y\}$ denotes the fractional part of y.

In 1812, Gauss examined the distribution function [1]

$$F_n(x) = \text{probability that } x_n \leq x$$

and believed that he possessed a proof of a remarkable limiting result:

$$\lim_{n \to \infty} F_n(x) = \frac{\ln(1 + x)}{\ln(2)}, \quad 0 \leq x \leq 1.$$

The first published proof is due to Kuzmin [2], with subsequent improvements in error bounds by Lévy [3] and Szüsz [4]. Wirsing [5] went farther and gave a proof that

$$\lim_{n \to \infty} \frac{F_n(x) - \frac{\ln(1+x)}{\ln(2)}}{(-c)^n} = \Psi(x),$$

where $c = 0.3036630028\ldots$ and Ψ is an analytic function satisfying $\Psi(0) = \Psi(1) = 0$. A graph in [6] suggests that Ψ is convex and $-0.1 < \Psi(x) < 0$ for $0 < x < 1$. The constant c is apparently unrelated to more familiar constants and is computed as an eigenvalue of a certain infinite-dimensional linear operator [2.17.1], with $\Psi(x)$ as the corresponding eigenfunction. The key to this analysis is the identity

$$F_{n+1}(x) = T[F_n](x) = \sum_{k=1}^{\infty} \left[F_n\left(\frac{1}{k}\right) - F_n\left(\frac{1}{k+x}\right) \right].$$

Babenko & Jurev [7–9] went even farther in establishing that a certain eigenvalue/eigenfunction expansion,

$$F_n(x) - \frac{\ln(1 + x)}{\ln(2)} = \sum_{k=2}^{\infty} \lambda_k^n \cdot \Psi_k(x), \quad 1 = \lambda_1 > |\lambda_2| \geq |\lambda_3| \geq \ldots,$$

is valid for all x and all $n > 0$. Building upon the work of others [1, 5, 6, 10, 11], Sebah [12] computed the Gauss–Kuzmin–Wirsing constant c to 100 digits, as well as the eigenvalues λ_k for $3 \leq k \leq 50$.

Some related paths of research are indicated in [13–19], but these are too far afield for us to discuss.

2.17.1 Ruelle–Mayer Operators

The operators examined here first arose in dynamical systems [20, 21]. Let Δ denote the open disk of radius $3/2$ with center at 1, and let $s > 1$. Let X denote the Banach space of functions f that are analytic on Δ and continuous on the closure of Δ, equipped with the supremum norm. Define a linear operator $G_s : X \to X$ by the formula [10, 11, 22, 23]

$$G_s[f](z) = \sum_{k=1}^{\infty} \frac{1}{(k + z)^s} f\left(\frac{1}{k + z}\right), \quad z \in \Delta.$$

We will examine only the case $s = 2$ here; the case $s = 4$ is needed in [2.19].

Note that the derivative $T[F]'(x) = G_2[f](x)$, where $F' = f$, hence an understanding of G_2 carries over to T. The first six eigenvalues [1, 6, 10–12] of G_2 after $\lambda_1 = 1$ are

$$\lambda_2 = -0.3036630028\ldots, \quad \lambda_3 = 0.1008845092\ldots, \quad \lambda_4 = -0.0354961590\ldots,$$
$$\lambda_5 = 0.0128437903\ldots, \quad \lambda_6 = -0.0047177775\ldots, \quad \lambda_7 = 0.0017486751\ldots.$$

On the one hand, it might be conjectured that

$$\lim_{n\to\infty} \frac{\lambda_{n+1}}{\lambda_n} = -1 - \varphi = -2.6180339887\ldots,$$

where φ is the Golden mean [1.2]. On the other hand, it has been proved that the trace of G_2 is exactly given by [11]

$$\tau_1 = \frac{1}{2} - \frac{1}{2\sqrt{5}} + \frac{1}{2}\sum_{k=1}^{\infty}(-1)^{k-1}\binom{2k}{k}(\zeta(2k) - 1) = 0.7711255236\ldots,$$

where $\tau_n = \sum_{j=1}^{\infty}\lambda_j^n$. The connection between G_s and zeta function values [1.6] is not surprising: Look at G_s applied to $f(z) = z^r$; then consider Maclaurin expansions of arbitrary functions f and the linearity of G_s.

Other interesting trace formulas include the following. Let [24, 25]

$$\xi_n = 0 + \frac{1|}{|n} + \frac{1|}{|n} + \frac{1|}{|n} + \cdots, \quad n = 1, 2, 3, \ldots.$$

Then

$$\tau_1 = \int_0^{\infty} \frac{J_1(2u)}{e^u - 1}du = \sum_{n=1}^{\infty} \frac{1}{1 + \xi_n^{-2}},$$

where

$$J_1(x) = \sum_{k=0}^{\infty} \frac{(-1)^k}{k!(k+1)!}\left(\frac{x}{2}\right)^{2k+1}$$

is the Bessel function of first order. In the same way, if

$$\xi_{m,n} = 0 + \frac{1|}{|m} + \frac{1|}{|n} + \frac{1|}{|m} + \frac{1|}{|n} + \cdots$$

then

$$\tau_2 = \int_0^{\infty}\int_0^{\infty} \frac{J_1(2\sqrt{uv})^2}{(e^u - 1)(e^v - 1)}du\,dv = \sum_{m=1}^{\infty}\sum_{n=1}^{\infty} \frac{1}{(\xi_{m,n}\xi_{n,m})^{-2} - 1} = 1.1038396536\ldots.$$

Generalization of these is possible.

It can be proved that the dominant eigenvalue $\lambda_1(s)$ of G_s (of largest modulus) is positive and unique, that the function $s \to \lambda_1(s)$ is analytic and strictly decreasing, and that [26]

$$\lim_{s\to 1^+}(s - 1)\lambda_1(s) = 1, \quad \lambda_1(2) = 1, \quad \lim_{s\to\infty}\frac{1}{s}\ln(\lambda_1(s)) = -\ln(\varphi).$$

A simple argument [22] shows that $\lambda_1'(2) = -\pi^2/(12\ln(2))$ is Lévy's constant [1.8]. Later, we will see that both $\lambda_1'(2)$ and $\lambda_1''(2)$ arise in connection with determining precisely the efficiency of the Euclidean algorithm [2.18]. Likewise, $\lambda_1(4)$ occurs in the analysis of certain comparison and sorting algorithms [2.19]. It is known that all eigenvalues $\lambda_j(s)$ are real, but questions of sign and uniqueness remain open for $j > 1$.

Here is an alternative definition of $\lambda_1(s)$. For any k-dimensional vector $w = (w_1, \ldots, w_k)$ of positive integers, let $\langle w \rangle$ denote the denominator of the continued fraction

$$0 + \frac{1|}{|w_1} + \frac{1|}{|w_2} + \frac{1|}{|w_3} + \cdots + \frac{1|}{|w_k}$$

and let $W(k)$ be the set of all such vectors. Then

$$\lambda_1(s) = \lim_{k \to \infty} \left(\sum_{w \in W(k)} \langle w \rangle^{-s} \right)^{\frac{1}{k}}$$

is true for all $s > 1$. This is the reason $\lambda_1(s)$ is often called a pseudo-zeta function associated with continued fractions.

2.17.2 Asymptotic Normality

We initially studied the denominator $Q_n(x)$ of the nth continued fraction convergent to x in [1.8]. With the machinery introduced in the previous section, more can now be said.

If x is drawn uniformly from $(0, 1)$, then the mean and variance of $\ln(Q_n(x))$ satisfy [22, 26]

$$\mathrm{E}(\ln(Q_n(x))) = An + B + O(c^n), \quad \mathrm{Var}(\ln(Q_n(x))) = Cn + D + O(c^n),$$

where $c = -\lambda_2(2) = 0.3036630028\ldots$, $A = -\lambda_1'(2) = 1.1865691104\ldots$, and [2.18]

$$C = \lambda_1''(2) - \lambda_1'(2)^2 = 0.8621470373\ldots = (0.9285187329\ldots)^2.$$

The constants B and D await numerical evaluation. Further, the distribution of $\ln(Q_n(x))$ is asymptotically normal:

$$\lim_{n \to \infty} \mathrm{P}\left(\frac{\ln(Q_n(x)) - An}{\sqrt{Cn}} \leq y \right) = \frac{1}{\sqrt{2\pi}} \int_{-\infty}^{y} \exp\left(-\frac{t^2}{2} \right) dt.$$

This is the first of several appearances of the Central Limit Theorem in this book.

2.17.3 Bounded Partial Denominators

A consequence of the Gauss–Kuzmin density is that almost all real numbers have unbounded partial denominators a_k. What does the set of all real numbers with only 1s and 2s for partial denominators "look like"? It is known [27–31] that this set has Hausdorff dimension between 0.53128049 and 0.53128051. Further discussion of this parameter is deferred until [8.20].

[1] D. E. Knuth, *The Art of Computer Programming*, v. 2, *Seminumerical Algorithms*, 3rd ed., Addison-Wesley, 1998; MR 44 #3531.

[2] R. Kuzmin, Sur un problème de Gauss, *Atti del Congresso Internazionale dei Matematici*, v. 6, Proc. 1928 Bologna conf., ed. N. Zanichelli, Societa Tipografica gia Compositori, 1929, pp. 83–89.

[3] P. Lévy, Sur les lois probabilité dont dépendent les quotients complets et incomplets d'une fraction continue, *Bull. Soc. Math. France* 57 (1929) 178–194; also in *Oeuvres*, v. 6, ed. D. Dugué, Gauthier-Villars, 1980, pp. 266–282.

[4] P. Szüsz, Über einen Kusminschen Satz, *Acta Math. Acad. Sci. Hungar.* 12 (1961) 447–453; MR 27 #124.

[5] E. Wirsing, On the theorem of Gauss-Kuzmin-Lévy and a Frobenius-type theorem for function spaces, *Acta Arith.* 24 (1974) 507–528; MR 49 #2637.

[6] A. J. MacLeod, High-accuracy numerical values in the Gauss-Kuzmin continued fraction problem, *Comput. Math. Appl. (Oxford)*, v. 26 (1993) n. 3, 37–44; MR 94h:11114.

[7] K. I. Babenko and S. P. Jurev, A problem of Gauss (in Russian), Institut Prikladnoi Mat. Akad. Nauk SSSR preprint n. 63 (1977); MR 58 #19017.

[8] K. I. Babenko, On a problem of Gauss (in Russian), *Dokl. Akad. Nauk SSSR* 238 (1978) 1021–1024; Engl. transl. in *Soviet Math. Dokl.* 19 (1978) 136–140; MR 57 #12436.

[9] K. I. Babenko and S. P. Jurev, On the discretization of a problem of Gauss (in Russian), *Dokl. Akad. Nauk SSSR* 240 (1978) 1273–1276; Engl. transl. in *Soviet Math. Dokl.* 19 (1978) 731–735; MR 81h:65015.

[10] H. Daudé, P. Flajolet, and B. Vallée, An average-case analysis of the Gaussian algorithm for lattice reduction, *Combin. Probab. Comput.* 6 (1997) 397–433; INRIA preprint RR2798; MR 99a:65196.

[11] P. Flajolet and B. Vallée, On the Gauss-Kuzmin-Wirsing constant, unpublished note (1995).

[12] P. Sebah, Computing eigenvalues of Wirsing's operator, unpublished note (2001).

[13] D. H. Mayer, On the thermodynamic formalism for the Gauss map, *Commun. Math. Phys.* 130 (1990) 311–333; MR 91g:58216.

[14] A. Durner, On a theorem of Gauss-Kuzmin-Lévy, *Arch. Math. (Basel)* 58 (1992) 251–256; MR 93c:11056.

[15] C. Faivre, The rate of convergence of approximations of a continued fraction, *J. Number Theory* 68 (1998) 21–28; MR 98m:11083.

[16] M. Iosifescu and S. Grigorescu, *Dependence with Complete Connections and Its Applications*, Cambridge Univ. Press, 1990; MR 91j:60098.

[17] M. Iosifescu, A very simple proof of a generalization of the Gauss-Kuzmin-Lévy theorem on continued fractions, and related questions, *Rev. Roumaine Math. Pures Appl.* 37 (1992) 901–914; MR 94j:40003.

[18] D. Hensley, Metric Diophantine approximation and probability, *New York J. Math.* 4 (1998) 249–257; MR 2000d:11102.

[19] K. Dajani and C. Kraaikamp, A Gauss-Kuzmin theorem for optimal continued fractions, *Trans. Amer. Math. Soc.* 351 (1999) 2055–2079; MR 99h:11089.

[20] D. Ruelle, *Dynamical Zeta Functions for Piecewise Monotone Maps of the Interval*, Amer. Math. Soc., 1994; MR 95m:58101.

[21] D. H. Mayer, Continued fractions and related transformations, *Ergodic Theory, Symbolic Dynamics and Hyperbolic Spaces*, ed. T. Bedford, M. Keane, and C. Series, Oxford Univ. Press, 1991, pp. 175–222; MR 93e:58002.

[22] P. Flajolet and B. Vallée, Continued fraction algorithms, functional operators, and structure constants, *Theoret. Comput. Sci.* 194 (1998) 1–34; INRIA preprint RR2931; MR 98j:11061.

[23] P. Flajolet, B. Vallée, and I. Vardi, Continued fractions from Euclid to the present day, École Polytechnique preprint (2000).

[24] D. Mayer and G. Roepstorff, On the relaxation time of Gauss' continued-fraction map. I: The Hilbert space approach (Koopmanism), *J. Stat. Phys.* 47 (1987) 149–171; MR 89a:28017.

[25] D. Mayer and G. Roepstorff, On the relaxation time of Gauss' continued-fraction map. II: The Banach space approach (Transfer operator method), *J. Stat. Phys.* 50 (1988) 331–344; MR 89g:58171.

[26] D. Hensley, The number of steps in the Euclidean algorithm, *J. Number Theory* 49 (1994) 142–182; MR 96b:11131.

[27] I. J. Good, The fractional dimensional theory of continued fractions, *Proc. Cambridge Philos. Soc.* 37 (1941) 199–228; corrigenda 105 (1989) 607; MR 3,75b and MR 90i:28013.

[28] R. T. Bumby, Hausdorff dimension of sets arising in number theory, *Number Theory: New York 1983-84*, ed. D. V. Chudnovsky, G. V. Chudnovsky, H. Cohn, and M. B. Nathanson, Lect. Notes in Math. 1135, Springer-Verlag, pp. 1–8, 1985; MR 87a:11074.

[29] D. Hensley, The Hausdorff dimensions of some continued fraction Cantor sets, *J. Number Theory* 33 (1989) 182–198; MR 91c:11043.

[30] D. Hensley, Continued fraction Cantor sets, Hausdorff dimension, and functional analysis, *J. Number Theory* 40 (1992) 336–358; MR 93c:11058.

[31] E. Cesaratto, On the Hausdorff dimension of certain sets arising in number theory, math.NT/9908043.

2.18 Porter–Hensley Constants

Given two nonnegative integers m and n, let $L(m, n)$ denote the number of division steps required to compute $\gcd(m, n)$ by the classical Euclidean algorithm. By definition, if $m \geq n$, then

$$L(m, n) = \begin{cases} 1 + L(n, m \bmod n) & \text{if } n \geq 1, \\ 0 & \text{if } n = 0, \end{cases}$$

and if $m < n$, then $L(m, n) = 1 + L(n, m)$. Equivalently, $L(m, n)$ is the length of the regular continued fraction representation of m/n. We are interested in determining precisely the efficiency of the Euclidean algorithm and will do so by examining three types of random variables:

$$X_n = L(m, n), \quad \text{where } 0 \leq m < n \text{ is chosen at random,}$$

$$Y_n = L(m, n), \quad \text{where } 0 \leq m < n \text{ is chosen at random and } m \text{ is coprime to } n,$$

$$Z_N = L(m, n), \quad \text{where both } 1 \leq m \leq N \text{ and } 1 \leq n \leq N \text{ are chosen at random.}$$

Of these three, the expected value of Y_n is best behaved and was the first to succumb to analysis. It is interesting to follow the progress in understanding these average values. In his first edition, Knuth [1] observed that, empirically, $E(Y_n) \sim 0.843 \ln(n) + 1.47$ and gave compelling reasons for

$$E(Y_n) \sim \frac{12 \ln(2)}{\pi^2} \ln(n) + 1.47, \quad E(Z_N) \sim \frac{12 \ln(2)}{\pi^2} \ln(N) + 0.06,$$

where the coefficient of $\ln(n)$ is Lévy's constant [1.8]. He decried the gaping theoretical holes in proving these asymptotics, however, and wrote, "The world's most famous algorithm deserves a complete analysis!"

By the second edition [2], remarkable progress had been achieved by Heilbronn [3], Dixon [4, 5], and Porter [6]. For any $\varepsilon > 0$, the following asymptotic formula is true:

$$E(Y_n) \sim \frac{12 \ln(2)}{\pi^2} \ln(n) + C + O\left(n^{-\frac{1}{6}+\varepsilon}\right),$$

and **Porter's constant** C is defined by

$$C = \frac{6\ln(2)}{\pi^2}\left(3\ln(2) + 4\gamma - \frac{24}{\pi^2}\zeta'(2) - 2\right) - \frac{1}{2} = 1.4670780794\ldots,$$

where γ is the Euler–Mascheroni constant [1.5],

$$\zeta'(2) = \left.\frac{d}{dx}\zeta(x)\right|_{x=2} = -\sum_{k=2}^{\infty}\frac{\ln(k)}{k^2} = -0.9375482543\ldots,$$

and $\zeta(x)$ is the Riemann zeta function [1.6]. This expression for C was discovered by Wrench [7], who also computed $\zeta'(2)$, and hence C, to 120 decimal places [8]. See [2.10] for more occurrences of $\zeta'(2)$.

What can be said of the other two average values? Norton [9] proved that, for any $\varepsilon > 0$,

$$E(Z_N) \sim \frac{12\ln(2)}{\pi^2}\ln(N) + B + O\left(N^{-\frac{1}{6}+\varepsilon}\right),$$

where

$$B = \frac{12\ln(2)}{\pi^2}\left(-\frac{1}{2} + \frac{6}{\pi^2}\zeta'(2)\right) + C - \frac{1}{2} = 0.0653514259\ldots.$$

The asymptotic expression for $E(X_n)$ is similar to that for $E(Y_n)$ minus a correction term [2, 9] based on the divisors of n:

$$E(X_n) \sim \frac{12\ln(2)}{\pi^2}\left(\ln(n) - \sum_{d|n}\frac{\Lambda(d)}{d}\right) + C + \frac{1}{n}\sum_{d|n}\varphi(d)\cdot O\left(d^{-\frac{1}{6}+\varepsilon}\right),$$

where φ is Euler's totient function [2.7] and Λ is von Mangoldt's function:

$$\Lambda(d) = \begin{cases} \ln(p) & \text{if } d = p^r \text{ for } p \text{ prime and } r \geq 1, \\ 0 & \text{otherwise.} \end{cases}$$

In the midst of the proof in [9], Norton mentioned the Glaisher–Kinkelin constant A, which we discuss in [2.15]. Porter's constant C can be written in terms of A as

$$C = \frac{6\ln(2)}{\pi^2}(48\ln(A) - 4\ln(\pi) - \ln(2) - 2) - \frac{1}{2}$$

Knuth [7] mentioned a long-forgotten paper [10] containing $(1 - 2B)/4 = 0.2173242870\ldots$ and proposed that C instead be called the Lochs–Porter constant.

It is far more difficult to compute the corresponding variance of $L(m, n)$. Let us focus only on Z_N. Hensley [11] proved that

$$\text{Var}(Z_N) = H\ln(N) + o(\ln(N)),$$

where

$$H = -\frac{\lambda_1''(2) - \lambda_1'(2)^2}{\pi^6\lambda_1'(2)^3} = 0.0005367882\ldots = (0.0231686908\ldots)^2.$$

and $\lambda_1'(2)$ and $\lambda_1''(2)$ are precisely as described in [2.17.1]. Numerical work by Flajolet & Vallée [12] yielded the estimate $4\lambda_1''(2) = 9.0803731646\ldots$ needed to evaluate H. Furthermore, the distribution of Z_N is asymptotically normal:

$$\lim_{N\to\infty} \mathrm{P}\left(\frac{Z_N - \frac{12\ln(2)}{\pi^2}\ln(N)}{\sqrt{H\ln(N)}} \leq w\right) = \frac{1}{\sqrt{2\pi}}\int_{-\infty}^{w} \exp\left(-\frac{t^2}{2}\right) dt.$$

A recent paper [13] contains several Porter-like constants in connection with the problem of sorting several real numbers via their continued fraction representations.

2.18.1 Binary Euclidean Algorithm

Assume m and n are positive odd integers. Let $e(m, n)$ be the largest integer such that $2^{e(m,n)}$ divides $m - n$. The number of subtraction steps required to compute $\gcd(m, n)$ by the binary Euclidean algorithm [14] is

$$K(m, n) = \begin{cases} 1 + K\left(\dfrac{m - n}{2^{e(m,n)}}, n\right) & \text{if } m > n, \\ 0 & \text{if } m = n, \\ K(n, m) & \text{if } m < n. \end{cases}$$

Define the random variable

$$W_N = K(m, n), \quad \text{where odd } 0 < m \leq N \text{ and } 0 < n \leq N \text{ are chosen at random.}$$

Computing the expected value of W_N is much more complicated than for Z_N. As in [2.17.1], study of a linear operator on function spaces [15, 16]

$$V_s[f](z) = \sum_{k \geq 1} \sum_{\substack{1 \leq j < 2^k \\ \text{odd}}} \frac{1}{(j + 2^k z)^s} f\left(\frac{1}{j + 2^k z}\right),$$

is needed. For $s = 2$, let ψ denote the unique fixed point of V_s (up to scaling) and define a constant

$$\kappa = \frac{2}{\pi^2 \psi(1)} \sum_{\substack{r \geq 1 \\ \text{odd}}} 2^{-\left\lfloor \frac{\ln(r)}{\ln(2)} \right\rfloor} \int_0^{\frac{1}{r}} \psi(x) dx;$$

then $\mathrm{E}(W_N) \sim \kappa \ln(N)$. Further, if a certain conjecture by Vallée is true [15, 16], then some heuristic formulas due to Brent [17–19] are applicable and

$$\kappa = 1.0185012157\ldots = \ln(2)^{-1} \cdot 0.7059712461\ldots.$$

A direct computation, based on the exact definition of κ, has yet to be carried out.

Other performance parameters [15, 16] and alternative algorithms [17] have been studied, giving more constants. There is a continued fraction interpretation of these results. A general framework for investigating Euclidean-like algorithms [20, 21] provides analyses of methods for evaluating the Jacobi symbol from number theory [22].

Even more constants emerge if we examine average bit complexity rather than arithmetical operation counts [23, 24]. Many related questions remain unanswered.

2.18.2 Worst-Case Analysis

It is known [14, 25, 26] that the maximum value of Z_N occurs when m and n are consecutive Fibonacci numbers f_k and f_{k+1}, and k is the largest integer with $f_{k+1} \leq N$. Therefore

$$\max(Z_N) = k \sim \frac{1}{\ln(\varphi)} \ln(N) = 2.0780869212 \ldots \cdot \ln(N),$$

where φ is the Golden mean [1.2]. In contrast [14],

$$\max(W_N) \sim \frac{1}{\ln(2)} \ln(N) = 1.4426950408 \ldots \cdot \ln(N),$$

and this occurs when m and n are of the form $2^{k-1} - 1$ and $2^{k-1} + 1$.

[1] D. E. Knuth, *The Art of Computer Programming*, v. 2, *Seminumerical Algorithms*, 1ˢᵗ ed., Addison-Wesley, 1969; MR 44 #3531.

[2] D. E. Knuth, *The Art of Computer Programming*, v. 2, *Seminumerical Algorithms*, 2ⁿᵈ ed., Addison-Wesley, 1981; MR 44 #3531.

[3] H. Heilbronn, On the average length of a class of finite continued fractions, *Number Theory and Analysis*, ed. P. Turán, Plenum Press, 1969, pp. 87–96; MR 41 #3406.

[4] J. D. Dixon, The number of steps in the Euclidean algorithm, *J. Number Theory* 2 (1970) 414–422; MR 42 #1791.

[5] J. D. Dixon, A simple estimate for the number of steps in the Euclidean algorithm, *Amer. Math. Monthly* 78 (1971) 374–376; MR 44 #2697.

[6] J. W. Porter, On a theorem of Heilbronn, *Mathematika* 22 (1975) 20–28; MR 58 #16567.

[7] D. E. Knuth, Evaluation of Porter's constant, *Comput. Math. Appl. (Oxford)*, v. 2 (1976) n. 1, 137–139; also in *Selected Papers on Analysis of Algorithms*, CSLI, 2000, pp. 189–194; MR 2001c:68066.

[8] B. C. Berndt, *Ramanujan's Notebooks: Part I*, Springer-Verlag, 1985, p. 225; MR 86c:01062.

[9] G. H. Norton, On the asymptotic analysis of the Euclidean algorithm, *J. Symbolic Comput.* 10 (1990) 53–58; MR 91k:11088.

[10] G. Lochs, Statistik der Teilnenner der zu den echten Brüchen gehörigen regelmässigen Kettenbrüche, *Monatsh. Math.* 65 (1961) 27–52; MR 23 #A1622.

[11] D. Hensley, The number of steps in the Euclidean algorithm, *J. Number Theory* 49 (1994) 142–182; MR 96b:11131.

[12] P. Flajolet and B. Vallée, Hensley's constant, unpublished note (1999).

[13] P. Flajolet and B. Vallée, Continued fractions, comparison algorithms, and fine structure constants, *Constructive, Experimental, and Nonlinear Analysis*, Proc. 1999 Limoges conf., ed. M. Théra, Amer. Math. Soc., 2000, pp. 53–82; INRIA preprint RR4072; MR 2001h:11161.

[14] D. E. Knuth, *The Art of Computer Programming*, v. 2, *Seminumerical Algorithms*, 3ʳᵈ ed., Addison-Wesley, 1997; MR 44 #3531.

[15] B. Vallée, The complete analysis of the binary Euclidean algorithm, *Proc. 1998 Algorithmic Number Theory Sympos. (ANTS-III)*, Portland, ed. J. P. Buhler, Lect. Notes in Comp. Sci. 1423, Springer-Verlag, 1998, pp. 77–94; MR 2000k:11143a.

[16] B. Vallée, Dynamics of the binary Euclidean algorithm: Functional analysis and operators, *Algorithmica* 22 (1998) 660–685; MR 2000k:11143b.

[17] R. P. Brent, Analysis of the binary Euclidean algorithm, *Algorithms and Complexity: New Directions and Recent Results*, ed. J. F. Traub, Academic Press, 1976, pp. 321–355; MR 55 #11701.

[18] R. P. Brent, The binary Euclidean algorithm, *Millennial Perspectives in Computer Science*, Proc. 1999 Oxford-Microsoft Symp., ed. J. Davies, B. Roscoe, and J. Woodcock, Palgrave, 2000, pp. 41–53.

[19] R. P. Brent, Further analysis of the binary Euclidean algorithm, Oxford Univ. PRG TR-7-99 (1999).

[20] B. Vallée, A unifying framework for the analysis of a class of Euclidean algorithms, *Proc. 2000 Latin American Theoretical Informatics Conf. (LATIN),* Punta del Este, ed. G. H. Gonnet, D. Panario, and A. Viola, Lect. Notes in Comp. Sci. 1776, Springer-Verlag, 2000, pp. 343–354.

[21] B. Vallée, Dynamical analysis of a class of Euclidean algorithms, *Theoret. Comput. Sci.,* submitted (2000).

[22] B. Vallée and C. Lemée, Average-case analyses of three algorithms for computing the Jacobi symbol, unpublished note (1998).

[23] A. Akhavi and B. Vallée, Average bit-complexity of Euclidean algorithms, *Proc. 2000 Int. Colloq. on Automata, Languages and Programming (ICALP)*, Geneva, ed. U. Montanari, J. D. P. Rolim, and E. Welzl, Lect. Notes in Comp. Sci. 1853, Springer-Verlag, pp. 373–387; MR 2001h:68052.

[24] B. Vallée, Digits and continuants in Euclidean algorithms, *J. Théorie Nombres Bordeaux* 12 (2000) 531–570; MR 2002b:11105.

[25] J. Shallit, Origins of the analysis of the Euclidean algorithm, *Historia Math.* 21 (1994) 401–419; MR 95h:01015.

[26] P. Schreiber, A supplement to J. Shallit's paper: "Origins of the analysis of the Euclidean algorithm," *Historia Math.* 22 (1995) 422–424; MR 96j:01010.

2.19 Vallée's Constant

Let x and y be random numbers drawn uniformly and independently from the interval $(0, 1)$. To **compare** x and y is to determine which of the following is true: $x < y$ or $x > y$. There is an obvious algorithm for comparing x and y: Search for where the decimal or binary expansions of x and y first disagree. In base b, the number L of iterations of this algorithm has mean value

$$E(L) = \frac{b}{b-1}$$

and a probability distribution given by

$$p_n = P(L \geq n + 1) = b^{-n}, \quad n = 0, 1, 2 \ldots.$$

Clearly

$$\lim_{n \to \infty} p_n^{\frac{1}{n}} = \frac{1}{b}$$

is a simply a way of expressing the (asymptotic) rate at which digits in the two base-b expansions coincide.

Here is a less obvious algorithm, proposed in [1], for comparing x and y. Write x and y (uniquely) as regular continued fractions:

$$x = 0 + \frac{1|}{|a_1} + \frac{1|}{|a_2} + \frac{1|}{|a_3} + \cdots, \quad y = 0 + \frac{1|}{|b_1} + \frac{1|}{|b_2} + \frac{1|}{|b_3} + \cdots,$$

where each a_j and b_j is a positive integer and search for where $a_k \neq b_k$ first occurs. If k is even, then $x < y$ if and only if $a_k < b_k$. If k is odd, then $x < y$ if and only if $a_k > b_k$. (There are other necessary provisions if x or y are rational, i.e., where a_j or b_j might be 0, which we do not discuss.)

The analysis of this algorithm is much more difficult and uses techniques and ideas discussed in [2.17.1]. Daudé, Flajolet & Vallée [2–5] proved that the mean number of iterations is

$$E(L) = \frac{3}{4} + \frac{180}{\pi^4} \sum_{i=1}^{\infty} \sum_{j=i+1}^{2i} \frac{1}{i^2 j^2} = \frac{17}{4} + \frac{360}{\pi^4} \sum_{i=1}^{\infty} \sum_{j=1}^{i} \frac{(-1)^i}{i^2 j^2}$$

$$= 17 - \frac{60}{\pi^4} \left[24 \operatorname{Li}_4 \left(\frac{1}{2} \right) - \pi^2 \ln(2)^2 + 21\zeta(3) \ln(2) + \ln(2)^4 \right]$$

$$= 1.3511315744\ldots,$$

where $\operatorname{Li}_4(z)$ is the tetralogarithm function [1.6.8] and $\zeta(3)$ is Apéry's constant [1.6]. This closed-form evaluation draws upon work in [6–8]. We also have

$$p_1 = \sum_{i=1}^{\infty} \frac{1}{i^2(i+1)^2} = \frac{\pi^2}{3} - 3 = 0.2898681336\ldots,$$

$$p_2 = \sum_{i=1}^{\infty} \sum_{j=1}^{\infty} \frac{1}{(ij+1)^2(ij+i+1)^2} = 0.0484808014\ldots$$

$$= -5 + \frac{2\pi^2}{3} - 2\zeta(3) + 2 \sum_{n=0}^{\infty} (-1)^n (n+1)\zeta(n+4) \left[\zeta(n+2) - 1 \right],$$

$$p_3 = \sum_{i=1}^{\infty} \sum_{j=1}^{\infty} \sum_{k=1}^{\infty} \frac{1}{(ijk+i+k)^2(ijk+ij+i+k+1)^2} = 0.0102781647\ldots,$$

but unlike earlier, a nice compact formula for p_n is not known. The elaborate recurrence giving rise to p_n appears later [2.19.1]. It can be deduced that [2–5]

$$v = \lim_{n \to \infty} p_n^{\frac{1}{n}} = 0.1994588183\ldots$$

using the fact that this is the largest eigenvalue of the linear operator G_4 defined in [2.17.1]. As with G_2, the eigenvalues of G_4 are real and seem to alternate in sign (the next one is $-0.0757395140\ldots$). A similar argument applies in the analysis of the Gaussian algorithm for finding a short basis of a lattice in two-dimensional space, given an initially skew basis. Vallée's constant v also appears in connection with the problem of sorting $n > 2$ real numbers via their continued fraction representations [9].

If, when comparing x and y, we instead use centered continued fractions, then the number $\hat{L}$ of iterations satisfy [2, 5]

$$E(\hat{L}) = \frac{360}{\pi^4} \sum_{i=1}^{\infty} \sum_{j=\lceil \varphi i \rceil}^{\lfloor (\varphi+1)i \rfloor} \frac{1}{i^2 j^2} = 1.0892214740\ldots,$$

$$\hat{v} = \lim_{n \to \infty} \hat{p}_n^{\frac{1}{n}} = 0.0773853773\ldots,$$

where φ is the Golden mean [1.2]. Since $1/v = 5.01\ldots$ and $1/\hat{v} = 12.92\ldots$, it follows that continued fractions behave roughly like base-5 and base-13 representations in this respect. Not much is known about the corresponding operator $\hat{G}_s$ and its spectrum. Flajolet & Vallée [5] also numerically computed values of the mock zeta function

$$\zeta_\theta(z) = \sum_{k=1}^{\infty} \frac{1}{\lfloor k\theta \rfloor^z}, \quad \text{Re}(z) > 1, \quad \theta > 1,$$

where $\theta > 1$ is irrational. For example, $\zeta_\varphi(2) = 1.2910603681\ldots$.

2.19.1 Continuant Polynomials

Define functions recursively by the rule [3]

$$f_k(x_1, x_2, \ldots, x_k) = x_k f_{k-1}(x_1, x_2, \ldots, x_{k-1}) + f_{k-2}(x_1, x_2, \ldots, x_{k-2}),$$
$$k = 2, 3, 4, \ldots,$$

where

$$f_0 = 1, \quad f_1(x_1) = x_1.$$

These are called **continuant polynomials** and can also be defined by taking the sum of monomials obtained from $x_1 x_2 \cdots x_k$ by crossing out in all possible ways pairs of adjacent variables $x_j x_{j+1}$. For example,

$$f_2(x_1, x_2) = x_1 x_2 + 1, \quad f_3(x_1, x_2, x_3) = x_1 x_2 x_3 + x_1 + x_3,$$
$$f_4(x_1, x_2, x_3, x_4) = x_1 x_2 x_3 x_4 + x_1 x_2 + x_1 x_4 + x_3 x_4 + 1.$$

The probability of interest to us is

$$p_k = \sum_{n_1=1}^{\infty} \sum_{n_2=1}^{\infty} \cdots \sum_{n_k=1}^{\infty} \frac{1}{f_k^2 (f_k + f_{k-1})^2}.$$

Each p_k can be expressed in terms of complicated series involving Riemann zeta function values and thus falls in the class of polynomial-time computable constants [5].

[1] M. Beeler, R. W. Gosper, and R. Schroeppel, Continued fraction arithmetic, HAKMEM, MIT AI Memo 239, item 101A.

[2] H. Daudé, P. Flajolet, and B. Vallée, An analysis of the Gaussian algorithm for lattice reduction, *Proc. 1994 Algorithmic Number Theory Sympos.* (ANTS-I), Ithaca, ed. L.
M. Adleman and M.-D. Huang, Lect. Notes in Comp. Sci. 877, Springer-Verlag, 1994,
pp. 144–158; MR 96a:11075.

[3] H. Daudé, P. Flajolet, and B. Vallée, An average-case analysis of the Gaussian algorithm for
lattice reduction, *Combin. Probab. Comput.* 6 (1997) 397–433; INRIA preprint RR2798;
MR 99a:65196.

[4] B. Vallée, Algorithms for computing signs of 2 × 2 determinants: Dynamics and average-
case analysis, *Proc. 1997 European Symp. on Algorithms (ESA)*, Graz Univ., ed. R. Burkard
and G. Woeginger, Lect. Notes in Comp. Sci. 1284, Springer-Verlag, pp. 486–499; MR
99d:68002.

[5] P. Flajolet and B. Vallée, Continued fractions, comparison algorithms, and fine structure
constants, *Constructive, Experimental, and Nonlinear Analysis*, Proc. 1999 Limoges conf.,
ed. M. Théra, Amer. Math. Soc., 2000, pp. 53–82; INRIA preprint RR4072; MR 2001h:
11161.

[6] R. Sitaramachandrarao, A formula of S. Ramanujan, *J. Number Theory* 25 (1987) 1–19;
MR 88c:11048.

[7] P. J. de Doelder, On some series containing $\psi(x) - \psi(y)$ and $(\psi(x) - \psi(y))^2$ for certain
values of x and y, *J. Comput. Appl. Math.* 37 (1991) 125–141; MR 92m:40002.

[8] G. Rutledge and R. D. Douglass, Evaluation of $\int_0^1 \frac{\log(u)}{u} \log(1 + u)^2 du$ and related definite
integrals, *Amer. Math. Monthly* 41 (1934) 29–36.

[9] P. Flajolet and B. Vallée, Continued fraction algorithms, functional operators, and structure constants, *Theoret. Comput. Sci.* 194 (1998) 1–34; INRIA preprint RR2931; MR 98j:
11061.

2.20 Erdös' Reciprocal Sum Constants

2.20.1 A-Sequences

An infinite sequence of positive integers $1 \le a_1 < a_2 < a_3 < \ldots$ is called an *A-sequence* if no a_k is the sum of two or more distinct earlier terms of the sequence
[1]. For example, the sequence of nonnegative powers of 2 is an *A*-sequence. Erdös [2]
proved that

$$S(A) = \sup_{A\text{-sequences}} \sum_{k=1}^{\infty} \frac{1}{a_k} < 103$$

and thus the largest reciprocal sum must be *finite* in particular. Levine & O'Sullivan
[3,4] proved that any *A*-sequence must satisfy what we call the χ-**inequality**:

$$(j + 1)a_j + a_i \ge (j + 1)i$$

for all i and j, and consequently $S(A) < 3.9998$. In the other direction, Abbott [5] and
Zhang [6] gave specific examples that demonstrate that $S(A) > 2.0649$. These are the
best-known bounds on $S(A)$ so far.

The χ-inequality is itself interesting. Levine & O'Sullivan [3,7] defined a specific
integer sequence by the greedy algorithm: $\chi_1 = 1$ and

$$\chi_i = \max_{1 \le j \le i-1} (j + 1)(i - \chi_j)$$

for $i > 1$, that is, $1, 2, 4, 6, 9, 12, 15, 18, 21, 24, 28, 32, 36, 40, 45, 50, 55, 60, 65, \ldots$.
They conjectured that

$$S(A) \le \sum_{k=1}^{\infty} \frac{1}{\chi_k} = 3.01 \ldots$$

and further that $\{\chi_k\}$ dominates the reciprocal sum of any other integer sequence satisfying the χ-inequality. Finch [8–10] wondered if this latter conjecture still holds for arbitrary (not necessarily integer) real sequences.

The authors of [3–5] used the phrase "sum-free sequence" to refer to A-sequences, which is unfortunate terminology since the word "sum-free" usually refers to an entirely different class of sequences [2.25]. We have adopted the phrase "A-sequence" from Guy [1]. See also [2.28] concerning sets with distinct subset sums.

2.20.2 B_2-Sequences

An infinite sequence of positive integers $1 \le b_1 < b_2 < b_3 < \ldots$ is called a B_2-sequence (or Sidon sequence) if all pairwise sums $b_i + b_j$, $i \le j$, are distinct [1]. For example, the greedy algorithm gives the Mian–Chowla [7, 11] sequence $1, 2, 4, 8, 13, 21, 31, 45, 66, 81, 97, 123, 148, 182, 204, 252, 290, \ldots$, which is known to have reciprocal sum [12] between 2.158435 and 2.158677. Zhang [13] proved that

$$S(B_2) = \sup_{B_2\text{-sequences}} \sum_{k=1}^{\infty} \frac{1}{b_k} > 2.1597$$

and thus is larger than the Mian–Chowla sum. An observation by Levine [1, 13] shows that $S(B_2)$ is necessarily finite; in fact, it is < 2.374. More recent work [12, 14] gives the improved bounds $2.16086 < S(B_2) < 2.247327$.

Erdös & Turán [15–17] asked if a finite B_2-sequence of positive integers $b_1 < b_2 < \ldots < b_m$ with $b_m \le n$ must satisfy $m \le n^{1/2} + C$ for some constant C. Lindström [18] demonstrated that $m < n^{1/2} + n^{1/4} + 1$. Zhang [19] computed that if such a C exists, it must be > 10.27. Lindström [20] improved the lower bound for C to 13.71. In a more recent paper [21], he concluded that C probably does not exist and conjectured that $m \le n^{1/2} + o(n^{1/4})$.

2.20.3 Nonaveraging Sequences

An infinite sequence of positive integers $1 \le c_1 < c_2 < c_3 < \ldots$ is said to be nonaveraging if it contains no three terms in arithmetic progression. Equivalently, $c + d \ne 2e$ for any three distinct terms c, d, e of the sequence [1]. For example, the greedy algorithm gives the Szekeres [7, 22] sequence $1, 2, 4, 5, 10, 11, 13, 14, 28, 29, 31, 32, 37, 38, 40, 41, 82, 83, \ldots$; that is, n is in the sequence if and only if the ternary expansion of $n - 1$ contains only 0s and 1s. This is known to have reciprocal sum between 3.00793 and 3.00794. Wróblewski [23], building upon [24, 25], constructed a special nonaveraging sequence to demonstrate that

$$S(C) = \sup_{\substack{\text{nonaveraging} \\ \text{sequences}}} \sum_{k=1}^{\infty} \frac{1}{c_k} > 3.00849.$$

A proof that $S(C)$ is necessarily finite is not known; the best lower bound [26] for c_k is only $O(k\sqrt{\ln(k)}/\ln(\ln(k)))$.

Some related studies of the density of $\{c_k\} \cap [1, n]$, constructed greedily with alternative formation rules or different initial values, appear in [27–31]. Under certain conditions, as n increases, the density oscillates with peaks and valleys (rather than falling smoothly) in roughly geometric progression. The ratio between two consecutive peaks seems, as $N \to \infty$, to approach a limit. This phenomenon deserves to be better understood.

[1] R. K. Guy, *Unsolved Problems in Number Theory*, 2nd ed., Springer-Verlag, 1994, sect. E10, E28; MR 96e:11002.

[2] P. Erdös, Remarks on number theory. III: Some problems in additive number theory, *Mat. Lapok* 13 (1962) 28–38; MR 26 #2412.

[3] E. Levine and J. O'Sullivan, An upper estimate for the reciprocal sum of a sum-free sequence, *Acta Arith.* 34 (1977) 9–24; MR 57 #5900.

[4] E. Levine, An extremal result for sum-free sequences, *J. Number Theory* 12 (1980) 251–257; MR 82d:10078.

[5] H. L. Abbott, On sum-free sequences, *Acta Arith.* 48 (1987) 93–96; MR 88g:11007.

[6] Z. Zhang, A sum-free sequence with larger reciprocal sum, unpublished note (1991).

[7] N. J. A. Sloane, On-Line Encyclopedia of Integer Sequences, A003278, A005282, A014011, and A046185.

[8] S. R. Finch, A convex maximization problem, *J. Global Optim.* 2 (1992) 419.

[9] S. R. Finch, A convex maximization problem: Discrete case, math.OC/9912035.

[10] S. R. Finch, A convex maximization problem: Continuous case, math.OC/9912036.

[11] A. M. Mian and S. Chowla, On the B_2 sequences of Sidon, *Proc. Nat. Acad. Sci. India. Sect. A.* 14 (1944) 3–4; MR 7,243a.

[12] R. Lewis, Mian-Chowla and B_2-sequences, unpublished note (1999).

[13] Z. Zhang, A B_2-sequence with larger reciprocal sum, *Math. Comp.* 60 (1993) 835–839; MR 93m:11012.

[14] G. S. Yovanof and H. Taylor, B_2-sequences and the distinct distance constant, *Comput. Math. Appl. (Oxford)* 39 (2000) 37–42; MR 2001j:11007.

[15] P. Erdös and P. Turán, On a problem of Sidon in additive number theory, and on some related problems, *J. London Math. Soc.* 16 (1941) 212–215; addendum 19 (1944) 208; also in *Collected Works of Paul Turán*, v. 1, ed. P. Erdös, Akadémiai Kiadó, pp. 257–261; MR 3,270e.

[16] H. Halberstam and K. F. Roth, *Sequences*, Springer-Verlag, 1983, pp. 84–88; MR 83m:10094.

[17] P. Erdös, On the combinatorial problems which I would most like to see solved, *Combinatorica* 1 (1981) 25–42; MR 82k:05001.

[18] B. Lindström, An inequality for B_2-sequences, *J. Combin. Theory* 6 (1969) 211–212; MR 38 #4436.

[19] Z. Zhang, Finding finite B_2-sequences with larger $m - a_m^{1/2}$, *Math. Comp.* 63 (1994) 403–414; MR 94i:11109.

[20] B. Lindström, An Erdös problem studied with the assistance of a computer, *Normat*, v. 45 (1997) n. 4, 145–149, 188; MR 98m:11140.

[21] B. Lindström, Recent results on Sidon sequences – A survey, Royal Institute of Technology report TRITA-MAT-1998-29.

[22] P. Erdös and P. Turán, On some sequences of integers, *J. London Math. Soc.* 11 (1936) 261–264.

[23] J. Wróblewski, A nonaveraging set of integers with a large sum of reciprocals, *Math. Comp.* 43 (1984) 261–262; MR 85k:11006.

[24] F. Behrend, On sets of integers which contain no three terms in an arithmetic progression, *Proc. Nat. Acad. Sci. USA* 32 (1946) 331–332; MR 8,317d.

[25] J. L. Gerver, The sum of the reciprocals of a set of integers with no arithmetic progression of *k* terms, *Proc. Amer. Math. Soc.* 62 (1977) 211–214; MR 55 #12678.

[26] J. Bourgain, On triples in arithmetic progression, *Geom. Funct. Anal.* 9 (1999) 968–984; MR 2001h:11132.

[27] A. M. Odlyzko and R. P. Stanley, Some curious sequences constructed with the greedy algorithm, unpublished note (1978).

[28] J. L. Gerver and L. Ramsey, Sets of integers with no long arithmetic progressions generated by the greedy algorithm, *Math. Comp.* 33 (1979) 1353–1360; MR 80k:10053.

[29] J. L. Gerver, Irregular sets of integers generated by the greedy algorithm, *Math. Comp.* 40 (1983) 667–676; MR 84d:10056.

[30] J. Gerver, J. Propp, and J. Simpson, Greedily partitioning the natural numbers into sets free of arithmetic progressions, *Proc. Amer. Math. Soc.* 102 (1988) 765–772; MR 89f:11026.

[31] S. C. Lindhurst, *An Investigation of Several Interesting Sets of Numbers Generated by the Greedy Algorithm*, AB thesis, Princeton Univ., 1990.

2.21 Stieltjes Constants

The Riemann zeta function $\zeta(z)$, as defined in [1.6], has a Laurent expansion in a neighborhood of its simple pole at $z = 1$:

$$\zeta(z) = \frac{1}{z-1} + \sum_{n=0}^{\infty} \frac{(-1)^n}{n!} \gamma_n (z-1)^n.$$

The coefficients γ_n can be proved to satisfy [1–9]

$$\gamma_n = \lim_{m \to \infty} \left(\sum_{k=1}^{m} \frac{\ln(k)^n}{k} - \frac{\ln(m)^{n+1}}{n+1} \right) = \begin{cases} 0.5772156649\ldots & \text{if } n = 0, \\ -0.0728158454\ldots & \text{if } n = 1, \\ -0.0096903631\ldots & \text{if } n = 2, \\ 0.0020538344\ldots & \text{if } n = 3, \\ 0.0023253700\ldots & \text{if } n = 4, \\ 0.0007933238\ldots & \text{if } n = 5, \end{cases}$$

and, in particular, $\gamma_0 = \gamma$, the Euler–Mascheroni constant [1.5].

Here is a sample application to number theory. Define a positive integer N to be **jagged** if its largest prime factor is $> \sqrt{N}$, and let $j(N)$ be the number of such integers not exceeding N. The first several jagged numbers are $2, 3, 5, 6, 7, 10, 11, 13, 14, \ldots$ and, asymptotically [10, 11],

$$j(N) = \ln(2)N - (1 - \gamma_0)\frac{N}{\ln(N)} - (1 - \gamma_0 - \gamma_1)\frac{N}{\ln(N)^2} + O\left(\frac{N}{\ln(N)^3}\right),$$

where $1 - \gamma_0 = 0.4227843351\ldots$ and $1 - \gamma_0 - \gamma_1 = 0.4956001805\ldots$. See the related discussion of smooth numbers in [5.4]. Other occurrences of γ_n include [12–17].

The signs of the Stieltjes constants γ_n follow a seemingly random pattern. Briggs [18] proved that infinitely many γ_n are positive and infinitely many are negative. Mitrovic [19] extended this result by demonstrating that each of the inequalities

$$\gamma_{2n} < 0, \quad \gamma_{2n} > 0, \quad \gamma_{2n-1} < 0, \quad \gamma_{2n-1} > 0$$

must hold for infinitely many n. In an elaborate analysis, Matsuoka [20, 21] proved that, for any $\varepsilon > 0$, there exist infinitely many integers n for which all of $\gamma_n, \gamma_{n+1}, \gamma_{n+2}, \ldots, \gamma_{n+\lfloor (2-\varepsilon)\ln(n) \rfloor}$ have the same sign, and there exist only finitely many integers n for which all of $\gamma_n, \gamma_{n+1}, \gamma_{n+2}, \ldots, \gamma_{n+\lfloor (2+\varepsilon)\ln(n) \rfloor}$ have the same sign. Also, if

$$f(n) = |\{0 \le k \le n : \gamma_n > 0\}|, \quad g(n) = |\{0 \le k \le n : \gamma_n < 0\}|$$

then $f(n) = n/2 + o(n)$ and $g(n) = n/2 + o(n)$.

The first few Stieltjes constants γ_n are close to 0, but this is deceptive. In fact, their magnitudes seem to $\to \infty$ as $n \to \infty$, although a proof is not known. Upper bounds for $|\gamma_n|$ were successively obtained by several authors [18, 22–26], culminating in

$$|\gamma_n| \le \frac{(3 + (-1)^n)(2n)!}{n^{n+1}(2\pi)^n}.$$

The last word again belongs to Matsuoka [20, 21], who proved that the lower bound

$$\exp(n \ln(\ln(n)) - \varepsilon n) < |\gamma_n|$$

holds for infinitely many n, while the upper bound

$$|\gamma_n| \le \frac{1}{10000} \exp(n \ln(\ln(n)))$$

holds for all $n \ge 10$.

We mentioned in [1.5] the following formula due to Vacca:

$$\gamma_0 = \sum_{k=1}^{\infty} \frac{(-1)^k}{k} \left\lfloor \frac{\ln(k)}{\ln(2)} \right\rfloor.$$

Hardy [27] gave an analog for γ_1:

$$\gamma_1 = \sum_{j=1}^{\infty} \frac{(-1)^j \ln(j)}{j} \left\lfloor \frac{\ln(j)}{\ln(2)} \right\rfloor - \frac{\ln(2)}{2} \sum_{k=1}^{\infty} \frac{(-1)^k}{k} \left\lfloor \frac{\ln(2k)}{\ln(2)} \right\rfloor \left\lfloor \frac{\ln(k)}{\ln(2)} \right\rfloor,$$

and Kluyver [28] presented more such series for higher-order constants. Also, if $\{x\}$ denotes the fractional part of x, then [29]

$$\int_1^{\infty} \frac{\{x\}}{x^2} dx = 1 - \gamma_0, \quad \int_1^{\infty} \int_x^{\infty} \frac{\{y\}}{xy^2} dy \, dx = 1 - \gamma_0 - \gamma_1.$$

Additional formulas for γ_n appear in [7, 8, 30–32].

We now discuss certain associated constants. An alternating series variant,

$$\tau_n = \sum_{k=1}^{\infty} (-1)^k \frac{\ln(k)^n}{k}$$

$$= \begin{cases} -\ln(2) = -0.6931471805\ldots & \text{if } n = 0, \\ -\frac{1}{2}\ln(2)^2 + \gamma_0 \ln(2) = 0.1598689037\ldots & \text{if } n = 1, \\ -\frac{1}{3}\ln(2)^3 + \gamma_0 \ln(2)^2 + 2\gamma_1 \ln(2) = 0.0653725925\ldots & \text{if } n = 2, \end{cases}$$

can be related to the Stieltjes constants via the formulas [1, 4, 8, 26]

$$\tau_n = -\frac{\ln(2)^{n+1}}{n+1} + \sum_{k=0}^{n-1} \binom{n}{k} \ln(2)^{n-k} \gamma_k, \quad \gamma_n = \frac{1}{n+1} \sum_{k=0}^{n+1} \binom{n+1}{k} B_{n+1-k} \ln(2)^{n-k} \tau_k,$$

where B_j is the jth Bernoulli number [1.6.1]. Consider also the Laurent expansion for $\zeta(z)$ at the origin (rather than at unity):

$$\zeta(z) = \frac{1}{z-1} + \sum_{n=0}^{\infty} \frac{(-1)^n}{n!} \delta_n z^n.$$

Sitaramachandrarao [33] proved that [3, 34]

$$\delta_n = \lim_{m \to \infty} \left(\sum_{k=1}^{m} \ln(k)^n - \int_1^m \ln(x)^n dx - \frac{1}{2}\ln(m)^n \right) = (-1)^n (\zeta^{(n)}(0) + n!)$$

$$= \begin{cases} \frac{1}{2} = 0.5 & \text{if } n = 0, \\ \frac{1}{2}\ln(2\pi) - 1 = -0.0810614667\ldots & \text{if } n = 1, \\ -\frac{\pi^2}{24} - \frac{1}{2}\ln(2\pi)^2 + \frac{\gamma_0^2}{2} + \gamma_1 + 2 = -0.0063564559\ldots & \text{if } n = 2, \end{cases}$$

and these, in turn, were helpful to Lehmer [35] in approximating sums of the form [7, 26]

$$\sigma_n = \sum_{\rho} \frac{1}{\rho^n} = \begin{cases} -\frac{1}{2}\ln(4\pi) + \frac{\gamma_0}{2} + 1 = 0.0230957089\ldots & \text{if } n = 1, \\ -\frac{\pi^2}{8} + \gamma_0^2 + 2\gamma_1 + 1 = -0.0461543172\ldots & \text{if } n = 2, \\ -\frac{7\zeta(3)}{8} + \gamma_0^3 + 3\gamma_0\gamma_1 + \frac{3\gamma_2}{2} + 1 = -0.0001111582\ldots & \text{if } n = 3, \end{cases}$$

where each sum is over all nontrivial zeros ρ of $\zeta(z)$. The constant σ_1 also appears in [1.6] and [2.32]. Keiper [36] and Kreminski [37] vastly extended Lehmer's computations.

The analog of γ_n corresponding to the arithmetic progression $a, a+b, a+2b, a+3b, \ldots$ was studied by Knopfmacher [38], Kanemitsu [39], and Dilcher [40]:

$$\gamma_{n,a,b} = \lim_{m \to \infty} \left(\sum_{\substack{0 < k \le m \\ k \equiv a \bmod b}} \frac{\ln(k)^n}{k} - \frac{1}{b} \frac{\ln(m)^{n+1}}{n+1} \right).$$

For example, $\sum_{a=0}^{b-1} \gamma_{n,a,b} = \gamma_n$ and

$$\gamma_{n,0,2} = \frac{1}{2}\left[\sum_{j=0}^{n}\binom{n}{j}\gamma_{n-j}\ln(2)^j - \frac{\ln(2)^{n+1}}{n+1}\right], \quad \gamma_{1,0,3} = \frac{1}{3}\left[\gamma_1 + \gamma_0\ln(3) - \frac{\ln(3)^2}{2}\right],$$

$$\gamma_{1,1,3} = \frac{1}{6}\left[2\gamma_1 - \gamma_0\ln(3) + \frac{\ln(3)^2}{2} - \left(\frac{\gamma_0+\ln(2\pi)}{3} - \ln\left[\Gamma(\tfrac{1}{3})^2\frac{\sqrt{3}}{2\pi}\right]\right)\pi\sqrt{3}\right].$$

Different extensions of γ_n are found in [23, 26, 41–46].

The reader should be warned that some authors define the Stieltjes constants to be $(-1)^n\gamma_n/n!$ rather than γ_n, so care is needed when reviewing the literature.

2.21.1 Generalized Gamma Functions

For complex z, the generalized gamma function $\Gamma_n(z)$ is defined by [47, 48]

$$\Gamma_n(z) = \lim_{m\to\infty}\frac{\exp\left(\dfrac{\ln(m)^{n+1}}{n+1}z\right)\displaystyle\prod_{k=1}^{m}\exp\left(\dfrac{\ln(k)^{n+1}}{n+1}\right)}{\displaystyle\prod_{k=0}^{m}\exp\left(\dfrac{\ln(k+z)^{n+1}}{n+1}\right)}$$

and is analytic over the complex plane slit along the negative x-axis. Clearly $\Gamma_0(z) = \Gamma(z)$ and $\Gamma_n(z)$ satisfies

$$\Gamma_n(1) = 1, \quad \Gamma_n(z+1) = \exp\left(\frac{\ln(z)^{n+1}}{n+1}\right)\Gamma_n(z).$$

The connection between $\Gamma_n(z)$ and γ_n is through the formula $\psi_n(1) = -\gamma_n$, where

$$\psi_n(x) = \frac{d}{dx}\ln(\Gamma_n(x)) = -\gamma_n - \sum_{k=0}^{\infty}\left(\frac{\ln(x+k)^n}{x+k} - \frac{\ln(k+1)^n}{k+1}\right)$$

is the generalized digamma function. A generalized Stirling formula includes

$$\Gamma_0(x) \sim \sqrt{2\pi}x^{x-\frac{1}{2}}e^{-x}, \quad \Gamma_1(x) \sim Cx^{\frac{1}{2}(x-\frac{1}{2})\ln(x)-x}e^x$$

as special cases, where [48, 49]

$$\ln(C) = \ln\left(\Gamma_1\left(\frac{1}{2}\right)\right) - \frac{1}{4}\ln(2)^2 - \frac{1}{2}\ln(2)\ln(2\pi)$$

$$= -\frac{\pi^2}{48} - \frac{1}{4}\ln(2\pi)^2 + \frac{\gamma_0^2}{4} + \frac{\gamma_1}{2} = -1.0031782279\ldots.$$

Many more formulas of this kind can be found.

[1] J. J. Y. Liang and J. Todd, The Stieltjes constants, *J. Res. Nat. Bur. Standards B* 76 (1972) 161–178; MR 48 #5316.

[2] A. Ivić, *The Riemann Zeta-Function*, Wiley, 1985, pp. 4–6, 49; MR 87d:11062.

[3] B. C. Berndt, *Ramanujan's Notebooks: Part I*, Springer-Verlag, 1985, pp. 164–165, 196–204; MR 86c:01062.

[4]   W. E. Briggs and S. Chowla, The power series coefficients of $\zeta(s)$, *Amer. Math. Monthly* 62 (1955) 323–325; MR 16,999f.

[5]   D. P. Verma, Laurent's expansion of Riemann's zeta-function, *Indian J. Math.* 5 (1963) 13–16; MR 28 #5046.

[6]   R. P. Ferguson, An application of Stieltjes integration to the power series coefficients of the Riemann zeta function, *Amer. Math. Monthly* 70 (1963) 60–61; MR 26 #2408.

[7]   M. I. Israilov, The Laurent expansion of the Riemann zeta function (in Russian), *Trudy Mat. Inst. Steklov* 158 (1981) 98–104, 229; Engl. transl. in *Proc. Steklov Inst. Math.* (1983) n. 4, 105–112; MR 83m:10069.

[8]   N. Y. Zhang, On the Stieltjes constants of the zeta function (in Chinese), *Beijing Daxue Xuebao* (1981) n. 4, 20–24; MR 84h:10056.

[9]   B. K. Choudhury, The Riemann zeta-function and its derivatives, *Proc. Royal Soc. London A* 450 (1995) 477–499; MR 97e:11095.

[10] N. J. A. Sloane, On-Line Encyclopedia of Integer Sequences, A064052.

[11] D. H. Greene and D. E. Knuth, *Mathematics for the Analysis of Algorithms*, 3rd ed., Birkhäuser, 1990, pp. 95–98; MR 92c:68067.

[12] N. G. de Bruijn, On Mahler's partition problem, *Proc. Konink. Nederl. Akad. Wetensch. Sci. Sect.* 51 (1948) 659–669; *Indag. Math.* 10 (1948) 210–220; MR 10,16d.

[13] W. B. Pennington, On Mahler's partition problem, *Annals of Math.* 57 (1953) 531–546; MR 14,846m.

[14] A. F. Lavrik, The principal term of the divisor problem and the power series of the Riemann zeta-function in a neighborhood of a pole (in Russian), *Trudy Mat. Inst. Steklov.* 142 (1976) 165–173, 269; Engl. transl. in *Proc. Steklov Inst. Math.* (1979) n. 3, 175–183; MR 58 #27836.

[15] A. F. Lavrik, M. I. Israilov, and Z. Ëdgorov, Integrals containing the remainder term of the divisor problem (in Russian), *Acta Arith.* 37 (1980) 381–389; MR 82e:10078.

[16] È. P. Stankus, A remark on the coefficients of Laurent series of the Riemann zeta function (in Russian), Studies in Number Theory, 8, *Zap. Nauchn. Sem. Leningrad Otdel. Mat. Inst. Steklov (LOMI)* 121 (1983) 103–107; MR 85d:11081.

[17] T. W. Cusick, Zaremba's conjecture and sums of the divisor function, *Math. Comp.* 61 (1993) 171–176; MR 93k:11063.

[18] W. E. Briggs, Some constants associated with the Riemann zeta-function, *Michigan Math. J.* 3 (1955–56) 117–121; MR 17,955c.

[19] D. Mitrovic, The signs of some constants associated with the Riemann zeta-function, *Michigan Math. J.* 9 (1962) 395–397; MR 29 #2232.

[20] Y. Matsuoka, On the power series coefficients of the Riemann zeta function, *Tokyo J. Math.* 12 (1989) 49–58; MR 90g:11116.

[21] Y. Matsuoka, Generalized Euler constants associated with the Riemann zeta function, *Number Theory and Combinatorics*, Proc. 1984 Tokyo conf., ed. J. Akiyama, Y. Ito, S. Kanemitsu, T. Kano, T. Mitsui, and I. Shiokawa, World Scientific, pp. 279–295; MR 87e:11105.

[22] E. Lammel, Ein Beweis, dass die Riemannsche Zetafunktion $\zeta(s)$ in $|s - 1| \leq 1$ keine Nullstelle besitzt, *Univ. Nacional de Tucumán Rev. Ser. A* 16 (1966) 209–217; MR 36 #5090.

[23] B. C. Berndt, On the Hurwitz zeta-function, *Rocky Mount. J. Math.* 2 (1972) 151–157; MR 44 #6622.

[24] K. Verma, Laurent expansions of Hurwitz and Riemann zeta functions about $s = 1$, *Ganita* 42 (1991) 65–70; MR 93i:11106.

[25] B. C. Yang and K. Wu, An inequality for the Stieltjes constants (in Chinese), *J. South China Normal Univ. Natur. Sci. Ed.* (1996) n. 2, 17–20; MR 97m:11163.

[26] N.-Y. Zhang and K. S. Williams, Some results on the generalized Stieltjes constants, *Analysis* 14 (1994) 147–162; MR 95k:11110.

[27] G. H. Hardy, Note on Dr. Vacca's series for γ, *Quart. J. Pure Appl. Math.* 43 (1912) 215–216; also in *Collected Papers*, v. 4, Oxford Univ. Press, 1966, pp. 475–476.

[28] J. C. Kluyver, On certain series of Mr. Hardy, *Quart. J. Pure Appl. Math.* 50 (1927) 185–192.

[29] P. Sebah, Correction to Ellison-Mendès-France example, ch. 1, sect. 5.2, unpublished note (2000).

[30] D. Andrica and L. Tóth, Some remarks on Stieltjes constants of the zeta function, *Stud. Cerc. Mat.* 43 (1991) 3–9; MR 93c:11066.

[31] M.-A. Coppo, Nouvelles expressions des constantes de Stieltjes, *Expos. Math.* 17 (1999) 349–358; MR 2000k:11097.

[32] M.-A. Coppo, Sur les sommes d'Euler divergentes, *Expos. Math.* 18 (2000) 297–308; MR 2001h:11158.

[33] R. Sitaramachandrarao, Maclaurin coefficients of the Riemann zeta function, *Abstracts Amer. Math. Soc.* 7 (1986) 280.

[34] T. M. Apostol, Formulas for higher derivatives of the Riemann zeta function, *Math. Comp.* 44 (1985) 223–232; MR 86c:11063.

[35] D. H. Lehmer, The sum of like powers of the zeros of the Riemann zeta function, *Math. Comp.* 50 (1988) 265–273; MR 88m:11073.

[36] J. B. Keiper, Power series expansions of Riemann's ξ function, *Math. Comp.* 58 (1992) 765–773; MR 92f:11116.

[37] R. M. Kreminski, Newton-Cotes integration for approximating Stieltjes (generalized Euler) constants, *Math. Comp.*, to appear.

[38] J. Knopfmacher, Generalised Euler constants, *Proc. Edinburgh Math. Soc.* 21 (1978) 25–32; MR 57 #12432.

[39] S. Kanemitsu, On evaluation of certain limits in closed form, *Théorie des nombres*, Proc. 1987 Québec conf., ed. J.-M. De Koninck and C. Levesque, Gruyter, 1989, pp. 459–474; MR 90m:11127.

[40] K. Dilcher, Generalized Euler constants for arithmetical progressions, *Math. Comp.* 59 (1992) 259–282 and S21-S24; MR 92k:11145.

[41] J. R. Wilton, A note on the coefficients in the expansion of $\zeta(s, x)$ in powers of $s - 1$, *Quart. J. Pure Appl. Math.* 50 (1927) 329–332.

[42] W. E. Briggs and R. G. Buschman, The power series coefficients of functions defined by Dirichlet series, *Illinois J. Math.* 5 (1961) 43–44; MR 22 #10956.

[43] A. F. Lavrik, Laurent coefficients of a generalized zeta function (in Russian), *Theory of Cubature Formulas and Numerical Mathematics*, Proc. 1978 Novosibirsk conf., ed. S. L. Sobolev, Nauka Sibirsk. Otdel., 1980, pp. 160–164, 254; MR 82i:10050.

[44] M. I. Israilov, On the Hurwitz zeta function (in Russian), *Izv. Akad. Nauk UzSSR Ser. Fiz.-Mat. Nauk* (1981) n. 6, 13–18, 78; MR 83g:10031.

[45] U. Balakrishnan, On the Laurent expansion of $\zeta(s, a)$ at $s = 1$, *J. Indian Math. Soc.* 46 (1982) 181–187; MR 88f:11080.

[46] J. Bohman and C.-E. Fröberg, The Stieltjes function – Definition and properties, *Math. Comp.* 51 (1988) 281–289; MR 89i:11095.

[47] E. L. Post, The generalized gamma functions, *Annals of Math.* 20 (1919) 202–217.

[48] K. Dilcher, On generalized gamma functions related to the Laurent coefficients of the Riemann zeta function, *Aequationes Math.* 48 (1994) 55–85; MR 95h:11086.

[49] V. S. Adamchik, $\Gamma_n(1/2)$ and generalized Stirling formulas, unpublished note (2001).

2.22 Liouville–Roth Constants

We may study constants by means of other constants. Given a real number ξ, let R denote the set of all positive real numbers r for which the inequality

$$0 < \left| \xi - \frac{p}{q} \right| < \frac{1}{q^r}$$

has at most finitely many solutions (p, q), where p and $q > 0$ are integers. Define the

Liouville–Roth constant (or **irrationality measure**)

$$r(\xi) = \inf_{r \in R} r,$$

that is, the critical rate threshold above which ξ is **not approximable** by rational numbers [1–3]. It is known that

ξ is rational $\Rightarrow r(\xi) = 1$,
ξ is algebraic irrational $\Rightarrow r(\xi) = 2$ (Thue-Siegel-Roth theorem [4,5]),
ξ is transcendental $\Rightarrow r(\xi) \geq 2$.

If ξ is a Liouville number, for example,

$$\sum_{n=1}^{\infty} \frac{1}{2^{n!}} = \frac{1}{2^1} + \frac{1}{2^2} + \frac{1}{2^6} + \frac{1}{2^{24}} + \frac{1}{2^{120}} + \cdots = 0.7656250596\ldots,$$

then $r(\xi) = \infty$. Similarly, one can construct ξ so that $r(\xi)$ assumes any value, $2 < r(\xi) < \infty$ (from series of rationals with appropriately fast convergence). Among famous constants, it is known that [2]

$$r(e) = 2$$

(in fact, much more precise inequalities are possible, but e is somewhat atypical), and

$2 \leq r(\pi) \leq 8.016045\ldots$ (Hata [6,7]),
$2 \leq r(\ln(2)) \leq 3.89139978\ldots$ (Rukhadze [8,9]),
$2 \leq r(\pi^2) \leq 5.441243\ldots$ (Hata [10], Rhin & Viola [11]),
$2 \leq r(\zeta(3)) \leq 5.513891\ldots$ (Hata [12], Rhin & Viola [13]),

where $\zeta(3)$ is Apéry's constant [1.6]. Upper bounds for r corresponding to Catalan's constant G [1.7] or Khintchine's constant K [1.8] are not known. Whether G and K are even irrational remains open.

A consequence of Hata's work concerning π is that the two functions [14,15]

$$C(x) = \inf_{n>0 \text{ integer}} n^x |\sin(n)|, \quad D(x) = \sup_{n>0 \text{ integer}} n^{-x} |\tan(n)|$$

satisfy $C(7.02) > 0$, $D(7.02) = 0$. If a conjecture [16] that $r(\pi) = 2$ is true, then $C(1 + \varepsilon) > 0, D(1 + \varepsilon) = 0$ for all $\varepsilon > 0$. Numerical evidence suggests that $C(1) = 0$, $D(1) = \infty$.

One can also examine multidimensional analogs of these constants. For example, let $1, \xi_1, \xi_2, \ldots, \xi_n$ be linearly independent over the rationals, where $\xi_1, \xi_2, \ldots, \xi_n$ are real algebraic numbers. Let R denote the set of all positive real numbers r for which the simultaneous system of inequalities

$$0 < \left| \xi_i - \frac{p_i}{q} \right| < \frac{1}{q^r}, \quad i = 1, 2, \ldots, n,$$

has at most finitely many solutions $(p_1, p_2, \ldots, p_n, q)$, where each p_i and $q > 0$ are integers. Define $r(\xi_1, \xi_2, \ldots, \xi_n)$ exactly as before. Schmidt [5,17,18] extended the Thue–Siegel–Roth theorem to deduce that

$$r(\xi_1, \xi_2, \ldots, \xi_n) = \frac{n+1}{n}..$$

Clearly the joint irrationality measure $r(e, \pi)$ satisfies $r(e, \pi) \leq \max\{r(e), r(\pi)\}$, but no one has improved on this bound. Of course, we do not even know whether e and π are linearly independent over the rationals!

A related subject, concerning the simultaneous Diophantine approximation constants [2.23], is similar yet possesses a different focus than that here.

[1] G. H. Hardy and E. M. Wright, *An Introduction to the Theory of Numbers*, 5th ed., Oxford Univ. Press, 1985, pp. 154–169; MR 81i:10002.

[2] J. M. Borwein and P. B. Borwein, *Pi and the AGM: A Study in Analytic Number Theory and Computational Complexity*, Wiley, 1987, pp. 351–352, 362–371; MR 99h:11147.

[3] H. M. Stark, *An Introduction to Number Theory*, MIT Press, 1978, pp. 172–180; MR 80a:10001.

[4] K. F. Roth, Rational approximations to algebraic numbers, *Mathematika* 2 (1955) 1–20; corrigendum, 168; MR 17,242d.

[5] A. Baker, *Transcendental Number Theory*, Cambridge Univ. Press, 1975, pp. 66–84; MR 54 #10163.

[6] M. Hata, Improvement in the irrationality measures of π and π^2, *Proc. Japan Acad. Ser. A. Math. Sci.* 68 (1992) 283–286; MR 94b:11064.

[7] M. Hata, Rational approximations to π and some other numbers, *Acta Arith.* 63 (1993) 335–349; MR 94e:11082.

[8] E. A. Rukhadze, A lower bound for the rational approximation of ln 2 by rational numbers (in Russian), *Vestnik Moskov. Univ. Ser. I Mat. Mekh.* (1987) n. 6, 25–29, 97; Engl. transl. in *Moscow Univ. Math. Bull.*, v. 42 (1987) n. 6, 30–35; MR 89b:11064.

[9] M. Hata, Legendre type polynomials and irrationality measures, *J. Reine Angew. Math.* 407 (1990) 99–125; MR 91i:11081.

[10] M. Hata, A note on Beuker's integral, *J. Austral. Math. Soc.* 58 (1995) 143–153; MR 96c:11081.

[11] G. Rhin and C. Viola, On a permutation group related to $\zeta(2)$, *Acta Arith.* 77 (1996) 23–56; MR 97m:11099.

[12] M. Hata, A new irrationality measure for $\zeta(3)$, *Acta Arith.* 92 (2000) 47–57; MR 2001a:11123.

[13] G. Rhin and C. Viola, The group structure for $\zeta(3)$, *Acta Arith.* 97 (2001) 269–293; MR 2002b:11098.

[14] R. B. Israel, Approximability of π, unpublished note (1996).

[15] I. Rosenholtz, Tangent sequences, world records, π, and the meaning of life: Some applications of number theory to calculus, *Math. Mag.* 72 (1999) 367–376; MR 2000i:11109.

[16] J. M. Borwein, P. B. Borwein, and D. H. Bailey, Ramanujan, modular equations, and approximations to pi, or how to compute one billion digits of pi, *Amer. Math. Monthly* 96 (1989) 201–219; also in *Organic Mathematics*, Proc. 1995 Burnaby workshop, ed. J. Borwein, P. Borwein, L. Jörgenson, and R. Corless, Amer. Math. Soc., 1997, pp. 35–71; MR 90d:11143.

[17] K. B. Stolarsky, *Algebraic Numbers and Diophantine Approximation*, Dekker, 1974, pp. 308–309; MR 51 #10241.

[18] W. M. Schmidt, Simultaneous approximation to algebraic numbers by rationals, *Acta Math.* 125 (1970) 189–201; MR 42 #3028.

2.23 Diophantine Approximation Constants

In our essay on Liouville–Roth constants [2.22], we discussed rational approximations of a single irrational number ξ. Here we study the simultaneous rational approximation of n real numbers $\xi_1, \xi_2, \ldots, \xi_n$, of which at least one is irrational, by fractions all with the same denominator. Dirichlet's box principle [1,2] implies that, if $c \geq 1$, then the system of inequalities

$$\left| \xi_i - \frac{p_i}{q} \right| < c^{\frac{1}{n}} q^{-\frac{n+1}{n}}, \quad i = 1, 2, \ldots, n,$$

has infinitely many solutions $(p_1, p_2, \ldots, p_n, q)$, where $p_1, p_2, \ldots, p_n$ and $q > 0$ are integers. The focus of this essay is not on the exponent $(n+1)/n$ of the right-hand side, as it was earlier, but rather on the linear coefficient c.

As is traditional, rearrange the inequalities to

$$q \cdot |q\xi_i - p_i|^n < c$$

and define c_n to be the infimum of all $0 < c \leq 1$ for which the solution set $(p_1, p_2, \ldots, p_n, q)$ remains infinite. Then define the **n-dimensional simultaneous Diophantine approximation constant** γ_n to be the supremum of c_n over all such $\xi_1, \xi_2, \ldots, \xi_n$. So γ_n is not measuring the goodness of approximation of a *single* set of n numbers, but instead it is defined across *all* possible sets and thus depends only on the dimension n.

Here is a summary of what is known about the approximation constants γ_n:

$$\gamma_1 = \tfrac{1}{\sqrt{5}} = 0.4472135955\ldots \qquad \text{(Hurwitz [1])},$$

$$0.2857142857\ldots = \tfrac{2}{7} \leq \gamma_2 \leq \tfrac{64}{169} = 0.378\ldots \qquad \text{(Cassels [2], Nowak [3])},$$

$$0.120\ldots = \tfrac{2}{5\sqrt{11}} \leq \gamma_3 \leq \delta_2 = \tfrac{1}{2}\tfrac{1}{\pi-2} = 0.437\ldots \qquad \text{(Cusick [4], Spohn [5])},$$

$$0.044\ldots = \tfrac{16}{9\sqrt{1609}} \leq \gamma_4 \leq \delta_3 = \tfrac{27}{4}\tfrac{1}{8\sqrt{3\pi}-27} = 0.408\ldots \qquad \text{(Krass [6], Spohn [5])},$$

$$0.010\ldots = \tfrac{16}{207\sqrt{53}} \leq \gamma_5 \leq \delta_4 = 0.390\ldots \qquad [5\text{--}7],$$

$$0.004\ldots = \tfrac{16}{9\sqrt{184607}} \leq \gamma_6 \leq \delta_5 = 0.379\ldots \qquad [5\text{--}7],$$

where the upper bounds [5] are computed via the definite integrals

$$\frac{1}{\delta_k} = k2^{k+1} \int\limits_0^1 \frac{x^{k-1}}{(1+x^k)(1+x)^k} dx.$$

There is a wealth of computational [8] and theoretical evidence [9, 10] that $\gamma_2 = 2/7$ but this cannot yet be regarded as a theorem. Adams [9] proved that $2/7$ is the correct value if we impose the constraint that $\xi_1 = 1$, ξ_2, ξ_3 form a basis of a real cubic number field. Cusick [10, 11] proved additional results under the hypothesis that the regular continued fraction expansion of $2\cos(2\pi/7)$ has certain finite partial denominator patterns occurring infinitely often. See also [12, 13].

With regard to γ_3, Szekeres [14] indicated that its true value might be as high as 0.170, substantially greater than the lower bound given here.

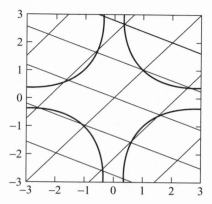

Figure 2.3. A star body S along with an S-admissible lattice L.

Nowak [15] obtained an improvement to Spohn's upper bounds, involving a function of δ_k, but numerical estimates are not possible at this time.

There is a remarkable connection between the values of γ_n and the geometry of numbers. We first illustrate this in the two-dimensional setting (see Figure 2.3). Consider the unbounded region S in the plane determined by $|xy| \leq 1$ (which is an example of what is called a **star body**). Consider as well the lattice L with basis vectors $(1, 1)$ and $((1 + \sqrt{5})/2, (1 - \sqrt{5})/2)$. It can be proved that the only vertex of L that lies within the interior of S is the origin $(0,0)$. Consequently L is said to be S-**admissible**.

The area of any single parallelogram cell of L is clearly $\sqrt{5}$. This is called the **determinant** of L, written $\det(L)$. It can be further proved that any other S-admissible lattice L must satisfy $\det(L) \geq \sqrt{5}$.

In the same way, consider the unbounded region S in $(n + 1)$-dimensional space determined by

$$|x_{n+1}| \cdot \max\{|x_1|^n, |x_2|^n, \ldots, |x_n|^n\} \leq 1$$

and consider all $(n + 1)$-dimensional S-admissible lattices L. Davenport [16, 17] proved that the volume, $\det(L)$, of any single parallelepiped cell of L satisfies $\det(L) \geq 1/\gamma_n$ and, moreover, equality must occur for some choice of L. Therefore

$$\frac{1}{\gamma_n} = \min_{\substack{S\text{-admissible} \\ \text{lattices } L}} \det(L)$$

is also known as the **critical determinant** or **lattice constant** for the star body S. This geometric insight unfortunately offers only limited help in computing γ_n. Some sample computations are given in [18–24].

Here is a similar problem from the geometry of numbers (having nothing to do with γ_n as far as is known). Again, we illustrate this in the two-dimensional setting (see Figure 2.4). Let Z denote the standard integer lattice in the plane, that is, with basis vectors $(1,0)$ and $(0,1)$. Consider an arbitrary parallelogram P centered at the origin $(0,0)$. P is called Z-**allowable** if the interior of P contains no other vertices of Z. Now,

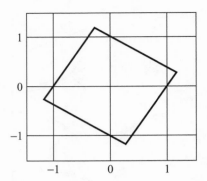

Figure 2.4. A Z-allowable parallelogram P.

given any basis v, w of the plane, there clearly exists a Z-allowable parallelogram P with sides perpendicular to v and w (just take P to have suitably small area). Define $\alpha(v, w)$ to be the supremum of the areas for all such P. Then define κ_2 to be the infimum of $\alpha(v, w)/4$ for all such bases v, w. Szekeres [25] proved that

$$\kappa_2 = \frac{1}{2}\left(1 + \frac{1}{\sqrt{5}}\right) = 0.7236067977\ldots.$$

The slopes of the "critical parallelogram," in this case a square, are $(1 + \sqrt{5})/2$ and $(1 - \sqrt{5})/2$. It is interesting that the Golden mean [1.2] occurs here as well as with the computation of γ_2 earlier.

For higher dimensions, let Z denote the standard n-dimensional integer lattice and consider n-dimensional Z-allowable parallelepipeds P with faces normal to a given basis $v_1, v_2, \ldots, v_n$. As before, $2^n \kappa_n$ is the largest possible volume of P in the sense that P can have volume $2^n \kappa_n$ independent of the prescribed directions $v_1, v_2, \ldots, v_n$, but this fails for P of volume $2^n \kappa_n + \varepsilon$ for any $\varepsilon > 0$. It is known [26–28] that $\kappa_3 > 1/4$, $\kappa_4 > 1/16$, and there is theoretical evidence [29] that possibly

$$\kappa_3 = \frac{8}{7}\cos\left(\frac{2\pi}{7}\right)\cos\left(\frac{\pi}{7}\right)^2 = 0.5784167628\ldots.$$

Moreover, it has been proved that asymptotically [28, 30]

$$\frac{n}{(n!)^2}\left(\frac{1}{2}\right)^{\frac{n(n+1)}{2}} < \kappa_n < \left[\frac{1}{2}\left(1 + \frac{1}{\sqrt{5}}\right)\right]^{\frac{n-1}{2}}.$$

One might call κ_2, κ_3, κ_4, ... the **Mordell constants** [31]; further discussion is found in [32–34].

Here is one more problem. Let K be a bounded convex body in n-space of volume $V(K)$ and symmetric with respect to the origin. Let $\Delta(K)$ denote the critical determinant of K and define

$$\rho_n = \inf_K \frac{V(K)}{\Delta(K)}.$$

For example, if $n = 2$ and K is a disk, then clearly $V(K)/\Delta(K) = 2\pi/\sqrt{3} = 3.627\ldots$. This is not optimal, for it is known [35–38] that

$$3.570624\ldots \le \rho_2 \le 4\frac{8 - 4\sqrt{2} - \ln(2)}{2\sqrt{2} - 1} = 3.6096567319\ldots$$

and further conjectured [39, 40] that ρ_2 is equal to its upper bound (corresponding to a smoothed octagon K obtained by rounding off each corner with a hyperbolic arc). It is also known [35, 41, 42] that $\rho_3 \ge 4.216$, $\rho_4 \ge 4.721$, and $\rho_n > r = 4.921553\ldots$ for $n \ge 5$, where r is the unique solution > 1 of the equation $r \ln(r) = 2(r - 1)$. Mahler [35], however, believed that $\rho_n \to \infty$ as $n \to \infty$, so there is considerable room for improvement. This theory is an outgrowth of the classical Minkowski–Hlawka theorem; by letting σ_n be the analog of ρ_n corresponding to bounded star bodies S, a parallel set of questions can be asked. For example [43], $\sigma_2 \le 3.5128\ldots$ (corresponding to S bounded by eight hyperbolic arcs), but no one appears to have conjectured an exact value for σ_2.

[1] G. H. Hardy and E. M. Wright, *An Introduction to the Theory of Numbers*, 5th ed., Oxford Univ. Press, 1985; MR 81i:10002.

[2] G. Szekeres, The n-dimensional approximation constant, *Bull. Austral. Math. Soc.* 29 (1984) 119–125; MR 85c:11056.

[3] W. G. Nowak, A note on simultaneous Diophantine approximation, *Manuscripta Math.* 36 (1981) 33–46; MR 83a:10062.

[4] T. W. Cusick, Estimates for Diophantine approximation constants, *J. Number Theory* 12 (1980) 543–556; MR 82j:10057.

[5] W. G. Spohn, Blichfeldt's theorem and simultaneous Diophantine approximation, *Amer. J. Math.* 90 (1968) 885–894; MR 38 #122.

[6] S. Krass, Estimates for n-dimensional Diophantine approximation constants for $n \ge 4$, *J. Number Theory* 20 (1985) 172–176; MR 86j:11070.

[7] G. Niklasch, Smallest absolute discriminants of number fields, unpublished notes (1997–1998).

[8] G. Szekeres, Computer examination of the 2-dimensional simultaneous approximation constant, *Ars Combin.* 19A (1985) 237–243; MR 86h:11051.

[9] W. W. Adams, The best two-dimensional Diophantine approximation constant for cubic irrationals, *Pacific J. Math.* 91 (1980) 29–30; MR 82i:10038.

[10] T. W. Cusick, The two-dimensional Diophantine approximation constant. II, *Pacific J. Math.* 105 (1983) 53–67; MR 84g:10060.

[11] T. W. Cusick and S. Krass, Formulas for some Diophantine approximation constants, *J. Austral. Math. Soc. Ser. A* 44 (1988) 311–323; MR 89c:11105.

[12] K. M. Briggs, Numbers approximating badly, unpublished note (1998).

[13] K. M. Briggs, On the Furtwängler algorithm for simultaneous rational approximation, BTexact Technologies preprint (2000).

[14] G. Szekeres, Search for the three-dimensional approximation constant, *Diophantine Analysis*, Proc. 1985 Number Theory Sect. Austral. Math. Soc. conf., ed. J. H. Loxton and A. J. van der Poorten, Cambridge Univ. Press, 1986, pp. 139–146; MR 88b:11041.

[15] W. G. Nowak, A remark concerning the s-dimensional simultaneous Diophantine approximation constants, *Österreichisch-Ungarisch-Slowakisches 1992 Kolloquium über Zahlentheorie*, ed. F. Halter-Koch and R. Tichy, Grazer Math. Ber. 318, 1993, pp. 105–110; MR 95f:11047.

[16] H. Davenport, On a theorem of Furtwängler, *J. London Math. Soc.* 30 (1955) 186–195; MR 16,803a.

[17] P. M. Gruber and C. G. Lekkerkerker, *Geometry of Numbers*, North-Holland 1987, pp. 427–429, 474–498, 546–548; MR 88j:11034.

[18] K. Ollerenshaw, Lattice points in a circular quadrilateral bounded by the arcs of four circles, *Quart. J. Math.* 17 (1946) 93–98; MR 7,506h.

[19] K. Ollerenshaw, On the region defined by $|xy| \leq 1$, $x^2 + y^2 \leq t$, *Proc. Cambridge Philos. Soc.* 49 (1953) 63–71; MR 14,624d.

[20] A. M. Cohen, Numerical determination of lattice constants, *J. London Math. Soc.* 37 (1962) 185–188; MR 25 #3422.

[21] W. G. Spohn, On the lattice constant for $|x^3 + y^3 + z^3| \leq 1$, *Math. Comp.* 23 (1969) 141–149; MR 39 #2706.

[22] W. G. Nowak, The critical determinant of the double paraboloid and Diophantine approximation in $\mathbb{R}^3$ and $\mathbb{R}^4$, *Math. Pannonica* 10 (1999) 111–122; MR 2000a:11102.

[23] R. J. Hans, Covering constants of some non-convex domains, *Indian J. Pure Appl. Math.* 1 (1970) 127–141; MR 42 #203.

[24] R. J. Hans-Gill, Covering constant of a star domain, *J. Number Theory* 2 (1970) 298–309; MR 42 #204.

[25] G. Szekeres, On a problem of the lattice plane, *J. London Math. Soc.* 12 (1937) 88–93.

[26] G. Szekeres, Note on lattice points within a parallelepiped, *J. London Math. Soc.* 12 (1937) 36–39.

[27] K. Chao, Note on the lattice points in a parallelepiped, *J. London Math. Soc.* 12 (1937) 40–47.

[28] P. M. Gruber and G. Ramharter, Beiträge zum Umkehrproblem für den Minkowskischen Linearformensatz, *Acta Math. Acad. Sci. Hungar.* 39 (1982) 135–141; MR 83m:10046.

[29] G. Ramharter, Über das Mordellsche Umkehrproblem für den Minkowskischen Linearformensatz, *Acta Arith.* 36 (1980) 27–41; MR 81k:10050.

[30] E. Hlawka, Über Gitterpunkte in Parallelepipeden, *J. Reine Angew. Math.* 187 (1950) 246–252; MR 12,161d.

[31] L. J. Mordell, Note on an arithmetical problem on linear forms, *J. London Math. Soc.* 12 (1937) 34–36.

[32] P. Erdös, P. M. Gruber, and J. Hammer, *Lattice Points*, Longman 1989, pp. 17–18, 97–102; MR 90g:11081.

[33] P. M. Gruber and C. G. Lekkerkerker, *Geometry of Numbers*, North-Holland, 1987, pp. 254–258, 263–266; MR 88j:11034.

[34] R. P. Bambah, V. C. Dumir, and R. J. Hans-Gill, On an analogue of a problem of Mordell, *Studia Sci. Math. Hungar.* 21 (1986) 135–142; MR 88i:11039.

[35] K. Mahler, The theorem of Minkowski-Hlawka, *Duke Math. J.* 13 (1946) 611–621; MR 8,444e.

[36] L. Fejes Tóth, On the densest packing of convex domains, *Proc. Konink. Nederl. Akad. Wetensch. Sci. Sect.* 51 (1948) 544–547; *Indag. Math.* 10 (1948) 188–192; MR 10,60a.

[37] V. Ennola, On the lattice constant of a symmetric convex domain, *J. London Math. Soc.* 36 (1961) 135–138; MR 28 #1177.

[38] P. Tammela, An estimate of the critical determinant of a two-dimensional convex symmetric domain (in Russian), *Izv. Vyssh. Uchebn. Zaved. Mat.* (1970) n. 12, 103–107; MR 44 #2707.

[39] K. Reinhardt, Über die dichteste gitterförmige Lagerung kongruenter Bereiche in der Ebene und eine besondere Art konvexer Kurven, *Abh. Math. Sem. Univ. Hamburg* 10 (1934) 216–230.

[40] K. Mahler, On the minimum determinant and the circumscribed hexagons of a convex domain, *Proc. Konink. Nederl. Akad. Wetensch. Sci. Sect.* 50 (1947) 692–703; *Indag. Math.* 9 (1947) 326–337; MR 9,10h.

[41] H. Davenport and C. A. Rogers, Hlawka's theorem in the geometry of numbers, *Duke Math. J.* 14 (1947) 367–375; MR 9,11a.

[42] C. G. Lekkerkerker, On the Minkowski-Hlawka theorem, *Proc. Konink. Nederl. Akad. Wetensch. Ser. A.* 59 (1956) 426–434; *Indag. Math.* 18 (1956) 426–434; MR 18,287a.

[43] K. Ollerenshaw, An irreducible non-convex region, *Proc. Cambridge Philos. Soc.* 49 (1953) 194–200; MR 14,850d.

2.24 Self-Numbers Density Constant

Any nonnegative integer n has a unique binary representation:

$$n = \sum_{k=0}^{\infty} n_k 2^k, \quad n_k = 0 \text{ or } 1.$$

What happens if we slightly perturb this formula, for example, by replacing the exponential 2^k by $2^k + 1$? Things become noticeably different: The integers $1, 4$, and 6 have *no* representations of the form

$$n_0 \cdot (2^0 + 1) + n_1 \cdot (2^1 + 1) + n_2 \cdot (2^2 + 1) = 2n_0 + 3n_1 + 5n_2, \quad n_k = 0 \text{ or } 1,$$

whereas 5 has *two* such representations, 5 and $2 + 3$.

Let us focus solely on the existence issue. Define S to be the set of all n for which a representation

$$n = \sum_{k=0}^{\infty} n_k (2^k + 1), \quad n_k = 0 \text{ or } 1$$

exists (including 0). Define T to be the complement of S relative to the nonnegative integers [1], thus $T = \{1, 4, 6, 13, 15, 18, 21, 23, 30, 32, 37, 39, \ldots\}$. These are known as **binary self numbers** (Kaprekar [2,3]) or **binary Columbian numbers** (Recamán [4]).

It can be proved that T is an infinite set. Let $\tau(N)$ denote the cardinality of binary self numbers not exceeding N. Zannier [5] proved that the limit

$$0 < \lambda = \lim_{N \to \infty} \frac{\tau(N)}{N} < 1$$

exists and moreover $\tau(N) = \lambda N + O(\ln(N)^2)$. The **self-numbers density constant** λ can be calculated by the formula

$$\lambda = \frac{1}{8} \left(\sum_{n \in S} \frac{1}{2^n} \right)^2 = 0.2526602590 \ldots$$

and was recently proved by Troi & Zannier [6,7] to be a transcendental number.

We can extend this discussion to any base $b > 1$. Define S_b to be the set of all n for which a representation

$$n = \sum_{k=0}^{\infty} n_k (b^k + 1), \quad n_k = 0, 1, \ldots, b-2 \text{ or } b-1,$$

exists. Define T_b and $\tau_b(N)$ similarly. We have $\tau_b(N) = \lambda_b N + O(\ln(N)^2)$ as before [5] and numerical approximations $\lambda_4 = 0.209 \ldots$ and $\lambda_{10} = 0.097 \ldots$ but no fast infinite series for λ_b (analogous to the formula for λ_2) has yet been established for any $b > 2$. Likewise, no one has yet proved that λ_b, $b \geq 3$, is even irrational.

There is also the issue of uniqueness. Let us focus on the binary case only. Define U to be the set of all n for which the representation

$$n = \sum_{k=0}^{\infty} n_k(2^k + 1), \quad n_k = 0 \text{ or } 1,$$

exists and is unique. Define V to be the complement of U relative to S. The set V is trivially infinite because, for all $k > 2$,

$$1 \cdot (2^k + 1) + 1 \cdot (2^2 + 1) = 1 \cdot (2^k + 1) + 1 \cdot (2^0 + 1) + 1 \cdot (2^1 + 1)$$

and the set U is trivially infinite because, for each integer t in T,

$$\sum_{k=0}^{t+1} (2^k + 1) = (2^{t+2} + 1) + t$$

has no other admissible representations. What can be said about the densities of U and V? See also [8] for the density of self numbers within arithmetic progressions, and [9] for related discussion of digitaddition series.

[1] N. J. A. Sloane, On-Line Encyclopedia of Integer Sequences, A003052, A010061, A010064, A010067, and A010070.
[2] D. R. Kaprekar, *Puzzles of the Self-Numbers*, unpublished manuscript, 1959; MR 20 #6381.
[3] M. Gardner, Mathematical games, *Sci. Amer.*, v. 232 (1975) n. 3, 113–114.
[4] B. Recamán and D. W. Bange, Columbian numbers, *Amer. Math. Monthly* 81 (1974) 407.
[5] U. Zannier, On the distribution of self-numbers, *Proc. Amer. Math. Soc.* 85 (1982) 10–14; MR 83i:10007.
[6] G. Troi and U. Zannier, Note on the density constant in the distribution of self-numbers, *Boll. Unione Mat. Ital. A* (7) 9 (1995) 143–148; MR 95k:11093.
[7] G. Troi and U. Zannier, Note on the density constant in the distribution of self-numbers. II, *Boll. Unione Mat. Ital. Sez. B Artic. Ric. Mat.* (8) 2 (1999) 397–399; MR 2000f:11093.
[8] M. B. S. Laporta and E. Laserra, Distribution of self-numbers in arithmetical progressions (in Italian), *Ricerche Mat.* 42 (1993) 307–313; MR 95e:11105.
[9] K. B. Stolarsky, The sum of a digitaddition series, *Proc. Amer. Math. Soc.* 59 (1976) 1–5; MR 53 #13099.

2.25 Cameron's Sum-Free Set Constants

A set S of positive integers is **sum-free** if the equation $x + y = z$ has no solutions $x, y, z \in S$. Equivalently, S is sum-free if and only if $(S + S) \cap S = \emptyset$, where $A + B$ denotes the set of all sums $a + b, a \in A, b \in B$. For example, the set of all odd positive integers is sum-free.

Consider now the collection of all sum-free sets. Cameron [1–3] defined a natural probability measure on this collection, which can informally be thought of as a recipe for constructing random sum-free sets S. The recipe is as follows:

- Set $S = \emptyset$ initially and look at each positive integer n one-by-one in order.
- If $n = a + b$ for some $a, b \in S$, then skip n and move ahead to $n + 1$.

- If $n = x + y$ has no solutions $x, y \in S$, then toss a fair coin; if heads, set $S = S \cup \{n\}$ and move ahead to $n + 1$; if tails, simply move ahead.

Observe, for example, that clearly

$$P(S \text{ consists entirely of even integers}) = 0.$$

In contrast, Cameron [1] proved the remarkable fact that the constant

$$c = P(S \text{ consists entirely of odd integers})$$

is *positive* and, in fact, $0.21759 \leq c \leq 0.21862$. Equivalently [2], if $N = \{0, 1, \ldots, n - 1\}$ and

$$F(n) = 2^{-2n} \sum_{X \subseteq N} 2^{|(X+X) \cap N|},$$

then $F(n)$ is decreasing and $\lim_{n \to \infty} F(n) = c$. The summation is over all subsets X of N and $|E|$ denotes the cardinality of a set E. An alternative proof was given by Calkin [4].

Cameron [2] proved a more general result, which bounds (from below) the probability that S is contained entirely within certain sum-free unions of arithmetic progressions. Rather than state his general theorem, we simply provide a sample application:

$$P(S \subseteq \{2, \ 7, \ 12, \ 17, \ 22, \ 27, \ldots\} \cup \{3, \ 8, \ 13, \ 18, \ 23, \ 28, \ldots\}) \geq \frac{c^2 d}{2} > 0.0066,$$

where $0.28295 \leq d = \lim_{n \to \infty} G(n) \leq 0.29484$ and the decreasing function $G(n)$ is defined by

$$G(n) = 2^{-3n} \sum_{X, Y \subseteq N} 2^{|(X+Y) \cap N|}.$$

This, however, is not close to his estimate of approximately 0.022 (based on computer simulation).

Calkin & Cameron [5] advanced our understanding of random sum-free sets even farther. Again, we do not present their theorem in general form, but merely give an example:

$$P(S \text{ contains 2 and } S \text{ contains no other even integers}) > 0.$$

Computer simulations provide an estimate for this probability of approximately 0.00016.

Let us now turn away from probability and consider instead the number s_n of sum-free subsets of $\{1, 2, \ldots, n\}$. The first several terms [6] of s_n are 1, 2, 3, 6, 9, 16, 24, ... Cameron & Erdös [7,8] conjectured that $s_n 2^{-n/2}$ is bounded and, moreover, the following two limits exist and are approximately

$$\lim_{k \to \infty} s_{2k+1} 2^{-(k+\frac{1}{2})} = c_o = 6.8 \ldots, \qquad \lim_{k \to \infty} s_{2k} 2^{-k} = c_e = 6.0 \ldots,$$

where

$$c_o = \sqrt{2} + \lim_{k \to \infty} H(2k+1), \quad c_e = 1 + \lim_{k \to \infty} H(2k),$$

$$H(n) = 2^{-n/2} \sum_{X \subseteq N'} 2^{-|(X+X) \cap N'|}, \quad N' = \{0, 1, \ldots, n\}.$$

Calkin [9], Alon [10], and Erdös & Granville independently demonstrated that

$$\lim_{n \to \infty} s_n 2^{-(\frac{1}{2}+\varepsilon)n} = 0$$

for every $\varepsilon > 0$. Additional evidence for boundedness appears in [11], and a generalization is found in [12–15].

We cannot resist presenting one more problem. A sum-free set S of positive integers is **complete** if, for all sufficiently large integers n, either $n \in S$ or there exist $s, t \in S$ such that $s + t = n$. Equivalently, S is complete if and only if it is constructed greedily from a finite set. A sum-free set S is **periodic** if there exists a positive integer m such that, for all sufficiently large integers n, $n \in S$ if and only if $n + m \in S$. Equivalently, S is periodic if and only if the elements of S, arranged in increasing order, give rise to an (eventually) periodic sequence of successive differences.

Is an arbitrary complete sum-free set necessarily periodic [16]? Cameron [3] gave the first potentially aperiodic example: the complete sum-free set starting with 3, 4, 13, 18, 24. Calkin & Finch [17] gave other potentially aperiodic examples, including 1, 3, 8, 20, 26, ... and 2, 15, 16, 23, 27, ... Calkin & Erdös [18] proved the existence of *incomplete* aperiodic sum-free sets – in fact, they exhibited uncountably many such sets, constructed in a natural way – but no one has yet established the existence of a single complete aperiodic sum-free set.

[1] P. J. Cameron, Cyclic automorphisms of a countable graph and random sum-free sets, *Graphs Combin.* 1 (1985) 129–135; MR 90b:05062.
[2] P. J. Cameron, On the structure of a random sum-free set, *Probab. Theory Relat. Fields* 76 (1987) 523–531; MR 89c:11018.
[3] P. J. Cameron, Portrait of a typical sum-free set, *Surveys in Combinatorics 1987*, ed. C. Whitehead, Cambridge Univ. Press, 1987, pp. 13–42; MR 88k:05138.
[4] N. J. Calkin, On the structure of a random sum-free set of positive integers, *Discrete Math.* 190 (1998) 247–257; MR 99f:11015.
[5] N. J. Calkin and P. J. Cameron, Almost odd random sum-free sets, *Combin. Probab. Comput.* 7 (1998) 27–32; MR 99c:11012.
[6] N. J. A. Sloane, On-Line Encyclopedia of Integer Sequences, A007865.
[7] P. J. Cameron and P. Erdös, On the number of sets of integers with various properties, *Number Theory*, Proc. 1990 Canad. Number Theory Assoc. Banff conf., ed. R. A. Mollin, Gruyter, pp. 61–79; MR 92g:11010.
[8] P. J. Cameron, The Cameron-Erdös constants, unpublished note (2002).
[9] N. J. Calkin, On the number of sum-free sets, *Bull. London Math. Soc.* 22 (1990) 141–144; MR 91b:11015.
[10] N. Alon, Independent sets in regular graphs and sum-free subsets of finite groups, *Israel J. Math.* 73 (1991) 247–256; MR 92k:11024.
[11] G. A. Freiman, On the structure and the number of sum-free sets, *Astérisque* 209 (1992) 195–201; MR 94a:11016.

[12] N. J. Calkin and A. C. Taylor, Counting sets of integers, no k of which sum to another, *J. Number Theory* 57 (1996) 323–327; MR 97d:11015.

[13] Y. Bilu, Sum-free sets and related sets, *Combinatorica* 18 (1998) 449–459; MR 2000j:11035.

[14] N. J. Calkin and J. M. Thomson, Counting generalized sum-free sets, *J. Number Theory* 68 (1998) 151–159; MR 98m:11010.

[15] T. Schoen, A note on the number of (k, l)-sum-free sets, *Elec. J. Combin.* 7 (2000) R30; MR 2001c:11030.

[16] R. K. Guy, *Unsolved Problems in Number Theory*, 2nd ed., Springer-Verlag, 1994, sect. E32; MR 96e:11002.

[17] N. J. Calkin and S. R. Finch, Some conditions on periodicity for a sum-free set, *Experim. Math.* 5 (1996) 131–137; MR 98c:11010.

[18] N. J. Calkin and P. Erdös, On a class of aperiodic sum-free sets, *Math. Proc. Cambridge Philos. Soc.* 120 (1996) 1–5; MR 97b:11030.

2.26 Triple-Free Set Constants

A set S of positive integers is called **double-free** if, for any integer x, the set $\{x, 2x\} \nsubseteq S$. Equivalently, S is double-free if $x \in S$ implies $2x \notin S$. Consider the function

$$r(n) = \max\{|S| : S \subseteq \{1, 2, \ldots, n\} \text{ is double-free}\},$$

that is, the maximum cardinality of double-free sets with no element exceeding n. It is not difficult to prove that

$$\lim_{n \to \infty} \frac{r(n)}{n} = \frac{2}{3};$$

that is, the asymptotic maximal density of double-free sets is $2/3$. Wang [1] obtained both recursive and closed-form expressions for $r(n)$ and, moreover, demonstrated that $r(n) = 2n/3 + O(\ln(n))$ as $n \to \infty$.

Let us now discuss a much harder problem. Define a set S of positive integers to be

- **weakly triple-free** (or **triple-free**) if, for any integer x, the set $\{x, 2x, 3x\} \nsubseteq S$, and
- **strongly triple-free** if $x \in S$ implies $2x \notin S$ and $3x \notin S$.

Unlike the double-free case, the weak and strong senses of triple-free do not coincide. Consider the functions

$$p(n) = \max\{|S| : S \subseteq \{1, 2, \ldots, n\} \text{ is weakly triple-free}\},$$

$$q(n) = \max\{|S| : S \subseteq \{1, 2, \ldots, n\} \text{ is strongly triple-free}\}.$$

We wish to calculate the constants

$$\lambda = \lim_{n \to \infty} \frac{p(n)}{n}, \quad \mu = \lim_{n \to \infty} \frac{q(n)}{n}.$$

Define an infinite set

$$A = \{2^i 3^j : i, j \geq 0\} = \{a_1 < a_2 < a_3 < \ldots\}$$
$$= \{1, 2, 3, 4, 6, 8, 9, 12, 16, 18, 24, 27, \ldots\}$$

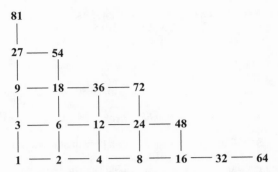

Figure 2.5. Grid graph associated with A_{19}, for which $g_{19} = 10$, $A_{19,0} = \{1, 4, 6, 9, 16, 24, 36,$ $54, 64, 81\}$, $f_{19} = 6 = h_{19}$, $B_{19,0} = \{1, 6, 8, 27, 36, 48, 64\}$, and $\tilde{B}_{19,0} = \{64\}$.

and A_n to be the first n terms of A; then λ and μ can be written as

$$\lambda = \frac{1}{3} \sum_{n=1}^{\infty} (n - f_n) \left(\frac{1}{a_n} - \frac{1}{a_{n+1}} \right), \quad \mu = \frac{1}{3} \sum_{n=1}^{\infty} g_n \left(\frac{1}{a_n} - \frac{1}{a_{n+1}} \right),$$

where the integer sequences

$$\{f_n\} = \{0, 0, 1, 1, 1, 1, 2, 2, 2, 3, 3, 4, 4, 4, 4, 5, 5, 5, 6, 6, 7, 7, 7, 8, 8, \ldots\},$$
$$\{g_n\} = \{1, 1, 2, 2, 3, 3, 4, 4, 5, 5, 6, 6, 7, 7, 8, 8, 9, 9, 10, 11, \ldots\}$$

will be defined momentarily.

The constant μ has not attracted as much attention as λ. Eppstein [2] showed that g_n is the size of the largest set of nonadjacent vertices in the grid graph A_n (called an **independence number**). For each $k = 0, 1$, define $A_{n,k} \subseteq A_n$ to consist of all elements $2^i 3^j$ satisfying $i + j \equiv k \bmod 2$. Then $\{A_{n,0}, A_{n,1}\}$ is a partition of A_n and at least one of these is a maximal independent set, as found by Cassaigne [3]. (See Figure 2.5). From here, Zimmermann [3] computed the **triple-free set constant** to be $\mu = 0.6134752692\ldots$.

By way of contrast, the constant λ has intrigued people for over twenty-five years [4]. Graham, Spencer & Witsenhausen [5] were concerned with general conditions on sets, contained in $\{1, 2, \ldots, n\}$, that avoid the values of linear forms $\sum_{v=1}^{w} c_{uv} x_v$. Among many things, they asked whether λ is irrational. Starting from a table of f_n values in [5], Cassaigne [6] proved that $\lambda \geq 4/5$. Chung, Erdös & Graham [7] showed that f_n is the size of the smallest set of vertices in A_n that intersects every L-shaped vertex configuration of the form $\{2^i 3^j, 2^{i+1} 3^j, 2^i 3^{j+1}\} \subseteq A_n$ (called an **L-hitting number**). For each $k = 0, 1, 2$, define $B_{n,k} \subseteq A_n$ to consist of all elements $2^i 3^j$ satisfying $i - j \equiv k \bmod 3$. Then $\{B_{n,0}, B_{n,1}, B_{n,2}\}$ is a partition of A_n. Define also $\tilde{B}_{n,k} \subseteq B_{n,k}$ to consist of all elements 2^i, $1 \leq i \equiv k \bmod 3$, for which $2^{i-1} 3 \notin A_n$. It is known that

$$f_n \leq h_n = \min_{0 \leq k \leq 2} |B_{n,k}| - |\tilde{B}_{n,k}| \leq \left\lfloor \frac{n}{3} \right\rfloor,$$

and consequently $0.800319 < \lambda < 0.800962$. It is conjectured that $f_n = h_n$ for all n, which if true would imply that $\lambda = 0.8003194838\ldots = 1 - 0.1996805161\ldots$.

Given fixed $s > 1$, consider sets S of positive integers for which $\{x, 2x, 3x, \ldots, s\,x\} \not\subseteq S$ for all integers x. Denote the corresponding asymptotic maximal density by λ_s. What can be said about the asymptotics of λ_s as $s \to \infty$? Spencer & Erdös [8] proved that there exist constants c and C for which

$$1 - \frac{C}{s \ln(s)} < \lambda_s < 1 - \frac{c}{s \ln(s)}$$

for all suitably large s, although specific numerical values were not presented. Also, consider sets T of positive integers for which $\{x, 2x, 3x, 6x\} \not\subseteq T$ for all integers x. The corresponding asymptotic maximal density is exactly $11/12$ [7], which is surprising since the case $s = 3$ was so much more difficult.

More instances of the interplay between the numbers 2 and 3 occur in [2.30.1], which is concerned with powers of $3/2$ modulo 1.

[1] E. T. H. Wang, On double-free sets of integers, *Ars Combin.* 28 (1989) 97–100; MR 91d:11011.
[2] D. Eppstein, Triple-free set asymptotics and independence numbers of grid graphs, unpublished note (1996).
[3] J. Cassaigne and P. Zimmermann, Numerical evaluation of the strongly triple-free constant, unpublished note (1996).
[4] P. Erdös and R. Graham, *Old and New Problems and Results in Combinatorial Number Theory*, Enseignement Math. Monogr. 28, 1980, p. 20; MR 82j:10001.
[5] R. Graham, J. Spencer, and H. Witsenhausen, On extremal density theorems for linear forms, *Number Theory and Algebra*, ed. H. Zassenhaus, Academic Press, 1977, pp. 103–109; MR 58 #569.
[6] J. Cassaigne, Lower bound on triple-free constant λ, unpublished note (1996).
[7] F. Chung, P. Erdös, and R. Graham, On sparse sets hitting linear forms, *Number Theory for the Millennium*, v. 1, Proc. 2000 Urbana conf., ed. M. A. Bennett, B. C. Berndt, N. Boston, H. G. Diamond, A. J. Hildebrand, and W. Philipp, A. K. Peters, to appear.
[8] J. Spencer and P. Erdös, A problem in covering progressions, *Stud. Sci. Math. Hung.* 30 (1995) 149–154; MR 96f:11018.

2.27 Erdös–Lebensold Constant

A strictly increasing sequence of positive integers $a_1, a_2, a_3, \ldots$ is **primitive** [1–3] if $a_i \nmid a_j$ for any $i \neq j$. That is, no term of the sequence divides any other. An example of a finite primitive sequence is the set of all integers m in the interval $\left\lceil \frac{n+1}{2} \right\rceil \leq m \leq n$, where n is a positive integer. An example of an infinite primitive sequence consists of all positive integers composed of exactly r prime factors, where r is fixed. We discuss the finite and infinite cases separately. See also [5.5] for a related note.

2.27.1 Finite Case

For each positive integer n, define

$$M(n) = \sup_{\substack{\text{primitive} \\ A \subseteq \{1,2,\ldots,n\}}} \sum_i 1$$

as the maximum possible number of terms, and

$$L(n) = \sup_{\substack{\text{primitive} \\ A \subseteq \{1,2,\ldots,n\}}} \sum_i \frac{1}{a_i}$$

as the maximum possible reciprocal sum. Clearly $M(n) = \lfloor \frac{n+1}{2} \rfloor$ and thus $\lim_{n \to \infty} M(n)/n = 1/2$. It is more difficult to establish [4, 5] that

$$\lim_{n \to \infty} \frac{\sqrt{\ln(\ln(n))}}{\ln(n)} L(n) = \frac{1}{\sqrt{2\pi}},$$

which is an unexpected appearance of Archimedes' constant [1.4].

2.27.2 Infinite Case

Any infinite primitive sequence satisfies

$$0 = \liminf_{n \to \infty} \frac{1}{n} \sum_{a_i \leq n} 1 \leq \limsup_{n \to \infty} \frac{1}{n} \sum_{a_i \leq n} 1 < \frac{1}{2}.$$

Besicovitch [1, 6] proved that, for each $\varepsilon > 0$, there exists a primitive sequence such that

$$\limsup_{n \to \infty} \frac{1}{n} \sum_{a_i \leq n} 1 > \frac{1}{2} - \varepsilon.$$

In particular, a primitive sequence need not possess an asymptotic density! Maybe the limiting value 1/2 is not so surprising, given the earlier result about $M(n)$.

In contrast, Erdös, Sárközy & Szemerédi [7] proved that

$$\lim_{n \to \infty} \frac{\sqrt{\ln(\ln(n))}}{\ln(n)} \sum_{a_i \leq n} \frac{1}{a_i} = 0,$$

which is drastically different from the earlier result about $L(n)$. The finite and infinite cases behave independently in this respect.

Forging a new trail, Erdös [1, 8] proved that the series

$$\sum_i \frac{1}{a_i \ln(a_i)}$$

is convergent (except for the trivial primitive sequence $\{1\}$) and is, moreover, bounded by some absolute constant. He conjectured that

$$\sum_i \frac{1}{a_i \ln(a_i)} \leq \sum_i \frac{1}{p_i \ln(p_i)} = 1.6366163233\ldots,$$

where the latter summation is over all primes. Several partial results are known. Zhang [9, 10] proved that the inequality is true for all primitive sequences whose terms contain at most four prime factors. Zhang [11] did likewise, hypothesizing a different, more technical set of conditions. Erdös & Zhang [12] proved that, for any primitive sequence,

$$\sum_i \frac{1}{a_i \ln(a_i)} \le 1.84$$

and Clark [13] strengthened this to

$$\sum_i \frac{1}{a_i \ln(a_i)} \le e^\gamma = 1.7810724179\ldots,$$

where γ is Euler's constant [1.5].

Incidently, the estimate $1.6366163233\ldots$ given here for the prime series is due to Cohen [14].

2.27.3 Generalizations

Let k be a positive integer. A strictly increasing sequence of positive integers a_1, a_2, a_3, ... is k-**primitive** if no term of the sequence divides k others. (This phraseology is new.) Let us consider only the finite case. Define $M(n, k)$ and $L(n, k)$ as before. An example of a 2-primitive sequence is the set of all integers m in the interval $\lceil \frac{n+1}{3} \rceil \le m \le n$; thus $\lim_{n \to \infty} M(n, 2)/n \ge 2/3$, but here improvement is possible. Lebensold [15] proved that

$$0.6725 \le \lim_{n \to \infty} \frac{M(n, 2)}{n} \le 0.6736$$

and observed that more accurate bounds could be achieved by additional computation in exactly the same manner. Erdös asked if the limit is irrational [10]. No one has examined $L(n, 2)$ or the case $k > 2$, as far as is known.

A strictly increasing sequence of positive integers b_1, b_2, b_3, ... is **quasi-primitive** [16] if the equation $\gcd(b_i, b_j) = b_r$ is not solvable with $r < i < j$. An example of an infinite quasi-primitive sequence consists of all prime powers

$$q_1 = 2, q_2 = 3, q_3 = 2^2, q_4 = 5, q_5 = 7, q_6 = 2^3, q_7 = 3^2, q_8 = 11, \ldots.$$

Erdös & Zhang [16] conjectured that, for any quasi-primitive sequence,

$$\sum_i \frac{1}{b_i \ln(b_i)} \le \sum_i \frac{1}{q_i \ln(q_i)} = 2.006\ldots.$$

Clark [17] corrected a false claim in [16] and proved that

$$\sum_i \frac{1}{b_i \ln(b_i)} < 4.2022.$$

A more accurate estimate for the prime-power series is an unsolved problem.

The topics of k-primitive sequences and quasi-primitive sequences appear to be wide open areas for research, as are the allied topics of triple-free set constants [2.26] and Erdös' reciprocal sum constants [2.20].

[1]   H. Halberstam and K. F. Roth, *Sequences*, Springer-Verlag, 1983, pp. 238–254; MR 83m:10094.

[2]   P. Erdös, A. Sárközy, and E. Szemerédi, On divisibility properties of sequences of integers, *Number Theory*, Proc. 1968 Debrecen conf., ed. P. Turán, Colloq. Math. Soc. János Bolyai 2, North-Holland, 1970, pp. 35–49; MR 43 #4790.

[3]   R. Ahlswede and L. H. Khachatrian, Classical results on primitive and recent results on cross-primitive sequences, *The Mathematics of Paul Erdös*, v. 1, ed. R. L. Graham and J. Nesetril, Springer-Verlag, 1997, pp. 104–116; MR 97j:11012.

[4]   P. Erdös, On the integers having exactly k prime factors, *Annals of Math.* 49 (1948) 53–66; MR 9,333b.

[5]   P. Erdös, A. Sárközy, and E. Szemerédi, On an extremal problem concerning primitive sequences, *J. London Math. Soc.* 42 (1967) 484–488; MR 36 #1412.

[6]   A. S. Besicovitch, On the density of certain sequences of integers, *Math. Annalen* 110 (1934) 336–341.

[7]   P. Erdös, A. Sárközy, and E. Szemerédi, On a theorem of Behrend, *J. Austral. Math. Soc.* 7 (1967) 9–16; MR 35 #148.

[8]   P. Erdös, Note on sequences of integers no one of which is divisible by any other, *J. London Math. Soc.* 10 (1935) 126–128.

[9]   Z. Zhang, On a conjecture of Erdös on the sum $\sum_{p \leq n} 1/(p \log p)$, *J. Number Theory* 39 (1991) 14–17; MR 92f:11131.

[10] R. K. Guy, *Unsolved Problems in Number Theory*, 2nd ed., Springer-Verlag, 1994, sect. B24, E4; MR 96e:11002.

[11] Z. Zhang, On a problem of Erdös concerning primitive sequences, *Math. Comp.* 60 (1993) 827–834; MR 93k:11120.

[12] P. Erdös and Z. Zhang, Upper bound of $\sum 1/(a_i \log a_i)$ for primitive sequences, *Proc. Amer. Math. Soc.* 117 (1993) 891–895; MR 93e:11018.

[13] D. A. Clark, An upper bound of $\sum 1/(a_i \log a_i)$ for primitive sequences, *Proc. Amer. Math. Soc.* 123 (1995) 363–365; MR 95c:11026.

[14] H. Cohen, High precision computation of Hardy-Littlewood constants, unpublished note (1999).

[15] K. Lebensold, A divisibility problem, *Studies in Appl. Math.* 56 (1976–77) 291–294; MR 58 #21639.

[16] P. Erdös and Z. Zhang, Upper bound of $\sum 1/(a_i \log a_i)$ for quasi-primitive sequences, *Comput. Math. Appl. (Oxford)* v. 26 (1993) n. 3, 1–5; MR 94f:11013.

[17] D. A. Clark, An upper bound of $\sum 1/(a_i \log a_i)$ for quasi-primitive sequences, *Comput. Math. Appl. (Oxford)*, v. 35 (1998) n. 4, 105–109; MR 99a:11021.

2.28 Erdös' Sum-Distinct Set Constant

A set $a_1 < a_2 < a_3 < \ldots < a_n$ of positive integers is called **sum-distinct** if the 2^n sums

$$\sum_{k=1}^{n} \varepsilon_k a_k \quad (\text{each } \varepsilon_k = 0 \text{ or } 1, \, 1 \leq k \leq n)$$

are all different. Equivalently, sum-distinctness holds if and only if any two subset sums are never equal [1–4]. The set of nonnegative powers of 2 is clearly sum-distinct and serves as a baseline for comparison. In 1931, Erdös examined the ratio

$$\alpha_n = \inf_A \frac{a_n}{2^n},$$

where the infimum is over all sum-distinct sets A of cardinality n, and conjectured that $\alpha = \inf_n \alpha_n$ is positive. No one knows whether this is true, but in 1955, Erdös and Moser [2, 5, 6] proved that, for all $n \geq 2$,

$$\alpha_n \geq \max\left(\frac{1}{n}, \frac{1}{4\sqrt{n}}\right),$$

and Elkies [7] proved that, for sufficiently large n,

$$\alpha_n \geq \frac{1}{\sqrt{\pi n}}.$$

Gleason & Elkies [8] subsequently removed the factor of π via a variance reduction technique. See also [9]. It is probably true that $\alpha > 1/8 = 0.125$. Significant progress in resolving Erdös' conjecture will almost certainly require a brand-new idea or as-yet-unseen insight.

Several interesting constructions provide upper bounds on α. In 1986, Atkinson, Negro & Santoro [10, 11] defined a sequence

$$u_0 = 0, \quad u_1 = 1, \quad u_{k+1} = 2u_k - u_{k-m}, \quad m = \left\lfloor \tfrac{1}{2}k + 1 \right\rfloor$$

that gives rise to a sum-distinct set $a_k = u_n - u_{n-k}$, $1 \leq k \leq n$, for each n. Clearly $a_n = u_n$. Lunnon [11] calculated that

$$\lim_{n \to \infty} \frac{u_n}{2^n} = 0.3166841737\ldots = \frac{1}{2}(0.6333683473\ldots).$$

A smaller ratio is obtained via a sequence due to Conway & Guy [2, 11–13]:

$$v_0 = 0, \quad v_1 = 1, \quad v_{k+1} = 2v_k - v_{k-m}, \quad m = \left\lfloor \tfrac{1}{2} + \sqrt{2k} \right\rfloor.$$

Only recently Bohman [14] proved that this sequence gives rise to a sum-distinct set $a_k = v_n - v_{n-k}$, $1 \leq k \leq n$, for each n. (Prior to 1996, we knew this claim to be true for only $n < 80$.) Lunnon [11] calculated that

$$\lim_{n \to \infty} \frac{v_n}{2^n} = 0.2351252848\ldots = \frac{1}{2}(0.4702505696\ldots).$$

Although the Atkinson–Negro–Santoro and Conway–Guy limiting ratios are interesting constants, they do not provide the best-known upper bounds on α. A frequently used trick for doing so is as follows: If $a_1 < a_2 < a_3 < \ldots < a_n$ is a sum-distinct set with n elements, then clearly $1 < 2a_1 < 2a_2 < 2a_3 < \ldots < 2a_n$ is a sum-distinct set with $n + 1$ elements. Enlarging as such can be continued indefinitely, of course. Thus if one has found a sum-distinct set with n elements and small ratio ρ, we immediately have an upper bound $\alpha \leq \rho$. For example, Lunnon [11] found a sum-distinct set with $n = 67$ and $\rho = 0.22096$ via computer search, which improves on the Conway–Guy bound. Generalizing the work of Conway, Guy, and Lunnon, Bohman [15] established the best-known upper bound $\alpha \leq 0.22002$. Additionally, Maltby [16] has shown, given a sum-distinct set, how to construct a larger sum-distinct set with a smaller ratio. Hence Erdös' constant α is not realized by any sum-distinct set; that is, the infimum is never achieved!

Bae [17] studied sum-distinct sets whose sums avoid r mod q, for given r and q. Also, consider the inequality

$$\sum_{k=1}^{n} \frac{1}{a_k} < 2 = \sum_{k=1}^{\infty} \frac{1}{2^{k-1}},$$

which is true for all sum-distinct sets A. It is curious that the upper bound 2 is sharp and elementary proofs are possible [9, 18, 19]. (Actually much more is known!) Elsewhere we discuss other such reciprocal sums [2.20], which are often exceedingly difficult to evaluate.

[1]   R. K. Guy, *Unsolved Problems in Number Theory*, 2nd ed., Springer-Verlag, 1994, sect. C8; MR 96e:11002.
[2]   R. K. Guy, Sets of integers whose subsets have distinct sums, *Theory and Practice of Combinatorics*, ed. A. Rosa, G. Sabidussi, and J. Turgeon, Annals of Discrete Math. 12, North-Holland, 1982, pp. 141–154; MR 86m:11009.
[3]   M. Gardner, Mathematical games: On the fine art of putting players, pills and points into their proper pigeonholes, *Sci. Amer.*, v. 243 (1980) n. 2, 14–18.
[4]   P. Smith, Solutions to problem on sum-distinct sets, *Amer. Math. Monthly* 83 (1976) 484 and 88 (1981) 538–539.
[5]   P. Erdös, Problems and results in additive number theory, *Colloq. Théorie des Nombres, Bruxelles 1955*, Liege and Paris, 1956, pp. 127–137; MR 18,18a.
[6]   N. Alon and J. Spencer, *The Probabilistic Method*, Wiley, 1992, pp. 47–48; MR 93h: 60002.
[7]   N. D. Elkies, An improved lower bound on the greatest element of a sum-distinct set of fixed order, *J. Combin. Theory A* 41 (1986) 89–94; MR 87b:05012.
[8]   A. M. Gleason and N. D. Elkies, Further improvements on a lower bound, unpublished note (1985).
[9]   J. Bae, On subset-sum-distinct sequences, *Analytic Number Theory*, Proc. 1995 Allerton Park conf., v. 1, ed. B. C. Berndt, H. G. Diamond, and A. J. Hildebrand, Birkhäuser, 1996, pp. 31–37; MR 97d:11016.
[10] M. D. Atkinson, A. Negro, and N. Santoro, Sums of lexicographically ordered sets, *Discrete Math.* 80 (1990) 115–122; MR 91m:90136.
[11] W. F. Lunnon, Integer sets with distinct subset-sums, *Math. Comp.* 50 (1988) 297–320; MR 89a:11019.
[12] J. H. Conway and R. K. Guy, Sets of natural numbers with distinct sums, *Notices Amer. Math. Soc.* 15 (1968) 345.
[13] J. H. Conway and R. K. Guy, Solution of a problem of P. Erdös, *Colloq. Math.* 20 (1969) 307.
[14] T. Bohman, A sum packing problem of Erdös and the Conway-Guy sequence, *Proc. Amer. Math. Soc.* 124 (1996) 3627–3636; MR 97b:11027.
[15] T. Bohman, A construction for sets of integers with distinct subset sums, *Elec. J. Combin.* 5 (1997) R3; MR 98k:11014.
[16] R. Maltby, Bigger and better subset-sum-distinct sets, *Mathematika* 44 (1997) 56–60; MR 98i:11012.
[17] J. Bae, An extremal problem for subset-sum-distinct sequences with congruence conditions, *Discrete Math.* 189 (1998) 1–20; MR 99h:11018.
[18] R. Honsberger, *Mathematical Gems III*, Math. Assoc. Amer., 1985, pp. 215–223.
[19] P. E. Frenkel, Integer sets with distinct subset sums, *Proc. Amer. Math. Soc.* 126 (1998) 3199–3200; MR 99a:11012.

2.29 Fast Matrix Multiplication Constants

Everyone knows that multiplying two arbitrary $n \times n$ matrices requires n^3 multiplications, at least if we do it using standard formulas.

In the mid 1960s, Pan and Winograd [1] discovered a way to reduce this to approximately $n^3/2$ multiplications for large n, and for a few years people believed that this might be the best possible reduction.

Define the **exponent of matrix multiplication** ω as the infimum of all real numbers τ such that multiplication of $n \times n$ matrices may be achieved with $O(n^\tau)$ multiplications. Clearly $\omega \leq 3$ and it can be proved that $\omega \geq 2$.

Strassen [2] discovered a surprising base algorithm to compute the product of 2×2 matrices with only seven multiplications. The technique can be recursively extended to large matrices via a tensor product construction. In this case, the construction is very simple: Large matrices are broken down recursively by partitioning the matrices into quarters, sixteenths, etc. This gives $\omega \leq \ln(7)/\ln(2) < 2.808$.

More sophisticated base algorithms and tensor product constructions permit further improvements. Many researchers have contributed to this problem, including Pan [3, 4] who found $\omega < 2.781$ and Strassen [5] who found $\omega < 2.479$. See [6, 7] for an overview and history.

Coppersmith & Winograd [8] presented a new method, based on a combinatorial theorem of Salem & Spencer [9], which gives dense sets of integers containing no three terms in arithmetic progression. They consequently obtained $\omega < 2.376$, which is the best-known upper bound today.

Is $\omega = 2$? Bürgisser [10] called this the central problem of algebraic complexity theory. Here is a closely related combinatorial problem [8, 11].

Given an abelian additive group G of order n, find the least integer $f(n, G)$ with the following property. If a subset S of G has cardinality $\geq f(n, G)$, then there exist three subsets A, B, C of S, pairwise disjoint and not all empty, such that

$$\sum_{a \in A} a = \sum_{b \in B} b = \sum_{c \in C} c.$$

(Clearly $f(n, G)$ exists for $n \geq 5$, because if $S = G$, then consider $A = \{0\}$, $B = \{g, -g\}$, $C = \{h, -h\}$, where nonzero elements g and h satisfy $g \neq h$ and $g \neq -h$.) Now define another function

$$F(n) = \max_G f(n, G),$$

the maximum taken over all abelian groups G of order n, and examine the ratio

$$\rho = \lim_{n \to \infty} \frac{\ln(n)}{F(n)}.$$

Coppersmith & Winograd [8] demonstrated that if $\rho = 0$, then $\omega = 2$. A proof that $\rho = 0$, however, is still unknown. What (if any) numerical evidence exists in support of $\rho = 0$?

Coppersmith [12] further gave a constant $\alpha > 0.294$ and, for any $\varepsilon > 0$, an algorithm for multiplying an $n \times n$ matrix by an $n \times n^\alpha$ matrix with complexity $O(n^{2+\varepsilon})$. An improvement in the lower bound for α would provide more hope that $\omega = 2$. Research in this area continues [13, 14].

[1] S. Winograd, A new algorithm for inner product, *IEEE Trans. Comput.* C-17 (1968) 693–694.

[2] V. Strassen, Gaussian elimination is not optimal, *Numer. Math.* 13 (1969) 354–356; MR 40 #2223.

[3] V. Pan, Strassen's algorithm is not optimal: Trilinear technique of aggregating, uniting and canceling for constructing fast algorithms for matrix operations, *Proc. 19th Symp. on Foundations of Computer Science (FOCS)*, Ann Arbor, IEEE, 1978, pp. 166–176; MR 80e:68118.

[4] V. Pan, New fast algorithms for matrix operations, *SIAM J. Comput.* 9 (1980) 321–342; MR 81f:65037.

[5] V. Strassen, The asymptotic spectrum of tensors and the exponent of matrix multiplication, *Proc. 27th Symp. on Foundations of Computer Science (FOCS)*, Toronto, IEEE, 1986, pp. 49–54.

[6] D. E. Knuth, *The Art of Computer Programming*, v. 2, *Seminumerical Algorithms*, 2nd ed., Addison-Wesley, 1981, pp. 481–482, 503–505, 654–655; MR 44 #3531.

[7] V. Pan, *How to Multiply Matrices Faster*, Lect. Notes in Comp. Sci. 179; Springer-Verlag, 1984; MR 86g:65006.

[8] D. Coppersmith and S. Winograd, Matrix multiplication via arithmetic progressions, *J. Symbolic Comput.* 9 (1990) 251–280; MR 91i:68058.

[9] R. Salem and D. C. Spencer, On sets of integers which contain no three terms in arithmetical progression, *Proc. Nat. Acad. Sci. USA* 28 (1942) 561–563; MR 4,131e.

[10] P. Bürgisser, Algebraische Komplexitätstheorie II – Schnelle Matrixmultiplikation und Kombinatorik, *Sémin. Lothar. Combin.* 36 (1996) B36b; MR 98d:68110.

[11] G. Chiaselotti, Sums of distinct elements in finite abelian groups, *Boll. Un. Mat. Ital. A* 7 (1993) 243–251; MR 94j:20053.

[12] D. Coppersmith, Rectangular matrix multiplication revisited, *J. Complexity* 13 (1997) 42–49; MR 98b:65028.

[13] X. Huang and V. Pan, Fast rectangular matrix multiplication and applications, *J. Complexity* 14 (1998) 257–299; MR 99i:15002.

[14] L. N. Trefethen, Predictions for scientific computing fifty years from now, *Mathematics Today* (Apr. 2000) 53–57; Oxford Univ. Computing Lab. report NA-98/12.

2.30 Pisot–Vijayaraghavan–Salem Constants

Given any positive real number x, let $\{x\} = x \bmod 1$ denote the fractional part of x. For any positive integer n, clearly $\{n + x\} = x$ for all x, and the sequence $\{nx\}$ is periodic if x is rational. A consequence of Weyl's criterion [1–4] is that the sequence $\{nx\}$ is dense in the interval $[0, 1]$ if x is irrational. Moreover, it is **uniformly distributed** in $[0, 1]$, meaning that the probability of finding an arbitrary element ω in any subinterval is proportional to the subinterval length.

Having discussed addition and multiplication, let us turn to exponentiation. It can be proved [5, 6] that the sequence $\{x^n\}$ is uniformly distributed for *almost all* real numbers $x > 1$ (curiously, no specific such values x were known until recently [7, 8]). It is believed that the sequence for $x = 3/2$ is a typical example [2.30.1]. The measure-zero, uncountable set E of exceptions x to this behavior [9–12] includes the numbers 2, 3, 4, ... and $1 + \sqrt{2}$. What else can be said about E?

First, we review some terminology. A **monic polynomial** is a polynomial with a leading coefficient equal to 1. An **algebraic integer** α is a zero of a monic polynomial with integer coefficients. The **conjugates** of α are all zeros of the minimal polynomial of α. Define the set U to be all real algebraic integers $\alpha > 1$ whose conjugates $\gamma \neq \alpha$ each satisfy $|\gamma| \leq 1$. It is known that $U \subseteq E$ and that U is countably infinite. Let us study the exceptional behavior in more detail.

Define the set S of **Pisot–Vijayaraghavan (P-V) numbers** to be all real algebraic integers $\theta > 1$ whose conjugates $\gamma \neq \theta$ each satisfy $|\gamma| < 1$. Define the set T of **Salem numbers** to be all real algebraic integers $\tau > 1$ whose conjugates $\gamma \neq \tau$ each satisfy $|\gamma| \leq 1$ with at least one case of equality. Then clearly S and T determine a partition of U. Moreover, if θ is a P-V number, then

$$\lim_{n \to \infty} \{\theta^n\} = 0 \bmod 1,$$

whereas, if τ is a Salem number, then $\{\tau^n\}$ is dense but not uniformly distributed in the interval $[0, 1]$. There are many related results and we give an example [11]. Suppose we are given an algebraic real $\alpha > 1$ and a real $\lambda > 0$ for which $\{\lambda\alpha^n\}$ has at most finitely many limit points modulo one. Then α must be in S. Additionally, the limit points must each be rational. It is unknown whether anyone has exhibited explicitly a number that is in E but not in U (e.g., a transcendental exceptional x).

We turn attention to the set S, which is known to be countably infinite and closed, and which possesses an isolated minimum point $\theta_0 > 1$. Salem [13] and Siegel [14] proved that $\theta_0 = 1.3247179572\ldots$ is the real zero of the polynomial $x^3 - x - 1$, that is,

$$\theta_0 = \left(\tfrac{1}{2} + \tfrac{\sqrt{69}}{18}\right)^{\frac{1}{3}} + \tfrac{1}{3}\left(\tfrac{1}{2} + \tfrac{\sqrt{69}}{18}\right)^{-\frac{1}{3}} = \tfrac{2\sqrt{3}}{3}\cos\left(\tfrac{1}{3}\arccos\left(\tfrac{3\sqrt{3}}{2}\right)\right).$$

This constant also appears in [1.2.2].

In fact, a complete listing of all P-V numbers up to $\varphi + \varepsilon$ is possible [15], where $\varphi = 1.6180339887\ldots$ is the Golden mean [1.2] and $0 < \varepsilon < 0.0004$. Also, let $S^{<1>}$ denote the set of all limit points of S, that is, the derived set of S. The minimum point of $S^{<1>}$ is φ and is isolated. More generally, let $S^{<k>}$ denote the derived set of $S^{<k-1>}$ for all $k \geq 2$. The minimum point of $S^{<2>}$ is 2, and the minimum point of $S^{<k>}$ is between $\sqrt{k}$ and $k + 1$, but no exact values of these points for $k \geq 3$ are known.

The set T is more difficult to study. We know that T is countably infinite and that U is a proper subset of the closure of T. The existence of a minimum Salem number remains an open problem, but it is conjectured to be $\tau_0 = 1.1762808182\ldots$, which is one of the zeros of **Lehmer's polynomial** [16]

$$x^{10} + x^9 - x^7 - x^6 - x^5 - x^4 - x^3 + x + 1.$$

It has been proved [17–20] that there are exactly forty-five Salem numbers less than 1.3 with degree at most 40. (There are only two known Salem numbers less than 1.3 with degree exceeding 40, but conceivably there may be more.) Is θ_0 the smallest limit point of T? The answer is not known to this question either.

The constants θ_0 and τ_0 appear in connection with a related conjecture, due to Lehmer, about Mahler's measure of a nonzero algebraic integer α. If α is of degree n with conjugates $\alpha_1 = \alpha, \alpha_2, \alpha_3, \ldots, \alpha_n$, define $M(\alpha)$ to be the absolute value of the product of all α_j satisfying $|\alpha_j| > 1$. Kronecker [21, 22] proved that if $M(\alpha) = 1$, then α is a root of unity. Is it true that for every $\varepsilon > 0$, there exists α such that $1 < M(\alpha) < 1 + \varepsilon$?

If α is **non-reciprocal**, that is, if α and $1/\alpha$ are not conjugate, then Smyth [11, 23] proved that the answer is no. More precisely, either $M(\alpha) \geq \theta_0 = 1.324\ldots$ or α is a root of unity.

For arbitrary α, Lehmer [16] conjectured that the answer remains no. More precisely, either $M(\alpha) \geq \tau_0 = 1.176\ldots$ or α is a root of unity. Despite extensive searches, no counterexamples to this inequality have been found. The best-known relevant estimate, if α is not a root of unity, is [24–30]

$$M(\alpha) > 1 + \left(\frac{9}{4} - \varepsilon\right)\left(\frac{\ln(\ln(n))}{\ln(n)}\right)^3$$

for sufficiently large n. For more about Mahler's measure, see [3.10]. We mention a related inequality [21, 30–32] involving what is called the **house** of α:

$$\overline{|\alpha|} = \max_{1 \leq k \leq n} |\alpha_k| > 1 + \frac{1}{n}\left(\frac{64}{\pi^2} - \varepsilon\right)\left(\frac{\ln(\ln(n))}{\ln(n)}\right)^3$$

and a corresponding conjecture [33]: $\overline{|\alpha|} \geq 1 + \frac{3}{2}\ln(\theta_0)/n = 1 + (0.4217993614\ldots)/n$. See also [34, 35].

2.30.1 Powers of 3/2 Modulo One

Pisot [9] and Vijayaraghavan [36] proved that $\{(3/2)^n\}$ has infinitely many accumulation points, that is, infinitely many convergent subsequences with distinct limits. The sequence is believed to be uniformly distributed, but no one has even proved that it is dense in $[0, 1]$.

Here is a somewhat less ambitious problem: Prove that $\{(3/2)^n\}$ has infinitely many accumulation points in both $[0, 1/2)$ and $[1/2, 1]$. In other words, prove that the sequence does not **prefer** one subinterval over the other. This problem remains unsolved, but Flatto, Lagarias & Pollington [37] recently made some progress. They proved that any subinterval of $[0, 1]$ containing all but perhaps finitely many accumulation points of $\{(3/2)^n\}$ must have length at least $1/3$. Therefore, the sequence cannot prefer $[0, 1/3 - \varepsilon)$ over $[1/3 - \varepsilon, 1]$ for any $\varepsilon > 0$. Likewise, it cannot prefer $[2/3 + \varepsilon, 1]$ over $[0, 2/3 + \varepsilon)$. To extend the proof to $[0, 1/2)$ and $[1/2, 1]$ would be a significant but formidable achievement.

Lagarias [38] mentioned the sequence $\{(3/2)^n\}$ and its loose connections with ergodic-theoretic aspects of the famous $3x + 1$ problem. The details are too elaborate to discuss here. What is fascinating is that the sequence is *also* fundamental to a seemingly distant area of number theory: Waring's problem on writing integers as sums of nth powers.

Let $g(n)$ denote the smallest integer k for which every positive integer can be expressed as the sum of k n^{th} powers of nonnegative integers. Hilbert [39] proved that $g(n) < \infty$ for each n. For $2 \le n \le 6$, it is known that [40–44]

$$g(n) = 2^n + \left\lfloor \left(\frac{3}{2}\right)^n \right\rfloor - 2.$$

Dickson [45, 46] and Pillai [47] independently proved that this formula is true for all $n > 6$, provided that the condition

$$\left\{\left(\frac{3}{2}\right)^n\right\} \le 1 - \left(\frac{3}{4}\right)^n$$

is satisfied. Hence it is sufficient to study this inequality, the last remaining obstacle in the solution of Waring's problem.

Kubina & Wunderlich [48], extending the work of Stemmler [49], verified computationally that the inequality is met for all $2 \le n \le 471600000$. Mahler [50] moreover proved that it fails for at most finitely many n, using the Thue–Siegel–Roth theorem on rational approximations to algebraic numbers [2.22]. The proof is non-constructive and thus a computer calculation that rules out failure altogether is still not possible.

It appears that the inequality can be strengthened to

$$\left(\frac{3}{4}\right)^n < \left\{\left(\frac{3}{2}\right)^n\right\} < 1 - \left(\frac{3}{4}\right)^n$$

for all $n > 7$ and generalized in certain ways [51, 52]. Again, no proof is known apart from Mahler's argument. (The best effective results are due to Beukers [53], Dubickas [54], and Habsieger [55], with $3/4$ replaced by 0.577.) The fact that so simple an inequality can defy all attempts at analysis is remarkable.

The calculation of $g(n)$ is sometimes called the "ideal" part of Waring's problem. Let $G(n)$ denote the smallest integer k for which all *sufficiently large* integers can be expressed as the sum of k n^{th} powers of nonnegative integers. Clearly $G(n) \le g(n)$, and Hurwitz [56] and Maillet [57] proved that $G(n) \ge n + 1$. In other words, there are arbitrarily large integers that are not the sum of n n^{th} powers. It is known [43, 58–60] that $G(2) = 4$, $4 \le G(3) \le 7$, $G(4) = 16$, $6 \le G(5) \le 17$, and $9 \le G(6) \le 24$. See [61–63] for numerical evidence supporting a conjecture that $G(3) = 4$. See also [64, 65] for the asymptotics of the number of representations of n as a sum of four cubes, which interestingly turns out to involve $\Gamma(4/3)$, where $\Gamma(x)$ is Euler's gamma function [1.5.4].

Here are several unrelated facts. Infinitely many integers of the form $\lfloor x^n \rfloor$ are composite [66, 67] when $x = 3/2$. This is also true when $x = 4/3$. Are infinitely many such integers prime? What can be said for other values of x?

A conjecture is that, if t is a real number for which 2^t and 3^t are both integers, then t is rational. This would follow from the so-called four-exponentials conjecture [68, 69]. A weaker result, the six-exponentials theorem, is known to be true.

Define an infinite sequence by $x_0 = 1$ and $x_n = \lceil \frac{3}{2} x_{n-1} \rceil$ for $n \geq 1$. Odlyzko & Wilf [70] proved that

$$ x_n = \left\lfloor K \cdot \left(\frac{3}{2} \right)^n \right\rfloor $$

for all n, where the constant $K = 1.6222705028\ldots$ (in fact, they proved much more). Their work is connected to the solution of the ancient Josephus problem. The constant K is analogous to Mills' constant [2.13], in the sense that the formula is useless computationally (unless an exact value for K somehow became available), but its mere existence is remarkable.

A **3-smooth number** is a positive integer whose only prime divisors are 2 or 3. A positive integer n possesses a **3-smooth representation** if n can be written as a sum of 3-smooth numbers, where no summand divides another. Let $r(n)$ denote the number of 3-smooth representations of n. Some recent papers [71–73] answer the question of the maximal and average orders of $r(n)$. See also [5.4].

Let n be an integer larger than 8. Need the base-3 expansion of 2^n possess a digit equal to 2 somewhere? Erdös [74] conjectured that the answer is yes, and Vardi [75] verified this up to $n = 2 \cdot 3^{20}$. More instances of the interplay between the numbers 2 and 3 occur in [2.26].

[1] H. Weyl, Über die Gleichverteilung von Zahlen mod. Eins, *Math. Annalen* 77 (1916) 313–352.

[2] J. W. S. Cassels, *An Introduction to Diophantine Approximation*, Cambridge Univ. Press, 1965; MR 50 #2084.

[3] A. Miklavc, Elementary proofs of two theorems on the distribution of numbers $\{nx\}$ (mod 1), *Proc. Amer. Math. Soc.* 39 (1973) 279–280; MR 47 #4962.

[4] F. M. Dekking and M. Mendès France, Uniform distribution modulo one: A geometrical viewpoint, *J. Reine Angew. Math.* 329 (1981) 143–153; MR 83b:10062.

[5] G. H. Hardy and J. E. Littlewood, Some problems of Diophantine approximation, *Acta Math.* 37 (1914) 155–191; also in *Collected Papers of G. H. Hardy*, v. 1, Oxford Univ. Press, 1966, pp. 28–66.

[6] J. F. Koksma, Ein mengentheoretischer Satz über die Gleichverteilung modulo Eins, *Compositio Math.* 2 (1935) 250–258; Zbl. 12/14.

[7] M. B. Levin, On the complete uniform distribution of the fractional parts of the exponential function (in Russian), *Trudy Sem. Petrovsk.* 7 (1981) 245–256; Engl. transl. in *J. Soviet Math.* 31 (1985) 3247–3256; MR 83j:10059.

[8] M. Drmota and R. F. Tichy, *Sequences, Discrepancies and Applications*, Lect. Notes in Math. 1651, Springer-Verlag, 1997; MR 98j:11057.

[9] C. Pisot, La répartition modulo 1 et les nombres algébriques, *Annali Scuola Norm. Sup. Pisa* 7 (1938) 205–248.

[10] T. Vijayaraghavan, On the fractional parts of the powers of a number. IV, *J. Indian Math. Soc.* 12 (1948) 33–39; MR 10,433b.

[11] M.-J. Bertin, A. Decomps-Guilloux, M. Grandet-Hugot, M. Pathiaux-Delefosse, and J.-P. Schreiber, *Pisot and Salem Numbers*, Birkhäuser, 1992; MR 93k:11095.

[12] M. Mendes France, Book review of "Pisot and Salem Numbers," *Bull. Amer. Math. Soc.* 29 (1993) 274–278.

[13] R. Salem, A remarkable class of algebraic integers: Proof of a conjecture of Vijayaraghavan, *Duke Math. J.* 11 (1944) 103–108; MR 5,254a.

[14] C. L. Siegel, Algebraic integers whose conjugates lie in the unit circle, *Duke Math. J.* 11 (1944) 597–602; MR 6,39b.

[15] J. Dufresnoy and C. Pisot, Etude de certaines fonctions méromorphes bornées sur le cercle unité. Application à un ensemble fermé d'entiers algébriques, *Annales Sci. École Norm. Sup.* 72 (1955) 69–92; MR 17,349d.

[16] D. H. Lehmer, Factorization of certain cyclotomic functions, *Annals of Math.* 34 (1933) 461–479.

[17] D. W. Boyd, Small Salem numbers, *Duke Math. J.* 44 (1977) 315–328; MR 56 #11952.

[18] D. W. Boyd, Pisot and Salem numbers in intervals of the real line, *Math. Comp.* 32 (1978) 1244–1260; MR 58 #10812.

[19] M. J. Mossinghoff, Polynomials with small Mahler measure, *Math. Comp.* 67 (1998) 1697–1705, S11–S14; MR 99a:11119.

[20] V. Flammang, M. Grandcolas, and G. Rhin, Small Salem numbers, *Number theory in Progress*, Proc. 1997 Zakopane conf., ed. K. Győry, H. Iwaniec, and J. Urbanowicz, v. 1, de Gruyter, 1999, pp. 165–168; MR 2000e:11132.

[21] A. Schinzel and H. Zassenhaus, A refinement of two theorems of Kronecker, *Michigan Math. J.* 12 (1965) 81–85; MR 31 #158.

[22] D. W. Boyd, Variations on a theme of Kronecker, *Canad. Math. Bull.* 21 (1978) 129–133; MR 58 #5580.

[23] C. J. Smyth, On the product of the conjugates outside the unit circle of an algebraic integer, *Bull. London Math. Soc.* 3 (1971) 169–175; MR 44 #6641.

[24] E. Dobrowolski, On a question of Lehmer and the number of irreducible factors of a polynomial, *Acta Arith.* 34 (1979) 391–401; MR 80i:10040.

[25] D. C. Cantor and E. G. Straus, On a conjecture of D. H. Lehmer, *Acta Arith.* 42 (1982) 97–100; correction 42 (1983) 327; MR 84a:12004 and MR 85a:11017.

[26] R. Louboutin, Sur la mesure de Mahler d'un nombre algébrique, *C. R. Acad. Sci. Paris Sér. I Math.* 296 (1983) 707–708; MR 85b:11058.

[27] U. Rausch, On a theorem of Dobrowolski about the product of conjugate numbers, *Colloq. Math.* 50 (1985) 137–142; MR 87i:11144.

[28] P. Voutier, An effective lower bound for the height of algebraic numbers, *Acta Arith.* 74 (1996) 81–95. MR 96j:11098.

[29] A. Dubickas, Algebraic conjugates outside the unit circle, *New Trends in Probability and Statistics*, v. 4, *Analytic and Probabilistic Methods in Number Theory*, Proc. 1996 Palanga conf., ed. A. Laurincikas, E. Manstavicius, and V. Stakėnas, VSP, 1997, pp. 11–21; MR 99i:11096.

[30] A. Schinzel, *Polynomials with Special Regard to Reducibility*, Cambridge Univ. Press, 2000; MR 2001h:11135.

[31] A. Dubickas, On a conjecture of A. Schinzel and H. Zassenhaus, *Acta Arith.* 63 (1993) 15–20; MR 94a:11161.

[32] A. Dubickas, The maximal conjugate of a non-reciprocal algebraic integer (in Russian), *Liet. Mat. Rink.* 37 (1997) 168–174; Engl. transl. in *Lithuanian Math. J.* 37 (1997) 129–133; MR 98j:11083.

[33] D. W. Boyd, The maximal modulus of an algebraic integer, *Math. Comp.* 45 (1985) 243–249, S17–S20; MR 87c:11097.

[34] E. Dobrowolski, Mahler's measure of a polynomial in function of the number of its coefficients. *Canad. Math. Bull.* 34 (1991) 186–195; MR 92f:11138.

[35] J. H. Silverman, Small Salem numbers, exceptional units, and Lehmer's conjecture, *Rocky Mount. J. Math.* 26 (1996) 1099–1114; MR 97k:11152.

[36] T. Vijayaraghavan, On the fractional parts of the powers of a number. I, *J. London Math. Soc.* 15 (1940) 159–160; MR 2,33e.

[37] L. Flatto, J. C. Lagarias, and A. D. Pollington, On the range of fractional parts $\{\xi \, (p/q)^n\}$, *Acta Arith.* 70 (1995) 125–147; MR 96a:11073.

[38] J. C. Lagarias, The $3x + 1$ problem and its generalizations, *Amer. Math. Monthly* 92 (1985) 3–23; also in *Organic Mathematics*, Proc. 1995 Burnaby workshop, ed. J. Borwein,

P. Borwein, L. Jörgenson, and R. Corless, Amer. Math. Soc., 1997, pp. 305–334; MR 86i:11043.

[39] D. Hilbert, Beweis für die Darstellbarkeit der ganzen Zahlen durch eine feste Anzahl n^{ter} Potenzen (Waringsches Problem), *Nachr. Königlichen Ges. Wiss. Göttingen, Math.-Phys. Klasse* (1909) 17–36; *Math. Annalen* 67 (1909) 281–305; also in *Gesammelte Abhandlungen*, v. 1, Chelsea, 1965, pp. 510–527.

[40] G. H. Hardy and E. M. Wright, *An Introduction to the Theory of Numbers*, 5th ed., Oxford Univ. Press, 1985; MR 81i:10002.

[41] W. J. Ellison, Waring's problem, *Amer. Math. Monthly* 78 (1971) 10–36; MR 54 #2611.

[42] C. Small, Waring's problem, *Math. Mag.* 50 (1977) 12–16; MR 55 #5561.

[43] P. Ribenboim, *The New Book of Prime Number Records*, Springer-Verlag, 1996, pp. 300–309; MR 96k:11112.

[44] R. Balasubramanian, J.-M. Deshouillers, and F. Dress, Problème de Waring pour les bicarrés 1, 2, *C. R. Acad. Sci. Paris Sér. I Math.* 303 (1986) 85–88, 161–163; MR 87m:11099 and MR 88e:11095.

[45] L. E. Dickson, Proof of the ideal Waring theorem for exponents 7–180, *Amer. J. Math.* 58 (1936) 521–529.

[46] L. E. Dickson, Solution of Waring's problem, *Amer. J. Math.* 58 (1936) 530–535.

[47] S. S. Pillai, On Waring's problem, *J. Indian Math. Soc.* 2 (1936) 16–44; Zbl. 14/294.

[48] J. M. Kubina and M. C. Wunderlich, Extending Waring's conjecture to 471,600,000, *Math. Comp.* 55 (1990) 815–820; MR 91b:11101.

[49] R. M. Stemmler, The ideal Waring theorem for exponents 401–200,000, *Math. Comp.* 18 (1964) 144–146; MR 28 #3019.

[50] K. Mahler, On the fractional parts of the powers of a rational number. II, *Mathematica* 4 (1957) 122–124; MR 20 #33.

[51] M. A. Bennett, Fractional parts of powers of rational numbers, *Math. Proc. Cambridge Philos. Soc.* 114 (1993) 191–201; MR 94h:11062.

[52] M. A. Bennett, An ideal Waring problem with restricted summands, *Acta Arith.* 66 (1994) 125–132; MR 95k:11126.

[53] F. Beukers, Fractional parts of powers of rationals, *Math. Proc. Cambridge Philos. Soc.* 90 (1981) 13–20; MR 83g:10028.

[54] A. Dubickas, A lower bound for the quantity $\|(3/2)^n\|$ (in Russian), *Uspekhi Mat. Nauk*, v. 45 (1990) n. 4, 153–154; Engl. transl. in *Russian Math. Survey*, v. 45 (1990) n. 4, 163–164; MR 91k:11058.

[55] L. Habsieger, Explicit lower bounds for $\|(3/2)^k\|$, unpublished note (1998).

[56] A. Hurwitz, Über die Darstellung der ganzen Zahlen als Summen von n^{ter} Potenzen ganzer Zahlen, *Math. Annalen* 65 (1908) 424–427; also in *Mathematische Werke*, v. 2, Birkhäuser, 1933, pp. 422–426.

[57] E. Maillet, Sur la décomposition d'un entier en une somme de puissances huitièmes d'entiers (Problème de Waring), *Bull. Soc. Math. France* 36 (1908) 69–77.

[58] M. B. Nathanson, *Additive Number Theory: The Classical Bases*, Springer-Verlag, 1996; MR 97e:11004.

[59] R. C. Vaughan and T. D. Wooley, Further improvements in Waring's problem, *Acta Math.* 174 (1995) 147–240; MR 96j:11129a.

[60] R. C. Vaughan and T. D. Wooley, Further improvements in Waring's problem. IV: Higher powers, *Acta Arith.* 94 (2000) 203–285; MR 2001g:11154.

[61] J. Bohman and C.-E. Fröberg, Numerical investigation of Waring's problem for cubes, *BIT* 21 (1981) 118–122; MR 82k:10063.

[62] F. Romani, Computations concerning Waring's problem for cubes, *Calcolo* 19 (1982) 415–431; MR 85g:11088.

[63] J.-M. Deshouillers, F. Hennecart, and B. Landreau, 7,373,170,279,850, *Math. Comp.* 69 (2000) 421–439; MR 2000i:11150.

[64] J. Brüdern and N. Watt, On Waring's problem for four cubes, *Duke Math. J.* 77 (1995) 583–599; MR 96e:11121.

[65] K. Kawada, On the sum of four cubes, *Mathematika* 43 (1996) 323–348; MR 97m:11125.

[66] W. Forman and H. N. Shapiro, An arithmetic property of certain rational powers, *Commun. Pure Appl. Math.* 20 (1967) 561–573; MR 35 #2852.

[67] R. K. Guy, *Unsolved Problems in Number Theory*, 2nd ed., Springer-Verlag 1994, sect. E19; MR 96e:11002.

[68] M. Waldschmidt, *Transcendence Methods*, Queen's Papers in Pure and Appl. Math., n. 52, ed. A. J. Coleman and P. Ribenboim, Queen's Univ., 1979; MR 83a:10068.

[69] M. Waldschmidt, On the transcendence method of Gel'fond and Schneider in several variables, *New Advances in Transcendence Theory*, ed. A. Baker, Cambridge Univ. Press, 1988, pp. 375–398; MR 90d:11089.

[70] A. M. Odlyzko and H. S. Wilf, Functional iteration and the Josephus problem, *Glasgow Math. J.* 33 (1991) 235–240; MR 92g:05006.

[71] R. Blecksmith, M. McCallum, and J. L. Selfridge, 3-smooth representations of integers, *Amer. Math. Monthly* 105 (1998) 529–543; MR 2000a:11019.

[72] M. R. Avidon, On primitive 3-smooth partitions of *n*, *Elec. J. Combin.* 4 (1997) R2; MR 98a:11136.

[73] P. Erdös and M. Lewin, *d*-complete sequences of integers, *Math. Comp.* 65 (1996) 837–840; MR 96g:11008.

[74] P. Erdös and R. Graham, *Old and New Problems and Results in Combinatorial Number Theory*, Enseignement Math. Monogr. 28, 1980, p. 80; MR 82j:10001.

[75] I. Vardi, *Computational Recreations in Mathematica*, Addison-Wesley, 1991, pp. 20–25; MR 93e:00002.

2.31 Freiman's Constant

2.31.1 Lagrange Spectrum

In our essay on Diophantine approximation constants [2.23], we discussed Hurwitz's [1, 2] theorem that, for any irrational number ξ, the inequality

$$\left| \xi - \frac{p}{q} \right| < \frac{1}{\sqrt{5}} \frac{1}{q^2}$$

has infinitely many solutions (p, q), where p and q are integers. Can this result be improved? That is, can $\sqrt{5}$ be replaced by a larger quantity? The answer is no for certain special numbers ξ, but it is yes otherwise. We now elaborate.

For each number ξ, define $\lambda(\xi)$ to be the supremum of all quantities c for which the integer solution set (p, q) of

$$\left| \xi - \frac{p}{q} \right| < \frac{1}{c} \frac{1}{q^2}$$

remains infinite. The set of values L taken by the function $\lambda(\xi)$ is called the **Lagrange spectrum** [3]. Clearly the smallest value in L is $\sqrt{5}$. It can be proved that the set $L \cap [2, 3]$ is countably infinite, with 3 as its only limit point, but $[\theta, \infty) \subseteq L$ for some point $\theta > 4$. Much more will be said about L shortly.

2.31.2 Markov Spectrum

A two-variable quadratic form with real coefficients $f(x, y) = \alpha x^2 + \beta xy + \gamma y^2$ is **indefinite** if f assumes both positive and negative values. If the **discriminant**

$d(f) = \beta^2 - 4\alpha\gamma$ is positive, then the plot of $z = f(x, y)$ in real xyz-space is a saddle surface, that is, with no maximum or minimum points.

For each such f, define

$$\mu(f) = \frac{\sqrt{d(f)}}{\inf\limits_{(m,n)\neq(0,0)} |f(m, n)|},$$

where the infimum ranges over all nonzero integer pairs. The set of values M taken by the function $\mu(f)$ is called the **Markov spectrum** [3]. It can be proved that $L \subseteq M$ and further that $M \cap [2, 3] = L \cap [2, 3]$ and $[\theta, \infty) \subseteq M$ for the same point $\theta > 4$ mentioned for L. However, $M \cap [3, \theta] \neq L \cap [3, \theta]$; that is, L is a *proper* subset of M, which gives rise to some interesting unresolved issues.

2.31.3 Markov–Hurwitz Equation

Let us return to Hurwitz's theorem. First, define two numbers ξ and η to be **equivalent** if there are integers a, b, c, d such that

$$\xi = \frac{a\eta + b}{c\eta + d}, \quad |ad - bc| = 1.$$

This relation permits the partitioning of numbers into equivalence classes. Two irrational numbers ξ and η are equivalent if and only if, after some point, their respective sequences of continued fraction partial denominators are identical.

Now, it can be proved that $\lambda(\xi) = \sqrt{5}$ for all ξ equivalent to the Golden mean φ [1.2], that is, possessing partial denominators that are eventually all 1s. Such numbers can be thought of as "simplest," but from the point of view of rational approximations, the simplest numbers are the "worst" [1,4]. If we leave these out, the next level of approximation difficulty is given by $\lambda(\xi) = \sqrt{8}$ for all ξ equivalent to Pythagoras' constant $\sqrt{2}$ [1.1], that is, possessing partial denominators that are eventually all 2s. If we leave these out as well, the next level is $\lambda(\xi) = \sqrt{221}/5$ and so on. See [3] for a table of smallest numbers in the Lagrange spectrum, as well as an algorithm for computing a corresponding representative quadratic form $f(x, y)$.

The values $\sqrt{5}$, $\sqrt{8}$, $\sqrt{221}/5$, $\sqrt{1517}/13$, $\sqrt{7565}/29, \ldots$ are all of the form $\sqrt{9w^2 - 4}/w$, where u, v, w are positive integers satisfying the Diophantine equation

$$u^2 + v^2 + w^2 = 3uvw, \quad 1 \leq u \leq v \leq w.$$

The first several admissible triples are

$$(u, v, w) = (1, 1, 1), (1, 1, 2), (1, 2, 5), (1, 5, 13), (2, 5, 29), (1, 13, 34), \ldots$$

and the infinite sequence of ws

$$1, \ 2, \ 5, \ 13, \ 29, \ 34, \ 89, \ 169, \ 194, \ 233, \ 433, \ 610, \ 985, \ldots$$

are called **Markov numbers** [5]. It is unknown [6–12] whether every w_k determines a *unique* admissible triple (u_k, v_k, w_k). Note that, clearly, the limit of $\lambda(w_k)$ as $k \to \infty$ is 3. This proves that $L \cap [2, 3]$ accumulates at 3, as was to be shown.

Here is a side topic. The number $N(n)$ of admissible triples (u, v, w) with $w \leq n$ was proved by Zagier [7, 8] to be

$$N(n) = C \cdot \ln(n)^2 + O\left[\ln(n) \cdot \ln(\ln(n))^2\right],$$

where

$$C = \frac{3}{\pi^2} \frac{1}{2} \left(\frac{1}{g(1)^2} + \frac{2g(1) - g(2)}{g(1)^2 g(2)} \right) + \frac{3}{\pi^2} \sum_{\substack{\text{admissible} \\ (u,v,w) \text{ with} \\ u < v < w}} \frac{g(u) + g(v) - g(w)}{g(u)g(v)g(w)}$$

$$= 0.1807171047\ldots$$

and

$$g(x) = \ln\left(\frac{3x + \sqrt{9x^2 - 4}}{2} \right) = \text{arccosh}\left(\frac{3x}{2} \right), \quad x \geq \frac{2}{3}.$$

He conjectured that this asymptotic result can be strengthened to

$$N(n) = C \cdot \ln(3n)^2 + o\left(\ln(n)\right),$$

which, if the uniqueness conjecture is true, may be rewritten as

$$w_k = \left(\frac{1}{3} + o(1) \right) \exp\left(\sqrt{\frac{k}{C}} \right) = \left(\frac{1}{3} + o(1) \right) (10.5101504239\ldots)^{\sqrt{k}}.$$

Here is a generalization of the side topic. Let $m \geq 3$. Consider the **Markov–Hurwitz equation**

$$u_1^2 + u_2^2 + \cdots + u_m^2 = m u_1 u_2 \cdots u_m, \quad 1 \leq u_1 \leq u_2 \leq \cdots \leq u_m,$$

and define $N_m(n)$ to be the number of admissible m-tuples $(u_1, u_2, \ldots, u_m)$ of positive integers with $u_m \leq n$. It is surprising that the growth rate of $N_m(n)$ is not $O(\ln(n)^{m-1})$, but rather $O(\ln(n)^{\alpha(m)+\varepsilon})$ for any $\varepsilon > 0$, where the exponents $\alpha(m)$ satisfy [13–15]

$$\alpha(3) = 2, \quad 2.430 < \alpha(4) < 2.477, \quad 2.730 < \alpha(5) < 2.798, \quad 2.963 < \alpha(6) < 3.048$$

and $\lim_{m\to\infty} \alpha(m)/\ln(m) = 1/\ln(2)$. The analog of Zagier's constant C for $m \geq 4$ is not known.

2.31.4 Hall's Ray

Our knowledge of $L \cap [3, \infty)$ and $M \cap [3, \infty)$ is much less complete than the aforementioned information for $L \cap [2, 3]$. Each of L and M is a closed subset of the real line; hence the complement of each spectrum is a countable union of open intervals, that is, of **gaps**. A gap is **maximal** if its endpoints are in the spectrum under consideration. Here are several maximal gaps (with regard to both L and M):

$$\left(\sqrt{12}, \sqrt{13} \right) = (3.464101\ldots, 3.605551\ldots),$$

$$\left(\sqrt{13}, \frac{65 + 9\sqrt{3}}{22} \right) = (3.605551\ldots, 3.663111\ldots),$$

$$\left(\frac{\sqrt{480}}{7}, \sqrt{10} \right) = (3.129843\ldots, 3.162277\ldots).$$

The first two were discovered by Perron [16]; many others are listed in [3]. Evidently there is no "first" gap with left-hand endpoint ≥ 3.

Hall [17] proved that any real number in the interval $[\sqrt{2} - 1, 4\sqrt{2} - 4]$ can be written as a sum of two numbers whose continued fraction partial denominators never exceed 4. It follows that L and M contain all sufficiently large real numbers; this portion of these spectra is called **Hall's ray**. Freiman [18] succeeded in computing the precise point θ at which Hall's ray begins (which is the same for both L and M) and its exact expression is [3, 6]

$$\theta = 4 + \frac{253589820 + 283748\sqrt{462}}{491993569} = 4.5278295661\ldots.$$

In fact, the "last" gap with right-hand endpoint $< \infty$ is $(4.527829538\ldots, 4.527829566\ldots)$, true for both L and M.

By way of contrast, Bumby [3, 19] determined that $M \cap [3, 3.33437\ldots]$ has Lebesgue measure zero! Can the endpoint $3.33437\ldots$ be shifted any farther to the right and yet preserve the measure-zero property? Can an exact expression for this endpoint be found?

2.31.5 L and M Compared

This is perhaps the most mysterious area of this study, and we shall be very brief [3]. Freiman [20] constructed a quadratic irrational $\xi = 3.118120178\ldots$ that is in M but not in L. Freiman [21] later found another example: $\eta = 3.293044265\ldots$. Infinitely many more such examples are now known. Berstein [22, 23] determined the largest intervals containing Freiman's points ξ and η but not containing any elements of L. The interval for ξ has approximate length 1.7×10^{-10} whereas that for η has approximate length 2×10^{-7}. Freiman additionally showed that these intervals each contain countably infinite elements of M.

Cusick & Flahive [3] conjectured that L and M coincide above $\sqrt{12} = 3.464101\ldots$. The largest known number in M but not in L is $3.29304\ldots$. Much more on this fascinating subject is found in [24].

[1] G. H. Hardy and E. M. Wright, *An Introduction to the Theory of Numbers*, 5th ed., Oxford Univ. Press, 1985, pp. 141–143, 163–169; MR 81i:10002.

[2] J. W. S. Cassels, *An Introduction to Diophantine Approximation*, Cambridge Univ. Press, 1965; MR 50 #2084.

[3] T. W. Cusick and M. E. Flahive, *The Markoff and Lagrange Spectra*, Amer. Math. Soc., 1989; MR 90i:11069.

[4] A. M. Rockett and P. Szüsz, *Continued Fractions*, World Scientific, 1992, pp. 72–110; MR 93m:11060.

[5] N. J. A. Sloane, On-Line Encyclopedia of Integer Sequences, A002559.

[6] J. H. Conway and R. K. Guy, *The Book of Numbers*, Springer-Verlag, 1996, pp. 187–189; MR 98g:00004.

[7] R. K. Guy, *Unsolved Problems in Number Theory*, 2nd ed., Springer-Verlag, 1994, sect. D12; MR 96e:11002.

[8] D. Zagier, On the number of Markoff numbers below a given bound, *Math. Comp.* 39 (1982) 709–723; MR 83k:10062.

[9] P. Schmutz, Systoles of arithmetic surfaces and the Markoff spectrum, *Math. Annalen* 305 (1996) 191–203; MR 97b:11090.

[10] A. Baragar, On the unicity conjecture for Markoff numbers, *Canad. Math. Bull.* 39 (1996) 3–9; MR 97d:11110.

[11] J. O. Button, The uniqueness of the prime Markoff numbers, *J. London Math. Soc.* 58 (1998) 9–17; MR 2000c:11043.

[12] J. O. Button, Markoff numbers, principal ideals and continued fraction expansions, *J. Number Theory* 87 (2001) 77–95; MR 2002a:11074.

[13] Yu. N. Baulina, On the number of solutions of the equation $x_1^2 + \cdots + x_n^2 = nx_1 \cdots x_n$ that do not exceed a given limit (in Russian), *Mat. Zametki* 57 (1995) 297–300; Engl. transl. in *Math. Notes* 57 (1995) 208–210; MR 97b:11049.

[14] A. Baragar, Asymptotic growth of Markoff-Hurwitz numbers, *Compositio Math.* 94 (1994) 1–18; MR 95i:11025.

[15] A. Baragar, The exponent for the Markoff-Hurwitz equations, *Pacific J. Math.* 182 (1998) 1–21; MR 99e:11035.

[16] O. Perron, Über die Approximation irrationaler Zahler durch rationale. II, *Sitzungsberichte der Heidelberger Akademie der Wissenschaften* 8 (1921) 1–12.

[17] M. Hall, On the sum and product of continued fractions, *Annals of Math.* 48 (1947) 966–993; MR 9,226b.

[18] G. A. Freiman, *Diophantine Approximations and the Geometry of Numbers (Markov's Problem)* (in Russian), Kalininskii Gosudarstvennyi Universitet, 1975; MR 58 #5536.

[19] R. T. Bumby, Hausdorff dimensions of Cantor sets, *J. Reine Angew. Math.* 331 (1982) 192–206; MR 83g:10038.

[20] G. A. Freiman, Non-coincidence of the spectra of Markov and of Lagrange (in Russian), *Mat. Zametki* 3 (1968) 195–200; Engl. transl. in *Math. Notes* 3 (1968) 125–128; MR 37 #2695.

[21] G. A. Freiman, Non-coincidence of the Markov and Lagrange spectra (in Russian), *Number-Theoretic Studies in the Markov Spectrum and in the Structural Theory of Set Addition*, ed. G. A. Freiman, A. M. Rubinov, and E. V. Novoselov, Kalinin. Gos. Univ., 1973, pp. 10–15, 121–125; MR 55 #2777.

[22] A. A. Berstein, The connections between the Markov and Lagrange spectra, *Number-Theoretic Studies in the Markov Spectrum and in the Structural Theory of Set Addition*, Kalinin. Gos. Univ., 1973, pp. 16–49, 121–125; MR 55 #2778.

[23] A. A. Berstein, The structure of the Markov spectrum, *Number-Theoretic Studies in the Markov Spectrum and in the Structural Theory of Set Addition*, Kalinin. Gos. Univ., 1973, pp. 50–78, 121–125; MR 55 #2779.

[24] A. D. Pollington and W. Moran (eds.), *Number Theory with an Emphasis on the Markoff Spectrum*, Proc. 1991 Provo conf., Dekker, 1993; MR 93m:11002.

2.32 De Bruijn–Newman Constant

We discuss a constant here that is unlike any other in this collection: It is positive if and only if the notorious Riemann hypothesis [1.6.2] is false. It is, moreover, defined in a manner that permits the computer calculation of precise numerical bounds [1].

Starting with the Riemann zeta function $\zeta(z)$, define [2]

$$\xi(z) = \tfrac{1}{2}z(z-1)\pi^{-\frac{1}{2}z}\Gamma(\tfrac{1}{2}z)\zeta(z), \quad \Xi(z) = \xi(iz + \tfrac{1}{2}), \quad z \text{ complex.}$$

It is trivial to prove that the Riemann hypothesis is true if and only if the zeros of $\Xi(z)$ are all real. This restatement of the conjecture will be useful to us in what follows.

Think of $\Xi(z/2)/8$ as a complex frequency function, that is, as the Fourier cosine transform of a time signal $\Phi(t)$. The signal can be calculated to be

$$\Phi(t) = \sum_{n=1}^{\infty}(2\pi^2 n^4 e^{9t} - 3\pi n^2 e^{5t})\exp(-\pi n^2 e^{4t}), \quad t \text{ real}, t \geq 0.$$

Given a real parameter λ, consider the modified signal $\Phi(t)\exp(\lambda t^2)$ and then carry it back into the frequency domain, that is, returning to where we were initially. The resulting family of Fourier cosine transforms, $H_\lambda(z)$, contains $H_0(z) = \Xi(z/2)/8$ as a special case.

What is known about the zeros of $H_\lambda(z)$, for fixed λ? De Bruijn [3] proved, among other things, that H_λ has only real zeros for $\lambda \geq 1/2$. Newman [4] established further that there is a constant, Λ, such that H_λ has only real zeros if and only if $\lambda \geq \Lambda$. Of course, $\Lambda \leq 1/2$ follows immediately from de Bruijn's result. The Riemann hypothesis is equivalent to the conjecture that $\Lambda \leq 0$. Newman conjectured that $\Lambda \geq 0$, emphasizing nicely that the Riemann hypothesis, if it is true, is just barely so.

Lower bounds on Λ are clearly of enormous interest to everybody concerned. Elaborate computations in [1, 5–8] gave $\Lambda > -0.0991$. Csordas, Smith & Varga [9, 10] proved a theorem, involving certain "close" consecutive zeros of the Riemann xi function (known as Lehmer pairs), that dramatically sharpened estimates of the de Bruijn–Newman constant. The current best lower bound [11, 12] is $\Lambda > -2.7 \times 10^{-9}$. No progress has been made, as far as is known, on improving the upper bound $1/2$ on Λ.

As an aside, we mention one other criterion equivalent to the Riemann hypothesis. Define, for each positive integer n, the series

$$\lambda_n = \sum_{\rho}\left[1 - \left(1 - \frac{1}{\rho}\right)^n\right]$$

$$= \begin{cases} -\frac{1}{2}\ln(4\pi) + \frac{\gamma_0}{2} + 1 = 0.0230957089\ldots & \text{if } n = 1, \\ \frac{\pi^2}{8} - \ln(4\pi) + \gamma_0 - \gamma_0^2 - 2\gamma_1 + 1 = 0.0923457352\ldots & \text{if } n = 2, \\ 0.2076389205\ldots & \text{if } n = 3, \end{cases}$$

where each sum is over all nontrivial zeros ρ of $\zeta(z)$ and γ_k is the kth Stieltjes constant [2.21]. Li [13] proved that $\lambda_n \geq 0$ for all n if and only if the Riemann hypothesis is true. See the related constants σ_n in [2.21] and insightful discussion in [14, 15].

[1] R. S. Varga, *Scientific Computation on Mathematical Problems and Conjectures*, SIAM, 1990; MR 92b:65012.
[2] E. C. Titchmarsh, *The Theory of the Riemann Zeta Function*, 2nd ed., rev. by D. R. Heath-Brown, Oxford Univ. Press, 1986, pp. 16, 255; MR 88c:11049.
[3] N. G. de Bruijn, The roots of trigonometric integrals, *Duke Math. J.* 17 (1950) 197–226; MR 12,250a.
[4] C. M. Newman, Fourier transforms with only real zeros, *Proc. Amer. Math. Soc.* 61 (1976) 245–251; MR 55 #7944.
[5] G. Csordas, T. S. Norfolk, and R. S. Varga, A lower bound for the de Bruijn-Newman constant Λ, *Numer. Math.* 52 (1988) 483–497; MR 89m:30054.
[6] H. J. J. te Riele, A new lower bound for the de Bruijn-Newman constant, *Numer. Math.* 58 (1991) 661–667; MR 92c:30030.

[7] T. S. Norfolk, A. Ruttan, and R. S. Varga, A lower bound for the de Bruijn-Newman constant
     Λ. II, *Progress in Approximation Theory*, Proc. 1990 Tampa conf., ed. A. A. Gonchar and
     E. B. Saff, Springer-Verlag, 1992, pp. 403–418; MR 94k:30062.

[8] G. Csordas, A. Ruttan, and R. S. Varga, The Laguerre inequalities with applications to a
     problem associated with the Riemann hypothesis, *Numer. Algorithms* 1 (1991) 305–329;
     MR 93c:30041.

[9] G. Csordas, W. Smith, and R. S. Varga, Lehmer pairs of zeros and the Riemann ξ-function,
     Mathematics of Computation 1943–1993: A Half-Century of Computational Mathematics,
     Proc. 1993 Vancouver conf., ed. W. Gautschi, Amer. Math. Soc., 1994, pp. 553–556; MR
     96b:11119.

[10] G. Csordas, W. Smith, and R. S. Varga, Lehmer pairs of zeros, the de Bruijn-Newman
     constant and the Riemann hypothesis, *Constr. Approx.* 10 (1994) 107–129; MR 94k:30061.

[11] G. Csordas, A. Odlyzko, W. Smith, and R. S. Varga, A new Lehmer pair of zeros and a
     new lower bound for the de Bruijn-Newman constant, *Elec. Trans. Numer. Anal.* 1 (1993)
     104–111; MR 94k:11098.

[12] A. M. Odlyzko, An improved bound for the de Bruijn-Newman constant, *Numer. Algorithms*
     25 (2000) 293–303; MR 2002a:30046.

[13] X.-J. Li, The positivity of a sequence of numbers and the Riemann hypothesis, *J. Number
     Theory* 65 (1997) 325–333; MR 98d:11101.

[14] E. Bombieri and J. C. Lagarias, Complements to Li's criterion for the Riemann hypothesis,
     J. Number Theory 77 (1999) 274–287; MR 2000h:11092.

[15] P. Biane, J. Pitman, and M. Yor, Probability laws related to the Jacobi theta and Riemann
     zeta functions, and Brownian excursions, *Bull. Amer. Math. Soc.* 38 (2001) 435–465.

2.33 Hall–Montgomery Constant

A complex-valued function f defined on the positive integers is **completely
multiplicative** if $f(mn) = f(m)f(n)$ for all m and n. Clearly such a function is determined by its values on $1 \cup \{\text{primes}\}$. Simple examples include $f(n) = 0$, $f(n) = 1$,
and $f(n) = n^r$ for some fixed $r > 0$. A more complicated example, for a fixed odd
prime p, is the Legendre symbol

$$f_p(n) = \left(\frac{n}{p}\right) = \begin{cases} 0 & \text{if } p|n, \\ 1 & \text{if } p \nmid n \text{ and } n \text{ is a quadratic residue modulo } p, \\ -1 & \text{otherwise;} \end{cases}$$

for example, $(6/19) = 1$ since $5^2 \equiv 6 \bmod 19$, but $(39/47) = -1$ since the congruence
$x^2 \equiv 39 \bmod 47$ has no solution.

To illustrate, define $g(N)$ to be the cardinality of the set $\{1 \le n \le N : f_p(n) = 1\}$. It
is known [1] that, from the integers $\{1, 2, \ldots, p - 1\}$, $(p - 1)/2$ are quadratic residues
and $(p - 1)/2$ are nonresidues. Hence $g(N)/N \to 1/2$ as $N \to \infty$ through multiples
of p. It is natural to ask about other possible limiting values of $g(N)/N$ for different
choices of N. We will return to this issue shortly.

Consider the class F of all completely multiplicative functions whose values are
constrained to the closed real interval $[-1, 1]$. What numbers arise as mean values of
functions in F? More precisely, what is the set Γ of limit points of

$$\mu_N(f) = \frac{1}{N} \sum_{n=1}^{N} f(n)$$

as f varies over F and as $N \to \infty$? The set Γ is called the **multiplicative spectrum** of $[-1, 1]$, and an understanding of its structure has been reached only recently.

Granville & Soundararajan [2, 3], building upon independent work by Hall & Montgomery [4], proved that Γ is a closed interval and, in fact,

$$\Gamma = [\delta_1, 1] = [-0.6569990137\ldots, 1],$$

where $\delta_1 = 2\delta_0 - 1$,

$$\delta_0 = 1 - \frac{\pi^2}{6} - \ln(1 + \sqrt{e}) \ln\left(\frac{e}{1 + \sqrt{e}}\right) + 2\operatorname{Li}_2\left(\frac{1}{1 + \sqrt{e}}\right) = 0.1715004931\ldots,$$

and $\operatorname{Li}_2(x)$ is the dilogarithm function [1.6.8]. By analytic continuation, the expression for δ_0 can be simplified to $1 + \pi^2/6 + 2\operatorname{Li}_2(-\sqrt{e})$. This remarkable formula is only the tip of a larger theory: Much can also be said about $\Gamma(S)$, where S is an arbitrary subset of the unit disk D in the complex plane (rather than just the interval $[-1, 1]$). An important role in the proofs is played by differential and integral equations with delay [5.4].

Returning to the special case of $f_p(n)$, by the aforementioned theorem,

$$g(N) - (N - g(N)) \geq (\delta_1 + o(1))N;$$

that is, $g(N) \geq (\delta_0 + o(1))N$. In other words, the proportion of integers not exceeding N that are quadratic residues mod p is at least δ_0, independent of the choice of p:

$$\delta_0 \leq \liminf_{N \to \infty} \frac{g(N)}{N} \leq \frac{1}{2} \leq \limsup_{N \to \infty} \frac{g(N)}{N} \leq 1.$$

This proves a 1994 conjecture of Heath-Brown [4]. Additionally, the constant δ_0 is the best possible and, in fact, the limit inferior is equal to δ_0 for infinitely many primes p.

Likewise, the limit superior is equal to 1 for infinitely many primes p. Here is a proof. For fixed N, select a prime $p \equiv 1 \bmod M$, where M is $8 \times$ the product of all odd primes $\leq N$. This is possible by Dirichlet's theorem on primes in arithmetic progressions. Thus $(2/p) = 1$ and, if q is an odd prime $\leq N$, then $(q/p) = (p/q) = (1/q) = 1$ by the law of quadratic reciprocity. Any $n \leq N$ is the product of primes $\leq N$; hence $(n/p) = 1$. Therefore, all $n \leq N$ are quadratic residues mod p. Infinitely many choices of p are possible, of course, so the result follows.

Let us examine a generalization. A complex-valued function f defined on the positive integers is **multiplicative** if $f(mn) = f(m)f(n)$ whenever m and n are relatively prime. (If f is completely multiplicative, then clearly f is multiplicative.) Assume that $-1 \leq f(n) \leq 1$ for all n (as before); then its mean value exists and is equal to [5–9]

$$\lim_{N \to \infty} \mu_N(f) = \prod_p \left(1 - \frac{1}{p}\right)\left(1 + \sum_{k=1}^{\infty} \frac{f(p^k)}{p^k}\right),$$

where the product is over all primes p. For example, if $f(n) = \varphi(n)/n$, where φ is the Euler totient function [2.7], then $\lim_{N \to \infty} \mu_N(f) = 6/\pi^2$. Note that, in this example, $f(p^k) = f(p)$ for any $k \geq 1$. Complicated conditions for the existence of $\lim_{N \to \infty} \mu_N(f)$ arise if we weaken our assumption to only $f(n) \in D$ for all n.

Here is an (unrelated) asymptotic result corresponding to a rather artificial example [10]. Define a multiplicative function f by the recursive formula

$$f(n) = \begin{cases} 1 & \text{if } n = 1, \\ pf(k) & \text{if } n = p^k \text{ for any prime } p; \end{cases}$$

then

$$\lim_{N \to \infty} \frac{1}{N^2} \sum_{n=1}^{N} f(n) = \frac{1}{2} \prod_{p} \left(1 - \frac{1}{p^2} + (p-1) \sum_{n=2}^{\infty} \frac{f(n)}{p^{2n}} \right)$$

$$= \frac{1}{2}(0.8351076361\ldots).$$

By way of contrast, the **completely additive** function $\Omega(n)$ introduced in [2.2] satisfies $\Omega(p^k) = k\Omega(p)$ for any prime p and has quite dissimilar asymptotics.

[1] K. Ireland and M. Rosen, *A Classical Introduction to Modern Number Theory*, 2nd ed., Springer-Verlag, 1990, pp. 50–65; MR 92e:11001.
[2] A. Granville and K. Soundararajan, Motivating the multiplicative spectrum, *Topics in Number Theory*, Proc. 1997 Penn. State Univ. conf., ed. S. D. Ahlgren, G. E. Andrews, and K. Ono, Kluwer, 1999, pp. 1–15; math.NT/9909190; MR 2000m:11088.
[3] A. Granville and K. Soundararajan, The spectrum of multiplicative functions, *Annals of Math.* 153 (2001) 407–470; MR 2002g:11127.
[4] R. R. Hall, Proof of a conjecture of Heath-Brown concerning quadratic residues, *Proc. Edinburgh Math. Soc.* 39 (1996) 581–588; MR 97m:11119.
[5] E. Wirsing, Das asymptotische Verhalten von Summen über multiplikative Funktionen. II, *Acta Math. Acad. Sci. Hungar.* 18 (1967) 411–467; MR 36 #6366.
[6] G. Halász, Über die Mittelwerte multiplikativer zahlentheoretischer Funktionen, *Acta Math. Acad. Sci. Hungar.* 19 (1968) 365–403; MR 37 #6254.
[7] A. Hildebrand, On Wirsing's mean value theorem for multiplicative functions, *Bull. London Math. Soc.* 18 (1986) 147–152; MR 87f:11075.
[8] P. D. T. A. Elliott, *Probabilistic Number Theory*. I: *Mean-Value Theorems*, Springer-Verlag, 1979, pp. 225–256; MR 82h:10002a.
[9] A. Granville and K. Soundararajan, Decay of mean-values of multiplicative functions, math.NT/9911246.
[10] R. A. Gillman and R. Tschiersch, The average size of a certain arithmetic function, *Amer. Math. Monthly* 100 (1993) 296–298; numerical calculation of C due to K. Ford.

3

Constants Associated with Analytic Inequalities

3.1 Shapiro–Drinfeld Constant

Consider the cyclic sum

$$f_n(x_1, x_2, \ldots, x_n) = \frac{x_1}{x_2 + x_3} + \frac{x_2}{x_3 + x_4} + \cdots + \frac{x_{n-1}}{x_n + x_1} + \frac{x_n}{x_1 + x_2},$$

where each x_j is nonnegative and each denominator is positive. Shapiro [1] asked if $f_n(x_1, x_2, \ldots, x_n) \geq n/2$ for all n. Lighthill [2] gave a counterexample for $n = 20$. Other counterexamples were subsequently discovered for $n = 14$ [3,4] and for $n = 25$ [5,6]. See [7–9] for a history of progress in understanding cyclic sums. We will only summarize: Shapiro's inequality is true for even $n \leq 12$ and odd $n \leq 23$ (using a computer-based proof [10]) and is false otherwise. This result has been analytically proved in the even case [11] but not yet for odd $13 \leq n \leq 23$.

It is interesting to examine the tools mathematicians used to unravel Shapiro's inequality early on. We look at just one. Let

$$f(n) = \inf_{x \geq 0} f_n(x_1, x_2, \ldots, x_n).$$

Rankin [12] studied the expression

$$\lambda = \lim_{n \to \infty} \frac{f(n)}{n} = \inf_{n \geq 1} \frac{f(n)}{n}$$

and proved that $\lambda < 0.49999993 < 1/2$. From this he deduced immediately that Shapiro's inequality is false for all sufficiently large n. Others took interest in the constant λ and attempted to calculate it to increasing accuracy [7]. Note that such efforts had no bearing on the truth of Shapiro's inequality for finite n. As is often the case, a tool for one person's use becomes the object of study for another.

Drinfeld [13] discovered a *geometric* interpretation of λ that also provides means for computing λ to arbitrary precision. Consider the two curves

$$y = \frac{1}{\exp(x)}, \quad y = \frac{2}{\exp(x) + \exp(x/2)}$$

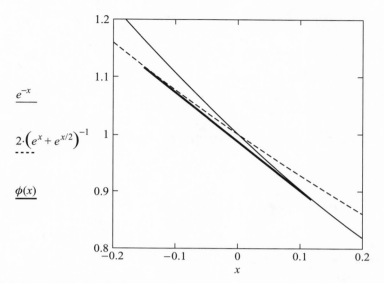

$\dfrac{e^{-x}}{\rule{1.2cm}{0.4pt}}$

$2\cdot\left(e^x+e^{x/2}\right)^{-1}$

$\underline{\phi(x)}$

Figure 3.1. In a neighborhood of $x = 0$, the graph of $y = \varphi(x)$ is a joint tangent to the other two curves.

in the xy-plane. Let $\varphi(x)$ be the convex support of these two functions. That is, $\varphi(x)$ is the largest concave up function not exceeding the others (see Figure 3.1). Then

$$\lambda = \frac{\varphi(0)}{2} = 0.4945668172\ldots = \frac{1}{2}(0.9891336344\ldots).$$

Many modifications of Shapiro's sum have been studied [7]. We mention only two. Consider first the cyclic sum

$$g_n(x_1, x_2, \ldots, x_n) = \frac{x_1 + x_3}{x_1 + x_2} + \frac{x_2 + x_4}{x_2 + x_3} + \cdots + \frac{x_{n-1} + x_1}{x_{n-1} + x_n} + \frac{x_n + x_2}{x_n + x_1}$$

under the same conditions for x_j. The inequality $g_n(x_1, x_2, \ldots, x_n) \geq n$ is, like Shapiro's inequality, false in general. Elbert [14] studied the expression

$$\mu = \lim_{n\to\infty} \frac{g(n)}{n}, \quad \text{where } g(n) = \inf_{x\geq 0} g_n(x_1, x_2, \ldots, x_n).$$

Using Drinfeld's method, he found that $\mu = \psi(0) = 0.9780124781\ldots$, where $y = \psi(x)$ is the convex support of the two functions

$$y = \frac{1 + \exp(x)}{2}, \quad y = \frac{1 + \exp(x)}{1 + \exp(x/2)}.$$

Recent computations of λ and μ include [15, 16]; generalizations are found in [17, 18]. Consider also the difference of cyclic sums $\Delta_n = f_n - h_n$, where f_n is as before and

$$h_n(x_1, x_2, \ldots, x_n) = \frac{x_1}{x_1 + x_2} + \frac{x_2}{x_2 + x_3} + \cdots + \frac{x_{n-1}}{x_{n-1} + x_n} + \frac{x_n}{x_n + x_1}.$$

Gauchman [19, 20] obtained that

$$\inf_{n \geq 1} \inf_{x \geq 0} \frac{\Delta_n(x_1, x_2, \ldots, x_n)}{n} = -0.0219875218\ldots,$$

and the corresponding two curves are

$$y = \frac{1 - \exp(x/2)}{\exp(x) + \exp(x/2)}, \quad y = \frac{\exp(-x) - 1}{2}.$$

We mention one other (non-cyclic) sum, due to Shallit [15, 21]:

$$s_n(x_1, x_2, \ldots, x_n) = \sum_{i=1}^{n} x_i + \sum_{1 \leq i \leq k \leq n} \prod_{j=i}^{k} \frac{1}{x_k},$$

which can be proved to satisfy

$$\lim_{n \to \infty} \inf_{x > 0} s_n(x_1, x_2, \ldots, x_n) - 3n = -1.3694514039\ldots$$

by numerical (non-geometric) means. Many variations of these sums f_n, Δ_n, and s_n suggest themselves.

3.1.1 Djokovic's Conjecture

Djokovic's conjecture, like Shapiro's, began as a *Monthly* problem and ultimately gave rise to an interesting constant. Assuming $x_1 < x_2 < \ldots < x_n$, define

$$P(x_1, x_2, \ldots, x_n) = \frac{1}{M} \int_{x_1}^{x_n} \left(\prod_{k=1}^{n} (t - x_k) \right) dt, \text{ where } M = \max_{x_1 \leq t \leq x_n} \left| \prod_{k=1}^{n} (t - x_k) \right|.$$

Djokovic [22] conjectured that $(-1)^{n+1-k}(\partial P/\partial x_k) > 0$ for each k. It is now known that this is not generally valid [23, 24], even for $n = 3$. Let $a_1 = 0.1824878875\ldots$ be the unique real zero of the cubic $12a^3 - 16a^2 + 8a - 1$ and $a_2 = 1 - a_1 = 0.8175121124\ldots$. Then Djokovic's inequality is true if $a_1(x_3 - x_1) < x_2 - x_1 < a_2(x_3 - x_1)$ and false otherwise. Similarly, for $n \geq 4$, the validity of the inequality depends on the distribution of the xs. If the xs are uniformly spaced, then for $n \leq 6$, the inequality is true, but for sufficiently large n, it is false.

[1] H. S. Shapiro, Problem 4603, *Amer. Math. Monthly* 61 (1954) 571.
[2] M. J. Lighthill, Note on problem 4603: An invalid inequality, *Amer. Math. Monthly* 63 (1956) 191–192; also *Math. Gazette* 40 (1956) 266.
[3] A. Zulauf, On a conjecture of L. J. Mordell, *Abh. Math. Sem. Univ. Hamburg* 22 (1958) 240–241; MR 23 #A1575.
[4] M. Herschorn and J. E. L. Peck, Partial solution of problem 4603: An invalid inequality, *Amer. Math. Monthly* 67 (1960) 87–88.
[5] D. E. Daykin, Inequalities for functions of a cyclic nature, *J. London Math. Soc.* 3 (1971) 453–462; MR 44 #1622a.
[6] M. A. Malcolm, A note on a conjecture of L. J. Mordell, *Math. Comp.* 25 (1971) 375–377; MR 44 #1622b.

[7] D. S. Mitrinovic, J. E. Pecaric, and A. M. Fink, *Classical and New Inequalities in Analysis*, Kluwer, 1993; MR 94c:00004.

[8] A. Clausing, A review of Shapiro's cyclic inequality, *General Inequalities 6*, Proc. 1990 Oberwolfach conf., ed. W. Walter, Birkhäuser, 1992, pp. 17–31; MR 94g:26030.

[9] P. J. Bushell, Shapiro's cyclic sum, *Bull. London Math. Soc.* 26 (1994) 564–574; MR 96f:26022.

[10] B. A. Troesch, The validity of Shapiro's cyclic inequality, *Math. Comp.* 53 (1989) 657–664; MR 90f:26025.

[11] P. J. Bushell and J. B. McLeod, Shapiro's cyclic inequality for even n, *J. Inequal. Appl.* 7 (2002) 331–348; Univ. of Sussex CMAIA report 2000–08.

[12] R. A. Rankin, An inequality, *Math. Gazette* 42 (1958) 39–40.

[13] V. G. Drinfeld, A certain cyclic inequality (in Russian), *Mat. Zametki* 9 (1971) 113–119; Engl. transl. in *Math. Notes Acad. Sci. USSR* 9 (1971) 68–71; MR 43 #6379.

[14] A. Elbert, On a cyclic inequality, *Period. Math. Hungar.* 4 (1973) 163–168; MR 50 #2424.

[15] A. MacLeod, Three constants, unpublished note (1996).

[16] D. Radcliffe, Calculating Shapiro's constant to 5000 digits, unpublished note (1999).

[17] E. K. Godunova and V. I. Levin, Exactness of a nontrivial estimate in a cyclic inequality (in Russian), *Mat. Zametki* 20 (1976) 203–205; Engl. transl. in *Math. Notes Acad. Sci. USSR* 20 (1976) 673–675; MR 54 #13007.

[18] E. K. Godunova and V. I. Levin, Lower bound for a cyclic sum (in Russian), *Mat. Zametki* 32 (1982) 3–7, 124; Engl. transl. in *Math. Notes Acad. Sci. USSR* 32 (1982) 481–483; MR 84c:26021.

[19] V. Cârtoaje, J. Dawson, and H. Volkmer, Solution of problem 10528a: Cyclic sum inequalities, *Amer. Math. Monthly* 105 (1998) 473–474.

[20] H. Gauchman, Solution of problem 10528b: Cyclic sum inequalities, unpublished note (1998).

[21] J. Shallit, C. C. Grosjean, and H. E. De Meyer, Solution of problem 94–15: A minimization problem, *SIAM Rev.* 37 (1995) 451–458.

[22] D. Z. Djokovic, The integral of a normalized polynomial with real roots, *Amer. Math. Monthly* 72 (1965) 794–795; 73 (1966) 788.

[23] G. C. Hu and J. K. Tang, The Djokovic's conjecture on an integral inequality, *J. Math. Res. Expos.* 10 (1990) 271–278; MR 91g:26024.

[24] D. S. Mitrinovic, J. E. Pecaric, and A. M. Fink, *Inequalities Involving Functions and Their Integrals and Derivatives*, Kluwer, 1991; MR 93m:26036.

3.2 Carlson–Levin Constants

Let f be a nonnegative real-valued function on $[0, \infty)$. We wish to determine bounds for the integral of $f(x)$, given the existence of the integrals of $x^a f(x)^p$ and $x^b f(x)^q$. In the special case $a = 0$, $b = 2$, $p = q = 2$, Carlson [1–3] determined that

$$\int_0^\infty f(x)dx \le \sqrt{\pi} \left(\int_0^\infty f(x)^2 dx \right)^{1/4} \left(\int_0^\infty x^2 f(x)^2 dx \right)^{1/4}$$

and that the constant $\sqrt{\pi}$ is the best possible. By "best possible" we mean that $\sqrt{\pi}$ is the smallest real coefficient for which the inequality is true. (If we attempt to sharpen the inequality by making the coefficient less than $\sqrt{\pi}$, then there is an admissible function f that will be a counterexample.)

For the general case, with $p > 1, q > 1, \lambda > 0$, and $\mu > 0$, Levin [2–4] discovered that

$$\int\limits_0^\infty f(x)dx \leq C \left(\int\limits_0^\infty x^{p-1-\lambda} f(x)^p dx \right)^s \left(\int\limits_0^\infty x^{q-1+\mu} f(x)^q dx \right)^t$$

and the best constant is

$$C = \frac{1}{(ps)^s} \frac{1}{(qt)^t} \left[\frac{\Gamma(\frac{s}{r})\Gamma(\frac{t}{r})}{(\lambda + \mu)\Gamma(\frac{s+t}{r})} \right]^r,$$

where

$$r = 1 - s - t, \quad s = \frac{\mu}{p\mu + q\lambda}, \quad t = \frac{\lambda}{p\mu + q\lambda},$$

and $\Gamma(x)$ is Euler's gamma function [1.5.4]. It is interesting that such a closed-form expression for the best constant even *exists*: Many inequalities cannot be evaluated so completely. See extensions in [5–8].

[1]   F. Carlson, Une inégalité, *Ark. Mat. Astron. Fysik*, v. 25B (1934) n. 1, 1–5.
[2]   E. F. Beckenbach and R. Bellman, *Inequalities*, Springer-Verlag, 1965; MR 33 #236.
[3]   D. S. Mitrinovic, J. E. Pecaric, and A. M. Fink, *Inequalities Involving Functions and Their Integrals and Derivatives*, Kluwer, 1991; MR 93m:26036.
[4]   V. I. Levin, Exact constants in inequalities of the Carlson type (in Russian), *Dokl. Akad. Nauk SSSR* 59 (1948) 635–638; MR 9,415b.
[5]   B. Kjellberg, Ein Momentenproblem, *Ark. Mat. Astron. Fysik*, v. 29A (1943) n. 2, 1–33; MR 6,203a.
[6]   B. Kjellberg, A note on an inequality, *Ark. Mat.* 3 (1956) 293–294; MR 17,950a.
[7]   V. I. Levin and S. B. Steckin, Inequalities, *Amer. Math. Soc. Transl.* 14 (1960) 1–29; MR 22 #3771.
[8]   V. I. Levin and E. K. Godunova, A generalization of Carlson's inequality (in Russian), *Mat. Sbornik* 67 (1965) 643–646; Engl. transl. in *Amer. Math. Soc. Transl.* 86 (1970) 133–136; MR 32 #5824.

3.3 Landau–Kolmogorov Constants

There is a vast literature on inequalities involving the norms of a function f and its derivatives $f^{(k)}$. We state just enough here to define certain constants $C(n, k)$ in four separate cases. The constants correspond to the inequality (to be explained in each case)

$$\|f^{(k)}\| \leq C(n, k)\|f\|^{1-\frac{k}{n}}\|f^{(n)}\|^{\frac{k}{n}}, \quad 1 \leq k < n,$$

which is henceforth called "inequality I."

3.3.1 $L_\infty(0, \infty)$ Case

Let $\|f\|$ here denote the supremum of $|f(x)|$, where the real-valued function f is defined on $(0, \infty)$. Landau [1] proved that if f is twice-differentiable and both f and

f'' are bounded, then

$$\|f'\| \le 2\|f\|^{\frac{1}{2}}\|f''\|^{\frac{1}{2}}$$

and the constant 2 is the best possible. By this, we mean that replacing 2 by $2 - \varepsilon$ for any positive number ε would necessarily lead to a counterexample f.

Schoenberg & Cavaretta [2, 3] extended this inequality to a setting where the nth derivative of f exists and both f and $f^{(n)}$ are bounded. They determined best constants $C(n, k)$, $1 \le k < n$, for inequality I and characterized $C(n, k)$ in terms of norms of Euler splines. For example,

$$C(3, 1) = \left(\tfrac{243}{8}\right)^{\frac{1}{3}} = 4.35622\ldots, \quad C(3, 2) = 24^{\frac{1}{3}} = 2.88449\ldots,$$
$$C(4, 1) = 4.288\ldots, \qquad\qquad C(4, 2) = 5.750\ldots, \qquad\qquad C(4, 3) = 3.708\ldots.$$

An explicit formula for all n and k is not available [4, 5].

3.3.2 $L_\infty(-\infty, \infty)$ *Case*

Let $\|f\|$ here denote the supremum of $|f(x)|$, where the real-valued function f is defined on $(-\infty, \infty)$. Hadamard [6] proved that if f is twice-differentiable and both f and f'' are bounded, then

$$\|f'\| \le \sqrt{2}\|f\|^{\frac{1}{2}}\|f''\|^{\frac{1}{2}}$$

and the constant $\sqrt{2}$ is the best possible.

Kolmogorov [7] determined best constants $C(n, k)$, $1 \le k < n$, for inequality I in terms of Favard constants [4.3]:

$$C(n, k) = a_{n-k}a_n^{-1+\frac{k}{n}}, \quad \text{where } a_n = \frac{4}{\pi}\sum_{j=0}^{\infty}\left[\frac{(-1)^j}{2j+1}\right]^{n+1}.$$

These formulas include special cases discovered by Shilov [8]:

$$C(3, 1) = \left(\tfrac{9}{8}\right)^{\frac{1}{3}}, \qquad C(3, 2) = 3^{\frac{1}{3}},$$
$$C(4, 1) = \left(\tfrac{512}{375}\right)^{\frac{1}{4}}, \qquad C(4, 2) = \left(\tfrac{6}{5}\right)^{\frac{1}{2}}, \quad C(4, 3) = \left(\tfrac{24}{5}\right)^{\frac{1}{4}},$$
$$C(5, 1) = \left(\tfrac{1953125}{1572864}\right)^{\frac{1}{5}}, \quad C(5, 2) = \left(\tfrac{125}{72}\right)^{\frac{1}{5}}.$$

Observe that this case, involving functions on the whole line, is easier than the previous case involving functions on the half line [4, 5].

3.3.3 $L_2(-\infty, \infty)$ *Case*

Given a real-valued function f defined on $(-\infty, \infty)$, define

$$\|f\| = \left(\int_{-\infty}^{\infty} f(x)^2 dx\right)^{\frac{1}{2}}.$$

Hardy, Littlewood & Pólya [9] proved, assuming the nth derivative of f exists and both f and $f^{(n)}$ are square-integrable, that $C(n, k) = 1$ is the best possible for $1 \leq k < n$.

3.3.4 $L_2(0, \infty)$ Case

As before, the half-line case is more difficult than the corresponding whole-line case. Given a real-valued function f defined on $(0, \infty)$, define

$$||f|| = \left(\int_0^\infty f(x)^2 dx \right)^{\frac{1}{2}}.$$

Hardy & Littlewood [9] proved, assuming f is twice-differentiable and both f and f'' are square-integrable, that

$$||f'|| \leq \sqrt{2} ||f||^{\frac{1}{2}} ||f''||^{\frac{1}{2}}$$

and the constant $\sqrt{2}$ is the best possible.

Ljubic [10] and Kupcov [11] extended this inequality to I and gave a remarkable algorithm for finding best constants $C(n, k)$ in terms of zeros of certain explicit polynomials. For example [12, 13],

$$C(3, 1) = C(3, 2) = 3^{\frac{1}{2}} \left[2 \left(2^{\frac{1}{2}} - 1 \right) \right]^{-\frac{1}{3}} = 1.84420\ldots,$$

$$C(4, 1) = C(4, 3) = \left[\frac{1}{a} \left(3^{\frac{1}{4}} + 3^{-\frac{3}{4}} \right) \right]^{\frac{1}{2}} = 2.27432\ldots,$$

$$C(4, 2) = \left(\frac{2}{b} \right)^{\frac{1}{2}} = 2.97963\ldots,$$

where a is the least positive root of $x^8 - 6x^4 - 8x^2 + 1 = 0$ and b is the least positive root of $x^4 - 2x^2 - 4x + 1 = 0$, and

$$C(5, 1) = C(5, 4) = 2.70247\ldots, \quad C(5, 2) = C(5, 3) = 4.37800\ldots.$$

In the special case $k = 1$, it can also be shown that

$$C(n, 1) = \left[\frac{(n-1)^{\frac{1}{n}} + (n-1)^{-1+\frac{1}{n}}}{c} \right]^{\frac{1}{2}},$$

where c is the least positive root of

$$\int_0^c \int_0^\infty \frac{1}{(x^{2n} - yx^2 + 1)\sqrt{y}} dx dy = \frac{\pi^2}{2n}.$$

A similar formula for $k > 1$ is not known. A consequence of Ljubic and Kupcov's work is that all $C(n, k)$ for this case must be algebraic numbers. This assertion appears to be true for the $L_\infty(0, \infty)$ case as well.

Among the topics we have omitted are:

- best constants associated with the $L_p(0, \infty)$ and $L_p(-\infty, \infty)$ norms, where $p \neq 2$ and $p \neq \infty$, or the same over a finite interval [14, 15];
- best constants in the discrete case, specifically, those associated with one-way and two-way infinite real sequences with the l_p norm and where derivatives are replaced by differences [16, 17].

It turns out that $p = 1, 2, \infty$ are the only cases for which best constants have exact formulas. For all other values of p, numerical approximation is evidently required.

Here is an unsolved problem, which concerns a slight variant of $L_2(0, \infty)$. Assuming f to be twice-differentiable and both f and f'' to be square-integrable with respect to a weighting function $w(x) = x$, Everitt & Guinand [5, 18] proved that

$$\left(\int\limits_0^\infty x f'(x)^2 dx \right)^2 \leq K \cdot \int\limits_0^\infty x f(x)^2 dx \cdot \int\limits_0^\infty x f''(x)^2 dx,$$

where the best possible constant satisfies $2.35070 < K < 2.35075$. An exact expression for K remains undiscovered.

[1] E. Landau, Einige Ungleichungen für zweimal differenzierbare Funktionen, *Proc. London Math. Soc.* 13 (1914) 43–49.

[2] I. J. Schoenberg, The elementary cases of Landau's problem of inequalities between derivatives, *Amer. Math. Monthly* 80 (1973) 121–158; MR 47 #3619.

[3] I. J. Schoenberg and A. Cavaretta, *Solution of Landau's Problem Concerning Higher Derivatives on the Halfline*, MRC TSR 1050 (1970), Univ. of Wisconsin; available through the National Technical Information Service, Springfield VA 22161; MR 51 #5868.

[4] M. K. Kwong and A. Zettl, *Norm Inequalities for Derivatives and Differences*, Lect. Notes in Math 1536, Springer-Verlag, 1992; MR 94f:26011.

[5] D. S. Mitrinovic, J. E. Pecaric, and A. M. Fink, *Inequalities Involving Functions and Their Integrals and Derivatives*, Kluwer, 1991; MR 93m:26036.

[6] J. Hadamard, Sur le module maximum d'une fonctioin et de ses dérivées, *Bull. Soc. Math. de France* 42 (1914) *C. R. Séances*, pp. 68–72; also in *Oeuvres*, t. 1, Centre Nat. Recherche Sci., 1968, pp. 379–382.

[7] A. N. Kolmogorov, On inequalities between upper bounds of consecutive derivatives of an arbitrary function defined on an infinite interval (in Russian), *Uchenye Zapiski Moskov. Gos. Univ. Matematika* 30 (1939) 3–16; Engl. transl. in *Amer. Math. Soc. Transl.* 2 (1962) 233–242; also in *Selected Works*, v. 1., ed. V. M. Tikhomirov, Kluwer, 1991, pp. 277–290; MR 1,298c.

[8] G. E. Shilov, On inequalities between derivatives (in Russian), *Sbornik Rabot Studencheskikh Nauchnykh Kruzhov Moskovskogo Gosudarstvennogo Universiteta* (1937) 17–27.

[9] G. H. Hardy, J. E. Littlewood, and G. Pólya, *Inequalities*, Cambridge Univ. Press, 1934; MR 89d:26016.

[10] J. I. Ljubic, On inequalities between the powers of a linear operator (in Russian), *Izv. Akad. Nauk SSSR Ser. Mat.* 24 (1960) 825–864; Engl. transl. in *Amer. Math. Soc. Transl.* 40 (1964) 39–84; MR 24 #A436.

[11] N. P. Kupcov, Kolmogorov estimates for derivatives in $L_2(0, \infty)$ (in Russian), *Trudy Mat. Inst. Steklov.* 138 (1975) 94–117, 199; Engl. transl. in *Proc. Steklov Inst. Math.* 138 (1975) 101–125; MR 52 #14198.

[12] B. Neta, On determination of best possible constants in integral inequalities involving derivatives, *Math. Comp.* 35 (1980) 1191–1193; MR 81m:26014.

[13] Z. M. Franco, H. G. Kaper, M. K. Kwong, and A. Zettl, Best constants in norm inequalities for derivatives on a half line, *Proc. Royal Soc. Edinburgh* 100A (1985) 67–84; MR 87a:47050.

[14] Z. M. Franco, H. G. Kaper, M. K. Kwong, and A. Zettl, Bounds for the best constant in Landau's inequality on the line, *Proc. Royal Soc. Edinburgh* 95A (1983) 257–262; MR 85m:26018.

[15] B.-O. Eriksson, Some best constants in the Landau inequality on a finite interval, *J. Approx. Theory* 94 (1998) 420–454; MR 99f:41013.

[16] Z. Ditzian, Discrete and shift Kolmogorov type inequalities, *Proc. Royal Soc. Edinburgh* 93A (1983) 307–317; MR 84m:47038.

[17] H. Kaper and B. E. Spellman, Best constants in norm inequalities for the difference operator, *Trans. Amer. Math. Soc.* 299 (1987) 351–372; MR 88d:39012.

[18] W. N. Everitt and A. P. Guinand, On a Hardy-Littlewood type integral inequality with a monotonic weight function, *General Inequalities 5*, Proc. 1986 Oberwolfach conf., ed. W. Walter, Birkhäuser, 1987, pp. 29–63; MR 91g:26023.

3.4 Hilbert's Constants

Let $p > 1$ and $q = p/(p-1)$. If $\{a_n\}, \{b_n\}$ are nonnegative sequences and $f(x), g(x)$ are nonnegative integrable functions, then Hilbert's inequality [1–3] for series is

$$\sum_{m=1}^{\infty} \sum_{n=1}^{\infty} \frac{a_m b_n}{m+n} < \pi \csc\left(\frac{\pi}{p}\right) \left(\sum_{m=1}^{\infty} a_m^p\right)^{\frac{1}{p}} \left(\sum_{n=1}^{\infty} b_n^q\right)^{\frac{1}{q}},$$

unless all a_n are zero or all b_n are zero, and Hilbert's inequality for integrals is

$$\int_0^{\infty} \int_0^{\infty} \frac{f(x)g(y)}{x+y} dx dy < \pi \csc\left(\frac{\pi}{p}\right) \left(\int_0^{\infty} f(x)^p dx\right)^{\frac{1}{p}} \left(\int_0^{\infty} g(y)^q dy\right)^{\frac{1}{q}},$$

unless f is identically zero or g is identically zero. The constant $\pi \csc(\pi/p)$ is the best possible in the sense that, if one replaces it by a smaller constant, then there exist counterexamples.

We are concerned with the following two-parameter extension of Hilbert's inequality. Let $p > 1, q > 1$ and

$$\tfrac{1}{p} + \tfrac{1}{q} \geq 1, \quad \text{so that } 0 < \lambda = 2 - \tfrac{1}{p} - \tfrac{1}{q} \leq 1.$$

Levin [4], Steckin [5], and Bonsall [6] showed that

$$\sum_{m=1}^{\infty} \sum_{n=1}^{\infty} \frac{a_m b_n}{(m+n)^\lambda} \leq \left[\pi \csc\left(\frac{\pi(q-1)}{\lambda q}\right)\right]^\lambda \left(\sum_{m=1}^{\infty} a_m^p\right)^{\frac{1}{p}} \left(\sum_{n=1}^{\infty} b_n^q\right)^{\frac{1}{q}},$$

$$\int_0^{\infty} \int_0^{\infty} \frac{f(x)g(y)}{(x+y)^\lambda} dx dy \leq \left[\pi \csc\left(\frac{\pi(q-1)}{\lambda q}\right)\right]^\lambda \left(\int_0^{\infty} f(x)^p dx\right)^{\frac{1}{p}} \left(\int_0^{\infty} g(y)^q dy\right)^{\frac{1}{q}},$$

but it is not known whether the indicated constant is the best possible.

There appears to be some confusion on the last point. Boas [7] indicated in 1949 that Steckin had proved the constant is the best possible in the discrete case; in 1950 Boas corrected himself and wrote that the bound is *not* exact. Mitrinovic, Pecaric & Fink [1] wrote that Steckin had established the constant to be the best possible. However, both Levin & Steckin [8] and Walker [9] wrote that the problem is still open.

As far as is known, no one has calculated the best constant even for the case $\lambda = 1/2$ and $p = q = 4/3$. Is a computation possible analogous to that discussed with the Copson–de Bruijn constant [3.5]?

[1] D. S. Mitrinovic, J. E. Pecaric, and A. M. Fink, *Inequalities Involving Functions and Their Integrals and Derivatives*, Kluwer, 1991; MR 93m:26036.
[2] G. H. Hardy, J. E. Littlewood, and G. Pólya, *Inequalities*, Cambridge Univ. Press, 1934; MR 89d:26016.
[3] K. Oleszkiewicz, An elementary proof of Hilbert's inequality, *Amer. Math. Monthly* 100 (1993) 276–280; MR 94a:51032.
[4] V. I. Levin, On the two-parameter extension and analogue of Hilbert's inequality, *J. London Math. Soc.* 11 (1936) 119–124.
[5] S. B. Steckin, On positive bilinear forms (in Russian), *Dokl. Akad. Nauk SSSR* 65 (1949) 17–20; MR 10,515e and MR 11,870 errata/addenda.
[6] F. F. Bonsall, Inequalities with non-conjugate parameters, *Quart. J. Math.* 2 (1951) 135–150; MR 12,807e.
[7] R. P. Boas, Review of "On positive bilinear forms," MR 10,515e, errata in MR 11,870.
[8] V. I. Levin and S. B. Steckin, Inequalities, *Amer. Math. Soc. Transl.* 14 (1960) 1–29; MR 22 #3771.
[9] P. L. Walker, A note on an inequality with non-conjugate parameters, *Proc. Edinburgh Math. Soc.* 18 (1973) 293–294; MR 48 #8723.

3.5 Copson–de Bruijn Constant

The interplay between series and integrals is sometimes very natural, but sometimes not. Let $\{a_n\}$ be a nonnegative sequence and $f(x)$ a nonnegative integrable function. Define

$$A_n = \sum_{k=1}^{n} a_k, \qquad B_n = \sum_{k=n}^{\infty} a_k,$$

$$F(x) = \int_0^x f(t)dt, \quad G(x) = \int_x^{\infty} f(t)dt.$$

Assume throughout that all infinite series and improper integrals under consideration are convergent and finite. We will examine two examples, the first for which all is as expected and the second for which all is not. Given $p > 1$, Hardy's inequality [1] is of the form

$$\sum_{n=1}^{\infty} \left(\frac{A_n}{n} \right)^p < \left(\frac{p}{p-1} \right)^p \sum_{n=1}^{\infty} a_n^p,$$

which always holds unless all a_n are zero. The corresponding theorem for integrals is

$$\int\limits_0^\infty \left(\frac{F(x)}{x}\right)^p dx < \left(\frac{p}{p-1}\right)^p \int\limits_0^\infty f(x)^p dx,$$

which always holds unless f is identically zero. The constant $(p/(p-1))^p$ is the best possible in the sense that, if one replaces it by a smaller constant, then there exist $\{a_n\}$ and $f(x)$ that are counterexamples.

Given $0 < p < 1$, one of Copson's integral inequalities [2,3] is of the form

$$\int\limits_0^\infty \left(\frac{G(x)}{x}\right)^p dx > \left(\frac{p}{1-p}\right)^p \int\limits_0^\infty f(x)^p dx,$$

unless f is identically zero. The corresponding theorem for series, curiously, is

$$\left(1 + \frac{1}{p-1}\right)\left(\frac{B_1}{1}\right)^p + \sum_{n=2}^\infty \left(\frac{B_n}{n}\right)^p > \left(\frac{p}{1-p}\right)^p \sum_{n=1}^\infty a_n^p,$$

unless all a_n are zero. The constant is the best possible, as found by Elliott. What is surprising is the correction term (or "gloss" as described in [2]) required to achieve the correspondence.

If one removes the correction term, the following inequality emerges [2,4]:

$$\sum_{n=1}^\infty \left(\frac{B_n}{n}\right)^p > p^p \sum_{n=1}^\infty a_n^p,$$

unless all a_n are zero. The constant p^p is, however, *not* the best possible. Hence by removing the "gloss" we have wrecked the precision of the inequality.

Levin & Steckin [5] proved, for $0 < p < 1/3$, that the best constant is $(p/(1-p))^p$, but they could not do likewise for $p > 1/3$.

Consider the special case when $p = 1/2$:

$$\sum_{n=1}^\infty \left(\frac{a_n + a_{n+1} + a_{n+2} + \cdots}{n}\right)^{\frac{1}{2}} \geq C \sum_{n=1}^\infty a_n^{\frac{1}{2}}$$

and rearrange the inequality by replacing a_n by a_n^2:

$$\sum_{n=1}^\infty a_n \leq c \sum_{n=1}^\infty \left(\frac{a_n^2 + a_{n+1}^2 + a_{n+2}^2 + \cdots}{n}\right)^{\frac{1}{2}}.$$

Steckin [6] proved that $c \leq 2/\sqrt{3}$ and Boas & de Bruijn [7] improved this to $1.08 < c < 17/15$. To estimate c more accurately, de Bruijn [8] defined a sequence of complex numbers via the recurrence

$$u_1 = x, \quad u_n = n^{-\frac{1}{2}}x + \left(u_{n-1}^2 - 1\right)^{\frac{1}{2}} \quad \text{for } n \geq 2.$$

It can be proved that $c = 1.1064957714\ldots$ is the smallest real number for which $x \geq c$ implies $u_n \geq 1$ (in particular, $\text{Im}(u_n) = 0$) for all $n \geq 1$. Further, if $x \geq c$, then

$$\lim_{n \to \infty} n^{-\frac{1}{2}} u_n = \begin{cases} x + \left(x^2 - 1\right)^{\frac{1}{2}} & \text{if } x > c, \\ c - \left(c^2 - 1\right)^{\frac{1}{2}} & \text{if } x = c. \end{cases}$$

Whether de Bruijn's procedure can be applied for other values of $p > 1/3$ is open.

[1] D. S. Mitrinovic, J. E. Pecaric, and A. M. Fink, *Inequalities Involving Functions and Their Integrals and Derivatives*, Kluwer, 1991; MR 93m:26036.

[2] G. H. Hardy, J. E. Littlewood, and G. Pólya, *Inequalities*, Cambridge Univ. Press, 1934, Thms. 337, 338, 345; MR 89d:26016.

[3] E. T. Copson, Some integral inequalities, *Proc. Royal Soc. Edinburgh* 75A (1975/76) 157–164, Thm. 4; MR 56 #559.

[4] E. T. Copson, Note on series of positive terms, *J. London Math. Soc.* 3 (1928) 49–51, Thm. 2.3.

[5] V. I. Levin and S. B. Steckin, Inequalities, *Amer. Math. Soc. Transl.* 14 (1960) 1–29; MR 22 #3771.

[6] S. B. Steckin, On absolute convergence of orthogonal series, I (in Russian), *Mat. Sbornik* 29 (1951) 225–232; MR 13,229g.

[7] R. P. Boas and N. G. de Bruijn, Solution for problem 83, *Wiskundige Opgaven met de Oplossingen* 20 (1957) 2–4.

[8] N. G. de Bruijn, *Asymptotic Methods in Analysis*, Dover, 1981; MR 83m:41028.

3.6 Sobolev Isoperimetric Constants

The area A enclosed by a simple closed curve C in the plane with perimeter P satisfies $4\pi A \leq P^2$, and equality holds if and only if C is a circle. We first generalize this **isoperimetric property** from two to n dimensions and then relate it to a certain **Sobolev inequality**.

Let Ω be the closure of a bounded, open, connected set in Euclidean space $\mathbb{R}^n$ with piecewise continuously differentiable boundary and surface area S. Let f be a continuously differentiable function defined on $\mathbb{R}^n$ with compact support, meaning that $f = 0$ identically outside of a ball, and let ∇f denote the gradient of f. Also define $\omega_n = \pi^{n/2} \Gamma(n/2 + 1)^{-1}$, the volume enclosed by the unit sphere in $\mathbb{R}^n$. The following two statements are equivalent [1–4]:

- The volume V of Ω satisfies $n^n \omega_n V^{n-1} \leq S^n$ with equality if and only if Ω is a ball.
- The $L_{n/(n-1)}$ norm of f is related to the L_1 norm of its gradient via

$$\left(\int_{\mathbb{R}^n} |f(x)|^{\frac{n}{n-1}} dx \right)^{\frac{n-1}{n}} \leq \frac{1}{n \omega_n^{1/n}} \int_{\mathbb{R}^n} |\nabla f(x)| dx$$

and the constant $n^{-1} \omega_n^{-1/n}$ is sharp.

The former is geometric in nature, whereas the latter falls within functional analysis. As a consequence, there is an extended interpretation of the phrase "isoperimetric problem" to encompass Sobolev inequalities and hence eigenvalues of differential equations with boundary conditions. We cannot even hope to summarize such a massive field [5–7] but attempt only to introduce a few constants.

Several authors [8,9] have commented that Sobolev inequalities act as uncertainty principles: The size of the gradient of a function f is bounded from below in terms of the size of f. Note that the constants ω_n are interesting in themselves; for example, $\lim_{n\to\infty} n^{1/2}\omega_n^{1/n} = \sqrt{2\pi e} = 4.1327313541\ldots$ by Stirling's formula. We turn to four sample exercises from physics.

3.6.1 String Inequality

If smooth functions f are constrained to satisfy $f(0) = f(1) = 0$, then

$$\int_0^1 f(x)^2 dx \leq \frac{1}{\pi^2} \int_0^1 \left(\frac{df}{dx}\right)^2 dx$$

and the constant $1/\pi^2 = 0.1013211836\ldots$ is the best possible [10]. This corresponds, via the calculus of variations, to the fact that the smallest eigenvalue of the ordinary differential equation (ODE)

$$\frac{d^2g}{dx^2} + \lambda g(x) = 0, \quad g(0) = g(\pi) = 0,$$

is $\lambda = 1$. This ODE, in turn, arises from the study of a vibrating, homogeneous string that is pulled taut on the x-axis and is fastened at the endpoints [11,12]. The value $\lambda = 1$ has the physical interpretation as the principal frequency of the sound one hears when the string is plucked.

A generalization of this is due to Talenti [3]:

$$\left(\int_0^1 |f(x)|^q dx\right)^{\frac{1}{q}} \leq \frac{q}{2}\left(1 + \frac{r}{q}\right)^{\frac{1}{p}}\left(1 + \frac{q}{r}\right)^{-\frac{1}{q}} \frac{\Gamma(\frac{1}{q} + \frac{1}{r})}{\Gamma(\frac{1}{q})\Gamma(\frac{1}{r})} \left(\int_0^1 \left|\frac{df}{dx}\right|^p dx\right)^{\frac{1}{p}},$$

where $f(0) = f(1) = 0$, $p > 1$, $q \geq 1$, and $r = p/(p-1)$. The indicated constant is sharp.

3.6.2 Rod Inequality

A second-order version of the "string inequality" follows. If suitably smooth f are constrained to satisfy

$$f(0) = \frac{df}{dx}(0) = f(1) = \frac{df}{dx}(1) = 0,$$

then

$$\int_0^1 f(x)^2 dx \leq \mu \int_0^1 \left(\frac{d^2f}{dx^2}\right)^2 dx,$$

where $\mu = 1/\theta^4 = 0.0019977469\ldots$ and $\theta = 4.7300407448\ldots$ is the smallest positive root of the equation

$$\cos(\theta)\cosh(\theta) = 1.$$

Moreover, the constant μ is the best possible [12–14]. This corresponds to the fact that the smallest eigenvalue of the ODE

$$\frac{d^4g}{dx^4} - \lambda g(x) = 0, \quad g(0) = \frac{dg}{dx}(0) = g(\pi) = \frac{dg}{dx}(\pi) = 0,$$

is $\lambda = \theta^4/\pi^4 = 5.1387801326\ldots$. This ODE, in turn, arises from the study of a vibrating, homogeneous rod or bar that is clamped at the endpoints.

3.6.3 Membrane Inequality

A two-dimensional version of the "string inequality" follows. If smooth f are constrained to vanish on the boundary C of the unit disk D, then

$$\int_D f^2 dx dy \leq \mu \int_D \left[\left(\frac{\partial f}{\partial x}\right)^2 + \left(\frac{\partial f}{\partial y}\right)^2 \right] dx\, dy,$$

where $\mu = 1/\theta^2 = 0.1729150690\ldots$ and $\theta = 2.4048255576\ldots$ is the smallest positive zero of the zeroth Bessel function

$$J_0(z) = \sum_{j=0}^{\infty} \frac{(-1)^j}{(j!)^2} \left(\frac{z}{2}\right)^{2j}.$$

Moreover, the constant μ is the best possible [11, 12, 15]. This corresponds to the fact that the smallest eigenvalue of the ODE

$$r^2 \frac{d^2g}{dr^2} + r\frac{dg}{dr} + \lambda r^2 g(r) = 0, \quad g(0) = 1, \quad g(1) = 0,$$

is $\lambda = \theta^2 = 5.7831859629\ldots$. This ODE, in turn, arises from the study of a vibrating, homogeneous membrane that is uniformly stretched across D and fastened at the boundary C. The value $\lambda = \theta^2$ is the principal frequency of the sound one hears when a kettledrum is struck.

Consider the Laplace partial differential equation (PDE)

$$\frac{\partial^2 u}{\partial x^2} + \frac{\partial^2 u}{\partial y^2} + \Lambda u = 0$$

for a vibrating membrane on an arbitrary region D of fixed area A with $u = 0$ on the boundary C. Rayleigh [16, 17] conjectured in 1877 that the first eigenvalue Λ is least when C is a circle. This conjecture was proved independently in 1923 by Faber [18] and Krahn [19]: $\Lambda \geq (\pi/A)\theta^2$ with equality if and only if C is a circle. Interestingly, the same is *not* true for the second eigenvalue: The critical boundary is not a circle, but a figure-eight [20–22].

3.6.4 Plate Inequality

A two-dimensional, second-order version of the "string inequality" follows. Assume that suitably smooth f and its outward normal derivative $\partial f / \partial n$ are both constrained to vanish on the boundary C of the unit disk D. Then

$$\int_D f^2 dxdy \le \mu \int_D \left(\frac{\partial^2 f}{\partial x^2} + \frac{\partial^2 f}{\partial y^2} \right)^2 dx\,dy$$

where $\mu = 1/\theta^4 = 0.0095819302\ldots$, $\theta = 3.1962206165\ldots$ is the smallest positive root of the equation

$$J_0(\theta)I_1(\theta) + I_0(\theta)J_1(\theta) = 0,$$

and $I_0(z)$ is the zeroth modified Bessel function

$$I_0(z) = \sum_{j=0}^{\infty} \frac{1}{(j!)^2} \left(\frac{z}{2} \right)^{2j}, \quad I_1(z) = \frac{dI_0}{dz}, \quad J_1(z) = -\frac{dJ_0}{dz}.$$

Moreover, the constant μ is the best possible [12, 14–16, 23]. This is associated with the study of a vibrating, homogeneous plate clamped at the boundary C.

As with the membrane case, we state a related isoperimetric inequality. Consider the PDE

$$\frac{\partial^2}{\partial x^2} \left(\frac{\partial^2 u}{\partial x^2} + \frac{\partial^2 u}{\partial y^2} \right) + \frac{\partial^2}{\partial y^2} \left(\frac{\partial^2 u}{\partial x^2} + \frac{\partial^2 u}{\partial y^2} \right) - \Lambda u = 0$$

for a vibrating plate on an arbitrary region of fixed area A with $u = \partial u / \partial n = 0$ on the boundary. Rayleigh [16] conjectured that $\Lambda \ge (\pi^2 / A^2)\theta^4$ and Szegö [24–26] proved this to be true under a special hypothesis. The general conjecture was proved only recently [27, 28].

3.6.5 Other Variations

Let $||f||$ denote the supremum of $|f(x, y)|$, where the function f is defined on all of $\mathbb{R}^2$ and is twice continuously differentiable. Then $||f||$ is related to the integral of the sum of squares of all partial derivatives of f via

$$||f|| \le \alpha_{2,2} \left[\int_{\mathbb{R}^2} \left(f^2 + f_x^2 + f_y^2 + f_{xx}^2 + f_{xy}^2 + f_{yy}^2 \right) dxdy \right]^{\frac{1}{2}},$$

where the best constant $\alpha_{2,2} = 0.3187590609\ldots$ is given by [29]

$$\alpha_{2,2} = \left(\frac{1}{\pi^2} \int_0^{\infty} \int_0^{\infty} \frac{dxdy}{1 + x^2 + y^2 + x^4 + x^2y^2 + y^4} \right)^{\frac{1}{2}} = \left(\frac{1}{2\pi} \int_1^{\infty} \frac{dt}{\sqrt{t^2 + 2\sqrt{t^2 + 3}}} \right)^{\frac{1}{2}}.$$

Such formulation is naturally extended to m-times continuously differentiable functions f defined on all of $\mathbb{R}^n$, with corresponding constant $\alpha_{m,n}$. For example,

$$\alpha_{1,1} = \left(\frac{1}{\pi} \int\limits_0^\infty \frac{dx}{1+x^2} \right)^{\frac{1}{2}} = \frac{\sqrt{2}}{2}, \quad \alpha_{2,3} = 0.231522\ldots, \quad \alpha_{3,3} = 0.142892\ldots.$$

If instead f is defined only on the unit cube in $\mathbb{R}^n$, then among the associated constants $\tilde{\alpha}_{m,n}$, we have [30–32]

$$\tilde{\alpha}_{1,1} = \tanh(1)^{-\frac{1}{2}} = 1.1458775176\ldots, \quad \tilde{\alpha}_{2,2} = 1.24796\ldots.$$

In fact, for arbitrary $m \geq 1$,

$$\alpha_{m,1} = \left[\frac{1}{m+1} \frac{\cos(\frac{\pi}{2m+2})}{\sin(\frac{3\pi}{2m+2})} \right]^{\frac{1}{2}}, \quad \tilde{\alpha}_{m,1} = \left[\frac{2}{m+1} \sum_{k=1}^m \frac{\sin(\frac{\pi k}{m+1})^3}{\tanh(\sin(\frac{\pi k}{m+1}))} \right]^{\frac{1}{2}}.$$

These inequalities are useful in the study of the finite element method in numerical analysis.

A related idea is Friedrichs' inequality [33], which involves continuously differentiable functions f on the closed interval $[0, 1] \subseteq \mathbb{R}$:

$$\left[\int\limits_0^1 \left(f(x)^2 + f'(x)^2 \right) dx \right]^{\frac{1}{2}} \leq \beta \left[f(0)^2 + f(1)^2 + \int\limits_0^1 f'(x)^2 dx \right]^{\frac{1}{2}}.$$

The best constant $\beta = 1.0786902162\ldots$ satisfies $\beta = \sqrt{1 + \theta^{-2}}$, where $\theta = 2.4725480752\ldots$ is the unique solution of the equation

$$\cos(\theta) - \theta(\theta^2 + 1)^{-1} \sin(\theta) = -1, \quad 0 < \theta < \pi.$$

Many more examples are possible [34–45].

Let us return to geometry for one more problem. Consider a simple closed curve C in $\mathbb{R}^3$ with perimeter P. Let V denote the volume of its convex hull, that is, the intersection of all convex sets in $\mathbb{R}^3$ containing C. Then $V \leq \gamma_3 P^3$ and the best constant is $\gamma_3 = 0.0031816877\ldots$ (obtained in [46, 47] via numerical solution of a system of ODEs). No closed-form expression for γ_3 is known. If the setting is changed from $\mathbb{R}^3$ to $\mathbb{R}^n$, where the integer n is even, then curiously the best constant [48] is exactly given by $\gamma_n = [(\pi n)^{n/2} n! (n/2)!]^{-1}$. The case for odd $n \geq 5$ remains open.

A deeper connection between Sobolev inequalities and isoperimetric properties within Riemannian manifolds ($\mathbb{R}^n$ being the simplest example) is beyond the scope of this book.

[1] H. Federer and W. H. Fleming, Normal and integral currents, *Annals of Math.* 72 (1960) 458–520; MR 23 #A588.
[2] V. G. Mazya, Classes of domains and imbedding theorems for function spaces (in Russian), *Dokl. Akad. Nauk SSSR* 133 (1960) 527–530; Engl. transl. in *Soviet Math. Dokl.* 1 (1960) 882–885; MR 23 #A3448.

[3] G. Talenti, Best constant in Sobolev inequality, *Annali Mat. Pura Appl.* 110 (1976) 353–372; MR 57 #3846.

[4] R. Osserman, The isoperimetric inequality, *Bull. Amer. Math. Soc.* 84 (1978) 1182–1238; MR 58 #18161.

[5] D. S. Mitrinovic, J. E. Pecaric, and A. M. Fink, *Inequalities Involving Functions and Their Integrals and Derivatives*, Kluwer, 1991; MR 93m:26036.

[6] Y. D. Burago and V. A. Zalgaller, *Geometric Inequalities*, Springer-Verlag, 1988; MR 89b:52020.

[7] P. R. Beesack, Integral inequalities involving a function and its derivative, *Amer. Math. Monthly* 78 (1971) 705–741; MR 48 #4235.

[8] E. F. Beckenbach and R. Bellman, *Inequalities*, 2nd ed., Springer-Verlag, 1965, pp. 177–188; MR 33 #236.

[9] E. H. Lieb and M. Loss, *Analysis*, Amer. Math. Soc., 1997, pp. 183–199; MR 98b:00004.

[10] G. H. Hardy, J. E. Littlewood, and G. Pólya, *Inequalities*, Cambridge Univ. Press, 1934; MR 89d:26016.

[11] G. F. Simmons, *Differential Equations with Applications and Historical Notes*, McGraw-Hill, 1972; MR 58 #17258.

[12] R. Courant and D. Hilbert, *Methods of Mathematical Physics*, v. 1, Interscience, 1953; MR 16,426a.

[13] N. Anderson, A. M. Arthurs, and R. R. Hall, Extremum principle for a nonlinear problem in magneto-elasticity, *Proc. Cambridge Philos. Soc.* 72 (1972) 315–318; MR 45 #7151.

[14] C. O. Horgan, A note on a class of integral inequalities, *Proc. Cambridge Philos. Soc.* 74 (1973) 127–131; MR 48 #9486.

[15] G. Pólya and G. Szegö, *Isoperimetric Inequalities in Mathematical Physics*, Princeton Univ. Press, 1951; MR 13,270d.

[16] J. W. S. Rayleigh, *The Theory of Sound*, v. 1, 2nd rev. ed., Dover, 1945.

[17] C. Bandle, *Isoperimetric Inequalities and Applications*, Pitman, 1980; MR 81e:35095.

[18] G. Faber, Beweis dass unter allen homogenen Membranen von gleicher Fläche und gleicher Spannung die kreisförmige den tiefsten Grundton gibt, *Sitzungsberichte Bayerische Akademie der Wissenschaften* (1923) 169–172.

[19] E. Krahn, Über eine von Rayleigh formulierte Minimaleigenschaft des Kreises, *Math. Annalen* 94 (1925) 97–100.

[20] E. Krahn, Über Minimaleigenschaften der Kugel in drei und mehr Dimensionen, *Acta et Commentationes Universitatis Tartuensis (Dorpatensis)* A9 (1926) 1–44; Engl. transl. in *Edgar Krahn 1894-1961: A Centenary Volume*, ed. U. Lumiste and J. Peetre, IOS Press, 1994, pp. 139–174.

[21] I. Hong, On an inequality concerning the eigenvalue problem of a membrane, *Kôdai Math. Sem. Rep.* (1954) 113–114; MR 16,1116b and MR 16,1337 errata/addenda.

[22] G. Pólya, On the characteristic frequencies of a symmetric membrane, *Math. Z.* 63 (1955) 331–337; also in *Collected Papers*, v. 3, ed. J. Hersch and G.-C. Rota, MIT Press, 1984, pp. 413–419, 519–521; MR 17,372e.

[23] P. M. Morse, *Vibration and Sound*, 2nd ed., McGraw-Hill, 1948.

[24] G. Szegö, On membranes and plates, *Proc. Nat. Acad. Sci. USA* 36 (1950) 210–216; 44 (1958) 314–316; also in *Collected Papers*, v. 3, ed. R. Askey, Birkhäuser, 1982, pp. 185–194 and 479–483; MR 11,757g and MR 20 #2924.

[25] L. E. Payne, Some comments on the past fifty years of isoperimetric inequalities, *Inequalities: Fifty Years on from Hardy, Littlewood and Pólya*, ed. W. N. Everitt, Dekker, 1991, pp. 143–161; MR 92f:26042.

[26] G. Talenti, On isoperimetric theorems of mathematical physics, *Handbook of Convex Geometry*, ed. P. M. Gruber and J. M. Wills, Elsevier, 1993, pp. 1131–1147; MR 94i:49002.

[27] N. S. Nadirashvili, Rayleigh's conjecture on the principal frequency of the clamped plate, *Arch. Rational Mech. Anal.* 129 (1995) 1–10; MR 97j:35113.

[28] M. S. Ashbaugh and R. D. Benguria, On Rayleigh's conjecture for the clamped plate and its generalization to three dimensions, *Duke Math. J.* 78 (1995) 1–17; MR 97j:35111.

[29] M. Hegland and J. T. Marti, Numerical computation of least constants for the Sobolev inequality, *Numer. Math.* 48 (1986) 607–616; MR 87k:65136.

[30] J. T. Marti, Evaluation of the least constant in Sobolev's inequality for $H^1(0, s)$, *SIAM J. Numer. Anal.* 20 (1983) 1239–1242; MR 85d:46044.

[31] W. Richardson, Steepest descent and the least C for Sobolev's inequality, *Bull. London Math. Soc.* 18 (1986) 478–484; MR 87i:46078.

[32] J. T. Marti, On the norm of the Sobolev imbedding of $H^2(G)$ into $C(G)$ for square domains in $\mathbb{R}^2$, *The Mathematics of Finite Elements and Applications* V (MAFELAP V), Proc. 1984 Uxbridge conf., ed. J. R. Whiteman, Academic Press, 1985, pp. 441–450; MR 87a:46055.

[33] J. T. Marti, The least constant in Friedrichs' inequality in one dimension, *SIAM J. Math. Anal.* 16 (1985) 148–150; MR 86e:46026.

[34] G. Rosen, Minimum value for c in the Sobolev inequality $||\varphi^3|| \le c||\nabla\varphi||^3$, *SIAM J. Appl. Math* 21 (1971) 30–32; MR 44 #6927.

[35] G. Rosen, Sobolev-type lower bounds on $||\nabla\psi||^2$ for arbitrary regions in two-dimensional Euclidean space, *Quart. Appl. Math.* 34 (1976/77) 200–202; MR 57 #12803.

[36] G. F. D. Duff, A general integral inequality for the derivative of an equimeasurable rearrangement, *Canad. J. Math.* 28 (1976) 793–804; MR 53 #13497.

[37] P. S. Crooke, An isoperimetric bound for a Sobolev constant, *Colloq. Math.* 38 (1978) 263–267; MR 58 #6115.

[38] E. J. M. Veling, Optimal lower bounds for the spectrum of a second order linear differential equation with a p-integrable coefficient, *Proc. Royal Soc. Edinburgh* 92A (1982) 95–101; MR 84h:34050.

[39] P. L. Lions, F. Pacella, and M. Tricarico, Best constants in Sobolev inequalities for functions vanishing on some part of the boundary and related questions, *Indiana Math. J.* 37 (1988) 301–324; MR 89i:46036.

[40] E. H. Lieb, Sharp constants in the Hardy-Littlewood-Sobolev and related inequalities, *Annals of Math.* 118 (1983) 349–374; MR 86i:42010.

[41] J. T. Marti, New upper and lower bounds for the eigenvalues of the Sturm-Liouville problem, *Computing* 42 (1989) 239–243; MR 90g:34028.

[42] C. O. Horgan, Eigenvalue estimates and the trace theorem, *J. Math. Anal. Appl.* 69 (1979) 231–242; MR 80f:49029.

[43] C. O. Horgan and L. E. Payne, Lower bounds for free membrane and related eigenvalues, *Rend. Mat. Appl.* 10 (1990) 457–491; MR 91h:35237.

[44] S. Waldron, Schmidt's inequality, *East J. Approx.* 3 (1997) 117–135; MR 98g:41013.

[45] A. A. Ilyin, Best constants in Sobolev inequalities on the sphere and in Euclidean space, *J. London Math. Soc.* 59 (1999) 263–286; MR 2000f:46043.

[46] Z. A. Melzak, The isoperimetric problem of the convex hull of a closed space curve, *Proc. Amer. Math. Soc.* 11 (1960) 265–274; MR 22 #7058.

[47] Z. A. Melzak, Numerical evaluation of an isoperimetric constant, *Math. Comp.* 22 (1968) 188–190; MR 36 #7023.

[48] I. J. Schoenberg, An isoperimetric inequality for closed curves convex in even-dimensional Euclidean spaces, *Acta Math.* 91 (1954) 143–164; MR 16,508b.

3.7 Korn Constants

Let $u(x)$ be a smooth vector field defined on the closure of a bounded, open, connected set Ω in n-dimensional space. Then $\nabla u(x)$ is the $n \times n$ matrix made up of partial derivatives of $u(x)$. By the norm $|M|$ of a matrix M, we mean the Euclidean norm of M, that is, the square root of the sum of squares of all entries. Let also M^{T} denote the transpose of M.

Consider the so-called **second case of Korn's inequality** [1–3]

$$\int_\Omega |\nabla u(x)|^2 dx \le K \int_\Omega \left| \frac{\nabla u(x) + \nabla u(x)^{\mathrm{T}}}{2} \right|^2 dx$$

with the side condition

$$\int_\Omega \left(\nabla u(x) - \nabla u(x)^{\mathrm{T}}\right) dx = 0.$$

The best constants $K(\Omega)$ for various domains Ω are important in linear elasticity theory and in incompressible fluid dynamics. If B_n is an n-dimensional ball [4,5], then $K(B_2) = 4$ and $K(B_3) = 56/13$. The corresponding values for $n \geq 4$ are not known. Let P_m denote a two-dimensional m-sided regular polygonal region. For a square P_4, it can be proved that [2]

$$5 \leq K(P_4) \leq 4(2 + \sqrt{2}),$$

and Horgan & Payne [6] conjectured that $K(P_4) = 7$. For an equilateral triangle P_3, we have

$$6 \leq K(P_3) \leq 8(2 + \sqrt{3})$$

using Laplacian eigenvalue formulas in [7–9]. For arbitrary m, we have the upper bound [2]

$$K(P_m) \leq \frac{4}{1 - \sin(\pi/m)},$$

and a lower bound for $K(P_6)$ is possible using eigenvalue numerical estimates in [9]. Korn constants for ellipses and limacons are given in [2, 10]; for circular rings and spherical shells, see [11, 12].

Here is a related problem (for $n = 2$ only). Let $z = x + iy$, where i is the imaginary unit, and let $f(x, y)$ and $g(x, y)$ denote the real and imaginary parts of an analytic function $w(z)$. In other words, $f(x, y)$ and $g(x, y)$ are **harmonic conjugates**. Consider Friedrichs' inequality [6, 10, 13–15]

$$\int_\Omega f(x, y)^2 dx dy \leq \Gamma \int_\Omega g(x, y)^2 dx dy$$

with the side condition

$$\int_\Omega f(x, y) dx dy = 0.$$

The best constants Γ for various simply-connected domains Ω are related to the Korn constants K by $K = 2(1 + \Gamma)$, assuming Ω has a continuously differentiable boundary. In the event Ω is a square region, Horgan & Payne [6] conjectured that the optimizing functions are

$$f(x, y) = 2xy, \quad g(x, y) = y^2 - x^2$$

and hence $\Gamma = 5/2$. This would lead immediately to $K = 7$ if it were not for the smoothness requirement.

Horgan's survey [2] is a valuable starting point for research. Related topics appear in [16, 17].

[1] C. O. Horgan, On Korn's inequalities for incompressible media, *SIAM J. Appl. Math.* 28 (1975) 419–430; MR 52 #2356.

[2] C. O. Horgan, Korn's inequalities and their applications in continuum mechanics, *SIAM Rev.* 37 (1995) 491–511; MR 96h:73014.

[3] A. Tiero, On Korn's inequality in the second case, *J. Elasticity* 54 (1999) 187–191; MR 2001j:35061.

[4] B. Bernstein and R. A. Toupin, Korn inequalities for the sphere and circle, *Arch. Rational Mech. Anal.* 6 (1960) 51–64; MR 23 #B1719.

[5] L. E. Payne and H. F. Weinberger, On Korn's inequality, *Arch. Rational Mech. Anal.* 8 (1961) 89–98; MR 28 #1537.

[6] C. O. Horgan and L. E. Payne, On inequalities of Korn, Friedrichs and Babuska-Aziz, *Arch. Rational Mech. Anal.* 82 (1983) 165–179; MR 84d:73014.

[7] M. A. Pinsky, The eigenvalues of an equilateral triangle, *SIAM J. Math. Anal.* 11 (1980) 819–827; 16 (1985) 848–851; MR 82d:35077 and MR 86k:35115.

[8] P. Sjoberg, An investigation of eigenfunctions over the equilateral triangle and square, unpublished note (1995).

[9] L. M. Cureton and J. R. Kuttler, Eigenvalues of the Laplacian on regular polygons and polygons resulting from their dissection, *J. Sound Vibration* 220 (1999) 83–98; MR 99j:35025.

[10] C. O. Horgan, Inequalities of Korn and Friedrichs in elasticity and potential theory, *Z. Angew Math. Phys.* 26 (1975) 155–164; MR 51 #2399.

[11] C. M. Dafermos, Some remarks on Korn's inequality, *Z. Angew. Math. Phys.* 19 (1968) 913–920; MR 39 #1154.

[12] E. Andreou, G. Dassios, and D. Polyzos, Korn's constant for a spherical shell, *Quart. Appl. Math.* 46 (1988) 583–591; MR 89j:73014.

[13] K. O. Friedrichs, On certain inequalities and characteristic value problems for analytic functions and for functions of two variables, *Trans. Amer. Math. Soc.* 41 (1937) 321–364.

[14] K. O. Friedrichs, On the boundary-value problems of the theory of elasticity and Korn's inequality, *Annals of Math.* 48 (1947) 441–471; MR 9,255b.

[15] W. Velte, On inequalities of Friedrichs and Babuska-Aziz, *Meccanica* 31 (1996) 589–596; MR 97k:73022.

[16] V. A. Kondrat'ev and O. A. Oleinik, Boundary value problems for a system in elasticity theory in unbounded domains: Korn's inequalities (in Russian), *Uspekhi Mat. Nauk*, v. 43 (1988) n. 5, 55–98, 239, Engl. transl. in *Russian Math. Surveys* 43 (1988) 65–119; MR 89m:35061.

[17] K. Bhattacharya, Korn's inequality for sequences, *Proc. Royal Soc. London A* 434 (1991) 479–484; MR 92i:73030.

3.8 Whitney–Mikhlin Extension Constants

Let $B_{n,r}$ denote the n-dimensional closed ball of radius r centered at the origin. Assume throughout that $r > 1$ is fixed. A function F defined on all of n-dimensional space is called an r-**extension** of a given function f defined on $B_{n,1}$ if $F(x) = f(x)$ for all $|x| \leq 1$ and $F(x) = 0$ for all $|x| \geq r$.

We are interested in procedures for building F, given f, and we want to do this in such a way as to "minimize waste." Here are two ways (among many) to interpret the phrase "minimize waste":

- To every continuous f, construct a continuous r-extension F such that

$$\max_{x \in B_{n,r}} |F(x)| \leq c \cdot \max_{x \in B_{n,1}} |f(x)|,$$

where c is a constant (independent of f) and is the smallest possible.

- To every continuously differentiable f, construct a continuously differentiable r-extension F such that

$$\left[\int_{B_{n,r}} \left(F(x)^2 + \sum_{k=1}^{n} \left(\frac{\partial F}{\partial x_k} \right)^2 \right) dx \right]^{\frac{1}{2}} \leq \chi \cdot \left[\int_{B_{n,1}} \left(f(x)^2 + \sum_{k=1}^{n} \left(\frac{\partial f}{\partial x_k} \right)^2 \right) dx \right]^{\frac{1}{2}},$$

where (again) χ is a constant and is the smallest possible.

Another way of phrasing this is as follows: Given two Banach spaces of functions defined on $B_{n,1}$ and $B_{n,r}$, determine the r-extension operator from one to the other of minimal norm. In the first case, the Banach space norm is the L_∞ or supremum norm; in the second, it is the Sobolev W_2^1 integral norm, which penalizes misbehaved derivatives as well.

Whitney [1] proved that $c = 1$ in the first case by a partition-of-unity argument. The calculus of variations provides that [2,3]

$$\chi = \sqrt{1 + \coth(1)\coth(r - 1)}$$

when $n = 1$ for the second case (note that this depends on r).

Mikhlin [4–6] determined best constants $\chi = \chi(n,r)$ when $n \geq 2$ for the second case. Earlier relevant work included Hestenes [7], Calderón [8], and Stein [9]. Define, for convenience, $\nu = (n - 2)/2$ and modified Bessel functions

$$I_\nu(r) = \left(\frac{r}{2} \right)^\nu \sum_{j=0}^{\infty} \frac{1}{j!\Gamma(\nu + j + 1)} \left(\frac{r}{2} \right)^{2j}, \quad K_\nu(r) = \frac{\pi}{2} \frac{I_{-\nu}(r) - I_\nu(r)}{\sin(\nu\pi)}.$$

See [4] for a table of numerical estimates of $\chi(n,r)$, based on algebraic formulas involving $I_\nu(r)$ and $K_\nu(r)$. Our interest is solely in the asymptotic values

$$\chi_n = \lim_{r \to \infty} \chi(n,r) = \sqrt{1 + \frac{I_\nu(1)}{I_{\nu+1}(1)} \frac{K_{\nu+1}(1)}{K_\nu(1)}},$$

and clearly

$$\chi_1 = \sqrt{\frac{2e^2}{e^2-1}}, \quad \chi_3 = e, \quad \chi_5 = \sqrt{\frac{e^2}{e^2-7}}, \quad \chi_7 = \sqrt{\frac{2}{7}}\sqrt{\frac{e^2}{37-5e^2}}, \quad \chi_9 = \sqrt{\frac{1}{37}}\sqrt{\frac{e^2}{18e^2-133}}$$

for odd dimensions n, an unexpected occurrence of the natural logarithmic base e. Similar formulation, in terms not of e but of $I_0(1)$, $I_1(1)$, $K_0(1)$, and $K_1(1)$, can be written for even dimensions n.

[1] H. Whitney, Analytic extensions of differentiable functions defined in closed sets, *Trans. Amer. Math. Soc.* 36 (1934) 63–89.
[2] R. Johnson, Sharp Sobolev constants, unpublished note (2000).
[3] D. H. Luecking, Extension operator of minimal norm, unpublished note (2000).
[4] S. G. Mikhlin, *Konstanten in einigen Ungleichungen der Analysis*, Teubner, 1981; *Constants in Some Inequalities of Analysis,* Wiley, 1986; MR 84a:46076 and MR 87g:46057.

[5] S. G. Mikhlin, Equivalent norms in Sobolev spaces and norms of extension operators (in Russian), *Sibirskii Mat. Z.* 19 (1978) 1141–1153; Engl. transl. in *Siberian Math. J.* 19 (1978) 804–813; MR 81g:46043.

[6] S. G. Mikhlin, On the minimal extension constant for functions of Sobolev classes (in Russian), Numerical Methods and Questions in the Organization of Calculations, 3, *Zap. Nauchn. Sem. Leningrad Otdel. Mat. Inst. Steklov (LOMI)* 90 (1979) 150–185, 300; MR 81k:46034.

[7] M. R. Hestenes, Extension of the range of a differentiable function, *Duke Math. J.* 8 (1941) 183–292; MR 2,219c.

[8] A.-P. Calderón, Lebesgue spaces of differentiable functions and distributions, *Partial Differential Equations*, ed. C. B. Morrey, Proc. Symp. Pure Math. 4, Amer. Math. Soc., 1961, pp. 33–49; MR 26 #603.

[9] E. M. Stein, *Singular Integrals and Differentiability Properties of Functions*, Princeton Univ. Press, 1970; MR 44 #7280.

3.9 Zolotarev–Schur Constant

Let n be a positive integer. Define S_n to be the set of nth degree polynomials $p(x)$ with real coefficients satisfying $|p(x)| \leq 1$ for all $-1 \leq x \leq 1$.

Markov [1, 2] proved that, if $p \in S_n$, then $|p'(x)| \leq n^2$ for all $-1 \leq x \leq 1$, where p' is the derivative of p. Equality occurs if and only if $x = \pm 1$ and $p(x) = \pm T_n(x)$, the nth Chebyshev polynomial [4.9].

Let $-1 \leq \xi \leq 1$ be a real number and $n \geq 3$ be an integer. Define $S_{n,\xi}$ to be the subset of S_n characterized by the additional restriction $p''(\xi) = 0$. Note that $T_n \notin S_{n,\pm 1}$; hence maximizing the quantity $|p'(\pm 1)|$ over the set $S_{n,\pm 1}$ leads to quite different solutions than before.

Schur [3, 4] proved that, if $p \in S_{n,\xi}$, then $|p'(\xi)| < \frac{1}{2}n^2$. Further, letting

$$s_n = \sup_{-1 \leq \xi \leq 1} \sup_{p \in S_{n,\xi}} \frac{|p'(\xi)|}{n^2} \text{ and } \sigma = \limsup_{n \to \infty} s_n$$

he obtained the bounds $0.217 \leq \sigma \leq 0.465$.

It turns out that identifying the constant σ is an outcome of work performed by Zolotarev [5–12]. Just as $T_n(x)$ arise as extremal polynomials in Markov's theorem, a new set of polynomials $Z_n(x)$ are required to fully understand Schur's theorem. Zolotarev determined in 1877 a number of exact solutions to various polynomial approximation problems using elliptic functions, in research that was far ahead of its time.

Erdös & Szegö [4] established the connection between Schur's theorem and Zolotarev's polynomials. They proved that

$$\sigma = \frac{1}{c^2}\left(1 - \frac{E(c)}{K(c)}\right)^2 = 0.3110788667\ldots,$$

where $K(x)$ and $E(x)$ are complete elliptic integrals of the first and second kind [1.4.6], and c is the unique solution of the equation

$$[K(c) - E(c)]^3 + (1 - c^2)K(c) - (1 + c^2)E(c) = 0, \quad 0 < c < 1.$$

The extremum $s_n n^2$ is attained for $n > 3$ at $\xi = 1$ and $p(x) = \pm Z_n(x)$, or at $\xi = -1$ and $p(x) = \pm Z_n(-x)$. To discuss Zolotarev's polynomials and the associated differential equation would take us too far afield, so we stop here.

3.9.1 Sewell's Problem on an Ellipse

Here is an extension of Markov's problem. Let $p(z)$ be a complex polynomial of degree n in $z = x + iy$ and assume that $|p(z)| \leq 1$ on the elliptical region E given by $x^2 + (y/g)^2 \leq 1$, where $0 < g \leq 1$. What is the smallest constant $K(g)$, independent of n, for which $|p'(z)| \leq n \cdot K(g)$ over all of E?

It is known [13–16] that $K(1) = 1$ and $K(g) \leq 1/g$. From the quadratic example $p(z) = (8z^2 - 3)/5$, van Delden [17] deduced that $K(1/2) \geq 8/5$. He further utilized the generalized Chebyshev polynomial sequence [4.9]

$$T_n(z, g) = \cos(n \arccos(\tilde{z})) = \frac{(\tilde{z} + \sqrt{\tilde{z}^2 - 1})^n + (\tilde{z} - \sqrt{\tilde{z}^2 - 1})^n}{2}, \quad \tilde{z} = \frac{z}{\sqrt{1 - g^2}},$$

to suggest that $K(g)$ is equal to its upper bound $1/g$.

Analogous constants can be defined over other boundary curves as well [18–20]. See also [21–25].

[1] A. A. Markov, On a certain problem of D. I. Mendeleev (in Russian), *Zapiski Imperatorskoi Akademii Nauk* 62 (1877) 1–24.
[2] R. J. Duffin and A. C. Schaeffer, A refinement of an inequality of the brothers Markoff, *Trans. Amer. Math. Soc.* 50 (1941) 517–528; MR 3,235c.
[3] I. Schur, Über das Maximum des absoluten Betrages eines Polynoms in einem gegebenen Intervall, *Math. Z.* 4 (1919) 271–287.
[4] P. Erdös and G. Szegö, On a problem of I. Schur, *Annals of Math.* 43 (1942) 451–470; correction 74 (1961) 628; also in *Gabor Szegö: Collected Papers*, v. 2, ed. R. Askey, Birkhäuser, 1982, pp. 805–828; MR 4,41d and MR 24 #A1341.
[5] E. I. Zolotarev, Applications of elliptic functions to questions about functions deviating least or most from zero (in Russian), *Zapiski Imperatorskoi Akademii Nauk*, v. 30 (1877) n. 5; also in *Collected Works*, v. 2, Izdat. Akad. Nauk SSSR, 1932, pp. 1–59.
[6] N. I. Achieser, *Theory of Approximation*, F. Ungar, 1956; MR 3,234d and MR 10,33b.
[7] B. C. Carlson and J. Todd, Zolotarev's first problem – The best approximation by polynomials of degree $\leq n - 2$ to $x^n - \sigma x^{n-1}$ in $[-1, 1]$, *Aequationes Math.* 26 (1983) 1–33; MR 85c:41012.
[8] J. Todd, Applications of transformation theory: A legacy from E. I. Zolotarev (1847-1878), *Approximation Theory and Spline Functions*, Proc. 1983 St. John's conf., ed. S. P. Singh, J. W. H. Burry, and B. Watson, Reidel, 1984, pp. 207–245; MR 86g:41044.
[9] J. Todd, A legacy from E. I. Zolotarev (1847–1878), *Math. Intellig.* 10 (1988) 50–53; MR 89m:01057.
[10] P. P. Petrushev and V. A. Popov, *Rational Approximation of Real Functions*, Cambridge Univ. Press, 1987; MR 89i:41022.
[11] V. M. Tikhomirov, Approximation theory, *Analysis II*, ed. R. V. Gamkrelidze, Springer-Verlag, 1990, pp. 93–255; MR 91e:00001.
[12] F. Peherstorfer and K. Schiefermayr, Description of extremal polynomials on several intervals and their computation. II, *Acta Math. Hungar.* 83 (1999) 59–83; MR 99m:41010.
[13] S. N. Bernstein, Sur l'ordre de la meilleure approximation des fonctions continues par des polynômes de degré donné, *Mémoires de l'Académie Royale de Belgique. Classe des Sciences. Collection*, 2nd ser., 4 (1912) 1–103; Russian transl. in *Collected Works*,

v. 1, *Constructive Theory of Functions (1905-1930)*, Izdat. Akad. Nauk SSSR, 1952; MR 14,2c.

[14] M. Riesz, Eine trigonometrische Interpolationsformel und einige Ungleichungen für Polynome, *Jahresbericht Deutsch. Math.-Verein.* 23 (1914) 354–368.

[15] W. E. Sewell, On the polynomial derivative constant for an ellipse, *Amer. Math. Monthly* 44 (1937) 577–578.

[16] Q. I. Rahman, Some inequalities for polynomials, *Amer. Math. Monthly* 67 (1960) 847–851; 68 (1961) 349; MR 23 A1011.

[17] J. van Delden, Polynomial optimization over an ellipse, unpublished note (2001).

[18] W. E. Sewell, The derivative of a polynomial on various arcs of the complex domain, *National Math. Mag.* 12 (1938) 167–170.

[19] W. E. Sewell, The derivative of a polynomial on further arcs of the complex domain, *Amer. Math. Monthly* 46 (1939) 644–645.

[20] W. E. Sewell, The polynomial derivative at a zero angle, *Proc. Amer. Math. Soc.* 12 (1961) 224–228; MR 22 #12206.

[21] A. C. Schaeffer and G. Szegö, Inequalities for harmonic polynomials in two and three dimensions, *Trans. Amer. Math. Soc.* 50 (1941) 187–225; also in *Gabor Szegö: Collected Papers*, v. 2, ed. R. Askey, Birkhäuser, 1982, pp. 755–794; MR 3,111b.

[22] J. H. B. Kemperman, Markov type inequalities for the derivatives of a polynomial, *Aspects of Mathematics and Its Applications*, ed. J. A. Barroso, North-Holland, 1986, pp. 465–476; MR 87j:26020.

[23] A. Jonsson, On Markov's and Bernstein's inequalities in the unit ball in $\mathbb{R}^k$, *J. Approx. Theory* 78 (1994) 151–154; MR 95h:41026.

[24] G. V. Milovanovic, D. S. Mitrinovic, and T. M. Rassias, *Topics in Polynomials: Extremal Problems, Inequalities, Zeros*, World Scientific, 1994, pp. 404–407, 448–449, 527–723; MR 95m:30009.

[25] W. Plesniak, Recent progress in multivariate Markov inequality, *Approximation Theory: In Memory of A. K. Varma*, ed. N. K. Govil, R. N. Mohapatra, Z. Nashed, A. Sharma, and J. Szabados, Dekker, 1998, pp. 449–464; MR 99g:41016.

3.10 Kneser–Mahler Polynomial Constants

Given a polynomial, what can be said about the size of its factors? Let $||p||$ denote the supremum norm of an nth degree polynomial $p(x)$ with complex coefficients, defined on the closed real interval $[-1, 1]$. Suppose $p(x) = q(x)r(x)$, where $q(x)$ is of degree k and $r(x)$ is of degree $n - k$. Then Kneser [1], building upon the work of Aumann [2], proved that [3–5]

$$||q|| \cdot ||r|| \leq \frac{1}{2} C_{n,k} C_{n,n-k} \cdot ||p||,$$

where

$$C_{n,k} = 2^k \prod_{j=1}^{k} \left[1 + \cos\left(\frac{(2j-1)\pi}{2n} \right) \right].$$

Furthermore, for any n and $k \leq n$, the constant is the best possible. Observe that here, the right-hand "knows" the degree k of $q(x)$.

Suppose information on the degree k of $q(x)$ is not available. Borwein [4, 5] observed as a corollary of Kneser's result that $k = \lfloor n/2 \rfloor$ maximizes $C_{n,k}$ and thus

$$||q|| \cdot ||r|| \leq \delta^{2n} ||p||$$

asymptotically as $n \to \infty$, where

$$\delta = \exp\left(\frac{2G}{\pi}\right) = 1.7916228120\ldots$$

is the dimer constant [5.23] and G is Catalan's constant [1.7]. Moreover, the inequality is sharp, meaning

$$\limsup_{n \to \infty} \left(\frac{\|q\| \cdot \|r\|}{\|p\|}\right)^{\frac{1}{n}} = \delta^2 = 3.2099123007\ldots,$$

where the supremum is over all polynomials p of degree n and factors q and r.

The remarkable occurrence of δ in this expression was anticipated several years earlier by Boyd [6], working over a different domain. Henceforth, define $\|p\|$ to be the supremum norm of $p(z)$ defined on the unit disk D in the complex plane. Boyd proved, if $p(z) = q(z)r(z)$, then asymptotically

$$\|q\| \cdot \|r\| \leq \delta^n \|p\|$$

and this is sharp. It is interesting that δ^2 occurs for $[-1, 1]$ but δ occurs for D.

Suppose we remove $\|r\|$ from this inequality. To avoid frivolous multiplication of q by a large constant, we assume that p and q and hence r are monic. Boyd [6] proved here that asymptotically

$$\|q\| \leq \beta^n \|p\|$$

and this is sharp, where

$$\beta = \exp\left(\frac{1}{\pi}I(\frac{2}{3}\pi)\right) = 1.3813564445\ldots$$

and

$$I(\theta) = \int\limits_0^\theta \ln\left(2\cos(\frac{x}{2})\right) dx.$$

The integral is simply $Cl(\pi - \theta)$, where $Cl(\theta)$ is Clausen's integral [7, 8]. We note a similar representation [6, 9]

$$\delta = \exp\left(\frac{2}{\pi}I(\frac{1}{2}\pi)\right)$$

and also two series [10, 11]

$$\ln(\delta) = \frac{2}{\pi}\left(1 - \frac{1}{3^2} + \frac{1}{5^2} - \frac{1}{7^2} + \frac{1}{9^2} - \frac{1}{11^2} + - \cdots\right) = 0.5831218080\ldots,$$

$$\ln(\beta) = \frac{3\sqrt{3}}{4\pi}\left(1 - \frac{1}{2^2} + \frac{1}{4^2} - \frac{1}{5^2} + \frac{1}{7^2} - \frac{1}{8^2} + - \cdots\right) = 0.3230659472\ldots.$$

The constant β has occurred in several places in the literature, the first in Mahler [12] with regard to an apparently unrelated polynomial inequality. In [13, 14], it appears in the asymptotics of what are called binomial circulant determinants. In [15], $\ln(\beta)$ is the entropy of a simple two-dimensional shift and in [16], $\pi \ln(\beta) = 1.0149416064\ldots$ is the largest possible volume of a hyperbolic tetrahedron. See also [5.23] and [8.9]. An amusing recent account of $\pi \ln(\beta)$ is found in [17], where it is called **Gieseking's constant**.

Likewise, δ has occurred throughout the literature. We already mentioned the connection to the dimer packing of a two-dimensional integer lattice. In [18, 19], $\ln(\delta)$ appears with regard to Schmidt's Gaussian integer continued fractions. Other ways δ plays a role in mathematical physics include those described in [20, 21].

Boyd [9] extended this discussion from two factors to m factors. If $p(z) = p_1(z)p_2(z)\cdots p_m(z)$, with m fixed, then asymptotically

$$\|p_1\| \cdot \|p_2\| \cdots \|p_m\| \leq c_m^n \cdot \|p\|$$

and this is sharp, where

$$c_m = \exp\left(\frac{m}{\pi} I(\frac{1}{m}\pi)\right).$$

Observe that $c_2 = \delta$ and, since $I(\pi/3) = (2/3)I(2\pi/3)$, we have $c_3 = \beta^2 = 1.9081456268\ldots$ [8]. We also have $c_4 = 1.9484547890\ldots$, $c_5 = 1.9670449011\ldots$, and $c_6 = 1.9771268308\ldots$.

Boyd [9] considered the case when $p(z)$ and all $p_i(z)$ have real coefficients, but are defined on D. Here the constant c_m is simply replaced by δ and this is sharp. That is, in the real case, the best constant does not depend on m. Borwein [4, 5] considered the case of complex $p(x)$ and $p_i(x)$ defined on the interval $[-1, 1]$. Here the constant c_m is simply replaced by δ^2 and again this is sharp. Pritsker [22, 23] obtained a general formula for the analog, $B(a)$, of β for Boyd's inequality [6] on the interval $[-a, a]$. For example, $B(2) = \beta^2 = 1.90815\ldots$ and $B(1) = \sqrt{2}\delta = 2.53373\ldots$. See also [24, 25].

In [2.30], we discuss **Mahler's measure** $M(\alpha)$ for algebraic integers α. This is, in essence, equivalent to Mahler's measure $M(f)$ for univariate polynomials [26]

$$f(z) = \alpha_0 \prod_{j=1}^{n}(z - \alpha_j),$$

which is given by

$$M(f) = \exp\left(\int_0^1 \ln(|f(e^{2\pi i\theta})|)d\theta\right) = |\alpha_0| \prod_{j=1}^{n} \max(|\alpha_j|, 1)$$

as a consequence of Jensen's formula [27].

An important generalization to multivariate functions $f(z_1, z_2, \ldots, z_m)$ is given by

$$M(f) = \exp\left(\int_0^1 \int_0^1 \cdots \int_0^1 \ln(|f(e^{2\pi i\theta_1}, e^{2\pi i\theta_2}, \ldots, e^{2\pi i\theta_m})|)d\theta_1 d\theta_2 \cdots d\theta_m\right).$$

Some examples are

$$M(1 + x) = 1, \quad M(1 + x + y) = \beta = M(\max(1, |x + 1|)),$$

$$M(1 + x + y + z) = \exp\left(\frac{7\zeta(3)}{2\pi^2}\right),$$

$$M(1 + x + y - xy) = \delta = M(\max(|x - 1|, |x + 1|)),$$

where $\zeta(3)$ is Apéry's constant [1.6]. Two asymptotic results are [10]

$$\lim_{m \to \infty} \frac{M(z_1 + z_2 + \cdots + z_m)}{\sqrt{m}} = \exp\left(-\frac{1}{2}\gamma\right) = 0.7493060013\ldots,$$

involving the Euler–Mascheroni constant γ [1.5], and

$$\lim_{m \to \infty} M(z_1 + (1 + z_2)(1 + z_3) \cdots (1 + z_m))^{\frac{1}{\sqrt{m}}} = \exp\left(\sqrt{\frac{\pi}{24}}\right).$$

Finally, we discuss **Bombieri's supremum norm**: If $p(z) = \sum_{j=0}^{n} a_j z^j$, then

$$[p] = \max_{0 \le j \le n} |a_j| \frac{n!}{j!(n - j)!}.$$

If $p(z)$ and $q(z)$ are complex monic polynomials on D, $\deg(p) = n$, and q is a factor of p, we are interested in the size of $\|q\|$ relative to $[p]$. It is known that asymptotically [28–31]

$$\|q\| \le K^n \cdot [p],$$

where

$$K = M(1 + |x + 1|) = M\left((1 + x + x^2 + y)^2\right) = 2.1760161352\ldots,$$

but a proof that K is the best possible remains undiscovered.

[1] H. Kneser, Das Maximum des Produkts zweier Polynome, *Sitzungsber. Preuss. Akad. Wiss.* (1934) 426–431.
[2] G. Aumann, Satz über das Verhalten von Polynomen auf Kontinuen, *Sitzungsber. Preuss. Akad. Wiss.* (1933) 924–931.
[3] D. S. Mitrinovic, *Analytic Inequalities*, Springer-Verlag, 1970; MR 43 #448.
[4] P. B. Borwein, Exact inequalities for the norms of factors of polynomials, *Canad. J. Math.* 46 (1994) 687–698; MR 95k:26015.
[5] P. Borwein and T. Erdélyi, *Polynomials and Polynomial Inequalities*, Springer-Verlag, 1995; MR 97e:41001.
[6] D. W. Boyd, Two sharp inequalities for the norm of a factor of a polynomial, *Mathematika* 39 (1992) 341–349; MR 94a:11162.
[7] M. Abramowitz and I. A. Stegun, *Handbook of Mathematical Functions*, Dover, 1972; MR 94b:00012.
[8] L. Lewin, *Polylogarithms and Associated Functions*, North-Holland, 1981; MR 83b:33019.
[9] D. W. Boyd, Sharp inequalities for the product of polynomials, *Bull. London Math. Soc.* 26 (1994) 449–454; MR 95m:30008.
[10] C. J. Smyth, On measures of polynomials in several variables, *Bull. Austral. Math. Soc.* 23 (1981) 49–63; G. Myerson and C. J. Smyth, corrigendum 26 (1982) 317–319; MR 82k:10074 and MR 84g:10088.

[11] D. W. Boyd, Speculations concerning the range of Mahler's measure, *Canad. Math. Bull.* 24 (1981) 453–469; MR 83h:12002.

[12] K. Mahler, A remark on a paper of mine on polynomials, *Illinois J. Math.* 8 (1964) 1–4; MR 28 #2194.

[13] J. S. Frame, Factors of the binomial circulant determinant, *Fibonacci Quart.* 18 (1980) 9–23; MR 81j:10007.

[14] D. W. Boyd, The asymptotic behaviour of the binomial circulant determinant, *J. Math. Anal. Appl.* 86 (1982) 30–38; MR 83f:10007.

[15] D. Lind, K. Schmidt, and T. Ward, Mahler measure and entropy for commuting automorphisms of compact groups, *Invent. Math.* 101 (1990) 593–629; MR 92j:22013.

[16] J. Milnor, Hyperbolic geometry: The first 150 years, *Bull. Amer. Math. Soc.* 6 (1982) 9–24; MR 82m:57005.

[17] C. C. Adams, The newest inductee in the Number Hall of Fame, *Math. Mag.* 71 (1998) 341–349.

[18] A. L. Schmidt, Ergodic theory of complex continued fractions, *Number Theory with an Emphasis on the Markoff Spectrum*, Proc. 1991 Provo conf., ed. A. D. Pollington and W. Moran, Dekker, 1993, pp. 215–226; MR 95f:11055.

[19] H. Nakada, The metrical theory of complex continued fractions, *Acta Arith.* 56 (1990) 279–289; MR 92e:11081.

[20] P. Sarnak, Spectral behavior of quasiperiodic potentials, *Commun. Math. Phys.* 84 (1982) 377–401; MR 84g:35136.

[21] D. J. Thouless, Scaling for the discrete Mathieu equation, *Commun. Math. Phys.* 127 (1990) 187–193; MR 90m:82004.

[22] I. E. Pritsker, An inequality for the norm of a polynomial factor, *Proc. Amer. Math. Soc.* 129 (2001) 2283–2291; math.CV/0001124; MR 2002f:30005.

[23] I. E. Pritsker, Norms of products and factors polynomials, *Number Theory for the Millennium*, v. 2, Proc. 2000 Urbana conf., ed. M. A. Bennett, B. C. Berndt, N. Boston, H. G. Diamond, A. J. Hildebrand, and W. Philipp, A. K. Peters, to appear; math.CV/0101164.

[24] A. Kroó and I. E. Pritsker, A sharp version of Mahler's inequality for products of polynomials, *Bull. London Math. Soc.* 31 (1999) 269–278; MR 99m:30008.

[25] I. E. Pritsker, Products of polynomials in uniform norms, *Trans. Amer. Math. Soc.* 353 (2001) 3971–3993; MR 2002f:30006.

[26] G. Everest, Measuring the height of a polynomial, *Math. Intellig.*, v. 20 (1998) n. 3, 9–16; MR 2000b:11115.

[27] R. M. Young, On Jensen's formula and $\int_0^{2\pi} \log |1 - e^{i\theta}| d\theta$, *Amer. Math. Monthly* 93 (1986) 44–45.

[28] D. W. Boyd, Bounds for the height of a factor of a polynomial in terms of Bombieri's norms. I: The largest factor, *J. Symbolic Comput.* 16 (1993) 115–130; MR 94m:11032a.

[29] D. W. Boyd, Bounds for the height of a factor of a polynomial in terms of Bombieri's norms. II: The smallest factor, *J. Symbolic Comput.* 16 (1993) 131–145; MR 94m:11032b.

[30] D. W. Boyd, Large factors of small polynomials, *The Rademacher Legacy to Mathematics*, ed. G. E. Andrews, D. M. Bressoud, and L. Alayne Parson, Contemp. Math. 166, Amer. Math. Soc., 1994, pp. 301–308; MR 95e:11034.

[31] D. W. Boyd, Mahler's measure and special values of L-functions, *Experim. Math.* 7 (1998) 37–82; MR 99d:11070.

3.11 Grothendieck's Constants

For any integer $n \geq 2$, there is a constant $k(n)$ with the following property [1, 2]: Let A be any $m \times m$ matrix for which

$$\left| \sum_{i=1}^{m} \sum_{j=1}^{m} a_{ij} s_i t_j \right| \leq 1$$

is satisfied for all scalars $s_1, s_2, \ldots, s_m, t_1, t_2, \ldots, t_m$ with $|s_i| \leq 1$, $|t_j| \leq 1$. Then

$$\left| \sum_{i=1}^{m} \sum_{j=1}^{m} a_{ij} \langle x_i, y_j \rangle \right| \leq k(n)$$

for all vectors $x_1, x_2, \ldots, x_m, y_1, y_2, \ldots, y_m$ in an n-dimensional Hilbert space with $||x_i|| \leq 1$, $||y_j|| \leq 1$. As usual, $\langle x, y \rangle$ is the inner product of x and y and $||x|| = \sqrt{\langle x, x \rangle}$. The constant $k(n)$ is taken to be the least possible.

This definition actually covers two possible cases:

- Scalars and matrices are real, and vectors are in a real Hilbert space.
- Scalars and matrices are complex, and vectors are in a complex Hilbert space.

We denote the two corresponding constants by $k_R(n)$ and $k_C(n)$. It is known [3–6] that

$$k_R(2) = \sqrt{2}, \quad k_R(3) < 1.517, \quad k_R(4) \leq \pi/2$$

but

$$1.1526 \leq k_C(2) \leq 1.2157, \quad 1.2108 \leq k_C(3) \leq 1.2744, \quad 1.2413 \leq k_C(4) \leq 1.3048.$$

Each sequence clearly increases with n. For both real and complex cases, define $\kappa = \lim_{n \to \infty} k(n)$. It is not hard to show that [2], in the limit,

$$\frac{1}{2} \kappa_R \leq \kappa_C \leq 2\kappa_R.$$

The best-known numerical bounds are [3, 4, 7–9]

$$1.67696 \leq \kappa_R \leq \frac{\pi}{2 \ln(1 + \sqrt{2})} = 1.7822139781 \ldots,$$

$$1.33807 \leq \kappa_C \leq \frac{8}{\pi \cdot (x_0 + 1)} = 1.40491 \ldots,$$

where x_0 is the solution of a certain equation involving complete elliptic integrals $K(x)$ and $E(x)$ of the first and second kind [1.4.6]:

$$\psi(x) = \frac{\pi}{8}(x + 1), \quad -1 < x < 1,$$

where

$$\psi(x) = x \int_0^{\frac{\pi}{2}} \frac{\cos(\theta)^2}{\sqrt{1 - x^2 \sin(\theta)^2}} d\theta = \frac{1}{x} \left[E(x) - (1 - x^2) K(x) \right].$$

The upper estimate for κ_R was conjectured by Krivine [3, 4, 10] to be the exact value. In contrast, Haagerup [7] doubted whether 1.40491 is the exact value for κ_C and thought that

$$\frac{1}{|\psi(i)|} = \left(\int\limits_{0}^{\frac{\pi}{2}} \frac{\cos(\theta)^2}{\sqrt{1 + \sin(\theta)^2}} d\theta \right)^{-1} = 1.4045759346\ldots$$

is a more plausible candidate. His reasoning was by analogy: The function $\psi(x)$ for the complex case is like the function $\varphi(x)$ employed by Krivine for the real case,

$$\varphi(x) = \frac{2}{\pi} \arcsin(x),$$

and one sees that

$$\frac{1}{|\varphi(i)|} = \frac{\pi}{2 \operatorname{arcsinh}(1)} = \frac{\pi}{2 \ln(1 + \sqrt{2})}.$$

A different approach for bounding κ_R is given in [11].

[1] J. Lindenstrauss and A. Pelczynski, Absolutely summing operators in L_p spaces and their applications, *Studia Math.* 29 (1968) 275–326; MR 37 #6743.

[2] G. L. O. Jameson, *Summing and Nuclear Norms in Banach Space Theory*, Cambridge Univ. Press, 1987; MR 89c:46020.

[3] J.-L. Krivine, Sur la constante de Grothendieck, *C. R. Acad. Sci. Paris* 284 (1977) 445–446; MR 55 #1435.

[4] J.-L. Krivine, Constantes de Grothendieck et fonctions de type positif sur les spheres, *Adv. Math.* 31 (1979) 16–30; MR 80e:46015.

[5] H. König, On the complex Grothendieck constant in the n-dimensional case, *Geometry of Banach Spaces*, Proc. 1989 Strobl conf., ed. P. F. X. Müller and W. Schachermayer, Cambridge Univ. Press, 1990, pp. 181–198; MR 92g:46011.

[6] H. König, Some remarks on the Grothendieck inequality, *General Inequalities 6*, Proc. 1990 Oberwolfach conf., ed. W. Walter, Birkhäuser, 1992, pp. 201–206; MR 94h:46035.

[7] U. Haagerup, A new upper bound for the complex Grothendieck constant, *Israel J. Math.* 60 (1987) 199–224; MR 89f:47029.

[8] A. M. Davies, Lower bound for κ_C, unpublished note (1984).

[9] J. A. Reeds, A new lower bound on the real Grothendieck constant, unpublished note (1991).

[10] F. Le Lionnais, *Les Nombres Remarquables*, Hermann 1983.

[11] P. C. Fishburn and J. A. Reeds, Bell inequalities, Grothendieck's constant, and root two, *SIAM J. Discrete Math.* 7 (1994) 48–56; MR 95e:05013.

3.12 Du Bois Reymond's Constants

Abel's theorem from advanced calculus implies that if the series of real numbers $\sum_{n=0}^{\infty} a_n$ converges, then the corresponding power series satisfies

$$\lim_{r \to 1^-} \sum_{n=0}^{\infty} a_n r^n = \sum_{n=0}^{\infty} a_n.$$

This is a consequence of uniform convergence on the interval $[0, 1]$. We start with a question: What happens if $\sum_{n=0}^{\infty} a_n$ *diverges*?

Define the sequence of partial sums $s_n = \sum_{k=0}^{n} a_k$ and assume

$$s = \liminf_{n \to \infty} s_n, \quad S = \limsup_{n \to \infty} s_n$$

are both finite. That is, the series is bounded and oscillates between two finite limits. It is natural to believe here that

$$s \leq \lim_{r \to 1^-} \sum_{n=0}^{\infty} a_n r^n \leq S$$

and this is indeed true [1].

In fact, much more is true. Let $\varphi(x)$ be a continuously differentiable function for $x > 0$ that satisfies the conditions

$$\lim_{x \to 0^+} \varphi(x) = 1, \quad \lim_{x \to \infty} \varphi(x) = 0, \quad I = \int_{0}^{\infty} \left| \frac{d}{dx} \varphi(x) \right| dx < \infty$$

and

$$f(x) = \sum_{n=0}^{\infty} a_n \varphi(nx) \quad \text{is convergent for all } x > 0.$$

Then it can be proved that [1, 2]

$$\frac{1}{2}(S+s) - \frac{1}{2}(S-s) \cdot I \leq \lim_{x \to 0^+} f(x) \leq \frac{1}{2}(S+s) + \frac{1}{2}(S-s) \cdot I.$$

Moreover, this truly extends what was discussed before: Set $r = \varphi(x) = \exp(-x)$ to see why.

Another important case arises if we instead set $\varphi(x) = (\sin(x)/x)^m$ for an integer $m \geq 2$. Define the mth **Du Bois Reymond constant** by

$$c_m = I - 1 = \int_{0}^{\infty} \left| \frac{d}{dx} \left(\frac{\sin(x)}{x} \right)^m \right| dx - 1.$$

Watson [2–6] proved that

$$c_2 = \tfrac{1}{2}(e^2 - 7) = 0.1945280495\ldots, \quad c_4 = \tfrac{1}{8}(e^4 - 4e^2 - 25) = 0.0052407047\ldots,$$

$$c_6 = \tfrac{1}{32}(e^6 - 6e^4 + 3e^2 - 98) = 0.0002206747\ldots$$

and that c_{2k} is expressible as a polynomial of degree k in e^2 with rational coefficients. No such expression is known for c_{2k+1}, but there is an interesting series available for all c_m. Let $\xi_1, \xi_2, \xi_3, \ldots$ denote all positive solutions of the equation $\tan(x) = x$. Then

$$c_m = 2 \sum_{j=1}^{\infty} \frac{1}{(1 + \xi_j^2)^{m/2}}$$

and, in particular, $c_3 = 0.0282517642\ldots$. It is possible to numerically evaluate c_5, $c_7, \ldots$ as well. Watson also determined that

$$c_3 = -\frac{2}{\pi} \int\limits_1^\infty \frac{x}{\sqrt{x^2 - 1}} \frac{d}{dx} \left(\frac{\tanh(x)^2}{x - \tanh(x)} \right) dx,$$

but there appears to be no further simplification of this integral.

The sequence $\xi_1, \xi_2, \xi_3, \ldots$ arose in a recent *Monthly* problem:

$$\sum_{n=1}^\infty \frac{1}{\xi_n^2} = \frac{1}{10}$$

and attracted much attention [7]. This formula parallels that just discussed and Watson's other results, namely,

$$b_m = 2 \sum_{j=1}^\infty \frac{(-1)^{j+1}}{(1 + \xi_j^2)^{m/2}}, \quad b_3 = -\frac{1}{4}(e^3 - 3e - 12) = 0.0173271405\ldots,$$

and b_{2k+1} is expressible as a polynomial of degree $2k + 1$ in e with rational coefficients. Note that similar expressions in e appear in [3.8].

Here are other constants involving equations with the tangent function. The maximum value $M(n)$ of the function

$$\left(\sum_{k=1}^n \frac{x_k}{k} \right)^2 + \sum_{k=1}^n \left(\frac{x_k}{k} \right)^2,$$

subject to the constraint $\sum_{k=1}^n x_k^2 \leq 1$, satisfies the following asymptotic result [8]:

$$\lim_{n \to \infty} M(n) = \left(\frac{\pi}{\xi} \right)^2 = 2.3979455861\ldots,$$

where $\xi = 2.0287578381\ldots$ is the smallest positive solution of the equation $x + \tan(x) = 0$. Another example [9], described in [3.14], involves the equation $\pi + x = \tan(x)$.

[1] E. W. Hobson, *The Theory of Functions of a Real Variable and the Theory of Fourier's Series*, v. 2, Dover, 1957, pp. 221–225; MR 19,1166b.

[2] G. N. Watson, Du Bois Reymond's constants, *Quart. J. Math.* 4 (1933) 140–146.

[3] A. Fletcher, J. C. P. Miller, L. Rosenhead, and L. J. Comrie, *An Index of Mathematical Tables*, 2nd ed., v. 1, Addison-Wesley, 1962, p. 129; MR 26 #365a.

[4] H. P. Robinson and E. Potter, *Mathematical Constants*, UCRL-20418, Univ. of Calif. at Berkeley, 1971; available through the National Technical Information Service, Springfield VA 22151.

[5] F. Le Lionnais, *Les Nombres Remarquables*, Hermann, 1983.

[6] S. Plouffe, 2nd Du Bois Reymond constant (Plouffe's Tables).

[7] R. M. Young, A Rayleigh popular problem, *Amer. Math. Monthly* 93 (1986) 660–664.

[8] G. Szegö, Über das Maximum einer quadratischen Form von unendlich-vielen Veränderlichen, *Jahresbericht Deutsch. Math.-Verein.* 31 (1922) 85–88; also in *Collected Papers*, v. 1, ed. R. Askey, Birkhäuser, 1982; pp. 589–593.

[9] G. Brown and K.-Y. Wang, An extension of the Fejér-Jackson inequality, *J. Austral. Math. Soc. Ser. A* 62 (1997) 1–12; MR 98e:42003.

3.13 Steinitz Constants

3.13.1 Motivation

If $\sum x_i$ is an absolutely convergent series of real numbers, then any rearrangement of the terms x_i of the series will have no impact on the sum.

By contrast, if $\sum x_i$ is a conditionally convergent series of real numbers, then the terms x_i may be rearranged to produce a series that has any desired sum (even ∞ or $-\infty$). This is a well-known theorem due to Riemann.

Suppose instead that the terms x_i are elements of a finite-dimensional normed real space; that is, the x_i are real vectors but possibly with a different notion of length (choice of metric). Assume nothing about the nature of $\sum x_i$. Let C denote the set of all sums of convergent rearrangements of the terms x_i. Steinitz [1–3] proved that C is either empty or of the form $y + L$, for some vector y and some linear subspace L. (Note that $L = \{0\}$, the zero subspace, is one possibility.)

To prove this theorem, Steinitz needed bounds on certain constants $K(0, 0)$, defined in the next section. For details on the precise connection, see [4–6].

3.13.2 Definitions

Let a and b be nonnegative real numbers. In an m-dimensional normed real space, define a set $S = \{u, v_1, v_2, \ldots, v_{n-1}, v_n, w\}$ of $n + 2$ vectors satisfying $|u| \leq a$, $|v_j| \leq 1$ for each $1 \leq j \leq n$, $|w| \leq b$, and $u + \sum_{j=1}^{n} v_j + w = 0$ (see Figure 3.2).

Let π denote a permutation of the indices $\{1, 2, \ldots, n\}$ and define a function

$$F(\pi, n, S) = \max_{1 \leq k \leq n} \left| u + \sum_{j=1}^{k} v_{\pi(j)} \right|.$$

In words, F is the radius of the smallest sphere, with center at 0, circumscribing the

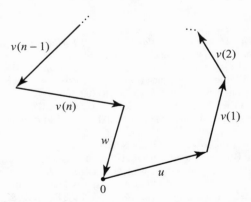

Figure 3.2. A set S of vectors satisfying $u + \sum_{j=1}^{n} v_j + w = 0$.

polygon with sides u, $v_{\pi(1)}$, $v_{\pi(2)}$, ..., $v_{\pi(n)}$. Of the vector orderings determined by all possible π, there is (at least) one that minimizes the spherical radius. Define

$$K_m(a, b) = \max_{n, S} \min_{\pi} F(\pi, n, S);$$

that is, $K_m(a, b)$ is the least number for which $|u + \sum_{j=1}^{k} v_{\pi(j)}| \leq K_m(a, b)$ for some permutation π, for all integers n and sets S.

3.13.3 Results

In the general setting just described (with no restrictions on the norm), the best-known upper bound on the m-**dimensional Steinitz constant** is

$$K_m(0, 0) \leq m - 1 + \frac{1}{m}$$

due to Banaszczyk [7], improving on the work in [8]. Further, Grinberg & Sevastyanov [8] observed that, for $m = 2$, the upper bound $3/2$ is the best possible. In other words, there exists a norm for which equality holds. Whether this observation holds for larger m is unknown.

Henceforth let us assume the norm is Euclidean. Banaszczyk [9] proved that

$$K_2(a, b) = \sqrt{1 + \max(a^2, b^2, 1/4)},$$

which extends the results $K_2(1, 0) = K_2(1, 1) = \sqrt{2}$, $K_2(0, 0) = \sqrt{5}/2 = 1.1180339887\ldots$ known to earlier authors. Damsteeg & Halperin [4] demonstrated that

$$K_m(0, 0) \geq \frac{1}{2}\sqrt{m + 3}$$

and, for $m \geq 2$,

$$K_m(1, 1) \geq K_m(1, 0) \geq \frac{1}{2}\sqrt{m + 6}.$$

Behrend [10] proved that

$$K_m(1, 0) \leq K_m(1, 1) < m, \quad K_3(1, 0) \leq K_3(1, 1) < \sqrt{5 + 2\sqrt{3}} = 2.9093129112\ldots,$$

but an exact value for any $m > 2$ remains unknown. (Note: There seems to be some confusion in [11] between $K(0, 0)$ and $K(1, 0)$, but not in the earlier reference [12].) Behrend believed it to be likely that the true order of these constants is $\sqrt{m}$. See also [13–18] for related ideas.

[1] E. Steinitz, Bedingt konvergente Reihen und konvexe Systeme, *J. Reine Angew. Math.* 143 (1913) 128–175; 144 (1914) 1–40.

[2] P. Rosenthal, The remarkable theorem of Lévy and Steinitz, *Amer. Math. Monthly* 94 (1987) 342–351; MR 88d:40005.

[3] M. I. Kadets and V. M. Kadets, *Series in Banach Spaces: Conditional and Unconditional Convergence*, Birkhäuser, 1997; MR 98a:46016.

[4] I. Damsteeg and I. Halperin, The Steinitz-Gross theorem on sums of vectors, *Trans. Royal Soc. Canada Ser. III* 44 (1950) 31–35; MR 12,419a.

[5] I. Halperin and N. Miller, An inequality of Steinitz and the limits of Riemann sums, *Trans. Royal Soc. Canada Ser. III* 48 (1954) 27–29l; MR 16,596a.

[6] I. Halperin, Sums of a series, permitting rearrangements, *C. R. Math. Rep. Acad. Sci. Canada* 8 (1986) 87–102; MR 87m:40004.

[7] W. Banaszczyk, The Steinitz constant of the plane, *J. Reine Angew. Math.* 373 (1987) 218–220; MR 88e:52016.

[8] V. S. Grinberg and S. V. Sevastyanov, O velicine konstanty Steinica, *Funkcional. Anal. i Prilozen.*, v. 14 (1980) n. 2, 56–57; Engl. transl. in *Functional Anal. Appl.* 14 (1980) 125–126; MR 81h:52008.

[9] W. Banaszczyk, A note on the Steinitz constant of the Euclidean plane, *C. R. Math. Rep. Acad. Sci. Canada* 12 (1990) 97–102; MR 91g:52005.

[10] F. A. Behrend, The Steinitz-Gross theorem on sums of vectors, *Canad. J. Math.* 6 (1954) 108–124; MR 15,551c.

[11] D. S. Mitrinovic, J. E. Pecaric, and A. M. Fink, *Classical and New Inequalities in Analysis*, Kluwer, 1993; MR 94c:00004.

[12] D. S. Mitrinovic, *Analytic Inequalities*, Springer-Verlag, 1970; MR 43 #448.

[13] W. Banaszczyk, The Dvoretzky-Hanani lemma for rectangles, *Period. Math. Hungar.* 31 (1995) 1–3; MR 96j:52011.

[14] S. Sevastjanov and W. Banaszczyk, To the Steinitz lemma in coordinate form, *Discrete Math.* 169 (1997) 145–152; MR 97m:05004.

[15] I. Bárány, M. Katchalski, and J. Pach, Quantitative Helly-type theorems, *Proc. Amer. Math. Soc.* 86 (1982) 109–114; MR 84h:52016.

[16] I. Bárány and A. Heppes, On the exact constant in the quantitative Steinitz theorem in the plane, *Discrete Comput. Geom.* 12 (1994) 387–398; MR 95g:52011.

[17] P. Brass, On the quantitative Steinitz theorem in the plane, *Discrete Comput. Geom.* 17 (1997) 111–117; MR 97h:52005.

[18] I. Halperin and T. Ando, *Bibliography: Series of Vectors and Riemann Sums*, Hokkaido Univ., Sapporo, Japan, 1989.

3.14 Young–Fejér–Jackson Constants

3.14.1 Nonnegativity of Cosine Sums

In the following, n is a positive integer, $0 \leq \theta \leq \pi$, and a is a parameter to be studied. Young [1] proved that the cosine sum

$$C(\theta, a, n) = \frac{1}{1 + a} + \sum_{k=1}^{n} \frac{\cos(k\theta)}{k + a} \geq 0$$

for $-1 < a \leq 0$. Rogosinski & Szegö [2] extended this result to $-1 < a \leq 1$ and proved that there is a best upper limit A, $1 \leq A \leq 2(1 + \sqrt{2})$, in the sense that

- $C(\theta, a, n) \geq 0$ for $-1 < a \leq A$, for all n and all θ,
- $C(\theta, a, n) < 0$ for $a > A$, for some n and some θ.

Gasper [3, 4] proved that $A = 4.5678018826\ldots$ and has minimal polynomial

$$9x^7 + 55x^6 - 14x^5 - 948x^4 - 3247x^3 - 5013x^2 - 3780x - 1134.$$

In fact, if $a > A$, then $C(\theta, a, 3) < 0$ for some θ. This completes the story for cosine sums.

3.14.2 Positivity of Sine Sums

Here, n is a positive integer, $0 < \theta < \pi$, and b is the parameter of interest. Fejér [5], Gronwall [6, 7], and Jackson [8] obtained that the corresponding sine series

$$S(\theta, b, n) = \sum_{k=1}^{n} \frac{\sin(k\theta)}{k + b} > 0$$

for $b = 0$. See [9] for a quick proof; see also [10–13]. Brown & Wang [14] extended this result to $-1 < b \leq B$ for odd integers n, where B is the best upper limit. For even integers n, the story is more complicated and we shall explain later.

Two intermediate constants need to be defined:

- $\lambda = 0.4302966531\ldots$, a solution of the equation $(1 + \lambda)\pi = \tan(\lambda\pi)$,
- $\mu = 0.8128252421\ldots$, a solution of the equation $(1 + \lambda)\sin(\mu\pi) = \mu\sin(\lambda\pi)$.

With these, define $B = 2.1102339661\ldots$ to be a solution of the equation [14, 15]

$$(1 + \lambda) \cdot \pi \cdot \left((B - 1)\psi(1 + \tfrac{B-1}{2}) - 2B\psi(1 + \tfrac{B}{2}) + (B + 1)\psi(1 + \tfrac{B+1}{2})\right) = 2\sin(\lambda\pi),$$

where $\psi(x)$ is the digamma function [1.5.4]. Is B algebraic? The answer is unknown.

We now discuss the case of even n. Define $c_n(x) = 1 - 2x/(4n + 1)$. If $-1 < b \leq B$ and n is even, then $S(\theta, b, n) > 0$ for $0 < \theta \leq \pi c_n(\mu)$. Further, the constant μ is the best possible, meaning that $0 < \nu < \mu$ implies $S(\pi c_n(\nu), b, n) < 0$ for some $b < B$ and infinitely many n.

Wilson [16] indicated that $S < 0$ can be expected on the basis of Belov's work [17].

3.14.3 Uniform Boundedness

Fix a parameter value $0 < r < 1$. Consider the sequence of functions

$$F_n(\theta, r) = \sum_{k=1}^{n} k^{-r} \cos(k\theta), \quad n = 1, 2, 3, \ldots.$$

This sequence is said to be **uniformly bounded below** if there exists a constant $m > -\infty$ such that $m < F_n(\theta, r)$ for all θ and all n. Note that m depends on the choice of r.

Zygmund [11] proved that there is a best lower limit $0 < R < 1$ for r, in the sense that

- $F_n(\theta, r)$ is uniformly bounded below for $r \geq R$ and
- $F_n(\theta, r)$ is not uniformly bounded below for $r < R$.

The constant $R = 0.3084437795 \ldots$ is the unique solution of the equation [15, 18–22]

$$\int_0^{\frac{3\pi}{2}} x^{-R} \cos(x) dx = 0$$

and this plays a role in Belov's papers [17, 23] as well. Interestingly, the sequence of functions

$$G_n(\theta, r) = \sum_{k=1}^n k^{-r} \sin(k\theta), \quad n = 1, 2, 3, \ldots,$$

is uniformly bounded below for all $r > 0$; hence there is no analog of R for the sequence $G_n(\theta, r)$.

[1]   W. H. Young, On a certain series of Fourier, *Proc. London Math. Soc.* 11 (1912) 357–366.
[2]   W. Rogosinski and G. Szegö, Über die Abschnitte von Potenzreihen, die in einem Kreise beschränkt bleiben, *Math. Z.* 28 (1928) 73–94; also in *Gabor Szegö: Collected Papers*, v. 2, ed. R. Askey, Birkhäuser, 1982, pp. 87–111.
[3]   G. Gasper, Nonnegative sums of cosine, ultraspherical and Jacobi polynomials, *J. Math. Anal. Appl.* 26 (1969) 60–68; MR 38 #6130.
[4]   D. S. Mitrinovic, J. E. Pecaric, and A. M. Fink, *Classical and New Inequalities in Analysis*, Kluwer, 1993, p. 615; MR 94c:00004.
[5]   L. Fejér, Lebesguesche Konstanten und divergente Fourierreihen, *J. Reine Angew. Math.* 138 (1910) 22–53.
[6]   T. H. Gronwall, Über die Gibbssche Erscheinung und die trigonometrischen Summen $\sin(x) + \frac{1}{2}\sin(2x) + \cdots + \frac{1}{n}\sin(nx)$, *Math. Annalen* 72 (1912) 228–243.
[7]   E. Hewitt and R. E. Hewitt, The Gibbs-Wilbraham phenomenon: An episode in Fourier analysis, *Arch. Hist. Exact Sci.* 21 (1979) 129–160; MR 81g:01015.
[8]   D. Jackson, Über eine trigonometrische Summe, *Rend. Circ. Mat. Palermo* 32 (1911) 257–262.
[9]   R. Askey, J. Fitch, and G. Gasper, On a positive trigonometric sum, *Proc. Amer. Math. Soc.* 19 (1968) 1507; MR 37 #6662.
[10] P. Turán, On a trigonometrical sum, *Annales Soc. Polonaise Math.* 25 (1952) 155–161; also in *Collected Works*, v. 1, ed. P. Erdös, Akadémiai Kiadó, pp. 661–667; MR 14,1080c.
[11] A. G. Zygmund, *Trigonometric Series,* v. 1, 2nd ed., Cambridge Univ. Press, 1959, pp. 8, 191–192; MR 89c:42001.
[12] R. Askey and J. Steinig, Some positive trigonometric sums, *Trans. Amer. Math. Soc.* 187 (1974) 295–307; MR 49 #3245.
[13] R. Askey and J. Steinig, A monotonic trigonometric sum, *Amer. J. Math.* 98 (1976) 357–365; MR 53 #11288.
[14] G. Brown and K.-Y. Wang, An extension of the Fejér-Jackson inequality, *J. Austral. Math. Soc. Ser. A* 62 (1997) 1–12; MR 98e:42003.
[15] J. Keane, Estimating Brown-Wang *B* and Zygmund *R* constants, unpublished note (2000).
[16] D. C. Wilson, Review of "An extension of the Fejér-Jackson inequality," MR 98e:42003.
[17] A. S. Belov, On the coefficients of trigonometric series with nonnegative partial sums (in Russian), *Mat. Zametki* 41 (1987) 152–158, 285; Engl. transl. in *Math. Notes* 41 (1987) 88–92; MR 88f:42001.
[18] R. P. Boas and V. C. Klema, A constant in the theory of trigonometric series, *Math. Comp.* 18 (1964) 674; MR 31 #558.
[19] R. F. Church, On a constant in the theory of trigonometric series, *Math. Comp.* 19 (1965) 501.

[20] Y. L. Luke, W. Fair, G. Coombs, and R. Moran, On a constant in the theory of trigonometric series, *Math. Comp.* 19 (1965) 501–502.
[21] R. D. Halbgewachs and S. M. Shah, Trigonometric sums and Fresnel-type integrals, *Proc. Indian Acad. Sci. Sect. A* 65 (1967) 227–232; MR 35 #3855.
[22] S. M. Shah, Trigonometric series with nonnegative partial sums, *Entire Functions and Related Parts of Analysis*, ed. J. Korevaar, S. S. Chern, L. Ehrenpreis, W. H. J. Fuchs, and L. A. Rubel, Proc. Symp. Pure Math. 11, Amer. Math. Soc., 1968, pp. 386–391; MR 38 #6293.
[23] A. S. Belov, Coefficients of trigonometric cosine series with nonnegative partial sums, *Theory of Functions* (in Russian), Proc. 1987 Amberd conf., ed. S. M. Nikolskii, *Trudy Mat. Inst. Steklov.* 190 (1989) 3–21; Engl. transl. in *Proc. Steklov Inst. Math.* 190 (1992) 1–19; MR 90m:42005.

3.15 Van der Corput's Constant

Let f be a real twice-continuously differentiable function on the interval $[a, b]$ with the property that $|f''(x)| \geq r$ for all x. There exists a smallest constant m, independent of a and b as well as f, such that

$$\left| \int_a^b \exp(i \cdot f(x)) dx \right| \leq \frac{m}{\sqrt{r}},$$

where i is the imaginary unit [1–3]. This inequality was first proved by van der Corput [1] and has several applications in analytic number theory. Kershner [4, 5], following a suggestion of Wintner, proved that the maximizing function f is the parabola $f(x) = rx^2/2 + c$, with domain endpoints given by

$$-a = b = \sqrt{\frac{\pi - 2c}{r}}$$

and coefficient $c = -0.7266432468\ldots$ given as the only solution of the equation

$$\int_0^{\sqrt{\frac{\pi}{2} - c}} \sin(x^2 + c) dx = 0, \quad -\frac{\pi}{2} \leq c \leq \frac{\pi}{2}.$$

From this, it follows that van der Corput's constant m is

$$m = 2\sqrt{2} \int_0^{\sqrt{\frac{\pi}{2} - c}} \cos(x^2 + c) dx = 3.3643175781\ldots.$$

[1] J. G. van der Corput, Zahlentheoretische Abschätzungen, *Math. Annalen* 84 (1921) 53–70.
[2] E. Landau, *Vorlesungen über Zahlentheorie*, v. 2, Verlag von S. Hirzel, 1927, p. 60.
[3] E. C. Titchmarsh, On van der Corput's method and the zeta-function of Riemann, *Quart. J. Math.* 2 (1932) 161–173.
[4] R. Kershner, Determination of a van der Corput-Landau absolute constant, *Amer. J. Math.* 57 (1935) 840–846.

[5] R. Kershner, Determination of a van der Corput absolute constant, *Amer. J. Math.* 60 (1938) 549–554.

3.16 Turán's Power Sum Constants

For fixed complex numbers $z_1, z_2, \ldots, z_n$, define [1]

$$S(z) = \max_{1 \leq k \leq n} \left| \sum_{j=1}^{n} z_j^k \right|$$

to be the maximum modulus of power sums of degree $\leq n$. Define also the $(n-1)$-dimensional complex region

$$K_n = \left\{ z \in \mathbb{C}^n : z_1 = 1 \text{ and } |z_j| \leq 1 \text{ for } 2 \leq j \leq n \right\}.$$

Consider the problem of minimizing $S(z)$ subject to $z \in K_n$. The optimal value σ_n of $S(z)$ is [2–4]

$$\frac{\sqrt{5}-1}{\sqrt{2}} = 0.8740320488\ldots \text{ if } n = 2, \text{ and } x = 0.8247830309\ldots \text{ if } n = 3,$$

where x has minimal polynomial [5]

$$x^{30} - 81x^{28} + 2613x^{26} - 43629x^{24} + 417429x^{22} - 2450985x^{20} + 9516137x^{18}$$
$$- 26203659x^{16} + 53016480x^{14} - 83714418x^{12} + 112601340x^{10} - 140002992x^{8}$$
$$+ 156204288x^{6} - 124361568x^{4} + 55427328x^{2} - 10077696.$$

Exact values of σ_n for $n \geq 4$ are not known, but we have bounds $0.3579 < \sigma_n < 1 - (250n)^{-1}$ for all sufficiently large n [1, 6, 7]. It is conjectured that $\lim_{n \to \infty} \sigma_n$ exists, but no one has numerically explored this issue, as far as is known.

Define instead [1, 8]

$$T(z) = \max_{2 \leq k \leq n+1} \left| \sum_{j=1}^{n} z_j^k \right|$$

and consider the problem of minimizing $T(z)$ subject to $z \in K_n$. The minimum value τ_n of $T(z)$ surprisingly satisfies $\tau_n < 1.321^{-n}$ for all sufficiently large n. This is very different behavior from that of σ_n. If we replace the exponent range $2 \leq k \leq n+1$ by $3 \leq k \leq n+2$, then the constant 1.321 can be replaced by 1.473.

Turán's book [1] is a gold mine of related theory and applications.

[1] P. Turán, *Über eine neue Methode der Analysis und ihre Anwendungen*, Akadémiai Kiadó, 1953 (original ed.); *On a New Method of Analysis and Its Applications*, Wiley, 1984 (revised ed.); MR 15,688c and MR 86b:11059.

[2] J. Lawrynowicz, Remark on a problem of P. Turán, *Bull. Soc. Sci. Lettres Lódz*, v. 11 (1960) n. 1, 1–4; MR 23 #3959.

[3] J. Lawrynowicz, Calculation of a minimum maximorum of complex numbers, *Bull. Soc.Sci. Lettres Lódz*, v. 11 (1960) n. 2, 1–9; MR 23 #3958.

[4] J. Lawrynowicz, Remark on power-sums of complex numbers, *Acta Math. Acad. Sci. Hungar.* 18 (1967) 279–281; MR 36 #379.

[5] P. Sebah, Minimal polynomial for Turán's constant, unpublished note (2000).

[6] F. V. Atkinson, Some further estimates concerning sums of powers of complex numbers, *Acta Math. Acad. Sci. Hungar.* 20 (1969) 193–210; MR 39 #443.

[7] J. Komlós, A. Sárkozy, and E. Szemerédi, On sums of powers of complex numbers (in Hungarian), *Mat. Lapok* 15 (1964) 337–347; MR 34 #2534.

[8] E. Makai, An estimation in the theory of diophantine approximations, *Acta Math. Acad. Sci. Hungar.* 9 (1958) 299–307; MR 21 #1293.

4

Constants Associated with the Approximation of Functions

4.1 Gibbs–Wilbraham Constant

Let f be a piecewise smooth function defined on the half-open interval $[-\pi, \pi)$, extended to the real line via periodicity, and possessing at most finitely many discontinuities (all finite jumps). Let

$$a_k = \frac{1}{\pi} \int_{-\pi}^{\pi} f(t) \cos(kt)\, dt, \quad b_k = \frac{1}{\pi} \int_{-\pi}^{\pi} f(t) \sin(kt)\, dt$$

denote the Fourier coefficients of f and let

$$S_n(f, x) = \frac{a_0}{2} + \sum_{k=1}^{n} (a_k \cos(kx) + b_k \sin(kx))$$

be the nth partial sum of the Fourier series of f. Let $x = c$ denote one of the discontinuities. Define

$$\delta = \left(\lim_{x \to c^-} f(x) \right) - \left(\lim_{x \to c^+} f(x) \right), \quad \mu = \frac{1}{2} \left[\left(\lim_{x \to c^-} f(x) \right) + \left(\lim_{x \to c^+} f(x) \right) \right]$$

and assume without loss of generality that $\delta > 0$. Let $x_n < c$ denote the first local maximum of $S_n(f, x)$ to the left of c, and let $\xi_n > c$ denote the first local minimum of $S_n(f, x)$ to the right of c. Then

$$\lim_{n \to \infty} S_n(f, x_n) = \mu + \frac{\delta}{\pi} G, \quad \lim_{n \to \infty} S_n(f, \xi_n) = \mu - \frac{\delta}{\pi} G,$$

where

$$G = \int_{0}^{\pi} \frac{\sin(\theta)}{\theta}\, d\theta = \sum_{n=0}^{\infty} \frac{(-1)^n \pi^{2n+1}}{(2n + 1)(2n + 1)!} = 1.8519370519\ldots$$

$$= \frac{\pi}{2}(1.1789797444\ldots)$$

is the **Gibbs–Wilbraham constant** [1–5].

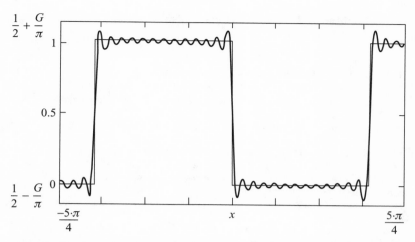

Figure 4.1. The Fourier series approximation of a square wave exhibits both overshooting and undershooting.

Consider the graph in Figure 4.1, with $f(x) = 1$ for $-\pi \leq x < 0$ and $f(x) = 0$ for $0 \leq x < \pi$. The limiting crest of the highest oscillation converges not to 1 but to $1/2 + G/\pi = 1.0894898722\ldots$. Similarly, the deepest trough converges not to 0 but to $1/2 - G/\pi = -0.0894898722\ldots$. In words, the Gibbs–Wilbraham constant quantifies the degree to which the Fourier series of a function overshoots or undershoots the function value at a jump discontinuity.

These phenomena were first observed by Wilbraham [6] and Gibbs [7]. Bôcher [8] generalized such observations to arbitrary functions f.

More generally, if $x_{n,2r-1} < c$ denotes the rth local maximum of $S_n(f, x)$ to the left of c, if $x_{n,2r} < c$ denotes the rth local minimum to the left of c, and if likewise for $\xi_{n,2r}$ and $\xi_{n,2r-1}$, then

$$\lim_{n \to \infty} S_n(f, x_{n,s}) = \mu + \frac{\delta}{\pi} \int_0^{s\pi} \frac{\sin(\theta)}{\theta}\, d\theta, \quad \lim_{n \to \infty} S_n(f, \xi_{n,s}) = \mu - \frac{\delta}{\pi} \int_0^{s\pi} \frac{\sin(\theta)}{\theta}\, d\theta.$$

The sine integral decreases to $\pi/2$ for increasing integer values of $s = 2r - 1$, but it increases to $\pi/2$ for $s = 2r$. For large enough r, the limiting values become $\mu \pm \delta/2$, which is consistent with intuition.

Fourier series are best L_2 (least-squares) trigonometric polynomial fits; Gibbs–Wilbraham phenomena appear in connection with splines [5, 9–11], wavelets [5, 12], and generalized Padé approximants [13] as well. Hence there are many Gibbs–Wilbraham constants! Moskona, Petrushev & Saff [5, 14] studied best L_1 trigonometric polynomial fits and determined the analog of $2G/\pi - 1 = 0.1789797444\ldots$ in this setting; its value is $\max_{x \geq 1} g(x) = 0.0657838882\ldots$, where

$$g(x) = -\frac{\sin(\pi x)}{\pi} \int_0^1 t^{x-1} \frac{1-t}{1+t}\, dt = -\frac{\sin(\pi x)}{\pi x} \sum_{k=1}^{\infty} \frac{k! \cdot 2^{-k}}{(x+1)(x+2) \cdots (x+k)}$$

for $x > 0$. The case of L_p approximation, where $1 < p \neq 2$, was investigated only recently [15].

[1] T. H. Gronwall, Über die Gibbssche Erscheinung und die trigonometrischen Summen $\sin(x) + \frac{1}{2}\sin(2x) + \cdots + \frac{1}{n}\sin(nx)$, *Math. Annalen* 72 (1912) 228–243.
[2] H. S. Carslaw, *Introduction to the Theory of Fourier's Series and Integrals*, 3rd ed., Dover, 1930.
[3] A. G. Zygmund, *Trigonometric Series*, v. 1, 2nd ed., Cambridge Univ. Press, 1959; MR 89c:42001.
[4] E. Hewitt and R. E. Hewitt, The Gibbs-Wilbraham phenomenon: An episode in Fourier analysis, *Arch. Hist. Exact Sci.* 21 (1979) 129–160; MR 81g:01015.
[5] A. J. Jerri, *The Gibbs Phenomenon in Fourier Analysis, Splines and Wavelet Approximations*, Kluwer, 1998; MR 99i:42001.
[6] H. Wilbraham, On a certain periodic function, *Cambridge and Dublin Math. J.* 3 (1848) 198–201.
[7] J. W. Gibbs, Fourier's series, *Nature* 59 (1898) 200 and 59 (1899) 606; also in *Collected Works*, v. 2, ed. H. A. Bumstead and R. G. Van Name, Longmans and Green, 1931, pp. 258–260.
[8] M. Bôcher, Introduction to the theory of Fourier's series, *Annals of Math.* 7 (1906) 81–152.
[9] J. Foster and F. B. Richards, The Gibbs phenomenon for piecewise-linear approximation, *Amer. Math. Monthly* 98 (1991) 47–49; MR 91m:41037.
[10] F. B. Richards, A Gibbs phenomenon for spline functions, *J. Approx. Theory* 66 (1991) 334–351; MR 92h:41025.
[11] J. Foster and F. B. Richards, Gibbs-Wilbraham splines, *Constr. Approx.* 11 (1995) 37–52; MR 96b:41018.
[12] S. E. Kelly, Gibbs phenomenon for wavelets, *Appl. Comput. Harmon. Anal.* 3 (1996) 72–81; MR 97f:42056.
[13] G. Németh and G. Páris, The Gibbs phenomenon in generalized Padé approximation, *J. Math. Phys.* 26 (1985) 1175–1178; MR 87a:41021.
[14] E. Moskona, P. Petrushev, and E. B. Saff, The Gibbs phenomenon for best L_1-trigonometric polynomial approximation. *Constr. Approx.* 11 (1995) 391–416; MR 96f: 42004.
[15] E. B. Saff and S. Tashev, Gibbs phenomenon for best L_p approximation by polygonal lines, *East J. Approx.* 5 (1999) 235–251; MR 2000i:41025.

4.2 Lebesgue Constants

4.2.1 Trigonometric Fourier Series

If a function f is integrable over the interval $[-\pi, \pi]$, let

$$a_k = \frac{1}{\pi} \int_{-\pi}^{\pi} f(t) \cos(kt)\,dt, \quad b_k = \frac{1}{\pi} \int_{-\pi}^{\pi} f(t) \sin(kt)\,dt$$

denote the Fourier coefficients of f and let

$$S_n(f, x) = \frac{a_0}{2} + \sum_{k=1}^{n} (a_k \cos(kx) + b_k \sin(kx))$$

be the nth partial sum of the Fourier series of f. Assuming further that $|f(x)| \leq 1$ for all x, it follows that

$$|S_n(f, x)| \leq \frac{1}{\pi} \int_0^\pi \frac{|\sin(\frac{2n+1}{2}\theta)|}{\sin(\frac{\theta}{2})} \, d\theta = L_n$$

for all x, where L_n is the nth **Lebesgue constant** [1,2]. The values of the first several Lebesgue constants are

$$L_0 = 1, \ L_1 = \tfrac{1}{3} + \tfrac{2\sqrt{3}}{\pi} = 1.4359911241\ldots, \ L_2 = 1.6421884352\ldots,$$

$$L_3 = 1.7783228615\ldots.$$

Several alternative formulas are due to Fejér [3,4] and Szegö [5]:

$$L_n = \frac{1}{2n+1} + \frac{2}{\pi} \sum_{k=1}^n \frac{1}{k} \tan\left(\frac{\pi k}{2n+1}\right) = \frac{16}{\pi^2} \sum_{k=1}^\infty \sum_{j=1}^{(2n+1)k} \frac{1}{4k^2 - 1} \frac{1}{2j-1}$$

The latter expression demonstrates that $\{L_n\}$ is monotonically increasing.

The Lebesgue constants are the best possible, in the sense that $L_n = \sup_f |S_n(f, 0)|$ and the supremum is taken over all continuous f satisfying $|f(x)| \leq 1$ for all x. It can be easily shown [6,7] that

$$\frac{4}{\pi^2} \ln(n) < L_n < 3 + \frac{4}{\pi^2} \ln(n).$$

This implies that $L_n \to \infty$ and, consequently, the Fourier series for f can be unbounded even if f is continuous [8–10]. It also implies that if the **modulus of continuity** of f,

$$\omega(f, \delta) = \sup_{|x-y|<\delta} |f(x) - f(y)|,$$

satisfies $\lim_{\delta \to 0} \omega(f, \delta) \ln(\delta) = 0$, then the Fourier series for f converges uniformly to f. This is known as the Dini–Lipschitz theorem [2,7]. In words, while mere continuity is not enough, continuity *plus* additional conditions (e.g., differentiability) ensure uniform convergence.

Much greater precision in estimating the Lebesgue constants is possible. Watson [11] proved that

$$\lim_{n \to \infty} \left(L_n - \frac{4}{\pi^2} \ln(2n+1) \right) = c,$$

where

$$c = \frac{8}{\pi^2} \left(\sum_{k=1}^\infty \frac{\ln(k)}{4k^2 - 1} \right) - \frac{4}{\pi^2} \psi(\tfrac{1}{2})$$

$$= \frac{8}{\pi^2} \left(\sum_{j=0}^\infty \frac{\lambda(2j+2) - 1}{2j+1} \right) + \frac{4}{\pi^2}(2\ln(2) + \gamma)$$

$$= 0.9894312738\ldots = \frac{4}{\pi^2}(2.4413238136\ldots),$$

γ is the Euler–Mascheroni constant [1.5], $\psi(x)$ is the digamma function [1.5.4], and $\lambda(x)$ appears in [1.7]. Higher-order coefficients in the asymptotic expansion of L_n can be written as finite combinations of Bernoulli numbers [1.6.1]. Galkin [12] further proved that

$$L_n - \frac{4}{\pi^2} \ln(2n+1) \text{ decreases to } c, \text{ whereas } L_n - \frac{4}{\pi^2} \ln(2n+2) \text{ increases to } c$$

as $n \to \infty$. More asymptotics appear in [13, 14]. We mention two integral formulas discovered by Hardy [15]:

$$L_n = 4 \int_0^\infty \frac{\tanh((2n+1)x)}{\tanh(x)} \frac{1}{\pi^2 + 4x^2} dx$$

$$= \frac{4}{\pi^2} \int_0^\infty \frac{\sinh((2n+1)x)}{\sinh(x)} \ln\left(\coth\left(\frac{2n+1}{2}x\right)\right) dx.$$

See a related discussion in our essay on Favard constants [4.3].

There are many possible extensions of L_n; it is interesting to ascertain which properties for Fourier series carry over to the case in question. For example, the monotonicity of Lebesgue constants for Legendre series has been proved [16], confirming a conjecture of Szegö.

Here is a related idea. If f is complex analytic inside the unit disk, continuous on the boundary, and $|f(z)| < 1$ for all $|z| < 1$, then [17]

$$f(z) = \sum_{k=0}^\infty a_k z^k \text{ implies that } \left| \sum_{k=0}^n a_k \right| \le G_n,$$

where

$$G_n = \sum_{m=0}^n \frac{1}{2^{4m}} \binom{2m}{m}^2 = 1 + \left(\frac{1}{2}\right)^2 + \left(\frac{1 \cdot 3}{2 \cdot 4}\right)^2 + \cdots + \left(\frac{1 \cdot 3 \cdots (2n-1)}{2 \cdot 4 \cdots (2n)}\right)^2$$

is the nth **Landau constant** (note the similarity with [1.5.4]). The constant G_n is the best possible for each n. It is known that [11]

$$\lim_{n \to \infty} \left(G_n - \frac{1}{\pi} \ln(n+1) \right) = \frac{1}{\pi}(4 \ln(2) + \gamma) = 1.0662758532\ldots,$$

$$G_{2n} \le L_n < \frac{4}{\pi} G_{2n},$$

and both sequences $\{G_n\}$ and $\{L_n/G_{2n}\}$ are monotonically increasing. More refinements are found in [18–21].

4.2.2 Lagrange Interpolation

Here is a different sense in which the same phrase "Lebesgue constants" is used. Given real-valued data $X = \{x_1, x_2, \ldots, x_n\}$, $Y = \{y_1, y_2, \ldots, y_n\}$ with $-1 \le x_1 < x_2 < \ldots <$

$x_n \leq 1$, there is a unique polynomial $p_{X,Y}(x)$ of degree at most $n - 1$ such that

$$p_{X,Y}(x_i) = y_i, \quad i = 1, 2, \ldots, n,$$

called the **Lagrange interpolating polynomial**, given X and Y. The formula for $p_{X,Y}(x)$ is

$$p_{X,Y}(x) = \sum_{k=1}^{n} \left(y_k \cdot \prod_{j \neq k} \frac{x - x_j}{x_k - x_j} \right).$$

We wish to understand the approximating power of interpolating polynomials as the spatial arrangement of $\{x_i\}$ varies or as n increases [6, 22]. The expression

$$\Lambda_n(X) = \max_{-1 \leq x \leq 1} \sum_{k=1}^{n} \left| \prod_{j \neq k} \frac{x - x_j}{x_k - x_j} \right|$$

is useful for this purpose and is called the nth **Lebesgue constant** corresponding to X. Note that Λ_n does not depend on Y. It can be easily shown that

$$\Lambda_n > \frac{4}{\pi^2} \ln(n) - 1$$

for all n and hence $\lim_{n \to \infty} \Lambda_n = \infty$, regardless of the choice of X. This means that, given any X, there exists a continuous function f such that $p_{X,f(X)}(x)$ does *not* converge uniformly to f as n increases. In words, there is no "universal" set X guaranteeing uniform convergence for all continuous functions f.

Erdös [23] further tightened the lower bound on the Lebesgue constants. He proved that there must exist a constant C such that

$$\Lambda_n > \frac{2}{\pi} \ln(n) - C$$

for all n, for arbitrary X. We will exhibit the smallest possible value of C shortly. Erdös' result cannot be improved because, if T consists of the n zeros

$$x_j = -\cos\left(\frac{(2j - 1)\pi}{2n} \right) \quad j = 1, 2, \ldots, n,$$

of the nth Chebyshev polynomial [4.9], then

$$\Lambda_n(T) = \frac{1}{n} \sum_{j=1}^{n} \cot\left(\frac{(2j - 1)\pi}{4n} \right) \leq \frac{2}{\pi} \ln(n) + 1.$$

In fact, $\{\Lambda_n(T) - \frac{2}{\pi} \ln(n)\}$ is monotonically decreasing with [24–26]

$$\lim_{n \to \infty} \left(\Lambda_n(T) - \frac{2}{\pi} \ln(n) \right) = \frac{2}{\pi}(3 \ln(2) - \ln(\pi) + \gamma) = 0.9625228267\ldots.$$

A complete asymptotic expansion (again involving Bernoulli numbers) was obtained in [27–30].

What is the optimal set X^* for which Λ_n is smallest [22]? Certainly the Chebyshev zeros are a good candidate for X^* but it can be shown that other choices of X will do even better. Kilgore [31] and de Boor & Pinkus [32] proved Bernstein's equioscillatory conjecture [33] regarding such X^*. A more precise, analytical description of X^* is not known.

A less hopeless problem is to estimate $\Lambda_n^* = \Lambda_n(X^*)$. Vértesi [34–36], building upon the work of Erdös [23], proved that

$$\lim_{n \to \infty} \left(\Lambda_n^* - \frac{2}{\pi} \ln(n) \right) = \frac{2}{\pi}(2\ln(2) - \ln(\pi) + \gamma) = 0.5212516264\ldots$$

This resolves the identity of C, but higher-order asymptotics and monotonicity issues remain open.

[1] H. Lebesgue, Sur la représentation trigonométrique approchée des fonctions satisfaisant à une condition de Lipschitz, *Bull. Soc. Math. France* 38 (1910) 184–210; also in *Oeuvres Scientifiques*, v. 3, L'Enseignement Math., 1972, pp. 363–389.

[2] A. G. Zygmund, *Trigonometric Series,* v. 1, 2nd ed., Cambridge Univ. Press, 1959; MR 89c:42001.

[3] L. Fejér, Sur les singularités de la série de Fourier des fonctions continues, *Annales Sci. École Norm. Sup.* 28 (1911) 64–103; also in *Gesammelte Arbeiten*, v. 1, Birkhäuser, 1970, pp. 654–689.

[4] L. Carlitz, Note on Lebesgue's constants, *Proc. Amer. Math. Soc.* 12 (1961) 932–935; MR 24 #A2791.

[5] G. Szegö, Über die Lebesgueschen Konstanten bei den Fourierschen Reihen, *Math. Z.* 9 (1921) 163–166; also in *Collected Papers*, v. 1, ed. R. Askey, Birkhäuser, 1982, pp. 307–313.

[6] T. J. Rivlin, *An Introduction to the Approximation of Functions*, Blaisdell, 1969; MR 83b:41001.

[7] E. W. Cheney, *Introduction to Approximation Theory*, McGraw-Hill, 1966; MR 99f:41001.

[8] R. L. Wheeden and A. G. Zygmund, *Measure and Integral: An Introduction to Real Analysis*, Dekker, 1977, pp. 222–229; MR 58 #11295.

[9] V. M. Tikhomirov, Approximation theory, *Analysis II*, ed. R. V. Gamkrelidze, Springer-Verlag, 1990, pp. 93–255; MR 91e:00001.

[10] N. Korneichuk, *Exact Constants in Approximation Theory*, Cambridge Univ. Press, 1991; MR 92m:41002.

[11] G. N. Watson, The constants of Landau and Lebesgue, *Quart. J. Math.* 1 (1930) 310–318.

[12] P. V. Galkin, Estimates for Lebesgue constants (in Russian), *Trudy Mat. Inst. Steklov.* 109 (1971) 3–5; Engl. transl. in *Proc. Steklov Inst. Math.* 109 (1971) 1–4; MR 46 #2338.

[13] L. Lorch, On Fejér's calculation of the Lebesgue constants, *Bull. Calcutta Math. Soc.* 37 (1945) 5–8; MR 7,59f.

[14] L. Lorch, The principal term in the asymptotic expansion of the Lebesgue constants, *Amer. Math. Monthly* 61 (1954) 245–249; MR 15,788d.

[15] G. H. Hardy, Note on Lebesgue's constants in the theory of Fourier series, *J. London Math. Soc.* 17 (1942) 4–13; also in *Collected Papers*, v. 3, Oxford Univ. Press, 1966, pp. 89–98; MR 4,36f.

[16] C. K. Qu and R. Wong, Szegö's conjecture on Lebesgue constants for Legendre series, *Pacific J. Math.* 135 (1988) 157–188; MR 89m:42025.

[17] E. Landau, Abschätzung der Koeffizientensumme einer Potenzreihe, *Archiv Math. Phys.* 21 (1913) 42–50, 250–255; also in *Collected Works*, v. 5–6, ed. L. Mirsky, I. J. Schoenberg, W. Schwarz, and H. Wefelscheid, Thales Verlag, 1985, pp. 432–440, 11–16.

[18] L. Brutman, A sharp estimate of the Landau constants, *J. Approx. Theory* 34 (1982) 217–220; MR 84m:41058.

[19] L. P. Falaleev, Inequalities for the Landau constants (in Russian), *Sibirskii Mat. Z.* 32 (1991) 194–195; Engl. transl. in *Siberian Math. J.* 32 (1992) 896–897; MR 93c:30001.

[20] J. E. Wilkins, The Landau constants, *Progress in Approximation Theory*, Proc. 1990 Tampa conf., ed. A. A. Gonchar and E. B. Saff, Academic Press, 1991, pp. 829–842; MR 92k:41045.

[21] D. Cvijovic and J. Klinowski, Inequalities for the Landau constants, *Math. Slovaca* 50 (2000) 159–164; MR 2001e:11125.

[22] L. Brutman, Lebesgue functions for polynomial interpolation – A survey, *Annals of Numer. Math.* 4 (1997) 111–127; MR 97m:41003.

[23] P. Erdös, Problems and results on the theory of interpolation. II, *Acta Math. Acad. Sci. Hungar.* 12 (1961) 235–244; MR 26 #2779.

[24] F. W. Luttmann and T. J. Rivlin, Some numerical experiments in the theory of polynomial interpolation, *IBM J. Res. Develop.* 9 (1965) 187–191; MR 31 #4147.

[25] H. Ehlich and K. Zeller, Auswertung der Normen von Interpolationsoperatoren, *Math. Annalen* 164 (1966) 105–112; MR 33 #3005.

[26] T. J. Rivlin, The Lebesgue constants for polynomial interpolation, *Functional Analysis and Its Applications*, Proc. 1973 Madras conf., ed. H. G. Garnir, K. R. Unni, and J. H. Williamson, Lect. Notes in Math. 399, Springer-Verlag, 1974, pp. 422–437; MR 53 #3549.

[27] R. Günttner, Evaluation of Lebesgue constants, *SIAM J. Numer. Anal.* 17 (1980) 512–520; MR 81i:41003.

[28] A. K. Pokalo and L. I. Sloma, On a representation of the Lebesgue constant by an asymptotic series (in Russian), *Dokl. Akad. Nauk BSSR* 25 (1981) 204–205, 284; MR 82i:41036.

[29] P. N. Shivakumar and R. Wong, Asymptotic expansion of the Lebesgue constants associated with polynomial interpolation, *Math. Comp.* 39 (1982) 195–200; MR 83i:41006.

[30] V. K. Dzjadik and V. V. Ivanov, On asymptotics and estimates for the uniform norms of the Lagrange interpolation polynomials corresponding to the Chebyshev nodal points, *Anal. Math.* 9 (1983) 85–97; MR 85d:41001.

[31] T. A. Kilgore, A characterization of the Lagrange interpolating projection with minimal Tchebyceff norm, *J. Approx. Theory* 24 (1978) 273–288; MR 80d:41002.

[32] C. de Boor and A. Pinkus, Proof of the conjectures of Bernstein and Erdös concerning the optimal nodes for polynomial interpolation, *J. Approx. Theory* 24 (1978) 289–303; MR 80d:41003.

[33] S. N. Bernstein, Sur la limitation des valeurs d'un polynome $P_n(x)$ de degré n sur tout un segment par ses valeurs en $n + 1$ points du segment, *Izv. Akad. Nauk SSSR* 8 (1931) 1025–1050; Russian transl. in *Collected Works*, v. 2, *Constructive Theory of Functions (1931–1953)*, Izdat. Akad. Nauk SSSR, 1954, pp. 107–126; MR 16,433o.

[34] P. Vértesi, On the optimal Lebesgue constants for polynomial interpolation, *Acta Math. Hungar.* 47 (1986) 165–178; MR 87i:41005.

[35] P. Vértesi, Optimal Lebesgue constant for Lagrange interpolation, *SIAM J. Numer. Anal.* 27 (1990) 1322–1331; MR 91k:41010.

[36] R. Günttner, Note on the lower estimate of optimal Lebesgue constants, *Acta Math. Hungar.* 65 (1994) 313–317; MR 95d:41051.

4.3 Achieser–Krein–Favard Constants

In this essay, we presuppose knowledge of the Lebesgue constants L_n [4.2]. Assume a function f to be integrable over the interval $[-\pi, \pi]$ and $S_n(f, x)$ to be the nth partial sum of the Fourier series of f. If $|f(x)| \leq 1$ for all x, then we know that

$$|S_n(f, x)| \leq L_n = \frac{4}{\pi^2} \ln(n) + O(1)$$

and, moreover, L_n is best possible (it is a maximum). If we restrict attention to continuous functions f, that is, a subclass of the integrable functions, then L_n is still best possible (although it is only a supremum).

This may be considered as an extreme case ($r = 0$) of the following result due to Kolmogorov [1–3]. Fix an integer $r \geq 1$. If a function f is r-times differentiable and satisfies $|f^{(r)}(x)| \leq 1$ for all x, then

$$|f(x) - S_n(f, x)| \leq L_{n,r} = \frac{4}{\pi^2} \frac{\ln(n)}{n^r} + O\left(\frac{1}{n^r}\right),$$

where

$$L_{n,r} = \begin{cases} \dfrac{1}{\pi} \displaystyle\int_{-\pi}^{\pi} \left| \sum_{k=n+1}^{\infty} \frac{\sin(k\theta)}{k^r} \right| d\theta & \text{if } r \geq 1 \text{ is odd,} \\[4mm] \dfrac{1}{\pi} \displaystyle\int_{-\pi}^{\pi} \left| \sum_{k=n+1}^{\infty} \frac{\cos(k\theta)}{k^r} \right| d\theta & \text{if } r \geq 2 \text{ is even} \end{cases}$$

is best possible.

All this is a somewhat roundabout way for introducing the **Achieser–Krein–Favard constants**, which are often simply called **Favard constants**. In the preceding, we focused solely on the quality of the Fourier estimate $S_n(f, x)$ of f. Suppose we replace $S_n(f, x)$ by an arbitrary trigonometric polynomial

$$P_n(x) = \frac{a_0}{2} + \sum_{k=1}^{n} (a_k \cos(kx) + b_k \sin(kx)),$$

where no conditions are placed on the coefficients (apart from being real). If, as before, the rth derivative of f is bounded between -1 and 1, then there *exists* a polynomial $P_n(x)$ for which

$$|f(x) - P_n(x)| \leq \frac{K_r}{(n+1)^r}$$

for all x, where the rth Favard constant [4–6]

$$K_r = \frac{4}{\pi} \sum_{j=0}^{\infty} \left[\frac{(-1)^j}{2j+1} \right]^{r+1}$$

is the smallest numerator possible. In other words, whereas Lebesgue constants are connected to approximations that are best in a least-squares sense (Fourier series), Favard constants are connected to approximations that are best in a pointwise sense.

Observe that

$$K_r = \begin{cases} \dfrac{4}{\pi} \lambda(r+1) & \text{if } r \text{ is odd,} \\[3mm] \dfrac{4}{\pi} \beta(r+1) & \text{if } r \text{ is even,} \end{cases}$$

where both the lambda and beta functions are discussed in [1.7]. Each Favard constant is hence a rational multiple of π^r, for example,

$$K_0 = 1, \quad K_1 = \frac{\pi}{2}, \quad K_2 = \frac{\pi^2}{8}, \quad K_3 = \frac{\pi^3}{24},$$

and $1 = K_0 < K_2 < \ldots < 4/\pi < \ldots < K_3 < K_1 = \pi/2$.

This is the first of many sharp results for various classes of functions and methods of approximation that involve the constants K_r. The theorems are rather technical and so will not be discussed here. We mention, however, the Bohr–Favard inequality [7–9] and the Landau–Kolmogorov constants [3.3]. See also [10, 11].

Here is an unsolved problem. For an arbitrary trigonometric polynomial $P_n(\theta)$, it is known that [12, 13]

$$\max_{-\pi \leq \theta \leq \pi} |P_n(\theta)| \leq C \frac{n}{2\pi} \int_{-\pi}^{\pi} |P_n(\theta)| \, d\theta,$$

and the best possible constant asymptotically satisfies $0.539 \leq C \leq 0.58$ as $n \to \infty$. An exact expression for C is not known.

[1] A. N. Kolmogorov, Zur Grössenordnung des Restgliedes Fourierscher reihen differenzierbarer Funktionen, *Annals of Math.* 36 (1935) 521–526; Engl. transl. in *Selected Works*, v. 1., ed. V. M. Tikhomirov, Kluwer, 1991, pp. 196–201; MR 93d:01096.

[2] S. Nikolsky, Approximations of periodic functions by trigonometrical polynomials (in Russian), *Travaux Inst. Math. Stekloff* 15 (1945) 1–76; MR 7,435c.

[3] A. G. Zygmund, *Trigonometric Series*, v. 1, 2nd ed., Cambridge Univ. Press, 1959; MR 89c:42001.

[4] J. Favard, Sur les meilleurs procédés d'approximation de certaines classes de fonctions par des polynomes trigonométriques, *Bull. Sci. Math.* 61 (1937) 209–224, 243–256.

[5] N. Achieser and M. Krein, Sur la meilleure approximation des fonctions périodiques dérivables au moyen de sommes trigonométriques, *C. R. (Dokl.) Acad. Sci. URSS* 15 (1937) 107–111.

[6] N. I. Achieser, *Theory of Approximation*, F. Ungar, 1956, pp. 187–199, 300–301; MR 3,234d and MR 10,33b.

[7] V. M. Tikhomirov, Approximation theory, *Analysis II*, ed. R. V. Gamkrelidze, Springer-Verlag, 1990, pp. 93–255; MR 91e:00001.

[8] D. S. Mitrinovic, J. E. Pecaric, and A. M. Fink, *Inequalities Involving Functions and Their Integrals and Derivatives*, Kluwer, 1991; MR 93m:26036.

[9] N. Korneichuk, *Exact Constants in Approximation Theory*, Cambridge Univ. Press, 1991; MR 92m:41002.

[10] B. C. Yang and Y. H. Zhu, Inequalities for the Hurwitz zeta-function on the real axis (in Chinese), *Acta Sci. Natur. Univ. Sunyatseni*, v. 36 (1997) n. 3, 30–35; MR 99h: 11101.

[11] B. C. Yang and K. Wu, Inequalities for Favard's constant (in Chinese), *J. South China Normal Univ. Natur. Sci. Ed.* (1998) n. 1, 12–17; MR 2001a:11031.

[12] L. V. Taikov, A group of extremal problems for trigonometric polynomials (in Russian), *Uspekhi Mat. Nauk*, v. 20 (1965) n. 3, 205–211; MR 32 #2829.

[13] G. V. Milovanovic, D. S. Mitrinovic, and T. M. Rassias, *Topics in Polynomials: Extremal Problems, Inequalities, Zeros*, World Scientific, 1994, pp. 495–496; MR 95m:30009.

4.4 Bernstein's Constant

For any real function $f(x)$ with domain $[-1, 1]$, let $E_n(f)$ denote the error of best uniform approximation to f by real polynomials of degree at most n. That is,

$$E_n(f) = \inf_{p \in P_n} \sup_{-1 \leq x \leq 1} |f(x) - p(x)|,$$

where $P_n = \{\sum_{k=0}^{n} a_k x^k : a_k \text{ real}\}$. Consider the special case $\alpha(x) = |x|$, for which Jackson's theorem [1,2] implies $E_n(\alpha) \leq 6/n$. Since $|x|$ is an even continuous function on $[-1, 1]$, then so is its (unique) best uniform approximation from P_n on $[-1, 1]$. It follows that $E_{2n}(\alpha) = E_{2n+1}(\alpha)$, so we consider only the even-subscript case henceforth. Bernstein [3] strengthened the Jackson inequality

$$2n E_{2n}(\alpha) \leq 6$$

to

$$2n E_{2n}(\alpha) \leq \frac{4n}{\pi(2n+1)} < \frac{2}{\pi} = 0.636\ldots$$

using Chebyshev polynomials [4.9]. He proved the existence of the following limit and obtained the indicated bounds:

$$0.278\ldots < \beta = \lim_{n \to \infty} 2n E_{2n}(\alpha) < 0.286\ldots.$$

Bernstein conjectured that $\beta = 1/(2\sqrt{\pi}) = 0.2821\ldots$. This conjecture remained unresolved for seventy years, owing to the difficulty in computing $E_{2n}(\alpha)$ for large n and to the slow convergence of $2n E_{2n}(\alpha)$ to β.

Varga & Carpenter [4, 5] computed $\beta = 0.2801694990\ldots$ to fifty decimal places, disproving Bernstein's conjecture. They required calculations of $2n E_{2n}(\alpha)$ up to $n = 52$ with accuracies of nearly 95 places and a number of other techniques. At the end of [4], they indicated that it is not implausible to believe that β might admit a closed-form expression in terms of the classical hypergeometric function or other known constants.

Since we have just discussed the problem of the best uniform *polynomial* approximation to $|x|$, it is natural to consider the problem of the best uniform *rational* approximation as well. Define, for arbitrary f on $[-1, 1]$,

$$E_{m,n}(f) = \inf_{r \in R_{m,n}} \sup_{-1 \leq x \leq 1} |f(x) - r(x)|,$$

where $R_{m,n} = \{p(x)/q(x) : p \in P_m, q \in P_n, q \neq 0\}$. Newman [6] proved that

$$\tfrac{1}{2} e^{-9\sqrt{n}} \leq E_{n,n}(\alpha) \leq 3 e^{-\sqrt{n}}, \quad n \geq 4,$$

equivalently, that $E_{n,n} \to 0$ incomparably faster than E_n. Newman's work created a sensation among researchers [5, 7]. Bulanov [8], extending results of Gonchar [9], proved that the lower bound could be improved to

$$e^{-\pi\sqrt{n+1}} \leq E_{n,n}(\alpha)$$

and Vjacheslavov [10] proved the existence of positive constants m and M such that

$$m \leq e^{\pi\sqrt{n}} E_{n,n}(\alpha) \leq M.$$

(Petrushev & Popov [7] remarked on the interesting juxtaposition of the constants e and π here in a seemingly unrelated setting.) As before, $E_{2n,2n}(\alpha) = E_{2n+1,2n+1}(\alpha)$, so we focus on the even-subscript case. Varga, Ruttan & Carpenter [11] conjectured, on the basis of careful computations, that

$$\lim_{n \to \infty} e^{\pi \sqrt{2n}} E_{2n,2n}(\alpha) = 8,$$

which Stahl [12, 13] recently proved. The contrast between the polynomial and rational cases is fascinating!

Gonchar [9] pointed out the relevance of Zolotarev's work [3.9] to this line of research.

[1] T. J. Rivlin, *An Introduction to the Approximation of Functions*, Blaisdell, 1969; MR 83b:41001.

[2] E. W. Cheney, *Introduction to Approximation Theory*, McGraw-Hill, 1966; MR 99f: 41001.

[3] S. N. Bernstein, Sur la meilleure approximation de |x| par les polynomes de degrés donnés, *Acta Math.* 37 (1913) 1–57; Russian transl. in *Collected Works*, v. 1, *Constructive Theory of Functions (1905–1930)*, Izdat. Akad. Nauk SSSR, 1952; MR 14,2c.

[4] R. S. Varga and A. J. Carpenter, A conjecture of S. Bernstein in approximation theory (in Russian), *Mat. Sbornik* 129 (1986) 535–548, 591–592; Engl. transl. in *Math. USSR Sbornik* 57 (1987) 547–560; MR 87g:41066.

[5] R. S. Varga, *Scientific Computation on Mathematical Problems and Conjectures*, SIAM, 1990; MR 92b:65012.

[6] D. J. Newman, Rational approximation to |x|, *Michigan Math. J.* 11 (1964) 11–14; MR 30 #1344.

[7] P. P. Petrushev and V. A. Popov, *Rational Approximation of Real Functions*, Cambridge Univ. Press, 1987; MR 89i:41022.

[8] A. P. Bulanov, Asymptotics for least deviations of |x| from rational functions (in Russian), *Mat. Sbornik* 76 (1968) 288–303; Engl. transl. in *Math. USSR Sbornik* 5 (1968) 275–290; MR 37 #4468.

[9] A. A. Gonchar, Estimates of the growth of rational functions and some of their applications (in Russian), *Mat. Sbornik* 72 (1967) 489–503; Engl. transl. in *Math. USSR Sbornik* 1 (1967) 445–456; MR 35 #4652.

[10] N. S. Vjacheslavov, The uniform approximation of |x| by rational functions (in Russian), *Dokl. Akad. Nauk SSSR* 220 (1975) 512–515; Engl. transl. in *Soviet Math. Dokl.* 16 (1975) 100–104; MR 52 #1114.

[11] R. S. Varga, A. Ruttan, and A. J. Carpenter, Numerical results on best uniform rational approximations to |x| on [−1, +1] (in Russian), *Mat. Sbornik* 182 (1991) 1523–1541; Engl. transl. in *Math. USSR Sbornik* 74 (1993) 271–290; MR 92i:65040.

[12] H. Stahl, Best uniform rational approximation of |x| on [−1, 1] (in Russian), *Mat. Sbornik* 183 (1992) 85–118; Engl. transl. in *Russian Acad. Sci. Sbornik Math.* 76 (1993) 461–487; MR 93i:41019.

[13] H. Stahl, Uniform rational approximation of |x|, *Methods of Approximation Theory in Complex Analysis and Mathematical Physics*, ed. A. A. Gonchar and E. B. Saff, Lect. Notes in Math. 1550, Springer-Verlag, 1993, pp. 110–130; MR 95m:41031.

4.5 The "One-Ninth" Constant

We are concerned here with the rational approximation of $\exp(-x)$ on the half-line $[0, \infty)$. Let $\lambda_{m,n}$ denote the error of best uniform approximation:

$$\lambda_{m,n} = \inf_{r \in R_{m,n}} \sup_{x \geq 0} |e^{-x} - r(x)|,$$

where $R_{m,n}$ is the set of real rational functions $p(x)/q(x)$ with $\deg(p) \leq m$, $\deg(q) \leq n$, and $q \neq 0$, as defined in [4.4].

There are two cases of special interest, when $m = 0$ and $m = n$, since clearly

$$0 < \lambda_{n,n} \leq \lambda_{n-1,n} \leq \lambda_{n-2,n} \leq \cdots \leq \lambda_{2,n} \leq \lambda_{1,n} \leq \lambda_{0,n}.$$

Many researchers [1–4] have studied these constants $\lambda_{m,n}$, referred to as **Chebyshev constants** in [4]. We mention the work of only a few. Schönhage [5] proved that

$$\lim_{n \to \infty} \lambda_{0,n}^{\frac{1}{n}} = \frac{1}{3},$$

which led several people to conjecture that

$$\lim_{n \to \infty} \lambda_{n,n}^{\frac{1}{n}} = \frac{1}{9}.$$

Numerical evidence uncovered by Schönhage [6] and Trefethen & Gutknecht [7] suggested that the conjecture is false. Carpenter, Ruttan & Varga [8] calculated the Chebyshev constants to an accuracy of 200 digits up to $n = 30$ and carefully obtained

$$\lim_{n \to \infty} \lambda_{n,n}^{\frac{1}{n}} = \frac{1}{9.2890254919\ldots} = 0.1076539192\ldots,$$

although a proof that the limit even *existed* was still to be found.

Building upon the work of Opitz & Scherer [9] and Magnus [10–12], Gonchar & Rakhmanov [4, 13] proved that the limit exists and that it equals

$$\Lambda = \exp\left(\frac{-\pi \; K(\sqrt{1 - c^2})}{K(c)}\right),$$

where $K(x)$ is the complete elliptic integral of the first kind [1.4.6] and the constant c is defined as follows. Let $E(x)$ be the complete elliptic integral of the second kind [1.4.6]; then $0 < c < 1$ is the unique solution of the equation $K(c) = 2E(c)$.

Gonchar and Rakhmanov's exact disproof of the "one-ninth" conjecture utilized ideas from complex potential theory, which seems far removed from the rational approximation of $\exp(-x)$! They also obtained a number-theoretic characterization of the "one-ninth" constant Λ. If

$$f(z) = \sum_{j=1}^{\infty} a_j z^j, \quad \text{where } a_j = \left|\sum_{d|j} (-1)^d d\right|,$$

then f is complex-analytic in the open unit disk. The unique positive root of the equation $f(z) = 1/8$ is the constant Λ. Another way of writing a_j is as follows [14]: If

$$j = 2^m p_1^{m_1} p_2^{m_2} \cdots p_k^{m_k}$$

is the prime factorization of the integer j, where $p_1 < p_2 < \ldots < p_k$ are odd primes, $m \geq 0$, and $m_i \geq 1$, then

$$a_j = |2^{m+1} - 3| \frac{p_1^{m_1+1} - 1}{p_1 - 1} \frac{p_2^{m_2+1} - 1}{p_2 - 1} \cdots \frac{p_k^{m_k+1} - 1}{p_k - 1}.$$

Carpenter [4] computed Λ to 101 digits using this equation.

Here is another expression due to Magnus [10]. The one-ninth constant Λ is the unique solution of the equation

$$\sum_{k=0}^{\infty}(2k+1)^2(-x)^{\frac{k(k+1)}{2}}=0, \quad 0 < x < 1,$$

which turns out to have been studied one hundred years earlier by Halphen [15]. Halphen was interested in theta functions and computed Λ to six digits, clearly unaware that this constant would become prominent a century later! Varga [4] suggested that Λ be renamed the Halphen constant. So many researchers have contributed to the solution of this approximation problem, however, that retaining the amusingly inaccurate "one-ninth" designation might be simplest.

The constant $c = 0.9089085575\ldots$ defining Λ arises in a completely unrelated field: the study of *Euler elasticae* [16–18]. A quotient of elliptic functions, similar to that discussed here, occurs in [7.8].

[1] W. J. Cody, G. Meinardus, and R. S. Varga, Chebyshev rational approximations to e^{-x} in $[0, +\infty)$ and applications to heat-conduction problems, *J. Approx. Theory* 2 (1969) 50–65; MR 39 #6536.

[2] R. S. Varga, *Topics in Polynomial and Rational Interpolation and Approximation*, Les Presses de l'Université de Montréal, 1982; MR 83h:30041.

[3] P. P. Petrushev and V. A. Popov, *Rational Approximation of Real Functions*, Cambridge Univ. Press, 1987; MR 89i:41022.

[4] R. S. Varga, *Scientific Computation on Mathematical Problems and Conjectures*, SIAM, 1990; MR 92b:65012.

[5] A. Schönhage, Zur rationalen Approximierbarkeit von e^{-x} über $[0, \infty)$, *J. Approx. Theory* 7 (1973) 395–398; MR 49 #3391.

[6] A. Schönhage, Rational approximation to e^{-x} and related L_2-problems, *SIAM J. Numer. Anal.* 19 (1982) 1067–1080; MR 83k:41016.

[7] L. N. Trefethen and M. H. Gutknecht, The Carathéodory-Fejér method for real rational approximation, *SIAM J. Numer. Anal.* 20 (1983) 420–436; MR 85g:41024.

[8] A. J. Carpenter, A. Ruttan, and R. S. Varga, Extended numerical computations on the "1/9" conjecture in rational approximation theory, *Rational Approximation and Interpolation*, ed. P. R. Graves-Morris, E. B. Saff, and R. S. Varga, Lect. Notes in Math. 1105, Springer-Verlag, 1984, pp. 383–411.

[9] H.-U. Opitz and K. Scherer, On the rational approximation of e^{-x} on $[0, \infty)$, *Constr. Approx.* 1 (1985) 195–216; MR 88f:41027.

[10] A. P. Magnus, On the use of the Carathéodory-Fejér method for investigating "1/9" and similar constants, *Nonlinear Numerical Methods and Rational Approximation*, ed. A. Cuyt, Reidel, 1988, pp. 105–132, MR 90j:65035.

[11] A. P. Magnus, Asymptotics and super asymptotics for best rational approximation error norms to the exponential function (the "1/9" problem) by the Carathéodory-Fejér method, *Nonlinear Numerical Methods and Rational Approximation II*, ed. A. Cuyt, Kluwer, 1994, pp. 173–185; MR 96b:41023.

[12] A. P. Magnus and J. Meinguet, The elliptic functions and integrals of the "1/9" problem, *Numer. Algorithms* 24 (2000) 117–139; MR 2001f:41017.

[13] A. A. Gonchar and E. A. Rakhmanov, Equilibrium distributions and degree of rational approximation of analytic functions (in Russian), *Mat. Sbornik* 134 (1987) 306–352, 447; Engl. transl. in *Math. USSR Sbornik* 62 (1989) 305–348; MR 89h:30054.

[14] A. A. Gonchar, Rational approximations of analytic functions (in Russian), *International Congress of Mathematicians*, v. 1, Proc. 1986 Berkeley conf., ed. A. M. Gleason, Amer.

Math. Soc., 1987, pp. 739–748; Engl. transl. in *Amer. Math. Soc. Transl.* 147 (1990) 25–34; MR 89e:30066.

[15]   G.-H. Halphen, *Traité des fonctions elliptiques et de leurs applications*, v. 1, Gauthier-Villars, 1886, p. 287.

[16]   D. A. Singer, Curves whose curvature depends on distance from the origin, *Amer. Math. Monthly* 106 (1999) 835–841; MR 2000j:53005.

[17]   T. A. Ivey and D. A. Singer, Knot types, homotopies and stability of closed elastic rods, *Proc. London Math. Soc.* 79 (1999) 429–450; MR 2000g:58015.

[18]   C. Truesdell, The influence of elasticity on analysis: The classic heritage, *Bull. Amer. Math. Soc.* 9 (1983) 293–310; MR 85f:01004.

4.6 Fransén–Robinson Constant

For increasing x, the **reciprocal gamma function** $1/\Gamma(x)$ decreases more rapidly than $\exp(-cx)$ for any constant c, and thus may be useful as a one-sided density function for certain probability models. As a consequence, the value

$$I = \int\limits_0^\infty \frac{1}{\Gamma(x)} dx = 2.8077702420\ldots$$

is needed for the sake of normalization.

One way to compute this integral is via the limit of Riemann sums I_n as $n \to \infty$, where [1]

$$I_n = \frac{1}{n} \sum_{k=1}^\infty \frac{1}{\Gamma(\frac{k}{n})} = \begin{cases} e = 2.7182818284\ldots & \text{if } n = 1, \\ \frac{1}{2}\left(\frac{1}{\sqrt{\pi}} + e\,\mathrm{erfc}(-1)\right) = 2.7865848321\ldots & \text{if } n = 2, \end{cases}$$

and

$$\mathrm{erf}(x) = \frac{2}{\sqrt{\pi}} \int\limits_0^x \exp(-t^2)dt = 1 - \mathrm{erfc}(x)$$

is the **error function**. This is, however, too slow a procedure for computing I to high precision.

Fransén [2] computed I to 65 decimal digits, using Euler–Maclaurin summation and the formula

$$\Gamma(x) = \frac{e^{-\gamma x}}{x} \prod_{n=1}^\infty \left(1 + \frac{x}{n}\right)^{-1} e^{\frac{x}{n}} = \frac{1}{x} \exp\left[\sum_{k=1}^\infty \frac{(-1)^k s_k}{k} x^k\right],$$

where $s_1 = \gamma$ and $s_k = \zeta(k)$, $k \geq 2$. Background on the Euler–Mascheroni constant γ appears in [1.5] and that on the Riemann zeta function $\zeta(z)$ in [1.6].

Robinson [2] independently obtained an estimate of I to 36 digits using an 11-point Newton–Coates approach. Fransén & Wrigge [3, 4], via Taylor series and other analytical tools, achieved 80 digits, and Johnson [5] subsequently achieved 300 decimal places.

Sebah [6] utilized the Clenshaw–Curtis method (based on Chebyshev polynomials) to compute the Fransén–Robinson constant to over 600 digits. He also noticed the elementary fact that

$$I = \int_1^2 \frac{f(x)}{\Gamma(x)} dx,$$

where $f(x)$ is defined by the fast converging series

$$f(x) = x + \sum_{k=0}^{\infty} \left(\prod_{j=0}^{k} \frac{1}{x+j} \right) = x + e \sum_{k=0}^{\infty} \frac{(-1)^k}{k!(x+k)}$$

and $f(1) = f(2) = e$, $f(3/2) = (1 + e\sqrt{\pi} \, \text{erf}(1))/2$. Using this, I is now known to 1025 digits.

Ramanujan [7, 8] observed that

$$\int_0^{\infty} \frac{w^x}{\Gamma(1+x)} dx = e^w - \int_{-\infty}^{\infty} \frac{\exp(-we^y)}{y^2 + \pi^2} dy,$$

which has value $2.2665345077\ldots$ when $w = 1$. Differentiating with respect to w gives the analogous expression that generalizes I:

$$\frac{1}{w} \int_0^{\infty} \frac{w^x}{\Gamma(x)} dx = e^w + \int_{-\infty}^{\infty} \frac{\exp(-we^y + y)}{y^2 + \pi^2} dy.$$

Such formulas play a role in the computation of moments for the reciprocal gamma distribution [5, 9].

The function x^x grows even more quickly than $\Gamma(x)$ and we compute [10]

$$\int_0^{\infty} \frac{1}{x^x} dx = 1.9954559575\ldots, \quad \int_1^{\infty} \frac{1}{x^x} dx = 0.7041699604\ldots.$$

More about iterated exponentials is found in [6.11]. Reciprocal distributions could be based on the multiple Barnes functions [2.15] or generalized gamma functions [2.21] as well.

[1] J. Spanier and K. B. Oldham, *An Atlas of Functions*, Hemisphere, 1987, p. 415, formula 43:5:12.
[2] A. Fransén, Accurate determination of the inverse gamma integral, *BIT* 19 (1979) 137–138; MR 80c:65047.
[3] A. Fransén and S. Wrigge, High-precision values of the gamma function and of some related coefficients, *Math. Comp.* 34 (1980) 553–566; addendum and corrigendum, 37 (1981) 233–235; MR 81f:65004 and MR 82m:65002.
[4] S. Plouffe, Fransén-Robinson constant (Plouffe's Tables).
[5] A. Fransén and S. Wrigge, Calculation of the moments and the moment generating function for the reciprocal gamma distribution, *Math. Comp.* 42 (1984) 601–616; MR 86f:65042a.
[6] P. Sebah, Several computations of the Fransén-Robinson constant, unpublished notes (2000–2001).
[7] G. H. Hardy, Another formula of Ramanujan, *J. London Math. Soc.* 12 (1937) 314–318; also in *Collected Papers*, v. 4, Oxford Univ. Press, 1966, pp. 544–548.

[8] G. H. Hardy, *Ramanujan: Twelve Lectures on Subjects Suggested by His Life and Work*, Chelsea, 1940, p. 196; MR 21 #4881.

[9] S. Wrigge, A note on the moment generating function for the reciprocal gamma distribution, *Math. Comp.* 42 (1984) 617–621; MR 86f:65042b.

[10] G. N. Watson, Theorems stated by Ramanujan. VIII: Theorems on divergent series, *J. London Math. Soc.* 4 (1929) 82–86.

4.7 Berry–Esseen Constant

Let $X_1, X_2, \ldots, X_n$ be independent random variables with moments

$$E(X_k) = 0, \quad E(X_k^2) = \sigma_k^2 > 0, \quad E(|X_k|^3) = \beta_k < \infty$$

for each $1 \leq k \leq n$. Let Φ_n be the probability distribution function of the random variable

$$X = \frac{1}{\sigma} \sum_{k=1}^{n} X_k, \quad \text{where } \sigma^2 = \sum_{k=1}^{n} \sigma_k^2.$$

Define the Lyapunov ratio

$$\lambda = \frac{\beta}{\sigma^3}, \quad \text{where } \beta = \sum_{k=1}^{n} \beta_k.$$

Let Φ denote the standard normal distribution function. Berry [1] and Esseen [2,3] proved that there exists a constant C such that

$$\sup_n \sup_{F_k} \sup_x |\Phi_n(x) - \Phi(x)| \leq C \lambda,$$

where, for all k, F_k denotes the distribution function of X_k. The smallest such constant C has bounds [4–12]

$$0.4097321837\ldots = \frac{3 + \sqrt{10}}{6\sqrt{2\pi}} \leq C < 0.7915$$

under the conditions given here. If $X_1, X_2, \ldots, X_n$ are identically distributed, then the upper bound for C can be improved to 0.7655. Furthermore, there is asymptotic evidence that C is equal to the indicated lower bound.

Related studies include [13–22]. In words, the Berry–Esseen inequality quantifies the rate of convergence in the Central Limit Theorem, that is, how close the normal distribution is to the distribution of a sum of independent random variables [23–26]. Hall & Barbour [27], by way of contrast, presented an inequality that describes how far apart the two distributions must be. Another constant arises here too, but little seems to be known about it.

[1] A. C. Berry, The accuracy of the Gaussian approximation to the sum of independent variates, *Trans. Amer. Math. Soc.* 49 (1941) 122–136; MR 2,228i.

[2] C.-G. Esseen, On the Liapounoff limit of error in the theory of probability, *Ark. Mat. Astron. Fysik*, v. 28A (1942) n. 9, 1–19; MR 6,232k.

[3] C.-G. Esseen, Fourier analysis of distribution functions: A mathematical study of the Laplace-Gaussian law, *Acta Math.* 77 (1945) 1–125; MR 7,312a.

[4] H. Bergström, On the central limit theorem, *Skand. Aktuarietidskr.* 27 (1944) 139–153; 28 (1945) 106–127; 32 (1949) 37–62; MR 7,458e, MR 7,459a, and MR 11,255b.

[5] C.-G. Esseen, A moment inequality with an application to the central limit theorem, *Skand. Aktuarietidskr* 39 (1956) 160–170; MR 19,777f.

[6] S. Ikeda, A note on the normal approximation to the sum of independent random variables, *Annals Inst. Statist. Math. Tokyo* 11 (1959) 121–130; MR 24 #A570.

[7] S. Zahl, Bounds for the central limit theorem error, *SIAM J. Appl. Math.* 14 (1966) 1225–1245; MR 35 #1077.

[8] V. M. Zolotarev, Absolute estimate of the remainder in the central limit theorem (in Russian), *Teor. Verojatnost. i Primenen.* 11 (1966) 108–119; Engl. transl. in *Theory Probab. Appl.* 11 (1966) 95–105; MR 33 #6686.

[9] V. M. Zolotarev, A sharpening of the inequality of Berry-Esseen, *Z. Wahrsch. Verw. Gebiete* 8 (1967) 332–342; MR 36 #4622.

[10] V. M. Zolotarev, Some inequalities from probability theory and their application to a refinement of A. M. Ljapunov's theorem (in Russian), *Dokl. Akad. Nauk SSSR* 177 (1967) 501–504; Engl. transl. in *Soviet Math. Dokl.* 8 (1967) 1427–1430; MR 36 #3398.

[11] P. van Beek, An application of Fourier methods to the problem of sharpening the Berry-Esseen inequality, *Z. Wahrsch. Verw. Gebiete* 23 (1972) 187–196; MR 48 #7342.

[12] I. S. Shiganov, Refinement of the upper bound of a constant in the remainder term of the central limit theorem (in Russian), *Problemy Ustoi Chivosti Stokhasticheskikh Modelei*, Proc. 1982 Moscow seminar, ed. V. M. Zolotarev and V. V. Kalashnikov, Vsesoyuz. Nauchno-Issled. Inst. Sistem. Issled., 1982, pp. 109–115; MR 85d:60008.

[13] U. V. Linnik, On the accuracy of the approximation to a Gaussian distribution of sums of independent random variables (in Russian), *Izv. Akad. Nauk SSSR* 11 (1947) 111–138; Engl. transl. in *Selected Transl. Math. Statist. and Probab.*, v. 2, Amer. Math. Soc., pp. 131–158; MR 8,591c.

[14] A. N. Kolmogorov, Some recent work on limit theorems in probability theory (in Russian), *Vestn. Moskov. Gos. Univ.* 10 (1953) 29–38; Engl. transl. in *Selected Works*, v. 2, ed. A. N. Shiryayev, Kluwer, 1992, pp. 406–418; MR 92j:01071.

[15] V. V. Petrov, On precise estimates in limit theorems (in Russian), *Vestnik Leningrad. Univ.*, v. 10 (1955) n. 11, 57–58; MR 17,753g.

[16] B. A. Rogozin, A remark on the paper "A moment inequality with an application to the central limit theorem" by C. G. Esseen (in Russian), *Teor. Verojatnost. i Primenen.* 5 (1960) 125–128; Engl. transl. in *Theory Probab. Appl.* 5 (1960) 114–117; MR 24 #A3683.

[17] H. Prawitz, On the remainder in the central limit theorem. I: One dimensional independent variables with finite absolute moments of third order, *Scand. Actuar. J.*, 1975, 145–156; MR 53 #1695.

[18] R. Michel, On the constant in the nonuniform version of the Berry-Esseen theorem, *Z. Wahrsch. Verw. Gebiete* 55 (1981) 109–117; MR 82c:60042.

[19] L. Paditz, On the analytical structure of the constant in the nonuniform version of the Esseen inequality, *Statistics* 20 (1989) 453–464; MR 90k:60046.

[20] A. Mitalauskas, On the calculation of the constant in the Berry-Esseen inequality for a class of distributions (in Russian), *Liet. Mat. Rink.* 32 (1992) 526–531; Engl. transl. in *Lithuanian Math. J.* 32 (1992) 410–413; MR 94i:60031.

[21] V. Bentkus, On the asymptotical behavior of the constant in the Berry-Esseen inequality, *J. Theoret. Probab.* 7 (1994) 211–224; MR 95d:60042.

[22] G. P. Chistyakov, Asymptotically proper constants in Lyapunov's theorem (in Russian), Probability and Statistics, 1, *Zap. Nauchn. Sem. S.-Peterburg. Otdel. Mat. Inst. Steklov (POMI)* 228 (1996) 349–355, 363–364; Engl. transl. in *J. Math. Sci.* 93 (1999) 480–483; MR 98g:60038.

[23] V. V. Petrov, *Sums of Independent Random Variables*, Springer-Verlag, 1975; MR 52 #9335.

[24]   V. V. Petrov, *Limit Theorems of Probability Theory: Sequences of Independent Random Variables*, Oxford Univ. Press, 1995; MR 96h:60048.

[25]   P. Hall, *Rates of Convergence in the Central Limit Theorem*, Pitman, 1982; MR 84k:60032.

[26]   R. N. Bhattacharya and R. Ranga Rao, *Normal Approximation and Asymptotic Expansions*, Wiley, 1976; MR 55 #9219.

[27]   P. Hall and A. D. Barbour, Reversing the Berry-Esseen inequality, *Proc. Amer. Math. Soc.* 90 (1984) 107–110; MR 86a:60028.

4.8 Laplace Limit Constant

Given real numbers M and ε, $|\varepsilon| \leq 1$, the accurate solution of **Kepler's equation**

$$M = E - \varepsilon \sin(E)$$

is critical in celestial mechanics [1–4]. It relates the **mean anomaly** M of a planet, in elliptical orbit around the sun, to the planet's **eccentric anomaly** E and to the eccentricity ε of the ellipse. It is a transcendental equation, that is, without an algebraic solution in terms of M and ε. Computing E is a commonly-used intermediate step to the calculation of planetary position as a function of time. Therefore it is not hard to see why hundreds of mathematicians from Newton to present have devoted thought to this problem.

We will not give the orbital mechanics underlying Kepler's equation but instead give a simple geometric motivational example. Pick an arbitrary point F inside the unit circle. Let P be the point on the circle closest to F and pick another point Q elsewhere on the circle. Define E and ε as pictured in Figure 4.2. Let M be twice the area of the shaded sector PFQ. Then

$$\frac{M}{2} = (\text{area of sector } POQ) - (\text{area of triangle } FOQ) = \frac{1}{2}E - \frac{1}{2}\varepsilon \sin(E).$$

So the solution of Kepler's equation allows us to compute the angle E, given the area M and the length ε.

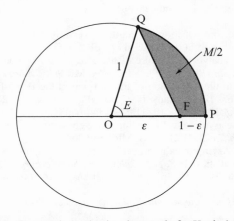

Figure 4.2. Geometric motivational example for Kepler's equation.

Kepler's equation has a unique solution, here given as a power series in ε (via the inversion method of Lagrange):

$$E = M + \sum_{n=1}^{\infty} a_n \varepsilon^n,$$

where [1, 5–7]

$$a_n = \frac{1}{n!2^{n-1}} \sum_{k=0}^{\lfloor n/2 \rfloor} (-1)^k \binom{n}{k} (n - 2k)^{n-1} \sin((n - 2k)M).$$

Power series solutions as such were the preferred way to do calculations in the pre-computer nineteenth century. So it perhaps came as a shock that this series diverges for $|\varepsilon| > 0.662$ as evidently first discovered by Laplace. Arnold [8] wrote, "This plays an important part in the history of mathematics ... The investigation of the origin of this mysterious constant led Cauchy to the creation of complex analysis."

In fact, the power series for E converges like a geometric series with ratio

$$f(\varepsilon) = \frac{\varepsilon}{1 + \sqrt{1 + \varepsilon^2}} \exp(\sqrt{1 + \varepsilon^2}).$$

The value $\lambda = 0.6627434193\ldots$ for which $f(\lambda) = 1$ is called the **Laplace limit**. A closed-form expression for λ in terms of elementary functions is not known. An infinite series or definite integral expression for λ is likewise not known.

The story does not end here. A Bessel function series for E is as follows [5, 6, 9]:

$$E = M + \sum_{n=1}^{\infty} \frac{2}{n} J_n(n\varepsilon) \sin(nM),$$

where

$$J_p(x) = \sum_{k=0}^{\infty} \frac{(-1)^k}{k!(p + k)!} \left(\frac{x}{2}\right)^{p+2k}.$$

This series is better than the power series since it converges like a geometric series with ratio

$$g(\varepsilon) = \frac{\varepsilon}{1 + \sqrt{1 - \varepsilon^2}} \exp(\sqrt{1 - \varepsilon^2}),$$

which satisfies $|g(\varepsilon)| \leq 1$ for all $|\varepsilon| \leq 1$.

Iterative methods, however, outperform both of these series expansion methods. Note that the function

$$T(E) = M + \varepsilon \sin(E) \quad \text{(for fixed } M \text{ and } \varepsilon\text{)}$$

is a contraction mapping; thus the method of successive approximations

$$E_0 = 0, \quad E_{i+1} = T(E_i) = M + \varepsilon \sin(E_i)$$

works well. Newton's method

$$E_0 = 0, \quad E_{i+1} = E_i + \frac{M + \varepsilon \sin(E_i) - E_i}{1 - \varepsilon \cos(E_i)}$$

converges even more quickly. Variations of these abound. Putting practicality aside, there are some interesting definite integral expressions [10–13] that solve Kepler's equation. These cannot be regarded as competitive in the race for quick accuracy, as far as is known.

An alternative representation of λ is as follows [7, 14, 15]: Let $\mu = 1.1996786402\ldots$ be the unique positive solution of $\coth(\mu) = \mu$, then $\lambda = \sqrt{\mu^2 - 1}$.

[1]   F. R. Moulton, *An Introduction to Celestial Mechanics*, 2nd ed., MacMillan, 1914.
[2]   H. Dörrie, *100 Great Problems of Elementary Mathematics: Their History and Solution*, Dover, 1965; MR 84b:00001.
[3]   J. B. Marion, *Classical Dynamics of Particles and Systems*, 2nd ed., Academic Press, 1970.
[4]   J. M. A. Danby, *Fundamentals of Celestial Mechanics*, 2nd ed., Willmann-Bell, 1988; MR 90b:70017.
[5]   A. Wintner, *The Analytical Foundations of Celestial Mechanics*, Princeton Univ. Press, 1941; MR 3,215b.
[6]   P. Henrici, *Applied and Computational Complex Analysis*, v. 1, *Power Series – Integration – Conformal Mapping – Location of Zeros*, Wiley, 1974; MR 90d:30002.
[7]   P. Colwell, *Solving Kepler's Equation over Three Centuries*, Willmann-Bell, 1993, p. 72.
[8]   V. I. Arnold, *Huygens and Barrow, Newton and Hooke*, Birkhäuser, 1990, p. 85; MR 91h:01014.
[9]   G. N. Watson, *A Treatise on the Theory of Bessel Functions*, 2nd ed., Cambridge Univ. Press, 1966; MR 96i:33010.
[10] C. E. Siewert and E. E. Burniston, An exact analytical solution of Kepler's equation, *Celest. Mech.* 6 (1972) 294–304; MR 51 #9596.
[11] N. I. Ioakimidis and K. E. Papadakis, A new simple method for the analytical solution of Kepler's equation, *Celest. Mech.* 35 (1985) 305–316; MR 86g:70001.
[12] N. I. Ioakimidis and K. E. Papadakis, A new class of quite elementary closed-form integral formulae for roots of nonlinear systems, *Appl. Math. Comput.*, v. 29 (1989) n. 2, 185–196; MR 89m:65050.
[13] S. Ferraz-Mello, The convergence domain of the Laplacian expansion of the disturbing function, *Celest. Mech. Dynam. Astron.* 58 (1994) 37–52; MR 94j:70011.
[14] E. Goursat, *A Course in Mathematical Analysis*, v. 2, Dover, 1959; MR 21 #4889.
[15] F. Le Lionnais, *Les Nombres Remarquables*, Hermann, 1983.

4.9 Integer Chebyshev Constant

Consider the class P_n of all real, monic polynomials of degree n. Which nonzero member of this class deviates least from zero in the interval $[0, 1]$? That is, what is the solution of the following optimization problem:

$$\min_{\substack{p \in P_n \\ p \neq 0}} \max_{0 \leq x \leq 1} |p(x)| = f(n)?$$

The unique answer is $p_n(x) = 2^{1-2n} T_n(2x - 1)$, where $[1, 2]$

$$T_n(x) = \cos(n \arccos(x)) = \frac{(x + \sqrt{x^2 - 1})^n + (x - \sqrt{x^2 - 1})^n}{2}$$

and

$$\lim_{n \to \infty} f(n)^{\frac{1}{n}} = \frac{1}{4}.$$

Table 4.1. *Real Chebyshev Polynomials*

n	$p_n(x)$	$f(n)$	$f(n)^{1/n}$
1	$x - \frac{1}{2}$	$\frac{2}{4^1} = \frac{1}{2}$	0.500
2	$x^2 - x + \frac{1}{8}$	$\frac{2}{4^2} = \frac{1}{8}$	0.353
3	$x^3 - \frac{3}{2}x^2 + \frac{9}{16}x - \frac{1}{32}$	$\frac{2}{4^3} = \frac{1}{32}$	0.314
4	$x^4 - 2x^3 + \frac{5}{4}x^2 - \frac{1}{4}x + \frac{1}{128}$	$\frac{2}{4^4} = \frac{1}{128}$	0.297
5	$x^5 - \frac{5}{2}x^4 + \frac{35}{16}x^3 - \frac{25}{32}x^2 + \frac{25}{256}x - \frac{1}{512}$	$\frac{2}{4^5} = \frac{1}{512}$	0.287

The first several polynomials $p_n(x)$, which we call **real Chebyshev polynomials** (defying tradition), are listed in Table 4.1. (The phrase "Chebyshev polynomial" is more customarily used to denote the polynomial $T_n(x)$.) In the definition of $f(n)$, note that we could just as well replace the word "monic" by the phrase "leading coefficient at least 1."

Consider instead the class Q_n of all integer polynomials of degree n, with positive leading coefficient. Again, which nonzero member of this class deviates least from zero in the interval [0, 1]? That is, what is the solution of

$$\min_{\substack{q \in Q_n \\ q \neq 0}} \max_{0 \leq x \leq 1} |q(x)| = g(n)?$$

Clearly this is a more restrictive version of the earlier problem. Here we do not have a complete solution nor do we have uniqueness. The first several polynomials $q_n(x)$, which we call **integer Chebyshev polynomials**, are listed in Table 4.2 [3,4]. Define the **integer Chebyshev constant** (or **integer transfinite diameter** or **integer logarithmic capacity** [4.9.1]) to be

$$\chi = \lim_{n \to \infty} g(n)^{\frac{1}{n}}.$$

What can be said about χ? On the one hand, we have a lower bound [3–5]

$$\exp(-0.8657725922\ldots) = \frac{1}{2.3768417063\ldots} = 0.4207263771\ldots = \alpha \leq \chi,$$

Table 4.2. *Integer Chebyshev Polynomials*

n	$q_n(x)$	$g(n)$	$g(n)^{1/n}$
1	x or $x - 1$ or $2x - 1$	1	1.000
2	$x(x - 1)$	$\frac{1}{4}$	0.500
3	$x(x - 1)(2x - 1)$	$\frac{\sqrt{3}}{18}$	0.458
4	$x^2(x - 1)^2$ or $x(x - 1)(2x - 1)^2$ or $x(x - 1)(5x^2 - 5x + 1)$	$\frac{1}{16}$	0.500
5	$x^2(x - 1)^2(2x - 1)$	$\frac{\sqrt{5}}{125}$	0.447
6	$x^2(x - 1)^2(2x - 1)^2$	$\frac{1}{108}$	0.458
7	$x^3(x - 1)^3(2x - 1)$	$\frac{27\sqrt{7}}{19208}$	0.449

where

$$\alpha_0 = 2, \quad \alpha_k = \alpha_{k-1} + \frac{1}{\alpha_{k-1}}, \ k \geq 1, \quad \alpha = \frac{1}{2} \prod_{j=0}^{\infty} \left(1 + \frac{1}{\alpha_j^2}\right)^{-\frac{1}{2^{j+1}}}.$$

This recursion was obtained with the help of what are known as Gorshkov–Wirsing polynomials [3,6]. It was conjectured [5] that $\chi = \alpha$ until Borwein & Erdélyi [4] proved to everyone's surprise that $\chi > \alpha$. On the other hand, we have an upper bound

$$\chi \leq \beta = 0.42347945 = \frac{1}{2.36138964} = \exp(-0.85925028)$$

due to Habsieger & Salvy [7], who succeeded in computing an integer Chebyshev polynomial for each degree up to 75. Better algorithms will be needed to find such polynomials to significantly higher degree and to determine β in this manner. By a different approach, however, Pritsker [8] recently obtained improved bounds $0.4213 < \chi < 0.4232$.

Thus far we have focused all attention on the interval $[0, 1]$, that is, on the constant $\chi = \chi(0, 1)$. What can be said about other intervals $[a, b]$? It is known [4,9] that

$$\chi(-1, 1)^4 = \chi(0, 1)^2 = \chi(0, \tfrac{1}{4});$$

hence the preceding bounds can be applied. The exact value of $\chi(a, b)$ for any $0 < b - a < 4$ remains an open question [4]. However, $\chi(a, b) = 1$ if $b - a \geq 4$ and $\chi(0, c) = \chi(0, 1)$ for all $1 - 0.17^2 \leq c < 1 + \varepsilon$ for some $\varepsilon > 0$, that is, $\chi(0, c)$ is locally constant at $c = 1$. Also [10], we have

$$\chi(0, 1) = \chi(1, 2) > 0.42,$$

but, from elementary considerations,

$$\chi(0, 2) \leq \tfrac{1}{\sqrt{2}} < 0.71 < 0.84 = 2(0.42);$$

that is, $\chi(0, 2)$ is not the same as either $2\chi(0, 1)$ or $\chi(0, 1) + \chi(1, 2)$. The relation $\chi(0, 1) = \chi(d, d + 1)$ also fails for non-integer d. So scaling, additivity, and translation-invariance do not hold for the integer Chebyshev case (unlike the real case).

There is an interesting connection between calculating $\chi(0, 1)$ and prime number theory [3,5] due to Gel'fond and Schnirelmann. If it were true that $\chi = 1/e = 0.36\ldots$, then one would have a new proof of the famous Prime Number Theorem. Unfortunately, this is false (as our bounds clearly indicate).

Finally, on the interval $[0, 1]$, Aparicio Bernardo [11] observed that integer Chebyshev polynomials $q_n(x)$ always have factors

$$x(x - 1), \ 2x - 1, \ \text{and} \ 5x^2 - 5x + 1$$

that tend to repeat and increase in power as n grows. The relative rates at which this occurs, that is, the asymptotic structure of the polynomial $q_n(x)$, gives rise to more interesting constants [4, 6, 8].

4.9.1 Transfinite Diameter

We utilized some language earlier from potential theory that deserves elaboration. Let E be a compact set in the complex plane. The **(real) transfinite diameter** or **(real) logarithmic capacity** is defined to be

$$\gamma(E) = \lim_{n \to \infty} \max_{z_1, z_2, \ldots, z_n \in E} \left(\prod_{j < k} |z_j - z_k| \right)^{\frac{2}{n(n-1)}},$$

that is, the maximal geometric mean of pairwise distances for n points in E, in the limit as $n \to \infty$. For example,

$$\gamma([0, 1]) = \frac{1}{4} = \lim_{n \to \infty} f(n)^{\frac{1}{n}},$$

and this equality is not an accidental coincidence. For arbitrary E, the phrases transfinite diameter, logarithmic capacity, and (real) Chebyshev constant are interchangeable [1, 12]. See [13–15] for sample computations. Relevant discussions of what are known as Robin constants appear in [16–18].

[1] P. Borwein and T. Erdélyi, *Polynomials and Polynomial Inequalities*, Springer-Verlag, 1995; MR 97e:41001.

[2] G. F. Simmons, *Differential Equations with Applications and Historical Notes*, McGraw-Hill, 1972; MR 58 #17258.

[3] H. L. Montgomery, *Ten Lectures on the Interface between Analytic Number Theory and Harmonic Analysis*, CBMS v. 84, Amer. Math. Soc., 1994, pp. 179–193; MR 96i:11002.

[4] P. Borwein and T. Erdélyi, The integer Chebyshev problem, *Math. Comp.* 65 (1996) 661–681; MR 96g:11077.

[5] G. V. Chudnovsky, Number theoretic applications of polynomials with rational coefficients defined by extremality conditions, *Arithmetic and Geometry: Papers Dedicated to I. R. Shafarevich*, v. 1, ed. M. Artin and J. Tate, Birkhäuser, 1983, pp. 61–105; MR 86c:11052.

[6] I. E. Pritsker, Chebyshev polynomials with integer coefficients, *Analytic and Geometric Inequalities and Applications*, ed. Th. M. Rassias and H. M. Srivastava, Kluwer, 1999, pp. 335–348; MR 2001h:30007.

[7] L. Habsieger and B. Salvy, On integer Chebyshev polynomials, *Math. Comp.* 66 (1997) 763–770; MR 97f:11053.

[8] I. E. Pritsker, Small polynomials with integer coefficients, math.CA/0101166.

[9] V. Flammang, Sur le diamètre transfini entier d'un intervalle à extrémités rationnelles, *Annales Inst. Fourier (Grenoble)* 45 (1995) 779–793; MR 96i:11083.

[10] V. Flammang, G. Rhin, and C. J. Smyth, The integer transfinite diameter of intervals and totally real algebraic integers, *J. Théorie Nombres Bordeaux* 9 (1997) 137–168; MR 98g:11119.

[11] E. Aparicio Bernardo, On the asymptotic structure of the polynomials of minimal Diophantic deviation from zero, *J. Approx. Theory* 55 (1988) 270–278; MR 90b:41010.

[12] E. Hille, *Methods in Classical and Functional Analysis*, Addison-Wesley, 1972; MR 57 #3802.

[13] N. S. Landkoff, *Foundations of Modern Potential Theory*, Springer-Verlag, 1972; MR 50 #2520.

[14] T. J. Ransford, *Potential Theory in the Complex Plane*, Cambridge Univ. Press, 1995; MR 96e:31001.

[15] J. Rostand, Computing logarithmic capacity with linear programming, *Experim. Math.* 6 (1997) 221–238; MR 98f:65032.

[16] L. V. Ahlfors, *Conformal Invariants: Topics in Geometric Function*, McGraw-Hill, 1973; MR 50 #10211.

[17] J. B. Conway, *Functions of One Complex Variable II*, Springer-Verlag, 1995; MR 96i:30001.

[18] P. K. Kythe, *Computational Conformal Mapping*, Birkhäuser, 1998; MR 99k:65027.

5

Constants Associated with Enumerating Discrete Structures

5.1 Abelian Group Enumeration Constants

Every finite abelian group is a direct sum of cyclic subgroups. A corollary of this fundamental theorem is the following. Given a positive integer n, the number $a(n)$ of non-isomorphic abelian groups of order n is given by [1, 2]

$$a(n) = P(\alpha_1)P(\alpha_2)P(\alpha_3) \cdots P(\alpha_r),$$

where $n = p_1^{\alpha_1} p_2^{\alpha_2} p_3^{\alpha_3} \cdots p_r^{\alpha_r}$ is the prime factorization of n, p_1, p_2, p_3, $\ldots$, p_r are distinct primes, each α_k is positive, and $P(\alpha_k)$ denotes the number of unrestricted partitions of α_k. For example, $a(p^4) = 5$ for any prime p since there are five partitions of 4:

$$4 = 1 + 3 = 2 + 2 = 1 + 1 + 2 = 1 + 1 + 1 + 1.$$

As another example, $a(p^4 q^4) = 25$ for any distinct primes p and q, but $a(p^8) = 22$. It is clear that

$$\liminf_{n \to \infty} a(n) = 1,$$

but it is more difficult to see that [3–6]

$$\limsup_{n \to \infty} \ln(a(n)) \frac{\ln(\ln(n))}{\ln(n)} = \frac{\ln(5)}{4}.$$

A number of authors have examined the average behavior of $a(n)$ over all positive integers. The most precise known results are [7–10]

$$\sum_{n=1}^{N} a(n) = A_1 N + A_2 N^{\frac{1}{2}} + A_3 N^{\frac{1}{3}} + O\left(N^{\frac{50}{199}+\varepsilon}\right),$$

273

where $\varepsilon > 0$ is arbitrarily small,

$$A_k = \prod_{\substack{j=1 \\ j \neq k}}^{\infty} \zeta\left(\frac{j}{k}\right) = \begin{cases} 2.2948565916\ldots & \text{if } k = 1, \\ -14.6475663016\ldots & \text{if } k = 2, \\ 118.6924619727\ldots & \text{if } k = 3, \end{cases}$$

and $\zeta(x)$ is Riemann's zeta function [1.6]. We cannot help but speculate about the following estimate:

$$\sum_{n=1}^{N} a(n) \sim \sum_{k=1}^{\infty} A_k N^{\frac{1}{k}} + \Delta(N),$$

but an understanding of the error $\Delta(N)$ has apparently not yet been achieved [11, 12]. Similar enumeration results for finite semisimple associative rings appear in [5.1.1].

If, instead, focus is shifted to the sum of the reciprocals of $a(n)$, then [13, 14]

$$\sum_{n=1}^{N} \frac{1}{a(n)} = A_0 N + O\left(N^{\frac{1}{2}} \ln(N)^{-\frac{1}{2}}\right),$$

where A_0 is an infinite product over all primes p:

$$A_0 = \prod_{p} \left[1 - \sum_{k=2}^{\infty} \left(\frac{1}{P(k-1)} - \frac{1}{P(k)}\right) \frac{1}{p^k}\right] = 0.7520107423\ldots.$$

In summary, the average number of non-isomorphic abelian groups of any given order is $A_1 = 2.2948$ if "average" is understood in the sense of arithmetic mean, and $A_0^{-1} = 1.3297$ if "average" is understood in the sense of harmonic mean. We cannot even hope to obtain analogous statistics for the general (not necessarily abelian) case at present. Some interesting bounds are known [15–19] and are based on the classification theorem of finite simple groups.

The constant A_1 also appears in [20] in connection with the arithmetical properties of class numbers of quadratic fields.

Erdös & Szekeres [21, 22] examined $a(n)$ and the following generalization: $a(n, i)$ is the number of representations of n as a product (of an arbitrary number of terms, with order ignored) of factors of the form p^j, where $j \geq i$. They proved that

$$\sum_{n=1}^{N} a(n, i) = C_i N^{\frac{1}{i}} + O\left(N^{\frac{1}{i+1}}\right), \quad \text{where } C_i = \prod_{k=1}^{\infty} \zeta\left(1 + \frac{k}{i}\right),$$

and surely someone has tightened this estimate by now. See also the discussion of square-full and cube-full integers in [2.6.1].

5.1.1 Semisimple Associative Rings

A finite associative ring R with identity element $1 \neq 0$ is said to be **simple** if R has no proper (two-sided) ideals and is **semisimple** if R is a direct sum of simple ideals.

Simple rings generalize fields. Semisimple rings, in turn, generalize simple rings. Every (finite) semisimple ring is, in fact, a direct sum of full matrix rings over finite fields. Consequently, given a positive integer n, the number $s(n)$ of non-isomorphic semisimple rings of order n is given by

$$s(n) = Q(\alpha_1)Q(\alpha_2)Q(\alpha_3) \cdots Q(\alpha_r),$$

where $n = p_1^{\alpha_1} p_2^{\alpha_2} p_3^{\alpha_3} \cdots p_r^{\alpha_r}$ is the prime factorization of n, $p_1, p_2, p_3, \ldots, p_r$ are distinct primes, each α_k is positive, and $Q(\alpha_k)$ denotes the number of (unordered) sets of integer pairs (r_j, m_j) for which

$$\alpha_k = \sum_j r_j m_j^2 \text{ and } r_j m_j^2 > 0 \text{ for all } j.$$

As an example, $s(p^5) = 8$ for any prime p since

$$5 = 1 \cdot 1^2 + 1 \cdot 2^2 = 5 \cdot 1^2 = 2 \cdot 1^2 + 3 \cdot 1^2 = 1 \cdot 1^2 + 4 \cdot 1^2$$
$$= 1 \cdot 1^2 + 1 \cdot 1^2 + 3 \cdot 1^2 = 1 \cdot 1^2 + 2 \cdot 1^2 + 2 \cdot 1^2$$
$$= 1 \cdot 1^2 + 1 \cdot 1^2 + 1 \cdot 1^2 + 2 \cdot 1^2 = 1 \cdot 1^2 + 1 \cdot 1^2 + 1 \cdot 1^2 + 1 \cdot 1^2 + 1 \cdot 1^2.$$

Asymptotically, there are extreme results [23, 24]:

$$\liminf_{n \to \infty} s(n) = 1,$$

$$\limsup_{n \to \infty} \ln(s(n)) \frac{\ln(\ln(n))}{\ln(n)} = \frac{\ln(6)}{4}$$

and average results [25–30]:

$$\sum_{n=1}^{N} s(n) = A_1 B_1 N + A_2 B_2 N^{\frac{1}{2}} + A_3 B_3 N^{\frac{1}{3}} + O\left(N^{\frac{50}{199}+\varepsilon}\right),$$

where $\varepsilon > 0$ is arbitrarily small, A_k is as defined in the preceding, and

$$B_k = \prod_{r=1}^{\infty} \prod_{m=2}^{\infty} \zeta\left(\frac{rm^2}{k}\right).$$

In particular, there are, on average,

$$A_1 B_1 = \prod_{rm^2 > 1} \zeta\left(rm^2\right) = 2.4996161129\ldots$$

non-isomorphic semisimple rings of any given order ("average" in the sense of arithmetic mean).

[1] D. G. Kendall and R. A. Rankin, On the number of abelian groups of a given order, *Quart. J. Math.* 18 (1947) 197–208; MR 9,226c.
[2] N. J. A. Sloane, On-Line Encyclopedia of Integer Sequences, A000688 and A004101.
[3] E. Krätzel, Die maximale Ordnung der Anzahl der wesentlich verschiedenen abelschen Gruppen n^{ter} Ordnung, *Quart. J. Math.* 21 (1970) 273–275; MR 42 #3171.

[4]   W. Schwarz and E. Wirsing, The maximal number of non-isomorphic abelian groups of order n, *Arch. Math. (Basel)* 24 (1973) 59–62; MR 47 #4953.

[5]   A. Ivić, The distribution of values of the enumerating function of non-isomorphic abelian groups of finite order, *Arch. Math. (Basel)* 30 (1978) 374–379; MR 58 #16562.

[6]   E. Krätzel, The distribution of values of $a(n)$, *Arch. Math. (Basel)* 57 (1991) 47–52; MR 92e:11097.

[7]   H.-E. Richert, Über die Anzahl Abelscher Gruppen gegebener Ordnung. I, *Math. Z.* 56 (1952) 21–32; MR 14,349e.

[8]   B. R. Srinivasan, On the number of abelian groups of a given order, *Acta Arith.* 23 (1973) 195–205; MR 49 #2610.

[9]   G. Kolesnik, On the number of abelian groups of a given order, *J. Reine Angew. Math.* 329 (1981) 164–175; MR 83b:10055.

[10] H.-Q. Liu, On the number of abelian groups of a given order, *Acta Arith.* 59 (1991) 261–277; supplement 64 (1993) 285–296; MR 92i:11103 and MR 94g:11073.

[11] E. Krätzel, *Lattice Points*, Kluwer, 1988, pp. 293–303; MR 90e:11144.

[12] A. Ivić, *The Riemann Zeta-Function*, Wiley, 1985, pp. 37–38, 413–420, 438–439; MR 87d:11062.

[13] J.-M. DeKoninck and A. Ivić, *Topics in Arithmetical Functions: Asymptotic Formulae for Sums of Reciprocals of Arithmetical Functions and Related Fields*, North-Holland, 1980; MR 82a:10047.

[14] P. Zimmermann, Estimating the infinite product A_0, unpublished note (1996).

[15] P. M. Neumann, An enumeration theorem for finite groups, *Quart. J. Math.* 20 (1969) 395–401; MR 40 #7344.

[16] L. Pyber, Enumerating finite groups of given order, *Annals of Math.* 137 (1993) 203–220; MR 93m:11097.

[17] M. Ram Murty, Counting finite groups, *Analysis, Geometry and Probability*, ed. R. Bhatia, Hindustan Book Agency, 1996, pp. 161–172; MR 98j:11076.

[18] L. Pyber, Group enumeration and where it leads us, *European Congress of Mathematics*, v. 2, Budapest, 1996, ed. A. Balog, G. O. H. Katona, A. Recski, and D. Szász, Birkhäuser, 1998, pp. 187–199; MR 99i:20037.

[19] B. Eick and E. A. O'Brien, Enumerating p-groups, *J. Austral. Math. Soc. Ser. A* 67 (1999) 191–205; MR 2000h:20033.

[20] H. Cohen, *A Course in Computational Algebraic Number Theory*, Springer-Verlag, 1993, pp. 290–293; MR 94i:11105.

[21] P. Erdös and G. Szekeres, Über die Anzahl der Abelschen Gruppen gegebener Ordnung und über ein verwandtes zahlentheoretisches Problem, *Acta Sci. Math. (Szeged)* 7 (1934-35) 95–102.

[22] I. Z. Ruzsa, Erdös and the integers, *J. Number Theory* 79 (1999) 115–163; MR 2002e:11002.

[23] J. Knopfmacher, Arithmetical properties of finite rings and algebras, and analytic number theory. IV, *J. Reine Angew. Math.* 270 (1974) 97–114; MR 51 #389.

[24] J. Knopfmacher, Arithmetical properties of finite rings and algebras, and analytic number theory. VI, *J. Reine Angew. Math.* 277 (1975) 45–62; MR 52 #3088.

[25] J. Knopfmacher, Arithmetical properties of finite rings and algebras, and analytic number theory. I, *J. Reine Angew. Math.* 252 (1972) 16–43; MR 47 #1769.

[26] J. Knopfmacher, *Abstract Analytic Number Theory*, North-Holland, 1975; MR 91d:11110.

[27] J. Duttlinger, Eine Bemerkung zu einer asymptotischen Formel von Herrn Knopfmacher, *J. Reine Angew. Math.* 266 (1974) 104–106; MR 49 #2605.

[28] C. Calderón and M. J. Zárate, The number of semisimple rings of order at most x, *Extracta Math.* 7 (1992) 144–147; MR 94m:11111.

[29] M. Kühleitner, Comparing the number of abelian groups and of semisimple rings of a given order, *Math. Slovaca* 45 (1995) 509–518; MR 97d:11143.

[30] W. G. Nowak, On the value distribution of a class of arithmetic functions, *Comment. Math. Univ. Carolinae* 37 (1996) 117–134; MR 97h:11104.

5.2 Pythagorean Triple Constants

The positive integers a, b, c are said to form a **primitive Pythagorean triple** if $a \leq b$, $\gcd(a, b, c) = 1$, and $a^2 + b^2 = c^2$. Clearly any such triple can be interpreted geometrically as the side lengths of a right triangle with commensurable sides. Define $P_h(n)$, $P_p(n)$, and $P_a(n)$ respectively as the number of primitive Pythagorean triples whose hypotenuses, perimeters, and areas do not exceed n. D. N. Lehmer [1] showed that

$$\lim_{n \to \infty} \frac{P_h(n)}{n} = \frac{1}{2\pi}, \quad \lim_{n \to \infty} \frac{P_p(n)}{n} = \frac{\ln(2)}{\pi^2}$$

and Lambek & Moser [2] showed that

$$\lim_{n \to \infty} \frac{P_a(n)}{\sqrt{n}} = C = \frac{1}{\sqrt{2\pi^5}} \Gamma\left(\frac{1}{4}\right)^2 = 0.5313399499\ldots,$$

where $\Gamma(x)$ is the Euler gamma function [1.5.4].

What can be said about the error terms? D. H. Lehmer [3] demonstrated that

$$P_p(n) = \frac{\ln(2)}{\pi^2} n + O\left(n^{\frac{1}{2}} \ln(n)\right),$$

and Lambek & Moser [2] and Wild [4] further demonstrated that

$$P_h(n) = \frac{1}{2\pi} n + O\left(n^{\frac{1}{2}} \ln(n)\right), \quad P_a(n) = C n^{\frac{1}{2}} - D n^{\frac{1}{3}} + O\left(n^{\frac{1}{4}} \ln(n)\right),$$

where

$$D = -\frac{1 + 2^{-\frac{1}{3}} \zeta(\frac{1}{3})}{1 + 4^{-\frac{1}{3}} \zeta(\frac{4}{3})} = 0.2974615529\ldots$$

and $\zeta(x)$ is the Riemann zeta function [1.6]. Sharper estimates for $P_a(n)$ were obtained in [5–8].

It is obvious that the hypotenuse c and the perimeter $a + b + c$ of a primitive Pythagorean triple a, b, c must both be integers. If ab was odd, then both a and b would be odd and hence $c^2 \equiv 2 \bmod 4$, which is impossible. Thus the area $ab/2$ must also be an integer. If $P_a'(n)$ is the number of primitive Pythagorean triples whose areas $\leq n$ are integers, then $P_a'(n) = P_a(n)$. Such an identity does not hold for non-right triangles, of course.

A somewhat related matter is the ancient **congruent number problem** [9], the solution of which Tunnell [10] has reduced to a weak form of the Birch–Swinnerton–Dyer conjecture from elliptic curve theory. In the congruent number problem, the right triangles are permitted to have rational sides (rather than just integer sides). For a prescribed integer n, does there exist a rational right triangle with area n?

There is also the problem of enumerating **primitive Heronian triples**, equivalently, coprime integers $a \leq b \leq c$ that are side lengths of an *arbitrary* triangle with commensurable sides. What can be said asymptotically about the numbers $H_h(n)$, $H_p(n)$, $H_a(n)$, and $H_a'(n)$ (analogously defined)? A starting point for answering this question might be [11, 12].

[1] D. N. Lehmer, Asymptotic evaluation of certain totient sums, *Amer. J. Math.* 22 (1900) 293–335.

[2] J. Lambek and L. Moser, On the distribution of Pythagorean triples, *Pacific J. Math.* 5 (1955) 73–83; MR 16,796h.

[3] D. H. Lehmer, A conjecture of Krishnaswami, *Bull. Amer. Math. Soc.* 54 (1948) 1185–1190; MR 10,431c.

[4] R. E. Wild, On the number of primitive Pythagorean triangles with area less than *n*, *Pacific J. Math.* 5 (1955) 85–91; MR 16,797a.

[5] J. Duttlinger and W. Schwarz, Über die Verteilung der pythagoräischen Dreiecke, *Colloq. Math.* 43 (1980) 365–372; MR 83e:10018.

[6] H. Menzer, On the number of primitive Pythagorean triangles, *Math. Nachr.* 128 (1986) 129–133; MR 87m:11022.

[7] W. Müller, W. G. Nowak, and H. Menzer, On the number of primitive Pythagorean triangles, *Annales Sci. Math. Québec* 12 (1988) 263–273; MR 90b:11020.

[8] W. Müller and W. G. Nowak, Lattice points in planar domains: Applications of Huxley's 'Discrete Hardy-Littlewood method,' *Number-Theoretic Analysis: Vienna 1988-89*, ed. E. Hlawka and R. F. Tichy, Lect. Notes in Math. 1452, Springer-Verlag, 1990, pp. 139–164; MR 92d:11113.

[9] N. Koblitz, *Introduction to Elliptic Curves and Modular Forms*, Springer-Verlag, 1984; MR 94a:11078.

[10] J. B. Tunnell, A classical Diophantine problem and modular forms of weight 3/2, *Invent. Math.* 72 (1983) 323–334; MR 85d:11046.

[11] C. P. Popovici, Heronian triangles (in Russian), *Rev. Math. Pures Appl.* 7 (1962) 439–457; MR 31 #121.

[12] D. Singmaster, Some corrections to Carlson's "Determination of Heronian triangles," *Fibonacci Quart.* 11 (1973) 157–158; MR 45 #156 and MR 47 #4922.

5.3 Rényi's Parking Constant

Consider the one-dimensional interval $[0, x]$ with $x > 1$. Imagine it to be a street for which parking is permitted on one side. Cars of unit length are one-by-one parked *completely at random* on the street and obviously no overlap is allowed with cars already in place. What is the mean number, $M(x)$, of cars that can fit?

Rényi [1–3] determined that $M(x)$ satisfies the following integrofunctional equation:

$$M(x) = \begin{cases} 0 & \text{if } 0 \leq x < 1, \\ 1 + \dfrac{2}{x-1} \displaystyle\int_0^{x-1} M(t)\, dt & \text{if } x \geq 1. \end{cases}$$

By a Laplace transform technique, Rényi proved that the limiting mean density, m, of cars in the interval $[0, x]$ is

$$m = \lim_{x \to \infty} \frac{M(x)}{x} = \int_0^\infty \beta(x)\, dx = 0.7475979202\ldots,$$

where

$$\beta(x) = \exp\left(-2\int_0^x \frac{1 - e^{-t}}{t}\, dt\right) = e^{-2(\ln(x) - \text{Ei}(-x) + \gamma)}, \quad \alpha(x) = m - \int_0^x \beta(t)\, dt,$$

γ is the Euler–Mascheroni constant [1.5], and Ei is the exponential integral [6.2.1]. Several alternative proofs appear in [4,5].

What can be said about the variance, $V(x)$, of the number of cars that can fit on the street? Mackenzie [6], Dvoretzky & Robbins [7], and Mannion [8,9] independently addressed this question and deduced that

$$v = \lim_{x \to \infty} \frac{V(x)}{x} = 4 \int_0^\infty \left[e^{-x}(1 - e^{-x})\frac{\alpha(x)}{x} - e^{-2x}(x + e^{-x} - 1)\frac{\alpha(x)^2}{\beta(x)x^2} \right] dx - m$$

$$= 0.0381563991\ldots.$$

A central limit theorem holds [7], that is, the total number of cars is approximately normally distributed with mean mx and variance vx for large enough x.

It is natural to consider the parking problem in a higher dimensional setting. Consider the two-dimensional rectangle of length $x > 1$ and width $y > 1$ and imagine cars to be unit squares with sides parallel to the sides of the parking rectangle. What is the mean number, $M(x, y)$, of cars that can fit? Palasti [10–12] conjectured that

$$\lim_{x \to \infty} \lim_{y \to \infty} \frac{M(x, y)}{xy} = m^2 = (0.7475979202\ldots)^2 = 0.558902\ldots.$$

Despite some determined yet controversial attempts at analysis [13, 14], the conjecture remains unproven. The mere existence of the limiting parking density was shown only recently [15]. Intensive computer simulation [16–18] suggests, however, that the conjecture is false and the true limiting value is $0.562009\ldots$.

Here is a variation in the one-dimensional setting. In Rényi's problem, a car that lands in a parking position overlapping with an earlier car is discarded. Solomon [14, 19–21] studied a revised rule in which the car "rolls off" the earlier car immediately to the left or to the right, whichever is closer. It is then parked if there exists space for it; otherwise it is discarded. The mean car density is larger:

$$m = \int_0^\infty (2x + 1) \exp\left[-2(x + e^{-x} - 1)\right] \beta(x)\, dx = 0.8086525183\ldots$$

since cars are permitted greater flexibility to park bumper to bumper. If Rényi's problem is thought of as a model for sphere packing in a three-dimensional volume, then Solomon's variation corresponds to packing with "shaking" allowed for the spheres to settle, hence creating more space for additional spheres.

Another variation involves random car lengths [22, 23]. If the left and right endpoints of the kth arriving car are taken as the smaller and larger of two independent uniform draws from $[0, x]$, then the asymptotic expected number of cars successfully parked is $C \cdot k^{(\sqrt{17}-3)/4}$, where [24, 25]

$$C = \left(1 - \frac{1}{2^{(\sqrt{17}-1)/4}}\right) \sqrt{\pi} \frac{\Gamma\left(\frac{\sqrt{17}}{2}\right)}{\Gamma\left(\frac{\sqrt{17}+1}{4}\right) \Gamma\left(\frac{\sqrt{17}+3}{4}\right)^2} = 0.9848712825\ldots$$

and Γ is the gamma function [1.5.4]. Note that x is only a scale factor in this variation and does not figure in the result.

Applications of the parking problem (or, more generally, the sequential packing or space-filling problem) include such widely separated disciplines as:

- Physics: models of liquid structure [26–29];
- Chemistry: adsorption of a fluid film on a crystal surface [5.3.1];
- Monte Carlo methods: evaluation of definite integrals [30];
- Linguistics: frequency of one-syllable, length-n English words [31];
- Sociology: models of elections in Japan and lengths of gaps generated in parking problems [32–35];
- Materials science: intercrack distance after multiple fracture of reinforced concrete [36];
- Computer science: optimal data placement on a CD [37] and linear probing hashing [38].

See also [39–41]. Note the similarities in formulation between the Golomb–Dickman constant [5.4] and the Rényi constant.

5.3.1 Random Sequential Adsorption

Consider the case in which the interval $[0, x]$ is replaced by the discrete finite linear lattice $1, 2, 3, \ldots, n$. Each car is a line segment of unit length and covers two lattice points when it parks. No car is permitted to touch points that have already been covered. The process stops when no adjacent pairs of lattice points are left uncovered. It can be proved that, as $n \to \infty$ [19, 42–45],

$$m = \frac{1 - e^{-2}}{2} = 0.4323323583\ldots, \quad v = e^{-4} = 0.0183156388\ldots,$$

both of which are smaller than their continuous-case counterparts. The two-dimensional discrete analog involves unit square cars covering four lattice points, and is analytically intractable just like the continuous case. Palasti's conjecture appears to be false here too: The limiting mean density in the plane is not $m^2 = 0.186911\ldots$ but rather $0.186985\ldots$ [46–48].

For simplicity's sake, we refer to the infinite linear lattice $1, 2, 3, \ldots$ as the $1 \times \infty$ strip. The $2 \times \infty$ strip is the infinite ladder lattice with two parallel lines and crossbeams, the $3 \times \infty$ strip is likewise with three parallel lines, and naturally the $\infty \times \infty$ strip is the infinite square lattice. Thus we have closed-form expressions for m and v on $1 \times \infty$, but only numerical corrections to Palasti's estimate on $\infty \times \infty$.

If a car is a unit line segment (**dimer**) on the $2 \times \infty$ strip, then the mean car density is $\frac{1}{2}(0.91556671\ldots)$. If instead the car is on the $\infty \times \infty$ strip, then the corresponding mean density is $\frac{1}{2}(0.90682\ldots)$ [49–55]. Can exact formulas be found for these two quantities?

If the car is a line segment of length two (linear **trimer**) on the $1 \times \infty$ strip, then the mean density of vacancies is $\mu(3) = 0.1763470368\ldots$, where [6, 56–58]

$$\mu(r) = 1 - r \int\limits_0^1 \exp\left(-2\sum_{k=1}^{r-1} \frac{1 - x^k}{k}\right) dx.$$

More generally, $\mu(r)$ is the mean density of vacancies for linear r-mers on the $1 \times \infty$ strip, for any integer $r \geq 2$. A corresponding formula for the variance is not known.

Now suppose that the car is a single particle and that no other cars are allowed to park in any adjacent lattice points (**monomer** with **nearest neighbor exclusion**). The mean car density for the $1 \times \infty$ strip is $m_1 = \frac{1}{2}(1 - e^{-2})$ as before, of course. The mean densities for the $2 \times \infty$ and $3 \times \infty$ strips are [59–61]

$$m_2 = \frac{2 - e^{-1}}{4} = 0.4080301397\ldots, \quad m_3 = \frac{1}{3} = 0.3333333333\ldots,$$

and the corresponding density for the $\infty \times \infty$ strip is $m_\infty = 0.364132\ldots$ [47, 48, 50, 53, 55, 62]. Again, can exact formulas for m_4 or m_∞ be found?

The continuous case can be captured from the discrete case by appropriate limiting arguments [6, 58, 63]. Exhaustive surveys of random sequential adsorption models are provided in [64–66].

[1] A. Rényi, On a one-dimensional problem concerning random space-filling (in Hungarian), *Magyar Tud. Akad. Mat. Kutató Int. Közl.* 3 (1958) 109–127; Engl. transl. in *Selected Transl. Math. Statist. and Probab.*, v. 4, Inst. Math. Stat. and Amer. Math. Soc., 1963, pp. 203–224; also in *Selected Papers of Alfréd Rényi*, v. 2, Akadémiai Kiadó, 1976, pp. 173–188; MR 21 #3039.

[2] M. Lal and P. Gillard, Evaluation of a constant associated with a parking problem, *Math. Comp.* 28 (1974) 561–564; MR 49 #6560.

[3] G. Marsaglia, A. Zaman, and J. C. W. Marsaglia, Numerical solution of some classical differential-difference equations, *Math. Comp.* 53 (1989) 191–201; MR 90h:65124.

[4] P. C. Hemmer, The random parking problem, *J. Stat. Phys.* 57 (1989) 865–869; MR 92e:82054.

[5] P. L. Krapivsky, Kinetics of random sequential parking on a line, *J. Stat. Phys.* 69 (1992) 135–150; MR 93h:82063.

[6] J. K. Mackenzie, Sequential filling of a line by intervals placed at random and its application to linear adsorption, *J. Chem. Phys.* 37 (1962) 723–728.

[7] A. Dvoretzky and H. Robbins, On the parking problem, *Magyar Tud. Akad. Mat. Kutató Int. Közl.* 9 (1964) 209–224; MR 30 #3488.

[8] D. Mannion, Random space-filling in one dimension, *Magyar Tud. Akad. Mat. Kutató Int. Közl.* 9 (1964) 143–154; MR 31 #1698.

[9] D. Mannion, Random packing of an interval, *Adv. Appl. Probab.* 8 (1976) 477–501; 11 (1979) 591–602; MR 55 #1401 and MR 80i:60014.

[10] I. Palasti, On some random space filling problems, *Magyar Tud. Akad. Mat. Kutató Int. Közl.* 5 (1960) 353–359; MR 26 #4466.

[11] I. Palasti, On a two-dimensional random space filling problem, *Studia Sci. Math. Hungar.* 11 (1976) 247–252; MR 81d:52011.

[12] I. Palasti, A two-dimensional case of random packing and covering, *Random Fields*, v. 2, ed. J. Fritz, J. L. Lebowitz, and D. Szász, Colloq. Math. Soc. János Bolyai 27, North-Holland, 1976, pp. 821–834; MR 84j:60022.

[13]   H. J. Weiner, Sequential random packing in the plane, *J. Appl. Probab.* 15 (1978) 803–814; letters to the editor and replies, 16 (1979) 697–707 and 17 (1980) 878–892; MR 80a:60015, MR 81b:60013, and MR 82m:60021.

[14]   H. Solomon and H. J. Weiner, A review of the packing problem, *Commun. Statist. Theory Methods* 15 (1986) 2571–2607; MR 88a:60028.

[15]   M. D. Penrose, Random parking, sequential adsorption, and the jamming limit, *Commun. Math. Phys.* 218 (2001) 153–176; MR 2002a:60015.

[16]   B. E. Blaisdell and H. Solomon, On random sequential packing in the plane and a conjecture of Palasti, *J. Appl. Probab.* 7 (1970) 667–698; MR 43 #8101.

[17]   B. J. Brosilow, R. M. Ziff, and R. D. Vigil, Random sequential adsorption of parallel squares, *Phys. Rev. A* 43 (1991) 631–638.

[18]   B. Bonnier, M. Hontebeyrie, and C. Meyers, On the random filling of $\mathbb{R}^d$ by nonoverlapping d-dimensional cubes, *Physica A* 198 (1993) 1–10; MR 94g:82045.

[19]   H. Solomon, Random packing density, *Proc. Fifth Berkeley Symp. Math. Stat. Probab.*, v. 3, ed. L. M. Le Cam and J. Neyman, Univ. of Calif. Press, 1967, pp. 119–134; MR 41 #1187.

[20]   J. Talbot and S. M. Ricci, Analytic model for a ballistic deposition process, *Phys. Rev. Lett.* 68 (1992) 958–961.

[21]   P. Viot, G. Tarjus, and J. Talbot, Exact solution of a generalized ballistic-deposition model, *Phys. Rev. E* 48 (1993) 480–488.

[22]   P. E. Ney, A random interval filling problem, *Annals of Math. Statist.* 33 (1962) 702–718; MR 25 #1561.

[23]   J. P. Mullooly, A one dimensional random space-filling problem, *J. Appl. Probab.* 5 (1968) 427–435; MR 38 #5261.

[24]   E. G. Coffman, C. L. Mallows, and B. Poonen, Parking arcs on the circle with applications to one-dimensional communication networks, *Annals of Appl. Probab.* 4 (1994) 1098–1111; MR 95k:60245.

[25]   E. G. Coffman, L. Flatto, P. Jelenkovic, and B. Poonen, Packing random intervals on-line, *Algorithmica* 22 (1998) 448–476; MR 2000h:60012.

[26]   J. D. Bernal, A geometrical approach to the structure of liquids, *Nature* 183 (1959) 141–147.

[27]   J. D. Bernal, Geometry of the structure of monatomic liquids, *Nature* 185 (1960) 68–70.

[28]   J. D. Bernal and J. Mason, Coordination of randomly packed spheres, *Nature* 188 (1959) 910–911.

[29]   J. D. Bernal, J. Mason, and K. R. Knight, Radial distribution of the random close packing of equal spheres, *Nature* 194 (1962) 956–958.

[30]   G. Bánkövi, Evaluation of integrals by Monte Carlo methods based on the one-dimensional random space filling, *Magyar Tud. Akad. Mat. Kutató Int. Közl.* 5 (1960) 339–352; MR 26 #4465.

[31]   J. Dolby and H. Solomon, Information density phenomena and random packing, *J. Appl. Probab.* 12 (1975) 364–370.

[32]   Y. Itoh and S. Ueda, A random packing model for elections, *Annals Inst. Statist. Math.* 31 (1979) 157–167.

[33]   G. Bánkövi, On gaps generated by a random space filling procedure, *Magyar Tud. Akad. Mat. Kutató Int. Közl.* 7 (1962) 395–407; MR 27 #6314.

[34]   Y. Itoh, On the minimum of gaps generated by one-dimensional random packing, *J. Appl. Probab.* 17 (1980) 134–144; MR 81a:60019.

[35]   J. A. Morrison, The minimum of gaps generated by random packing of unit intervals into a large interval, *SIAM J. Appl. Math.* 47 (1987) 398–410; MR 88g:60033.

[36]   A. C. Kimber, An application of random packing to the multiple fracture of composite materials, *J. Appl. Probab.* 31 (1994) 564–569; MR 94m:73093.

[37]   E. G. Coffman and G. S. Lueker, *Probabilistic Analysis of Packing and Partitioning Algorithms*, Wiley, 1991; MR 92h:68038.

[38]   P. Flajolet, P. Poblete, and A. Viola, On the analysis of linear probing hashing, *Algorithmica* 22 (1998) 490–515; MR 2000h:68056.

[39] J. M. F. Chamayou, On two cascade models, *Stochastic Process. Appl.* 7 (1978) 153–163; MR 58 #24621.

[40] M. Sibuya and Y. Itoh, Random sequential bisection and its associated binary tree, *Annals Inst. Statist. Math.* 39 (1987) 69–84; MR 88e:60120.

[41] F. Komaki and Y. Itoh, A unified model for Kakutani's interval splitting and Rényi's random packing, *Adv. Appl. Probab.* 24 (1992) 502–505; MR 93c:60009.

[42] P. J. Flory, Intramolecular reaction between neighboring substituents of vinyl polymers, *J. Amer. Chem. Soc.* 61 (1939) 1518–1521.

[43] E. S. Page, The distribution of vacancies on a line, *J. Royal Statist. Soc. Ser. B* 21 (1959) 364–374; MR 22 #9984.

[44] F. Downton, A note on vacancies on a line, *J. Royal Statist. Soc. Ser. B* 23 (1961) 207–214; MR 24 #A3672.

[45] J. Texter, Alternative solution to a discrete car parking problem, *J. Chem. Phys.* 91 (1989) 6295–6301; MR 92c:82118.

[46] V. Privman, J.-S. Wang, and P. Nielaba, Continuum limit in random sequential adsorption, *Phys. Rev. B* 43 (1991) 3366–3371.

[47] R. Dickman, J.-S. Wang, and I. Jensen, Random sequential adsorption: Series and virial expansions, *J. Chem. Phys.* 94 (1991) 8252–8257.

[48] A. Baram and M. Fixman, Random sequential adsorption: Long time dynamics, *J. Chem. Phys.* 103 (1995) 1929–1933.

[49] R. S. Nord and J. W. Evans, Irreversible immobile random adsorption of dimers, trimers, ... on 2D lattices, *J. Chem. Phys.* 82 (1985) 2795–2810.

[50] J. W. Evans and R. S. Nord, Random and cooperative sequential adsorption on infinite ladders and strips, *J. Stat. Phys.* 69 (1992) 151–162.

[51] M. J. de Oliveira, T. Tomé, and R. Dickman, Anisotropic random sequential adsorption of dimers on a square lattice, *Phys. Rev. A* 46 (1992) 6294–6299.

[52] J.-S. Wang and R. B. Pandey, Kinetics and jamming coverage in a random sequential adsorption of polymer chains, *Phys. Rev. Lett.* 77 (1996) 1773–1776.

[53] C. K. Gan and J.-S. Wang, Extended series expansions for random sequential adsorption, *J. Chem. Phys.* 108 (1998) 3010–3012.

[54] C. Fusco, P. Gallo, A. Petri, and M. Rovere, Random sequential adsorption and diffusion of dimers and k-mers on a square lattice, *J. Chem. Phys.* 114 (2001) 7563–7569.

[55] J.-S. Wang, Series expansion and computer simulation studies of random sequential adsorption, *Colloids and Surfaces A* 165 (2000) 325–343.

[56] M. Gordon and I. H. Hillier, Statistics of random placement, subject to restrictions, on a linear lattice, *J. Chem. Phys.* 38 (1963) 1376–1380.

[57] E. A. Boucher, Kinetics and statistics of occupation of linear arrays: A model for polymer reactions, *J. Chem. Phys.* 59 (1973) 3848–3852.

[58] J. J. González, P. C. Hemmer, and J. S. Høye, Cooperative effects in random sequential polymer reactions, *Chem. Phys.* 3 (1974) 228–238.

[59] A. Baram and D. Kutasov, Random sequential adsorption on a quasi-one-dimensional lattice: An exact solution, *J. Phys. A* 25 (1992) L493–L498.

[60] Y. Fan and J. K. Percus, Random sequential adsorption on a ladder, *J. Stat. Phys.* 66 (1992) 263–271; MR 92j:82075.

[61] A. Baram and D. Kutasov, Random sequential adsorption on a $3 \times \infty$ lattice: An exact solution, *J. Phys. A* 27 (1994) 3683–3687.

[62] P. Meakin, J. L. Cardy, E. Loh, and D. J. Scalapino, Maximal coverage in random sequential adsorption, *J. Chem. Phys.* 86 (1987) 2380–2382.

[63] M. C. Bartelt, J. W. Evans, and M. L. Glasser, The car-parking limit of random sequential adsorption: Expansions in one dimension, *J. Chem. Phys.* 99 (1993) 1438–1439.

[64] J. W. Evans, Random and cooperative sequential adsorption, *Rev. Mod. Phys.* 65 (1993) 1281–1329.

[65] J. Talbot, G. Tarjus, P. R. van Tassel, and P. Viot, From car parking to protein adsorption: An overview of sequential adsorption processes, *Colloids and Surfaces A* 165 (2000) 287–324.

[66] V. Privman, Recent theoretical results for nonequilibrium deposition of submicron particles, *J. Adhesion* 74 (2000) 421–440; cond-mat/0003062.

5.4 Golomb–Dickman Constant

Every permutation on n symbols can be uniquely expressed as a product of disjoint cycles. For example, the permutation π on $\{0, 1, 2, \ldots, 9\}$ defined by $\pi(x) = 3x$ mod 10 has cycle structure

$$\pi = (0)\,(1\ 3\ 9\ 7)\,(2\ 6\ 8\ 4)\,(5).$$

In this case, the permutation π has $\alpha_1(\pi) = 2$ cycles of length 1, $\alpha_2(\pi) = 0$ cycles of length 2, $\alpha_3(\pi) = 0$ cycles of length 3, and $\alpha_4(\pi) = 2$ cycles of length 4. The total number $\sum_{j=1}^{\infty} \alpha_j$ of cycles in π is equal to 4 in the example.

Assume that n is fixed and that the $n!$ permutations on $\{0, 1, 2, \ldots, n-1\}$ are assigned equal probability. Picking π at random, we have the classical results [1–4]:

$$\mathrm{E}\left(\sum_{j=1}^{\infty} \alpha_j\right) = \sum_{i=1}^{n} \frac{1}{i} = \ln(n) + \gamma + O\left(\frac{1}{n}\right),$$

$$\mathrm{Var}\left(\sum_{j=1}^{\infty} \alpha_j\right) = \sum_{i=1}^{n} \frac{i-1}{i^2} = \ln(n) + \gamma - \frac{\pi^2}{6} + O\left(\frac{1}{n}\right),$$

$$\lim_{n \to \infty} \mathrm{P}(\alpha_j = k) = \frac{1}{k!} \exp\left(-\frac{1}{j}\right)\left(\frac{1}{j}\right)^k \quad \text{(asymptotic Poisson distribution),}$$

$$\lim_{n \to \infty} \mathrm{P}\left(\frac{\sum_{j=1}^{\infty} \alpha_j - \ln(n)}{\sqrt{\ln(n)}} \leq x\right)$$

$$= \frac{1}{\sqrt{2\pi}} \int_{-\infty}^{x} \exp\left(-\frac{t^2}{2}\right) dt \quad \text{(asymptotic normal distribution),}$$

where γ is the Euler–Mascheroni constant [1.5].

What can be said about the limiting distribution of the **longest cycle** and the **shortest cycle**,

$$M(\pi) = \max\{j \geq 1 : \alpha_j > 0\}, \quad m(\pi) = \min\{j \geq 1 : \alpha_j > 0\},$$

given a random permutation π? Goncharov [1,2] and Golomb [5–7] both considered the average value of $M(\pi)$. Golomb examined the constant [8–10]

$$\lambda = \lim_{n \to \infty} \frac{\mathrm{E}(M(\pi))}{n} = 1 - \int_{1}^{\infty} \frac{\rho(x)}{x^2} dx = 0.6243299885\ldots,$$

where $\rho(x)$ is the unique continuous solution of the following delay-differential equation:

$$\rho(x) = 1 \text{ for } 0 \leq x \leq 1, \ x\rho'(x) + \rho(x-1) = 0 \ \text{ for } x > 1.$$

(Actually, he worked with the function $\rho(x-1)$.) Shepp & Lloyd [11] and others [6] discovered additional expressions:

$$\lambda = \int_0^\infty e^{-x+\mathrm{Ei}(-x)}\, dx = \int_0^1 e^{\mathrm{Li}(x)}\, dx = G(1,1),$$

where

$$G(a,r) = \frac{1}{a} \int_0^\infty \left(1 - \exp(a\,\mathrm{Ei}(-x)) \sum_{k=0}^{r-1} \frac{(-a)^k}{k!}\,\mathrm{Ei}(-x)^k\right) dx,$$

Ei is the exponential integral [6.2.1], and Li is the logarithmic integral [6.2.2]. Gourdon [12] determined the complete asymptotic expansion for $\mathrm{E}(M(\pi))$:

$$\mathrm{E}(M(\pi)) = \lambda n + \frac{\lambda}{2} - \frac{e^\gamma}{24}\frac{1}{n} + \left[\frac{e^\gamma}{48} - \frac{(-1)^n}{8}\right]\frac{1}{n^2}$$
$$+ \left[\frac{17e^\gamma}{3840} + \frac{(-1)^n}{8} + \frac{e^{\frac{2(2n+1)\pi}{3}i}}{6} + \frac{e^{\frac{2(n+2)\pi}{3}i}}{6}\right]\frac{1}{n^3} + O\left(\frac{1}{n^4}\right).$$

Note the periodic fluctuations involving roots of unity.

A similar integral formula for $\lim_{n\to\infty} \mathrm{Var}(M(\pi))/n^2 = 0.0369078300\ldots = H(1,1)$ holds, where [12]

$$H(a,r) = \frac{2}{a(a+1)} \int_0^\infty \left(1 - \exp(a\,\mathrm{Ei}(-x)) \sum_{k=0}^{r-1} \frac{(-a)^k}{k!}\,\mathrm{Ei}(-x)^k\right) x\, dx - G(a,r)^2.$$

We will need values of $G(a,r)$ and $H(a,r)$, $a \neq 1 \neq r$, later in this essay. An analog of λ appears in [13, 14] in connection with polynomial factorization.

The arguments leading to asymptotic average values of $m(\pi)$ are more complicated. Shepp & Lloyd [11] proved that

$$\lim_{n\to\infty} \frac{\mathrm{E}(m(\pi))}{\ln(n)} = e^{-\gamma} = 0.5614594835\ldots$$

as well as formulas for higher moments. A complete asymptotic expansion for $\mathrm{E}(m(\pi))$, however, remains open.

The mean and variance of the rth longest cycle (normalized by n and n^2, as $n \to \infty$) are given by $G(1,r)$ and $H(1,r)$. For example, $G(1,2) = 0.2095808742\ldots$, $H(1,2) = 0.0125537906\ldots$ and $G(1,3) = 0.0883160988\ldots$, $H(1,3) = 0.0044939231\ldots$ [11,12].

There is a fascinating connection between λ and prime factorization algorithms [15, 16]. Let $f(n)$ denote the largest prime factor of n. By choosing a random integer

n between 1 and N, Dickman [17–20] determined that

$$\lim_{N \to \infty} P(f(n) \leq n^x) = \rho(\tfrac{1}{x})$$

for $0 < x \leq 1$. With this in mind, what is the average value of x such that $f(n) = n^x$? Dickman obtained numerically that

$$\mu = \lim_{N \to \infty} E(x) = \lim_{N \to \infty} E\left(\frac{\ln(f(n))}{\ln(n)}\right) = \int_0^1 x \, d\rho\left(\tfrac{1}{x}\right) = 1 - \int_1^\infty \frac{\rho(y)}{y^2} dy = \lambda,$$

which is indeed surprising! Dickman's constant μ and Golomb's constant λ are identical! Knuth & Trabb Pardo [15] described this result as follows: λn is the *asymptotic average number of digits* in the largest prime factor of an n-digit number. More generally, if we are factoring a random n-digit number, the distribution of digits in its prime factors is approximately the same as the distribution of the cycle lengths in a random permutation on n elements. This remarkable and unexpected fact is explored in greater depth in [21,22].

Other asymptotic formulas involving the largest prime factor function $f(n)$ include [15,23,24]

$$E(f(n)^k) \sim \frac{\zeta(k+1)}{k+1} \frac{N^k}{\ln(N)}, \quad E(\ln(f(n))) \sim \lambda \ln(N) - \lambda(1 - \gamma),$$

where $\zeta(x)$ is the zeta function [1.6]. See also [25–29]. Note the curious coincidence [15] involving integral and sum:

$$\int_0^\infty \rho(x) \, dx = e^\gamma = \sum_{n=1}^\infty n\rho(n).$$

Dickman's function is important in the study of y-smooth numbers [24, 30–32], that is, integers whose prime divisors never exceed y. It appears in probability theory as the density function (normalized by e^γ) of [33, 34]

$$X_1 + X_1 X_2 + X_1 X_2 X_3 + \cdots, \quad X_j \text{ independent uniform random variables on } [0, 1].$$

See [35–40] for other applications of $\rho(x)$. A closely-allied function, due to Buchstab, satisfies [24, 34, 41–45]

$$\omega(x) = \frac{1}{x} \text{ for } 1 \leq x \leq 2, \; x\omega'(x) + \omega(x) - \omega(x - 1) = 0 \; \text{ for } x > 2,$$

which arises when estimating the frequency of integers n whose *smallest* prime factor $\geq n^x$. Both functions are positive everywhere, and special values include [46]

$$\rho(\tfrac{3+\sqrt{5}}{2}) = 1 - \ln(\tfrac{3+\sqrt{5}}{2}) + \ln(\tfrac{1+\sqrt{5}}{2})^2 - \tfrac{\pi^2}{60}, \quad \lim_{x \to \infty} \rho(x) = 0,$$

$$\tfrac{5+\sqrt{5}}{2}\omega(\tfrac{5+\sqrt{5}}{2}) = 1 + \ln(\tfrac{3+\sqrt{5}}{2}) + \ln(\tfrac{1+\sqrt{5}}{2})^2 - \tfrac{\pi^2}{60}, \quad \lim_{x \to \infty} \omega(x) = e^{-\gamma}.$$

Whereas $\rho(x)$ is nonincreasing, the difference $\omega(x) - e^{-\gamma}$ changes sign (at most twice) in every interval of length 1. Its oscillatory behavior plays a role in understanding irregularities in the distribution of primes.

Note the similarity in formulation between the Golomb–Dickman constant and Rényi's parking constant [5.3].

5.4.1 Symmetric Group

Here are several related questions. Given π, a permutation on n symbols, define its **order** $\theta(\pi)$ to be the least positive integer m such that $\pi^m = $ identity. Clearly $1 \leq \theta(\pi) \leq n!$. What is its mean value, $E(\theta(\pi))$? Goh & Schmutz [47], building upon the work of Erdös & Turán [48], proved that

$$\ln(E(\theta(\pi))) = B\sqrt{\frac{n}{\ln(n)}} + o(1),$$

where $B = 2\sqrt{2b} = 2.9904703993\ldots$ and

$$b = \int_0^\infty \ln\left(1 - \ln(1 - e^{-x})\right) dx = 1.1178641511\ldots.$$

Stong [49] improved the $o(1)$ estimate and gave alternative representations for b:

$$b = \int_0^\infty \frac{xe^{-x}}{(1 - e^{-x})(1 - \ln(1 - e^{-x}))}\, dx = \int_0^\infty \frac{\ln(x + 1)}{e^x - 1}\, dx = -\sum_{k=1}^\infty \frac{e^k}{k} \text{Ei}(-k).$$

A typical permutation π can be shown to satisfy $\ln(\theta(\pi)) \sim \frac{1}{2}\ln(n)^2$; hence a few exceptional permutations contribute significantly to the mean. What can be said about the variance of $\theta(\pi)$?

Also, define $g(n)$ to be the maximum order $\theta(\pi)$ of all n-permutations π. Landau [50, 51] proved that $\ln(g(n)) \sim \sqrt{n\ln(n)}$, and greatly refined estimates of $g(n)$ appeared in [52].

A natural equivalence relation can be defined on the symmetric group S_n via conjugacy. In the limit as $n \to \infty$, for almost all conjugacy classes C, the elements of C have order equal to $\exp(\sqrt{n}(A + o(1)))$, where [48, 53, 54]

$$A = \frac{2\sqrt{6}}{\pi} \sum_{j \neq 0} \frac{(-1)^{j+1}}{3j^2 + j} = 4\sqrt{2} - \frac{6\sqrt{6}}{\pi}.$$

Note that the summation involves reciprocals of nonzero pentagonal numbers.

Let s_n denote the probability that two elements of the symmetric group, S_n, chosen at random (with replacement) actually generate S_n. The first several values are $s_1 = 1$, $s_2 = 3/4$, $s_3 = 1/2$, $s_4 = 3/8$, $\ldots$ [55]. What can be said about the asymptotics of s_n? Dixon [56] proved an 1892 conjecture by Netto [57] that $s_n \to 3/4$ as $n \to \infty$. Babai [58] gave a more refined estimate.

5.4.2 Random Mapping Statistics

We now generalize the discussion from permutations (bijective functions) on n symbols to arbitrary mappings on n symbols. For example, the function φ on $\{0, 1, 2, \ldots, 9\}$

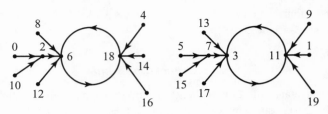

Figure 5.1. The functional graph for $\psi(x) = x^2 + 2 \bmod 20$ has two components, each containing a cycle of length 2.

defined by $\varphi(x) = 2x \bmod 10$ has cycles (0) and (2 4 8 6). The remaining symbols 1, 3, 5, 7, and 9 are transient in the sense that if one starts with 3, one is absorbed into the cycle (2 4 8 6) and never returns to 3. We can nevertheless define cycle lengths α_j as before; in this simple example, $\alpha_1(\varphi) = 1$, $\alpha_2(\varphi) = \alpha_3(\varphi) = 0$, and $\alpha_4(\varphi) = 1$.

The lengths of the longest and shortest cycles, $M(\varphi)$ and $m(\varphi)$, are clearly of interest in pseudo-random number generation. Purdom & Williams [59–61] found that

$$\lim_{n \to \infty} \frac{\mathrm{E}(M(\varphi))}{\sqrt{n}} = \lambda \sqrt{\frac{\pi}{2}} = 0.7824816009\ldots, \quad \lim_{n \to \infty} \frac{\mathrm{E}(m(\varphi))}{\ln(n)} = \frac{1}{2} e^{-\gamma}.$$

Observe that $\mathrm{E}(M(\varphi))$ grows on the order of only $\sqrt{n}$ rather than n as earlier.

As another example, consider the function ψ on $\{0, 1, 2, \ldots, 19\}$ defined by $\psi(x) = x^2 + 2 \bmod 20$. From Figure 5.1, clearly $\alpha_2(\psi) = 2$. Here are other interesting quantities [62]. Note that the transient symbols 0, 5, 10, and 15 each require 2 steps to reach a cycle, and this is the maximum such distance. Thus define the **longest tail** $L(\psi) = 2$. Note also that 4 is the number of vertices in the nonrepeating trajectory for each of 0, 5, 10, and 15, and this is the maximum such length. Thus define the **longest rho-path** $R(\psi) = 4$. Clearly, for the earlier example, $L(\varphi) = 1$ and $R(\varphi) = 5$. It can be proved that, for arbitrary n-mappings φ [61],

$$\lim_{n \to \infty} \frac{\mathrm{E}(L(\varphi))}{\sqrt{n}} = \sqrt{2\pi} \ln(2) = 1.7374623212\ldots,$$

$$\lim_{n \to \infty} \frac{\mathrm{E}(R(\varphi))}{\sqrt{n}} = \sqrt{\frac{\pi}{2}} \int_0^{\infty} (1 - e^{\mathrm{Ei}(-x) - I(x)}) \, dx = 2.4149010237\ldots,$$

where

$$I(x) = \int_0^x \frac{e^{-y}}{y} \left(1 - \exp\left(\frac{-2y}{e^{x-y} - 1} \right) \right) dy.$$

Another quantity associated with a mapping φ is the **largest tree** $P(\varphi)$. Each vertex in each cycle of φ is the root of a unique maximal tree [5.6]. Select the tree with the greatest number of vertices, and call this number $P(\varphi)$. For the two examples, clearly

$P(\varphi) = 2$ and $P(\psi) = 6$. It is known that, for arbitrary n-mappings φ [12,61],

$$\nu = \lim_{n \to \infty} \frac{E(P(\varphi))}{n} = 2 \int_0^\infty \left[1 - (1 - F(x))^{-1}\right] dx = 0.4834983471\ldots,$$

$$\lim_{n \to \infty} \frac{\text{Var}(P(\varphi))}{n^2} = \frac{8}{3} \int_0^\infty \left[1 - (1 - F(x))^{-1}\right] x \, dx - \nu^2 = 0.0494698522\ldots,$$

where

$$F(x) = \frac{-1}{2\sqrt{\pi}} \int_x^\infty e^{-t} t^{-\frac{3}{2}} \, dt = 1 - \frac{1}{\sqrt{\pi x}} \exp(-x) - \text{erf}(\sqrt{x})$$

and erf is the error function [4.6]. Gourdon [63] mentioned a coin-tossing game, the analysis of which yields the preceding two constants.

Finally, let us examine the connected component structure of a mapping. We have come full circle, in a sense, because components relate to mappings as cycles relate to permutations. For the two examples, the counting function is $\beta_2(\varphi) = 1$, $\beta_8(\varphi) = 1$ while $\beta_{10}(\psi) = 2$. In the interest of analogy, here are more details. The total number $\sum_{j=1}^{\infty} \beta_j$ of components is equal to 2 in both cases. Picking φ at random, we have [64–67]

$$E\left(\sum_{j=1}^{\infty} \beta_j\right) = \sum_{i=1}^{n} c_{n,0,i} = \frac{1}{2} \ln(n) + \frac{1}{2}(\ln(2) + \gamma) + o(1),$$

$$\text{Var}\left(\sum_{j=1}^{\infty} \beta_j\right) = \sum_{i=1}^{n} c_{n,0,i} - \left(\sum_{i=1}^{n} c_{n,0,i}\right)^2 + \sum_{i=1}^{n} c_{n,0,i} \sum_{j=1}^{n-i} c_{n,i,j}$$

$$= \frac{1}{2} \ln(n) + o(\ln(n)),$$

$$\lim_{n \to \infty} P(\beta_j = k) = \frac{1}{k!} \exp(-d_j) d_j^k, \quad \text{(asymptotic Poisson distribution)},$$

where

$$c_{n,p,q} = \binom{n-p}{q} \frac{(q-1)!}{n^q}, \quad d_j = \frac{e^{-j}}{j} \sum_{i=0}^{j-1} \frac{j^i}{i!},$$

and a corresponding Gaussian limit also holds. Define the **largest component** $Q(\varphi) = \max\{j \geq 1 : \beta_j > 0\}$; then [12,61,68]

$$\lim_{n \to \infty} \frac{E(Q(\varphi))}{n} = G(\tfrac{1}{2}, 1) = 0.7578230112\ldots,$$

$$\lim_{n \to \infty} \frac{\text{Var}(Q(\varphi))}{n^2} = H(\tfrac{1}{2}, 1) = 0.0370072165\ldots.$$

Such results answer questions raised in [69–71]. It seems fitting to call $0.75782\ldots$ the **Flajolet–Odlyzko constant**, owing to its importance. The mean and variance of the rth largest component (again normalized by n and n^2, as $n \to \infty$) are given by $G(\frac{1}{2}, r)$ and $H(\frac{1}{2}, r)$. For example, $G(\frac{1}{2}, 2) = 0.1709096198\ldots$ and $H(\frac{1}{2}, 2) = 0.0186202233\ldots$. A discussion of smallest components appears in [72].

[1] W. Goncharov, Sur la distribution des cycles dans les permutations, *C. R. (Dokl.) Acad. Sci. URSS* 35 (1942) 267–269; MR 4,102g.

[2] W. Goncharov, On the field of combinatory analysis (in Russian), *Izv. Akad. Nauk SSSR* 8 (1944) 3–48; Engl. transl. in *Amer. Math. Soc. Transl.* 19 (1962) 1–46; MR 6,88b and MR 24 A1221.

[3] R. E. Greenwood, The number of cycles associated with the elements of a permutation group, *Amer. Math. Monthly* 60 (1953) 407–409; MR 14,939b.

[4] H. S. Wilf, *generatingfunctionology*, Academic Press, 1990; MR 95a:05002.

[5] S. W. Golomb, Random permutations, *Bull. Amer. Math. Soc.* 70 (1964) 747.

[6] S. W. Golomb, *Shift Register Sequences*, Holden-Day, 1967; MR 39 #3906.

[7] S. W. Golomb and P. Gaal, On the number of permutations on n objects with greatest cycle length k, *Adv. Appl. Math.* 20 (1998) 98–107; *Probabilistic Methods in Discrete Mathematics*, Proc. 1996 Petrozavodsk conf., ed. V. F. Kolchin, V. Ya. Kozlov, Yu. L. Pavlov, and Yu. V. Prokhorov, VSP, 1997, pp. 211–218; MR 98k:05003 and MR 99j:05001.

[8] W. C. Mitchell, An evaluation of Golomb's constant, *Math. Comp.* 22 (1968) 411–415.

[9] D. E. Knuth, *The Art of Computer Programming*, v. 1, *Fundamental Algorithms*, Addison-Wesley, 1969, pp. 180–181, 519–520; MR 51 #14624.

[10] A. MacLeod, Golomb's constant to 250 decimal places, unpublished note (1997).

[11] L. A. Shepp and S. P. Lloyd, Ordered cycle lengths in a random permutation, *Trans. Amer. Math. Soc.* 121 (1966) 350–557; MR 33 #3320.

[12] X. Gourdon, *Combinatoire, Algorithmique et Géométrie des Polynômes*, Ph.D. thesis, École Polytechnique, 1996.

[13] P. Flajolet, X. Gourdon, and D. Panario, Random polynomials and polynomial factorization, *Proc. 1996 Int. Colloq. on Automata, Languages and Programming (ICALP)*, Paderborn, ed. F. Meyer auf der Heide and B. Monien, Lect. Notes in Comp. Sci. 1099, Springer-Verlag, pp. 232–243; MR 98e:68123.

[14] P. Flajolet, X. Gourdon, and D. Panario, The complete analysis of a polynomial factorization algorithm over finite fields, *J. Algorithms* 40 (2001) 37–81; INRIA report RR3370; MR 2002f:68193.

[15] D. E. Knuth and L. Trabb Pardo, Analysis of a simple factorization algorithm, *Theoret. Comput. Sci.* 3 (1976) 321–348; also in *Selected Papers on Analysis of Algorithms*, CSLI, 2000, pp. 303–339; MR 58 #16485.

[16] D. E. Knuth, *The Art of Computer Programming*, v. 2, *Seminumerical Algorithms*, 2nd ed., Addison-Wesley, 1981, pp. 367–368, 395, 611; MR 83i:68003.

[17] K. Dickman, On the frequency of numbers containing prime factors of a certain relative magnitude, *Ark. Mat. Astron. Fysik*, v. 22A (1930) n. 10, 1–14.

[18] S. D. Chowla and T. Vijayaraghavan, On the largest prime divisors of numbers, *J. Indian Math. Soc.* 11 (1947) 31–37; MR 9,332d.

[19] V. Ramaswami, On the number of positive integers less than x and free of prime divisors greater than x^c, *Bull. Amer. Math. Soc.* 55 (1949) 1122–1127; MR 11,233f.

[20] N. G. de Bruijn, On the number of positive integers $\leq x$ and free of prime factors $> y$, *Proc. Konink. Nederl. Acad. Wetensch. Ser. A* 54 (1951) 50–60; *Indag. Math.* 13 (1951) 50–60; MR 13,724e.

[21] R. Arratia, A. D. Barbour, and S. Tavaré, Random combinatorial structures and prime factorizations, *Notices Amer. Math. Soc.* 44 (1997) 903–910; MR 98i:60007.

[22] R. Arratia, A. D. Barbour, and S. Tavaré, *Logarithmic Combinatorial Structures: A Probabilistic Approach,* unpublished manuscript (2001).

[23] K. Alladi and P. Erdös, On an additive arithmetic function, *Pacific J. Math.* 71 (1977) 275–294; MR 56 #5401.

[24] G. Tenenbaum, *Introduction to Analytic and Probabilistic Number Theory*, Cambridge Univ. Press, 1995, pp. 365–366, 393, 399–400; MR 97e:11005b.

[25] P. Erdös and A. Ivić, Estimates for sums involving the largest prime factor of an integer and certain related additive functions, *Studia Sci. Math. Hungar.* 15 (1980) 183–199; MR 84a:10046.

[26] T. Z. Xuan, On a result of Erdös and Ivić, *Arch. Math. (Basel)* 62 (1994) 143–154; MR 94m:11109.

[27] H. Z. Cao, Sums involving the smallest prime factor of an integer, *Utilitas Math.* 45 (1994) 245–251; MR 95d:11126.

[28] S. R. Finch, Moments of the Smarandache function, *Smarandache Notions J.* 10 (1999) 95–96; 11 (2000) 140–141; MR 2000a:11129.

[29] K. Ford, The normal behavior of the Smarandache function, *Smarandache Notions J.* 10 (1999) 81–86; MR 2000a:11130.

[30] K. K. Norton, Numbers with small prime factors, and the least k^{th} power non-residue, *Memoirs Amer. Math. Soc.* 106 (1971) 1–106; MR 44 #3948.

[31] A. Hildebrand and G. Tenenbaum, Integers without large prime factors, *J. Théorie Nombres Bordeaux* 5 (1993) 411–484; MR 95d:11116.

[32] P. Moree, *On the Psixyology of Diophantine Equations*, Ph.D. thesis, Univ. of Leiden, 1993.

[33] J.-M.-F. Chamayou, A probabilistic approach to a differential-difference equation arising in analytic number theory, *Math. Comp.* 27 (1973) 197–203; MR 49 #1725.

[34] G. Marsaglia, A. Zaman, and J. C. W. Marsaglia, Numerical solution of some classical differential-difference equations, *Math. Comp.* 53 (1989) 191–201; MR 90h:65124.

[35] H. Davenport and P. Erdös, The distribution of quadratic and higher residues, *Publ. Math. (Debrecen)* 2 (1952) 252–265; MR 14,1063h.

[36] L. I. Pál and G. Németh, A statistical theory of lattice damage in solids irradiated by high-energy particles, *Nuovo Cimento* 12 (1959) 293–309; MR 21 #7630.

[37] G. A. Watterson, The stationary distribution of the infinitely-many neutral alleles diffusion model, *J. Appl. Probab.* 13 (1976) 639–651; correction 14 (1977) 897; MR 58 #20594a and b.

[38] D. Hensley, The convolution powers of the Dickman function, *J. London Math. Soc.* 33 (1986) 395–406; MR 87k:11097.

[39] D. Hensley, Distribution of sums of exponentials of random variables, *Amer. Math. Monthly* 94 (1987) 304–306.

[40] C. J. Lloyd and E. J. Williams, Recursive splitting of an interval when the proportions are identical and independent random variables, *Stochastic Process. Appl.* 28 (1988) 111–122; MR 89e:60025.

[41] A. A. Buchstab, Asymptotic estimates of a general number theoretic function (in Russian), *Mat. Sbornik* 2 (1937) 1239–1246.

[42] S. Selberg, The number of cancelled elements in the sieve of Eratosthenes (in Norwegian), *Norsk Mat. Tidsskr.* 26 (1944) 79–84; MR 8,317a.

[43] N. G. de Bruijn, On the number of uncancelled elements in the sieve of Eratosthenes, *Proc. Konink. Nederl. Acad. Wetensch. Sci. Sect.* 53 (1950) 803–812; *Indag. Math.* 12 (1950) 247–256; MR 12,11d.

[44] A. Y. Cheer and D. A. Goldston, A differential delay equation arising from the sieve of Eratosthenes, *Math. Comp.* 55 (1990) 129–141; MR 90j:11091.

[45] A. Hildebrand and G. Tenenbaum, On a class of differential-difference equations arising in analytic number theory, *J. d'Analyse Math.* 61 (1993) 145–179; MR 94i:11069.

[46] P. Moree, A special value of Dickman's function, *Math. Student* 64 (1995) 47–50.

[47] W. M. Y. Goh and E. Schmutz, The expected order of a random permutation, *Bull. London Math. Soc.* 23 (1991) 34–42; MR 93a:11080.

[48] P. Turán, Combinatorics, partitions, group theory, *Colloquio Internazionale sulle Teorie Combinatorie*, t. 2, Proc. 1973 Rome conf., Accad. Naz. Lincei, 1976, pp. 181–200; also in *Collected Works*, v. 3, ed. P. Erdös, Akadémiai Kiadó, pp. 2302–2321; MR 58 #21978.

[49] R. Stong, The average order of a permutation, *Elec. J. Combin.* 5 (1998) R41; MR 99f:11122.

[50] W. Miller, The maximum order of an element of a finite symmetric group, *Amer. Math. Monthly* 94 (1987) 497–506; MR 89k:20005.

[51] J.-L. Nicolas, On Landau's function $g(n)$, *The Mathematics of Paul Erdös*, v. 1, ed. R. L. Graham and J. Nesetril, Springer-Verlag, 1997, pp. 228–240; MR 98b:11096.

[52] J.-P. Massias, J.-L. Nicolas, and G. Robin, Effective bounds for the maximal order of an element in the symmetric group, *Math. Comp.* 53 (1989) 665–678; MR 90e:11139.

[53] D. H. Lehmer, On a constant of Turán and Erdös, *Acta Arith.* 37 (1980) 359–361; MR 82b:05014.

[54] W. Schwarz, Another evaluation of an Erdös-Turán constant, *Analysis* 5 (1985) 343–345; MR 86m:40003.

[55] N. J. A. Sloane, On-Line Encyclopedia of Integer Sequences, A040173 and A040174.

[56] J. D. Dixon, The probability of generating the symmetric group, *Math. Z.* 110 (1969) 199–205; MR 40 #4985.

[57] E. Netto, *The Theory of Substitutions and Its Applications to Algebra*, 2nd ed., Chelsea, 1964; MR 31 #184.

[58] L. Babai, The probability of generating the symmetric group, *J. Combin. Theory Ser. A* 52 (1989) 148–153; MR 91a:20007.

[59] P. W. Purdom and J. H. Williams, Cycle length in a random function, *Trans. Amer. Math. Soc.* 133 (1968) 547–551; MR 37 #3616.

[60] D. E. Knuth, *The Art of Computer Programming*, v. 2, *Seminumerical Algorithms*, 2nd ed., Addison-Wesley, 1981; pp. 7–8, 517–520; MR 83i:68003.

[61] P. Flajolet and A. M. Odlyzko, Random mapping statistics, *Advances in Cryptology – EUROCRYPT '89*, ed. J.-J. Quisquater and J. Vandewalle, Lect. Notes in Comp. Sci. 434, Springer-Verlag, 1990, pp. 329–354; MR 91h:94003.

[62] R. Sedgewick and P. Flajolet, *Introduction to the Analysis of Algorithms*, Addison-Wesley, 1996, pp. 357–358, 454–465.

[63] X. Gourdon, Largest components in random combinatorial structures, *Discrete Math.* 180 (1998) 185–209; MR 99c:60013.

[64] M. D. Kruskal, The expected number of components under a random mapping function, *Amer. Math. Monthly* 61 (1954) 392–397; MR 16,52b.

[65] S. M. Ross, A random graph, *J. Appl. Probab.* 18 (1981) 309–315; MR 81m:05124.

[66] P. M. Higgins and E. J. Williams, Random functions on a finite set, *Ars Combin.* 26 (1988) A, 93–102; MR 90g:60008.

[67] V. F. Kolchin, *Random Mappings*, Optimization Software Inc., 1986, pp. 46, 79, 164; MR 88a:60022.

[68] D. Panario and B. Richmond, Exact largest and smallest size of components, *Algorithmica* 31 (2001) 413–432; MR 2002j:68065.

[69] G. A. Watterson and H. A. Guess, Is the most frequent allele the oldest?, *Theoret. Populat. Biol.* 11 (1977) 141–160.

[70] P. J. Donnelly, W. J. Ewens, and S. Padmadisastra, Functionals of random mappings: Exact and asymptotic results, *Adv. Appl. Probab.* 23 (1991) 437–455; MR 92k:60017.

[71] P. M. Higgins, *Techniques of Semigroup Theory*, Oxford Univ. Press, 1992; MR 93d:20101.

[72] D. Panario and B. Richmond, Smallest components in decomposable structures: exp-log class, *Algorithmica* 29 (2001) 205–226.

5.5 Kalmár's Composition Constant

An **additive composition** of an integer n is a sequence $x_1, x_2, \ldots, x_k$ of integers (for some $k \geq 1$) such that

$$n = x_1 + x_2 + \cdots + x_k, \quad x_j \geq 1 \text{ for all } 1 \leq j \leq k.$$

A **multiplicative composition** of n is the same except

$$n = x_1 x_2 \cdots x_k, \quad x_j \geq 2 \text{ for all } 1 \leq j \leq k.$$

The number $a(n)$ of additive compositions of n is trivially 2^{n-1}. The number $m(n)$ of multiplicative compositions does not possess a closed-form expression, but asymptotically satisfies

$$\sum_{n=1}^{N} m(n) \sim \frac{-1}{\rho \zeta'(\rho)} N^\rho = (0.3181736521\ldots) \cdot N^\rho,$$

where $\rho = 1.7286472389\ldots$ is the unique solution of $\zeta(x) = 2$ with $x > 1$ and $\zeta(x)$ is Riemann's zeta function [1.6]. This result was first deduced by Kalmár [1,2] and refined in [3–8].

An **additive partition** of an integer n is a sequence $x_1, x_2, \ldots, x_k$ of integers (for some $k \geq 1$) such that

$$n = x_1 + x_2 + \cdots + x_k, \quad 1 \leq x_1 \leq x_2 \leq \cdots \leq x_k.$$

Partitions naturally represent equivalence classes of compositions under sorting. The number $A(n)$ of additive partitions of n is mentioned in [1.4.2], while the number $M(n)$ of **multiplicative partitions** asymptotically satisfies [9, 10]

$$\sum_{n=1}^{N} M(n) \sim \frac{1}{2\sqrt{\pi}} N \exp\left(2\sqrt{\ln(N)}\right) \ln(N)^{-\frac{3}{4}}.$$

Thus far we have dealt with *unrestricted* compositions and partitions. Of many possible variations, let us focus on the case in which each x_j is restricted to be a prime number. For example, the number $M_p(n)$ of **prime multiplicative partitions** is trivially 1 for $n \geq 2$. The number $a_p(n)$ of **prime additive compositions** is [11]

$$a_p(n) \sim \frac{1}{\xi f'(\xi)} \left(\frac{1}{\xi}\right)^n = (0.3036552633\ldots) \cdot (1.4762287836\ldots)^n,$$

where $\xi = 0.6774017761\ldots$ is the unique solution of the equation

$$f(x) = \sum_p x^p = 1, \quad x > 0,$$

and the sum is over all primes p. The number $m_p(n)$ of **prime multiplicative compositions** satisfies [12]

$$\sum_{n=1}^{N} m_p(n) \sim \frac{-1}{\eta g'(\eta)} N^{-\eta} = (0.4127732370\ldots) \cdot N^{-\eta},$$

where $\eta = -1.3994333287\ldots$ is the unique solution of the equation

$$g(y) = \sum_p p^y = 1, \quad y < 0.$$

Not much is known about the number $A_p(n)$ of **prime additive partitions** [13–16] except that $A_p(n + 1) > A_p(n)$ for $n \geq 8$.

Here is a related, somewhat artificial topic. Let p_n be the nth prime, with $p_1 = 2$, and define formal series

$$P(z) = 1 + \sum_{n=1}^{\infty} p_n z^n, \quad Q(z) = \frac{1}{P(z)} = \sum_{n=0}^{\infty} q_n z^n.$$

Some people may be surprised to learn that the coefficients q_n obey the following asymptotics [17]:

$$q_n \sim \frac{1}{\theta \, P'(\theta)} \left(\frac{1}{\theta}\right)^n = (-0.6223065745\ldots) \cdot (-1.4560749485\ldots)^n.$$

where $\theta = -0.6867778344\ldots$ is the unique zero of $P(z)$ inside the disk $|z| < 3/4$. By way of contrast, $p_n \sim n \ln(n)$ by the Prime Number Theorem. In a similar spirit, consider the coefficients c_k of the $(n-1)^{\text{st}}$ degree polynomial fit

$$c_0 + c_1(x-1) + c_2(x-1)(x-2) + \cdots + c_{n-1}(x-1)(x-2)(x-3)\cdots(x-n+1)$$

to the dataset [18]

$$(1, 2), (2, 3), (3, 5), (4, 7), (5, 11), (6, 13), \ldots, (n, p_n).$$

In the limit as $n \to \infty$, the sum $\sum_{k=0}^{n-1} c_k$ converges to $3.4070691656\ldots$.

Let us return to the counting of compositions and partitions, and merely mention variations in which each x_j is restricted to be square-free [12] or where the xs must be distinct [8]. Also, compositions/partitions $x_1, x_2, \ldots, x_k$ and $y_1, y_2, \ldots, y_l$ of n are said to be **independent** if proper subsequence sums/products of xs and ys never coincide. How many such pairs are there (as a function of n)? See [19] for an asymptotic answer.

Cameron & Erdös [20] pointed out that the number of sequences $1 \leq z_1 < z_2 < \cdots < z_k = n$ for which $z_i | z_j$ whenever $i < j$ is $2m(n)$. The factor 2 arises because we can choose whether or not to include 1 in the sequence. What can be said about the number $c(n)$ of sequences $1 \leq w_1 < w_2 < \cdots < w_k \leq n$ for which $w_i \nmid w_j$ whenever $i \neq j$? It is conjectured that $\lim_{n \to \infty} c(n)^{1/n}$ exists, and it is known that $1.55967^n \leq c(n) \leq 1.59^n$ for sufficiently large n. For more about such sequences, known as **primitive sequences**, see [2.27].

Finally, define $h(n)$ to be the number of ways to express 1 as a sum of $n+1$ elements of the set $\{2^{-i} : i \geq 0\}$, where repetitions are allowed and order is immaterial. Flajolet & Prodinger [21] demonstrated that

$$h(n) \sim (0.2545055235\ldots)\kappa^n,$$

where $\kappa = 1.7941471875\ldots$ is the reciprocal of the smallest positive root x of the equation

$$\sum_{j=1}^{\infty} (-1)^{j+1} \frac{x^{2^{j+1}-2-j}}{(1-x)(1-x^3)(1-x^7)\cdots(1-x^{2^j-1})} - 1 = 0.$$

This is connected to enumerating level number sequences associated with binary trees [5.6].

[1] L. Kalmár, A "factorisatio numerorum" problémájáról, *Mat. Fiz. Lapok* 38 (1931) 1–15.

[2] L. Kalmár, Über die mittlere Anzahl Produktdarstellungen der Zahlen, *Acta Sci. Math. (Szeged)* 5 (1930-32) 95–107.

[3] E. Hille, A problem in "Factorisatio Numerorum," *Acta Arith.* 2 (1936) 136–144.

[4] P. Erdös, On some asymptotic formulas in the theory of the "factorisatio numerorum," *Annals of Math.* 42 (1941) 989–993; MR 3,165b.

[5] P. Erdös, Corrections to two of my papers, *Annals of Math.* 44 (1943) 647–651; MR 5,172c.

[6] S. Ikehara, On Kalmár's problem in "Factorisatio Numerorum." II, *Proc. Phys.-Math. Soc. Japan* 23 (1941) 767–774; MR 7,365h.

[7] R. Warlimont, Factorisatio numerorum with constraints, *J. Number Theory* 45 (1993) 186–199; MR 94f:11098.

[8] H.-K. Hwang, Distribution of the number of factors in random ordered factorizations of integers, *J. Number Theory* 81 (2000) 61–92; MR 2001k:11183.

[9] A. Oppenheim, On an arithmetic function. II, *J. London Math. Soc.* 2 (1927) 123–130.

[10] G. Szekeres and P. Turán, Über das zweite Hauptproblem der "Factorisatio Numerorum," *Acta Sci. Math. (Szeged)* 6 (1932-34) 143–154; also in *Collected Works of Paul Turán*, v. 1, ed. P. Erdös, Akadémiai Kiadó, pp. 1–12.

[11] P. Flajolet, Remarks on coefficient asymptotics, unpublished note (1995).

[12] A. Knopfmacher, J. Knopfmacher, and R. Warlimont, Ordered factorizations for integers and arithmetical semigroups, *Advances in Number Theory*, Proc. 1991 Kingston conf., ed. F. Q. Gouvêa and N. Yui, Oxford Univ. Press, 1993, pp. 151–165; MR 97e:11118.

[13] P. T. Bateman and P. Erdös, Monotonicity of partition functions, *Mathematika* 3 (1956) 1–14; MR 18,195a.

[14] P. T. Bateman and P. Erdös, Partitions into primes, *Publ. Math. (Debrecen)* 4 (1956) 198–200; MR 18,15c.

[15] J. Browkin, Sur les décompositions des nombres naturels en sommes de nombres premiers, *Colloq. Math.* 5 (1958) 205–207; MR 21 #1956.

[16] N. J. A. Sloane, On-Line Encyclopedia of Integer Sequences, A000041, A000607, A001055, A002033, A002572, A008480, and A023360.

[17] N. Backhouse, Formal reciprocal of a prime power series, unpublished note (1995).

[18] F. Magata, Newtonian interpolation and primes, unpublished note (1998).

[19] P. Erdös, J.-L. Nicolas, and A. Sárközy, On the number of pairs of partitions of n without common subsums, *Colloq. Math.* 63 (1992) 61–83; MR 93c:11087.

[20] P. J. Cameron and P. Erdös, On the number of sets of integers with various properties, *Number Theory*, Proc. 1990 Canad. Number Theory Assoc. Banff conf., ed. R. A. Mollin, Gruyter, pp. 61–79; MR 92g:11010.

[21] P. Flajolet and H. Prodinger, Level number sequences for trees, *Discrete Math.* 65 (1987) 149–156; MR 88e:05030.

5.6 Otter's Tree Enumeration Constants

A **graph** of order n consists of a set of n **vertices** (points) together with a set of **edges** (unordered pairs of distinct points). Note that loops and multiple parallel edges are automatically disallowed. Two vertices joined by an edge are called **adjacent**.

A **forest** is a graph that is **acyclic**, meaning that there is no sequence of adjacent vertices $v_0, v_1, \ldots, v_m$ such that $v_i \neq v_j$ for all $i < j < m$ and $v_0 = v_m$.

A **tree** (or **free tree**) is a forest that is **connected**, meaning that for any two distinct vertices u and w, there is a sequence of adjacent vertices $v_0, v_1, \ldots, v_m$ such that $v_0 = u$ and $v_m = w$.

Two trees σ and τ are **isomorphic** if there is a one-to-one map from the vertices of σ to the vertices of τ that preserves adjacency (see Figure 5.2). Diagrams for all non-isomorphic trees of order < 11 appear in [1]. Applications are given in [2].

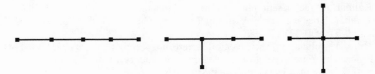

Figure 5.2. There exist three non-isomorphic trees of order 5.

What can be said about the asymptotics of t_n, the number of non-isomorphic trees of order n? Building upon the work of Cayley and Pólya, Otter [3–6] determined that

$$\lim_{n \to \infty} \frac{t_n n^{\frac{5}{2}}}{\alpha^n} = \beta,$$

where $\alpha = 2.9557652856\ldots = (0.3383218568\ldots)^{-1}$ is the unique positive solution of the equation $T(x^{-1}) = 1$ involving a certain function T to be defined shortly, and

$$\beta = \frac{1}{\sqrt{2\pi}} \left(1 + \sum_{k=2}^{\infty} \frac{1}{\alpha^k} T'\left(\frac{1}{\alpha^k}\right) \right)^{\frac{3}{2}} = 0.5349496061\ldots$$

where T' denotes the derivative of T. Although α and β can be calculated efficiently to great accuracy, it is not known whether they are algebraic or transcendental [6, 7].

A **rooted tree** is a tree in which precisely one vertex, called the **root**, is distinguished from the others (see Figure 5.3). We agree to draw the root as a tree's topmost vertex and that an isomorphism of rooted trees maps a root to a root. What can be said about the asymptotics of T_n, the number of non-isomorphic rooted trees of order n? Otter's corresponding result is

$$\lim_{n \to \infty} \frac{T_n n^{\frac{3}{2}}}{\alpha^n} = \left(\frac{\beta}{2\pi}\right)^{\frac{1}{3}} = 0.4399240125\ldots = \left(\frac{1}{4\pi\alpha}\right)^{\frac{1}{2}} (2.6811281472\ldots).$$

In fact, the generating functions

$$t(x) = \sum_{n=1}^{\infty} t_n x^n$$

$$= x + x^2 + x^3 + 2x^4 + 3x^5 + 6x^6 + 11x^7 + 23x^8 + 47x^9 + 106x^{10} + \cdots,$$

$$T(x) = \sum_{n=1}^{\infty} T_n x^n$$

$$= x + x^2 + 2x^3 + 4x^4 + 9x^5 + 20x^6 + 48x^7 + 115x^8 + 286x^9 + \cdots$$

are related by the formula $t(x) = T(x) - \frac{1}{2}(T(x)^2 - T(x^2))$, the constant α^{-1} is the radius of convergence for both, and the coefficients T_n can be computed using

$$T(x) = x \exp\left(\sum_{k=1}^{\infty} \frac{T(x^k)}{k}\right), \quad T_{n+1} = \frac{1}{n} \sum_{k=1}^{n} \left(\sum_{d|k} d T_d\right) T_{n-k+1}.$$

There are many varieties of trees and the elaborate details of enumerating them are best left to [4, 5]. Here is the first of many examples. A **weakly binary tree** is a rooted

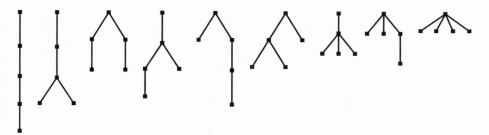

Figure 5.3. There exist nine non-isomorphic rooted trees of order 5.

tree for which the root is adjacent to at most two vertices and all non-root vertices are adjacent to at most three vertices. For instance, there exist six non-isomorphic weakly binary trees of order 5. The asymptotics of B_n, the number of non-isomorphic weakly binary trees of order n, were obtained by Otter [3, 8–10]:

$$\lim_{n\to\infty} \frac{B_n n^{\frac{3}{2}}}{\xi^n} = \eta,$$

where $\xi^{-1} = 0.4026975036\ldots = (2.4832535361\ldots)^{-1}$ is the radius of convergence for

$$B(x) = \sum_{n=0}^{\infty} B_n x^n$$

$$= 1 + x + x^2 + 2x^3 + 3x^4 + 6x^5 + 11x^6 + 23x^7 + 46x^8 + 98x^9 + \cdots$$

and

$$\eta = \sqrt{\frac{\xi}{2\pi}} \left(1 + \frac{1}{\xi}B(\frac{1}{\xi^2}) + \frac{1}{\xi^3}B'(\frac{1}{\xi^2})\right)^{\frac{1}{2}}$$

$$= 0.7916031835\ldots = (0.3187766258\ldots)\xi.$$

The series coefficients arise from

$$B(x) = 1 + \frac{1}{2}x \left(B(x)^2 + B(x^2)\right),$$

$$B_k = \begin{cases} \dfrac{B_i(B_i + 1)}{2} + \displaystyle\sum_{j=0}^{i-1} B_{k-j-1}B_j & \text{if } k = 2i + 1, \\ \displaystyle\sum_{j=0}^{i-1} B_{k-j-1}B_j & \text{if } k = 2i. \end{cases}$$

Otter showed, in this special case, that $\xi = \lim_{n\to\infty} c_n^{2^{-n}}$, where the sequence $\{c_n\}$ obeys the quadratic recurrence

$$c_0 = 2, \qquad c_n = c_{n-1}^2 + 2 \quad \text{for } n \geq 1,$$

and consequently

$$\eta = \frac{1}{2}\sqrt{\frac{\xi}{\pi}} \sqrt{3 + \frac{1}{c_1} + \frac{1}{c_1 c_2} + \frac{1}{c_1 c_2 c_3} + \frac{1}{c_1 c_2 c_3 c_4} + \cdots}.$$

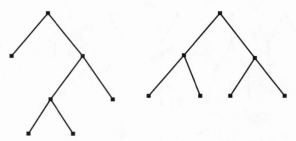

Figure 5.4. There exist two non-isomorphic strongly binary trees of order 7.

Here is a slight specialization of the preceding. Define a **strongly binary tree** to be a rooted tree for which the root is adjacent to either zero or two vertices, and all non-root vertices are adjacent to either one or three vertices (see Figure 5.4). These trees, also called **binary trees**, are discussed further in [5.6.9] and [5.13]. The number of non-isomorphic strongly binary trees of order $2n + 1$ turns out to be exactly B_n. The one-to-one correspondence is obtained, in the forward direction, by deleting all the **leaves** (terminal nodes) of a strongly binary tree. To go in reverse, starting with a weakly binary tree, add two leaves to any vertex of degree 1 (or to the root if it has degree 0), and add one leaf to any vertex of degree 2 (or to the root if it has degree 1). Hence the same asymptotics apply in both weak and strong cases.

Also, in a commutative non-associative algebra, the expression x^4 is ambiguous and could be interpreted as xx^3 or x^2x^2. The expression x^5 likewise could mean xxx^3, xx^2x^2, or x^2x^3. Clearly B_{n-1} is the number of possible interpretations of x^n; thus $\{B_n\}$ is sometimes called the Wedderburn-Etherington sequence [11–15].

5.6.1   Chemical Isomers

A **weakly ternary tree** is a rooted tree for which the root is adjacent to at most three vertices and all non-root vertices are adjacent to at most four vertices. For instance, there exist eight non-isomorphic weakly ternary trees of order 5. The asymptotics of R_n, the number of non-isomorphic weakly ternary trees of order n, were again obtained by Otter [3, 15–17]:

$$\lim_{n \to \infty} \frac{R_n n^{\frac{3}{2}}}{\xi_R^n} = \eta_R,$$

where $\xi_R^{-1} = 0.3551817423\ldots = (2.8154600332\ldots)^{-1}$ is the radius of convergence for

$$R(x) = \sum_{n=0}^{\infty} R_n x^n$$

$$= 1 + x + x^2 + 2x^3 + 4x^4 + 8x^5 + 17x^6 + 39x^7 + 89x^8 + 211x^9 + \cdots,$$

$$\eta_R = \sqrt{\frac{\xi_R}{2\pi}} \left(-1 + \rho + \frac{1}{\xi_R^3} R'\left(\frac{1}{\xi_R^2}\right) \rho + \frac{1}{\xi_R^4} R'\left(\frac{1}{\xi_R^3}\right) \right)^{\frac{1}{2}} \rho^{-\frac{1}{2}}$$

$$= 0.5178759064\ldots,$$

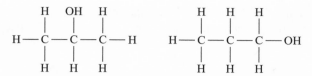

Figure 5.5. The formula C_3H_7OH (propanol) has two isomers.

and $\rho = R(\xi_R^{-1})$. The series coefficients arise from

$$R(x) = 1 + \frac{1}{6}x \left(R(x)^3 + 3R(x)R(x^2) + 2R(x^3) \right).$$

An application of this material involves organic chemistry [18–21]: R_n is the number of **constitutional isomers** of the molecular formula $C_n H_{2n+1}OH$ (alcohols – see Figure 5.5). Constitutional isomeric pairs differ in their atomic connectivity, but the relative positioning of the OH group is immaterial.

Further, if we define [18, 19, 22, 23]

$$r(x) = \frac{1}{24}x \left(R(x)^4 + 6R(x)^2 R(x^2) + 8R(x)R(x^3) + 3R(x^2)^2 + 6R(x^4) \right)$$

$$- \frac{1}{2}\left(R(x)^2 - R(x^2) \right) + R(x)$$

then

$$r(x) = \sum_{n=0}^{\infty} r_n x^n$$

$$= 1 + x + x^2 + x^3 + 2x^4 + 3x^5 + 5x^6 + 9x^7 + 18x^8 + 35x^9 + 75x^{10} + \cdots$$

and r_n is the number of constitutional isomers of the molecular formula $C_n H_{2n+2}$ (alkanes – see Figure 5.6). The series $r(x)$ is related to $R(x)$ as $t(x)$ is related to $T(x)$ (in the sense that r, t are free and R, T are rooted); its radius of convergence is likewise ξ_R^{-1} and

$$\lim_{n \to \infty} \frac{r_n n^{\frac{5}{2}}}{\xi_R^n} = 2\pi \frac{\eta_R^3}{\xi_R}\rho = 0.6563186958\ldots.$$

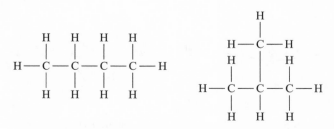

Figure 5.6. The formula C_4H_{10} (butane) has two isomers.

A carbon atom is **chiral** or **asymmetric** if it is attached to four distinct substituents (atoms or groups). If Q_n is the number of constitutional isomers of $C_nH_{2n+1}OH$ without chiral C atoms, then [18, 24]

$$\lim_{n \to \infty} \frac{Q_n}{\xi_Q^n} = \eta_Q,$$

where $\xi_Q^{-1} = 0.5947539639\ldots = (1.6813675244\ldots)^{-1}$ is the radius of convergence for

$$Q(x) = \sum_{n=0}^{\infty} Q_n x^n$$

$$= 1 + x + x^2 + 2x^3 + 3x^4 + 5x^5 + 8x^6 + 14x^7 + 23x^8 + 39x^9 + \cdots.$$

The coefficients arise from $Q(x) = 1 + x Q(x)Q(x^2)$, so that

$$Q(x) = \frac{1|}{|1} - \frac{x|}{|1} - \frac{x^2|}{|1} - \frac{x^4|}{|1} - \frac{x^8|}{|1} - \frac{x^{16}|}{|1} - \cdots,$$

which is an interesting continued fraction. From this, it easily follows that $Q(x) = \psi(x^2)/\psi(x)$ uniquely (assuming ψ is analytic and $\psi(0) = 1$) and hence

$$\eta_Q = -\xi_Q \psi\left(\frac{1}{\xi_Q^2}\right)\left(\psi'\left(\frac{1}{\xi_Q}\right)\right)^{-1} = 0.3607140971\ldots.$$

Let S_n denote the number of **stereoisomers** of $C_nH_{2n+1}OH$. The relative positioning of the hydroxyl group now matters as well [18, 19, 25]; for instance, the illustrated stereoisomeric pair (represented by two tetrahedra – see Figure 5.7) are non-superimposable. The generating function for S_n is

$$S(x) = \sum_{n=0}^{\infty} S_n x^n$$

$$= 1 + x + x^2 + 2x^3 + 5x^4 + 11x^5 + 28x^6 + 74x^7 + 199x^8 + 551x^9 + \cdots,$$

$$S(x) = 1 + \frac{1}{3}x\left(S(x)^3 + 2S(x^3)\right), \quad S_n \sim \eta_S\, n^{-\frac{3}{2}}\, \xi_S^n,$$

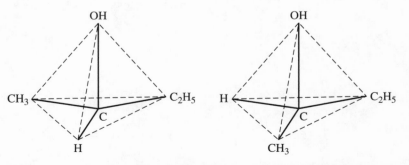

Figure 5.7. The simplest alcohol for which there are (nontrivial) stereoisomers is C_4H_9OH.

with radius of convergence $\xi_S^{-1} = 0.3042184090\ldots = (3.2871120555\ldots)^{-1}$. We omit the value of η_S for brevity's sake.

5.6.2 More Tree Varieties

An **identity tree** is a tree for which the only automorphism is the identity map. There clearly exist unique identity trees of orders 7 and 8 but no nontrivial cases of order ≤ 6. The generating function for identity trees is [4, 26]

$$u(x) = \sum_{n=1}^{\infty} u_n x^n$$
$$= x + x^7 + x^8 + 3x^9 + 6x^{10} + 15x^{11} + 29x^{12} + 67x^{13} + 139x^{14} + \cdots.$$

A **rooted identity tree** is a rooted tree for which the identity map is the only automorphism that fixes the root. With this additional condition, rooted identity trees exist of all orders, and the associated generating function is

$$U(x) = \sum_{n=1}^{\infty} U_n x^n = x + x^2 + x^3 + 2x^4 + 3x^5 + 6x^6 + 12x^7 + 25x^8 + 52x^9 + \cdots.$$

See the pictures of rooted identity trees in [6.11]. Such trees are also said to be **asymmetric**, in the sense that every vertex and edge is unique, that is, isomorphic siblings are forbidden. It can be proved that [5, 27]

$$\lim_{n \to \infty} \frac{U_n n^{\frac{3}{2}}}{\xi_U^n} = \eta_U = \frac{1}{\sqrt{2\pi}} \left(1 - \sum_{k=2}^{\infty} \frac{(-1)^k}{\xi_U^k} U'\left(\frac{1}{\xi_U^k}\right) \right)^{\frac{1}{2}} = 0.3625364234\ldots,$$

$$\lim_{n \to \infty} \frac{u_n n^{\frac{5}{2}}}{\xi_U^n} = 2\pi \eta_U^3 = 0.2993882877\ldots,$$

where $\xi_U^{-1} = 0.3972130965 = (2.5175403550\ldots)^{-1}$ is the radius of convergence for both $U(x)$ and $u(x)$, and further

$$U(x) = x \exp\left(\sum_{k=1}^{\infty} (-1)^{k+1} \frac{U(x^k)}{k} \right), \quad u(x) = U(x) - \tfrac{1}{2}(U(x)^2 + U(x^2)).$$

A tree is **homeomorphically irreducible** (or **series-reduced**) if no vertex is adjacent to exactly two other vertices. Clearly no such tree of order 3 exists, and the generating function is [4, 26, 28]

$$h(x) = \sum_{n=1}^{\infty} h_n x^n$$
$$= x + x^2 + x^4 + x^5 + 2x^6 + 2x^7 + 4x^8 + 5x^9 + 10x^{10} + 14x^{11} + \cdots.$$

A **planted homeomorphically irreducible tree** is a rooted tree that is homeomorphically irreducible and whose root is adjacent to exactly one other vertex. The associated generating function is

$$H(x) = \sum_{n=1}^{\infty} H_n x^n$$
$$= x^2 + x^4 + x^5 + 2x^6 + 3x^7 + 6x^8 + 10x^9 + 19x^{10} + 35x^{11} + \cdots = x\tilde{H}(x).$$

It can be proved that [5, 29]

$$\lim_{n\to\infty} \frac{H_n n^{\frac{3}{2}}}{\xi_H^n} = \eta_H = \frac{1}{\xi_H \sqrt{2\pi}} \left(\frac{\xi_H}{\xi_H + 1} + \sum_{k=2}^{\infty} \frac{1}{\xi_H^k} \tilde{H}'\left(\frac{1}{\xi_H^k}\right) \right)^{\frac{1}{2}} = 0.1924225474\ldots,$$

$$\lim_{n\to\infty} \frac{h_n n^{\frac{5}{2}}}{\xi_H^n} = 2\pi \xi_H^2 (\xi_H + 1)\eta_H^3 = 0.6844472720\ldots,$$

where $\xi_H^{-1} = 0.4567332095\ldots = (2.1894619856\ldots)^{-1}$ is the radius of convergence for both $H(x)$ and $h(x)$, and further

$$\tilde{H}(x) = \frac{x}{x+1} \exp\left(\sum_{k=1}^{\infty} \frac{\tilde{H}(x^k)}{k}\right),$$
$$h(x) = (x+1)\tilde{H}(x) - \frac{x+1}{2}\tilde{H}(x)^2 - \frac{x-1}{2}\tilde{H}(x^2).$$

If we take into account the ordering (from left to right) of the subtrees of any vertex, then **ordered trees** arise and different enumeration problems occur. For example, define two ordered rooted trees σ and τ to be **cyclically isomorphic** if σ and τ are isomorphic as rooted trees, and if τ can be obtained from σ by circularly rearranging all the subtrees of any vertex, or likewise for each of several vertices. The equivalence classes under this relation are called **mobiles**. There exist fifty-one mobiles of order 7 but only forty-eight rooted trees of order 7 (see Figure 5.8).

The generating function for mobiles is [22, 26, 30]

$$M(x) = \sum_{n=1}^{\infty} M_n x^n$$
$$= x + x^2 + 2x^3 + 4x^4 + 9x^5 + 20x^6 + 51x^7 + 128x^8 + 345x^9 + \cdots,$$

$$M(x) = x\left(1 - \sum_{k=1}^{\infty} \frac{\varphi(k)}{k} \ln(1 - M(x^k))\right), \quad M_n \sim \eta_M\, n^{-\frac{3}{2}} \xi_M^n,$$

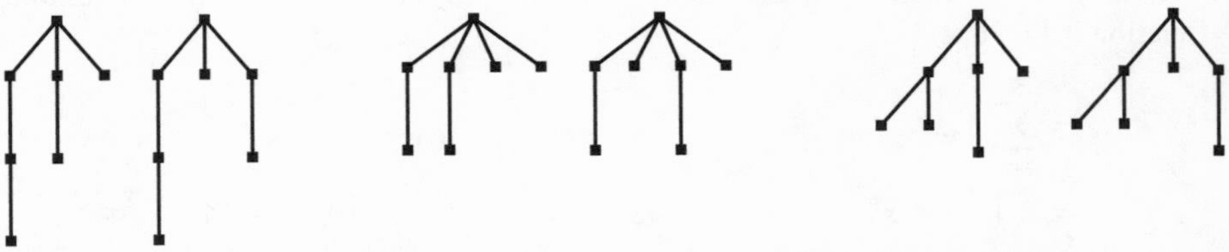

Figure 5.8. There exist three pairs of distinct mobiles (of order 7) that are identical as rooted trees.

where φ is the Euler totient function [2.7] and $\xi_M^{-1} = 0.3061875165\ldots =$ $(3.2659724710\ldots)^{-1}$.

If we **label** the vertices of a graph distinctly with the integers $1, 2, \ldots, n$, the corresponding enumeration problems often simplify; for example, there are exactly n^{n-2} labeled free trees and n^{n-1} labeled rooted trees. For labeled mobiles, the problem becomes quite interesting, with exponential generating function [31]

$$\hat{M}(x) = \sum_{n=1}^{\infty} \frac{\hat{M}_n}{n!} x^n$$

$$= x + \frac{2}{2!}x^2 + \frac{9}{3!}x^3 + \frac{68}{4!}x^4 + \frac{730}{5!}x^5 + \frac{10164}{6!}x^6 + \frac{173838}{7!}x^7 + \cdots,$$

$$\hat{M}(x) = x\,(1 - \ln(1 - \hat{M}(x))), \quad \hat{M}_n \sim \hat{\eta}\,\hat{\xi}^n n^{n-1},$$

where $\hat{\xi} = e^{-1}(1 - \mu)^{-1} = 1.1574198038\ldots$, $\hat{\eta} = \sqrt{\mu(1-\mu)} = 0.4656386467$ $\ldots$, and $\mu = 0.6821555671\ldots$ is the unique solution of the equation $\mu(1-\mu)^{-1} = 1 - \ln(1 - \mu)$.

An **increasing tree** is a labeled rooted tree for which the labels along any branch starting at the root are increasing. The root must be labeled 1. Again, for increasing mobiles, enumeration provides interesting constants [32]:

$$\tilde{M}(x) = \sum_{n=1}^{\infty} \frac{\tilde{M}_n}{n!} x^n$$

$$= x + \frac{1}{2!}x^2 + \frac{2}{3!}x^3 + \frac{7}{4!}x^4 + \frac{36}{5!}x^5 + \frac{245}{6!}x^6 + \frac{2076}{7!}x^7 + \cdots,$$

$$\tilde{M}'(x) = 1 - \ln(1 - \tilde{M}(x)), \quad \tilde{M}_n \sim \tilde{\xi}^{n-1}n!\left(\frac{1}{n^2} - \frac{1}{n^2\ln(n)} + O\left(\frac{1}{n^2\ln(n)^2}\right)\right)$$

where $\tilde{\xi}^{-1} = -e\,\mathrm{Ei}(-1) = 0.5963473623\ldots = e^{-1}(0.6168878482\ldots)^{-1}$ is the Euler–Gompertz constant [6.2]. See a strengthening of these asymptotics in [31,33].

5.6.3 Attributes

Thus far, we have discussed only enumeration issues. Otter's original constants α and β, however, appear in several asymptotic formulas governing other attributes of trees. By the **degree** (or **valency**) of a vertex, we mean the number of vertices that are adjacent to it. Given a random rooted tree with n vertices, the expected degree of the root is [34]

$$\theta = 1 + \sum_{i=1}^{\infty} T\left(\frac{1}{\alpha^i}\right) = 2 + \sum_{j=1}^{\infty} T_j \frac{1}{\alpha^j(\alpha^j - 1)} = 2.1918374031\ldots$$

as $n \to \infty$, and the variance of the degree of the root is

$$\sum_{i=1}^{\infty} i\,T\left(\frac{1}{\alpha^i}\right) = 1 + \sum_{j=1}^{\infty} T_j \frac{2\alpha^j - 1}{\alpha^j(\alpha^j - 1)^2} = 1.4741726868\ldots.$$

By the **distance** between two vertices, we mean the number of edges in the shortest path connecting them. The average distance between a vertex and the root is

$$\frac{1}{2}\left(\frac{2\pi}{\beta}\right)^{\frac{1}{3}} n^{\frac{1}{2}} = (1.1365599187\ldots)n^{\frac{1}{2}}$$

as $n \to \infty$, and the variance of the distance is

$$\frac{4-\pi}{4\pi}\left(\frac{2\pi}{\beta}\right)^{\frac{2}{3}} n = (0.3529622229\ldots)n.$$

Let v be an arbitrary vertex in a random free tree with n vertices and let p_m denote the probability, in the limit as $n \to \infty$, that v is of degree m. Then [35]

$$p_1 = \frac{\alpha^{-1} + \sum_{k=1}^{\infty} D_k \dfrac{\alpha^{-2k}}{1-\alpha^{-k}}}{1 + \sum_{k=1}^{\infty} k T_k \dfrac{\alpha^{-2k}}{1-\alpha^{-k}}} = 0.4381562356\ldots,$$

where $D_1 = 1$ and $D_{k+1} = \sum_{j=1}^{n} \left(\sum_{d\mid j} D_d\right) T_{k-j+1}$. Clearly $p_m \to 0$ as $m \to \infty$. More precisely, if

$$\omega = \prod_{i=1}^{\infty}\left(1-\frac{1}{\alpha^i}\right)^{-T_{i+1}} = \exp\left(\sum_{j=1}^{\infty}\frac{1}{j}\left[\alpha^j T(\frac{1}{\alpha^j})-1\right]\right) = 7.7581602911\ldots$$

then $\lim_{m\to\infty} \alpha^m p_m$ is given by [36, 37]

$$(2\pi\beta^2)^{-\frac{1}{3}}\omega = (1.2160045618\ldots)^{-1}\omega = 6.3800420942\ldots.$$

We will need both θ and ω later. See also [38, 39].

Let G be a graph and let $A(G)$ be the automorphism group of G. A vertex v of G is a **fixed point** if $\varphi(v) = v$ for every $\varphi \in A(G)$. Let q denote the probability, in the limit as $n \to \infty$, that an arbitrary vertex in a random tree of order n is a fixed point. Harary & Palmer [7, 40] proved that

$$q = (2\pi\beta^2)^{-\frac{1}{3}}\left(1 - E\left(\frac{1}{\alpha^2}\right)\right) = 0.6995388700\ldots,$$

where $E(x) = T(x)(1 + F(x) - F(x^2))$. Interestingly, the same value q applies for rooted trees as well.

For reasons of space, we omit discussion of constants associated with covering and packing [41–43], as well as counting maximally independent sets of vertices [44–47], games [48], and equicolorable trees [49].

5.6.4 Forests

Let f_n denote the number of non-isomorphic forests of order n; then the generating function [26]

$$f(x) = \sum_{n=1}^{\infty} f_n x^n$$

$$= x + 2x^2 + 3x^3 + 6x^4 + 10x^5 + 20x^6 + 37x^7 + 76x^8 + 153x^9 + 329x^{10} + \cdots$$

satisfies

$$1 + f(x) = \exp\left(\sum_{k=1}^{\infty} \frac{t(x^k)}{k}\right), \quad f_n = \frac{1}{n} \sum_{k=1}^{n} \left(\sum_{d|k} d\, t_d\right) f_{n-k}$$

and $f_0 = 1$ for the sake only of the latter formula. Palmer & Schwenk [50] showed that

$$f_n \sim c\, t_n = \left(1 + f\left(\frac{1}{\alpha}\right)\right) t_n = (1.9126258077\ldots) t_n.$$

If a forest is chosen at random, then as $n \to \infty$, the expected number of trees in the forest is

$$1 + \sum_{i=1}^{\infty} t\left(\frac{1}{\alpha^i}\right) = \frac{3}{2} + \frac{1}{2} T\left(\frac{1}{\alpha^2}\right) + \sum_{j=1}^{\infty} t_j \frac{1}{\alpha^j(\alpha^j - 1)} = 1.7555101394\ldots.$$

The corresponding number for rooted trees is $\theta = 2.1918374031\ldots$, a constant that unsurprisingly we encountered earlier [5.6.3]. The probability of exactly k rooted trees in a random forest is asymptotically $\omega\alpha^{-k} = (7.7581602911\ldots)\alpha^{-k}$. For free trees, the analogous probability likewise drops off geometrically as α^{-k} with coefficient

$$\frac{\alpha}{c} \prod_{i=1}^{\infty}\left(1 - \frac{1}{\alpha^i}\right)^{-t_{i+1}} = \frac{\alpha}{c} \exp\left(\sum_{j=1}^{\infty} \frac{1}{j}\left[\alpha^j t\left(\frac{1}{\alpha^j}\right) - 1\right]\right) = 3.2907434386\ldots.$$

Also, the asymptotic probability that two rooted forests of order n have no tree in common is [51]

$$\prod_{i=1}^{\infty}\left(1 - \frac{1}{\alpha^{2i}}\right)^{T_i} = \exp\left(-\sum_{j=1}^{\infty} \frac{1}{j} T\left(\frac{1}{\alpha^{2j}}\right)\right) = 0.8705112052\ldots.$$

5.6.5 Cacti and 2-Trees

We now examine graphs that are not trees but are nevertheless tree-like. A **cactus** is a connected graph in which no edge lies on more than one (minimal) cycle [52–54]. See Figure 5.9. If we further assume that every edge lies on exactly one cycle and that all cycles are polygons with m sides for a fixed integer m, the cactus is called an m-**cactus**. By convention, a 2-cactus is simply a tree. Discussions of 3-cacti appear in [4], 4-cacti in [55], and m-cacti with vertex coloring in [56]; we will not talk about such special

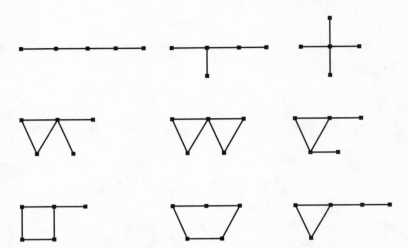

Figure 5.9. There exist nine non-isomorphic cacti of order 5.

cases. The generating functions for cacti and rooted cacti are [57]

$$c(x) = \sum_{n=1}^{\infty} c_n x^n$$
$$= x + x^2 + 2x^3 + 4x^4 + 9x^5 + 23x^6 + 63x^7 + 188x^8 + 596x^9 + 1979x^{10} + \cdots,$$

$$C(x) = \sum_{n=1}^{\infty} C_n x^n$$
$$= x + x^2 + 3x^3 + 8x^4 + 26x^5 + 84x^6 + 297x^7 + 1066x^8 + 3976x^9 + \cdots,$$

and these satisfy [58–60]

$$C(x) = x \exp\left[-\sum_{k=1}^{\infty} \frac{1}{k}\left(\frac{C(x^k)^2 - 2 + C(x^{2k})}{2(C(x^k) - 1)(C(x^{2k}) - 1)} + 1\right)\right],$$

$$c(x) = C(x) - \frac{1}{2}\sum_{k=1}^{\infty} \frac{\varphi(k)}{k}\ln(1 - C(x^k)) + \frac{(C(x) + 1)(C(x)^2 - 2C(x) + C(x^2))}{4(C(x) - 1)(C(x^2) - 1)},$$

with radius of convergence $0.2221510651\ldots$. For the labeled case, we have

$$\hat{c}(x) = \sum_{n=1}^{\infty} \frac{\hat{c}_n}{n!} x^n$$
$$= x + \frac{1}{2!}x^2 + \frac{4}{3!}x^3 + \frac{31}{4!}x^4 + \frac{362}{5!}x^5 + \frac{5676}{6!}x^6 + \frac{111982}{7!}x^7 + \cdots,$$

$$\hat{C}(x) = \sum_{n=1}^{\infty} \frac{\hat{C}_n}{n!} x^n$$
$$= x + \frac{2}{2!}x^2 + \frac{12}{3!}x^3 + \frac{124}{4!}x^4 + \frac{1810}{5!}x^5 + \frac{34056}{6!}x^6 + \frac{783874}{7!}x^7 + \cdots,$$

and these satisfy

$$\hat{C}(x) = x \exp\left(\frac{\hat{C}(x)}{2}\frac{2 - \hat{C}(x)}{1 - \hat{C}(x)}\right), \quad x\hat{c}'(x) = \hat{C}(x),$$

with radius of convergence $0.2387401436\ldots$.

A **2-tree** is defined recursively as follows [4]. A 2-tree of rank 1 is a triangle (a graph with three vertices and three edges), and a 2-tree of rank $n \geq 2$ is built from a 2-tree of rank $n - 1$ by creating a new vertex of degree 2 adjacent to each of two existing adjacent vertices. Hence a 2-tree of rank n has $n + 2$ vertices and $2n + 1$ edges. The generating function for 2-trees is [61]

$$w(x) = \sum_{n=0}^{\infty} w_n x^n$$

$$= 1 + x + x^2 + 2x^3 + 5x^4 + 12x^5 + 39x^6 + 136x^7 + 529x^8 + 2171x^9 + \cdots$$

$$w(x) = \frac{1}{2}\left[W(x) + \exp\left(\sum_{k=1}^{\infty}\frac{1}{2k}(2x^k W(x^{2k}) + x^{2k} W(x^{2k})^2 - x^{2k} W(x^{4k}))\right)\right]$$

$$+ \frac{1}{3}x\left(W(x^3) - W(x)^3\right),$$

where $W(x)$ is the generating function for 2-trees with a distinguished and oriented edge:

$$W(x) = \sum_{n=0}^{\infty} W_n x^n$$

$$= 1 + x + 3x^2 + 10x^3 + 39x^4 + 160x^5 + 702x^6 + 3177x^7 + 14830x^8 + \cdots$$

$$W(x) = \exp\left(\sum_{k=1}^{\infty}\frac{x^k W(x^k)^2}{k}\right), \quad w_n \sim \eta_w \, n^{-\frac{5}{2}} \, \xi_w^n.$$

Further, $w(x)$ has radius of convergence $\xi_w^{-1} = 0.1770995223\ldots = (5.6465426162\ldots)^{-1}$ and

$$\eta_w = \frac{1}{16\xi\sqrt{\pi}}\left(\xi + 2\tilde{w}'\left(\frac{1}{\xi}\right)\tilde{W}\left(\frac{1}{\xi}\right)^{-1}\right)^{\frac{3}{2}} = 0.0948154165\ldots,$$

$$\tilde{W}(x) = e^{-x W(x)^2} W(x).$$

5.6.6 Mapping Patterns

We studied labeled functional graphs on n vertices in [5.4]. Let us remove the labels and consider only graph isomorphism classes, called **mapping patterns**. Observe that the original Otter constants α and β play a crucial role here. The generating function of mapping patterns is [57, 62]

$$P(x) = \sum_{n=1}^{\infty} P_n x^n$$
$$= x + 3x^2 + 7x^3 + 19x^4 + 47x^5 + 130x^6 + 343x^7 + 951x^8 + 2615x^9 + \cdots,$$

$$1 + P(x) = \prod_{k=1}^{\infty} \left(1 - T(x^k)\right)^{-1}, \quad P_n \sim \eta_P \, n^{-\frac{1}{2}} \alpha^n,$$

where

$$\eta_P = \frac{1}{2\pi} \left(\frac{2\pi}{\beta}\right)^{\frac{1}{3}} \prod_{i=2}^{\infty} \left(1 - T(\frac{1}{\alpha^i})\right)^{-1} = 0.4428767697\ldots$$
$$= (1.2241663491\ldots)(4\pi^2 \beta)^{-\frac{1}{3}}.$$

From this, it follows that the expected length of an arbitrary cycle in a random mapping pattern is

$$\frac{1}{2} \left(\frac{2\pi}{\beta}\right)^{\frac{1}{3}} n^{\frac{1}{2}} = (1.1365599187\ldots)n^{\frac{1}{2}}, \quad n \to \infty$$

(an expression that we saw in [5.6.3], by coincidence) and the asymptotic probability that the mapping pattern is connected is

$$\frac{1}{2\eta_P} n^{-\frac{1}{2}} = (1.1289822228\ldots)n^{-\frac{1}{2}}.$$

It we further restrict attention to connected mapping patterns, the associated generating function is

$$K(x) = \sum_{n=1}^{\infty} K_n x^n$$
$$= x + 2x^2 + 4x^3 + 9x^4 + 20x^5 + 51x^6 + 125x^7 + 329x^8 + 862x^9 + \cdots$$

$$K(x) = -\sum_{j=1}^{\infty} \frac{\varphi(j)}{j} \ln(1 - T(x^j)), \quad K_n \sim \frac{1}{2} n^{-1} \alpha^n.$$

It follows that the expected length of the (unique) cycle in a random connected mapping pattern is

$$\frac{1}{\pi} \left(\frac{2\pi}{\beta}\right)^{\frac{1}{3}} n^{\frac{1}{2}} = (0.7235565167\ldots)n^{\frac{1}{2}}, \quad n \to \infty,$$

which is less than before. A comparison between such statistics for both unlabeled and labeled cases (the numerical results are indeed slightly different) appears in [62]. See [63, 64] for more recent work in this area.

5.6.7 *More Graph Varieties*

A graph G is an **interval graph** if it can be represented as follows: Each vertex of G corresponds to a subinterval of the real line in such a way that two vertices are adjacent if and only if their corresponding intervals have nonempty intersection. It is a **unit interval graph** if the intervals can all be chosen to be of length 1. The generating function of unit interval graphs, for example, is [65,66]

$$I(x) = \sum_{n=1}^{\infty} I_n x^n$$
$$= x + 2x^2 + 4x^3 + 9x^4 + 21x^5 + 55x^6 + 151x^7 + 447x^8 + 1389x^9 + \cdots,$$

$$1 + I(x) = \exp\left(\sum_{k=1}^{\infty} \frac{\psi(x^k)}{k}\right), \quad \psi(x) = \frac{1 + 2x - \sqrt{1 - 4x}\sqrt{1 - 4x^2}}{4\sqrt{1 - 4x^2}},$$

with asymptotics

$$I_n \sim \frac{1}{8\kappa\sqrt{\pi}} n^{-\frac{3}{2}} 4^n, \quad \kappa = \exp\left(-\frac{\sqrt{3}}{4}\right) \exp\left(-\sum_{j=2}^{\infty} \frac{\psi(4^{-j})}{j}\right) = 0.6231198963\ldots.$$

Interval graphs have found applications in genetics and other fields [67,68].

A graph is **2-regular** if every vertex has degree two. The number J_n of 2-regular graphs on n vertices is equal to the number of partitions of n into parts ≥ 3, whereas the exponential generating function of 2-regular labeled graphs is [69]

$$\hat{J}(x) = \sum_{n=0}^{\infty} \frac{\hat{J}_n}{n!} x^n = 1 + \frac{1}{3!} x^3 + \frac{3}{4!} x^4 + \frac{12}{5!} x^5 + \frac{70}{6!} x^6 + \cdots$$
$$= \frac{1}{\sqrt{1-x}} \exp\left(-\frac{1}{2}x - \frac{1}{4}x^2\right);$$

therefore

$$J_n \sim \frac{\pi^2}{12\sqrt{3}n^2} \exp\left(\pi\sqrt{\frac{2n}{3}}\right), \quad \hat{J}_n \sim \sqrt{2}e^{-\frac{3}{4}} \left(\frac{n}{e}\right)^n.$$

The latter has an interesting geometric interpretation [14,70]. Given n planar lines in general position with $\binom{n}{2}$ intersecting points, a **cloud** of size n is a (maximal) set of n intersecting points, no three of which are collinear. The number of clouds of size n is clearly $\hat{J}_n$.

A **directed graph** or **digraph** is a graph for which the edges are ordered pairs of distinct vertices (rather than unordered pairs). Note that loops are automatically disallowed. An **acyclic digraph** further contains no directed cycles; in particular, it has no multiple parallel edges. The (transformed) exponential generating function of labeled acyclic digraphs is [65, 71–74]

$$A(x) = \sum_{n=0}^{\infty} \frac{A_n}{n!2^{\binom{n}{2}}} x^n = 1 + x + \frac{3}{2! \cdot 2} x^2 + \frac{25}{3! \cdot 2^3} x^3 + \frac{543}{4! \cdot 2^6} x^4 + \frac{29281}{5! \cdot 2^{10}} x^5 + \cdots,$$

$$A'(x) = A(x)^2 A(\tfrac{1}{2}x)^{-1}, \quad A_n \sim \frac{n!2^{\binom{n}{2}}}{\eta_A \, \xi_A^n},$$

where $\xi_A = 1.4880785456\ldots$ is the smallest positive zero of the function

$$\lambda(x) = \sum_{n=0}^{\infty} \frac{(-1)^n}{n!2^{\binom{n}{2}}} x^n = A(x)^{-1}, \quad \lambda'(x) = -\lambda(\tfrac{1}{2}x),$$

and $\eta_A = \xi_A \lambda(\xi_A/2) = 0.5743623733\ldots = (1.7410611252\ldots)^{-1}$. It is curious that the function $\lambda(-x)$ was earlier studied by Mahler [75] with regard to enumerating partitions of integers into powers of 2. See [76, 77] for discussion of the unlabeled acyclic digraph analog.

5.6.8 Data Structures

To a combinatorialist, the phrase "(strongly) binary tree with $2n + 1$ vertices" means an isomorphism class of trees. To a computer scientist, however, the same phrase virtually always includes the word "ordered," whether stated explicitly or not. Hence the phrase "random binary tree" is sometimes ambiguous in the literature: The sample space has B_n elements for the former person but $\binom{2n}{n}/(n+1)$ elements for the latter! We cannot hope here to survey the role of trees in computer algorithms, only to provide a few constants.

A **leftist tree** of size n is an ordered binary tree with n leaves such that, in any subtree σ, the leaf closest to the root of σ is in the right subtree of σ. The generating function of leftist trees is [6, 65, 78, 79]

$$L(x) = \sum_{n=0}^{\infty} L_n x^n$$
$$= x + x^2 + x^3 + 2x^4 + 4x^5 + 8x^6 + 17x^7 + 38x^8 + 87x^9 + 203x^{10} + \cdots$$

$$L(x) = x + \frac{1}{2}L(x)^2 + \frac{1}{2}\sum_{m=1}^{\infty} l_m(x)^2 = \sum_{m=1}^{\infty} l_m(x),$$

where the auxiliary generating functions $l_m(x)$ satisfy

$$l_1(x) = x, \quad l_2(x) = xL(x), \quad l_{m+1}(x) = l_m(x)\left(L(x) - \sum_{k=1}^{m-1} l_k(x)\right), \quad m \geq 2.$$

It can be proved (with difficulty) that

$$L_n \sim (0.2503634293\ldots) \cdot (2.7494879027\ldots)^n n^{-\frac{3}{2}}.$$

Leftist trees are useful in certain sorting and merging algorithms.

A **2,3-tree** of size n is a rooted ordered tree with n leaves satisfying the following:

- Each non-leaf vertex has either 2 or 3 successors.
- All of the root-to-leaf paths have the same length.

The generating function of 2,3-trees (no relation to 2-trees!) is [65, 80, 81]

$$Z(x) = \sum_{n=0}^{\infty} Z_n x^n$$

$$= x + x^2 + x^3 + x^4 + 2x^5 + 2x^6 + 3x^7 + 4x^8 + 5x^9 + 8x^{10} + 14x^{11} + \cdots$$

$$Z(x) = x + Z(x^2 + x^3), \quad Z_n = \sum_{k=\lceil n/3 \rceil}^{\lfloor n/2 \rfloor} \binom{k}{3k-n} Z_k \sim \varphi^n n^{-1} f(\ln(n)),$$

where φ is the Golden mean [1.2] and $f(x)$ is a nonconstant, positive, continuous function that is periodic with period $\ln(4 - \varphi) = 0.867\ldots$, has mean $(\varphi \ln(4 - \varphi))^{-1} = 0.712\ldots$, and oscillates between $0.682\ldots$ and $0.806\ldots$. These are also a particular type of **B-trees**. A similar analysis [82] uncovers the asymptotics of what are known as AVL-trees (or height-balanced trees). Such trees support efficient database searches, deletions, and insertions; other varieties are too numerous to mention.

If τ is an ordered binary tree, then its **height** and **register functions** are recursively defined by [83]

$$\mathrm{ht}(\tau) = \begin{cases} 0 & \text{if } \tau \text{ is a point,} \\ 1 + \max(\mathrm{ht}(\tau_L), \mathrm{ht}(\tau_R)) & \text{otherwise,} \end{cases}$$

$$\mathrm{rg}(\tau) = \begin{cases} 0 & \text{if } \tau \text{ is a point,} \\ 1 + \mathrm{rg}(\tau_L) & \text{if } \mathrm{rg}(\tau_L) = \mathrm{rg}(\tau_R), \\ \max(\mathrm{rg}(\tau_L), \mathrm{rg}(\tau_R)) & \text{otherwise,} \end{cases}$$

where τ_L and τ_R are the left and right subtrees of the root. That is, $\mathrm{ht}(\tau)$ is the number of edges along the longest branch from the root, whereas $\mathrm{rg}(\tau)$ is the minimum number of registers needed to evaluate the tree (thought of as an arithmetic expression). If we randomly select a binary tree τ with $2n + 1$ vertices, then the asymptotics of $E(\mathrm{ht}(\tau))$ involve $2\sqrt{\pi n}$ as mentioned in [1.4], and those of $E(\mathrm{rg}(\tau))$ involve $\ln(n)/\ln(4)$ plus a zero mean oscillating function [2.16]. Also, define $\mathrm{ym}(\tau)$ to be the number of maximal subtrees of τ having register function exactly 1 less than $\mathrm{rg}(\tau)$. Prodinger [84], building upon the work of Yekutiele & Mandelbrot [85], proved that $E(\mathrm{ym}(\tau))$ is asymptotically

$$\frac{2G}{\pi \ln(2)} + \frac{5}{2} = 3.3412669407\ldots$$

plus a zero mean oscillating function, where G is Catalan's constant [1.7]. This is also known as the **bifurcation ratio** at the root, which quantifies the hierarchical complexity of more general branching structures.

5.6.9 Galton–Watson Branching Process

Thus far, by "random binary trees," it is meant that we select binary trees with n vertices from a population endowed with the uniform probability distribution. The integer n is fixed.

It is also possible, however, to *grow* binary trees (rather than to merely select them). Fix a probability $0 < p < 1$ and define recursively a (strongly) binary tree τ in terms of left and right subtrees of the root as follows: Take $\tau_L = \emptyset$ with probability $1 - p$, and independently take $\tau_R = \emptyset$ with probability $1 - p$. It can be shown [86–88] that this process terminates, that is, τ is a finite tree, with **extinction probability** 1 if $p \leq 1/2$ and $1/p - 1$ if $p > 1/2$. Of course, the number of vertices N is here a random variable, called the **total progeny**.

Much can be said about the Bienaymé–Galton–Watson process (which is actually more general than described here). We focus on just one detail. Let N_k denote the number of vertices at distance k from the root, that is, the size of the kth generation. Consider the subcritical case $p < 1/2$. Let a_k denote the probability that $N_k = 0$; then the sequence $a_0, a_1, a_2, \ldots$ obeys the quadratic recurrence [6.10]

$$a_0 = 0, \qquad a_k = (1 - p) + p a_{k-1}^2 \quad \text{for } k \geq 1, \qquad \lim_{k \to \infty} a_k = 1.$$

What can be said about the convergence rate of $\{a_k\}$? It can be proved that

$$C(p) = \lim_{k \to \infty} \frac{1 - a_k}{(2p)^k} = \prod_{l=0}^{\infty} \frac{1 + a_l}{2},$$

which has no closed-form expression in terms of p, as far as is known. This is over and beyond the fact, of greatest interest to us here, that $P(N_k > 0) \sim C(p)(2p)^k$ for $0 < p < 1/2$. Other interesting parameters are the **moment of extinction** $\min\{k : N_k = 0\}$ or tree height, and the **maximal generation size** $\max\{N_k : k \geq 0\}$ or tree width.

5.6.10 Erdös–Rényi Evolutionary Process

Starting with n initially disconnected vertices, define a random graph by successively adding edges between pairs of distinct points, chosen uniformly from $\binom{n}{2}$ candidates without replacement. Continue with this process until no candidate edges are left [89–92].

At some stage of the evolution, a **complex component** emerges, that is, the first component possessing more than one cycle. It is remarkable that this complex component will usually remain unique throughout the entire process, and the probability that this is true is $5\pi/18 = 0.8726\ldots$ as $n \to \infty$. In other words, the first component that acquires more edges than vertices is quite likely to become the **giant component** of the random graph. The probability that exactly two complex components emerge is $50\pi/1296 = 0.1212\ldots$, but the probability ($> 0.9938\ldots$) that the evolving graph never has more than two complex components at any time is not precisely known [93].

There are many related results, but we mention only one. Start with an $m \times n$ rectangular grid of rooms, each with four walls. Successively remove interior walls in a random manner such that, at some step in the procedure, the associated graph (with all *mn* rooms as vertices and all neighboring pairs of rooms with open passage as edges) becomes a tree. Stop when this condition is met; the result is a **random maze** [94]. The difficulty lies in detecting whether the addition of a new edge creates an unwanted cycle. An efficient way of doing this (maintaining equivalence classes that change over time) is found in QF and QFW, two of a class of **union-find algorithms** in computer science. Exact performance analyses of QF and QFW appear in [95–97], using random graph theory and a variant of the Erdös-Rényi process.

[1] F. Harary, *Graph Theory*, Addison-Wesley, 1969; MR 41 #1566.

[2] R. Sedgewick and P. Flajolet, *Introduction to the Analysis of Algorithms*, Addison-Wesley, 1996.

[3] R. Otter, The number of trees, *Annals of Math.* 49 (1948) 583–599; MR 10,53c.

[4] F. Harary and E. M. Palmer, *Graphical Enumeration*, Academic Press, 1973; MR 50 #9682.

[5] F. Harary, R. W. Robinson, and A. J. Schwenk, Twenty-step algorithm for determining the asymptotic number of trees of various species, *J. Austral. Math. Soc. Ser. A* 20 (1975) 483–503; corrigenda 41 (1986) 325; MR 53 #10644 and MR 87j:05091.

[6] A. M. Odlyzko, Asymptotic enumeration methods, *Handbook of Combinatorics*, ed. R. L. Graham, M. Groetschel, and L. Lovasz, MIT Press, 1995, pp. 1063–1229; MR 97b: 05012.

[7] D. J. Broadhurst and D. Kreimer, Renormalization automated by Hopf algebra, *J. Symbolic Comput.* 27 (1999) 581–600; hep-th/9810087; MR 2000h:81167.

[8] E. A. Bender, Asymptotic methods in enumeration, *SIAM Rev.* 16 (1974) 485–515; errata 18 (1976) 292; MR 51 #12545 and MR 55 #10276.

[9] D. E. Knuth, *The Art of Computer Programming*, v. 1, *Fundamental Algorithms*, Addison-Wesley, 1997, pp. 396–397, 588–589; MR 51 #14624.

[10] J. N. Franklin and S. W. Golomb, A function-theoretic approach to the study of nonlinear recurring sequences, *Pacific J. Math.* 56 (1975) 455–468; MR 51 #10212.

[11] J. H. M. Wedderburn, The functional equation $g(x^2) = 2ax + [g(x)]^2$, *Annals of Math.* 24 (1922-23) 121–140.

[12] I. M. H. Etherington, Non-associate powers and a functional equation, *Math. Gazette* 21 (1937) 36–39, 153.

[13] H. W. Becker, Genetic algebra, *Amer. Math. Monthly* 56 (1949) 697–699.

[14] L. Comtet, *Advanced Combinatorics: The Art of Finite and Infinite Expansions*, Reidel, 1974, pp. 52–55, 273–279; MR 57 #124.

[15] N. J. A. Sloane, On-Line Encyclopedia of Integer Sequences, A000055, A000081, A000598, A000602, A000621, A000625, and A001190.

[16] C. Bailey, E. Palmer, and J. Kennedy, Points by degree and orbit size in chemical trees. II, *Discrete Appl. Math.* 5 (1983) 157–164; MR 85b:05098.

[17] E. A. Bender and S. Gill Williamson, *Foundations of Applied Combinatorics*, Addison-Wesley, 1991, pp. 372–373, 395–396.

[18] G. Pólya and R. C. Read, *Combinatorial Enumeration of Groups, Graphs, and Chemical Compounds*, Springer-Verlag, 1987, pp. 4–8, 78–86, 130–134; MR 89f:05013.

[19] A. T. Balaban, *Chemical Applications of Graph Theory*, Academic Press, 1976; MR 58 #21870.

[20] N. Trinajstic, *Chemical Graph Theory*, v. 2, CRC Press, 1992; MR 93g:92034.

[21] D. H. Rouvray, Combinatorics in chemistry, *Handbook of Combinatorics*, ed. R. L. Graham, M. Groetschel, and L. Lovasz, MIT Press, 1995, pp. 1955–1981; MR 97e:92017.

[22] F. Bergeron, G. Labelle, and P. Leroux, *Combinatorial Species and Tree-Like Structures*, Cambridge Univ. Press, 1998; MR 2000a:05008.

[23] E. M. Rains and N. J. A. Sloane, On Cayley's enumeration of alkanes (or 4-valent trees), *J. Integer Seq.* 2 (1999) 99.1.1; math.CO/0207176; MR 99j:05010.

[24] P. Flajolet and R. Sedgewick, *Analytic Combinatorics*, unpublished manuscript, 2001.

[25] R. W. Robinson, F. Harary, and A. T. Balaban, The numbers of chiral and achiral alkanes and monosubstituted alkanes, *Tetrahedron* 32 (1976) 355–361.

[26] N. J. A. Sloane, On-Line Encyclopedia of Integer Sequences, A000014, A000220, A001678, A004111, A005200, A005201, A029768, A032200, A038037, A005195, and A059123.

[27] A. Meir, J. W. Moon, and J. Mycielski, Hereditarily finite sets and identity trees, *J. Combin. Theory Ser. B* 35 (1983) 142–155; MR 85h:05009.

[28] F. Harary and G. Prins, The number of homeomorphically irreducible trees, and other species, *Acta Math.* 101 (1959) 141–162; MR 21 #653.

[29] S. R. Finch, Counting topological trees, unpublished note (2001).

[30] C. G. Bower, Mobiles (cyclic trees), unpublished note (2001).

[31] I. M. Gessel, B. E. Sagan, and Y. N. Yeh, Enumeration of trees by inversions, *J. Graph Theory* 19 (1995) 435–459; MR 97b:05070.

[32] F. Bergeron, P. Flajolet, and B. Salvy, Varieties of increasing trees, *17th Colloq. on Trees in Algebra and Programming (CAAP)*, Proc. 1992 Rennes conf., ed. J.-C. Raoult, Lect. Notes in Comp. Sci. 581, Springer-Verlag, 1992, pp. 24–48; MR 94j:68233.

[33] W. Y. C. Chen, The pessimistic search and the straightening involution for trees, *Europ. J. Combin.* 19 (1998) 553–558; MR 99g:05103.

[34] A. Meir and J. W. Moon, On the altitude of nodes in random trees, *Canad. J. Math.* 30 (1978) 997–1015; MR 80k:05043.

[35] R. W. Robinson and A. J. Schwenk, The distribution of degrees in a large random tree, *Discrete Math.* 12 (1975) 359–372; MR 53 #10629.

[36] A. J. Schwenk, An asymptotic evaluation of the cycle index of a symmetric group, *Discrete Math.* 18 (1977) 71–78; MR 57 #9598.

[37] A. Meir and J. W. Moon, On an asymptotic evaluation of the cycle index of the symmetric group, *Discrete Math.* 46 (1983) 103–105; MR 84h:05071.

[38] C. K. Bailey, Distribution of points by degree and orbit size in a large random tree, *J. Graph Theory* 6 (1982) 283–293; MR 83i:05037.

[39] W. M. Y. Goh and E. Schmutz, Unlabeled trees: Distribution of the maximum degree, *Random Structures Algorithms* 5 (1994) 411–440; MR 95c:05111.

[40] F. Harary and E. M. Palmer, The probability that a point of a tree is fixed, *Math. Proc. Cambridge Philos. Soc.* 85 (1979) 407–415; MR 80f:05020.

[41] A. Meir and J. W. Moon, Packing and covering constants for certain families of trees. I, *J. Graph Theory* 1 (1977) 157–174; MR 57 #2965.

[42] A. Meir and J. W. Moon, Packing and covering constants for certain families of trees. II, *Trans. Amer. Math. Soc.* 233 (1977) 167–178; MR 57 #157.

[43] A. Meir and J. W. Moon, Path edge-covering constants for certain families of trees, *Utilitas Math.* 14 (1978) 313–333; MR 80a:05073.

[44] A. Meir and J. W. Moon, On maximal independent sets of nodes in trees, *J. Graph Theory* 12 (1988) 265–283; MR 89f:05064.

[45] P. Kirschenhofer, H. Prodinger, and R. F. Tichy, Fibonacci numbers of graphs. II, *Fibonacci Quart.* 21 (1983) 219–229; MR 85e:05053.

[46] P. Kirschenhofer, H. Prodinger, and R. F. Tichy, Fibonacci numbers of graphs. III: Planted plane trees, *Fibonacci Numbers and Their Applications*, Proc. 1984 Patras conf., ed. A. N. Philippou, G. E. Bergum, and A. F. Horadam, Reidel, 1986, pp. 105–120, MR 88k:05065.

[47] M. Drmota, On generalized Fibonacci numbers of graphs, *Applications of Fibonacci Numbers*, v. 3, Proc. 1988 Pisa conf., ed. G. E. Bergum, A. N. Philippou, and A. F. Horadam, Kluwer, 1990, pp. 63–76; MR 92e:05032.

[48] A. Meir and J. W. Moon, Games on random trees, *Proc. 15th Southeastern Conf. on Combinatorics, Graph Theory and Computing*, Baton Rouge, 1984, ed. F. Hoffman, K. B. Reid, R. C. Mullin, and R. G. Stanton, Congr. Numer. 44, Utilitas Math., 1984, pp. 293–303; MR 86h:05045.

[49] N. Pippenger, Enumeration of equicolorable trees, *SIAM J. Discrete Math.* 14 (2001) 93–115; MR 2001j:05073.

[50] E. M. Palmer and A. J. Schwenk, On the number of trees in a random forest, *J. Combin. Theory Ser. B* 27 (1979) 109–121; MR 81j:05071.

[51] S. Corteel, C. D. Savage, H. S. Wilf, and D. Zeilberger, A pentagonal number sieve, *J. Combin. Theory Ser. A* 82 (1998) 186–192; MR 99d:11111.

[52] K. Husimi, Note on Mayers' theory of cluster integrals, *J. Chem. Phys.* 18 (1950) 682–684; MR 12,467i.

[53] G. E. Uhlenbeck and G. W. Ford, *Lectures in Statistical Mechanics*, Lect. in Appl. Math., v. 1, Amer. Math. Soc., 1963; MR 27 #1241.

[54] G. E. Uhlenbeck and G. W. Ford, The theory of linear graphs with applications to the theory of the virial development of the properties of gases, *Studies in Statistical Mechanics*, v. 1, ed. J. de Boer and G. Uhlenbeck, North-Holland, 1962, pp. 119–211; MR 24 #B2420.

[55] F. Harary and G. E. Uhlenbeck, On the number of Husimi trees. I, *Proc. Nat. Acad. Sci. USA* 39 (1953) 315–322; MR 14,836a.

[56] M. Bóna, M. Bousquet, G. Labelle, and P. Leroux, Enumeration of m-ary cacti, *Adv. Appl. Math.* 24 (2000) 22–56; MR 2001c:05072.

[57] N. J. A. Sloane, On-Line Encyclopedia of Integer Sequences, A000083, A000237, A000314, A001205, A001372, A002861, A005750, A035351, and A054581.

[58] C. G. Bower, Cacti (mixed Husimi trees), unpublished note (2001).

[59] G. W. Ford and G. E. Uhlenbeck, Combinatorial problems in the theory of graphs. III, *Proc. Nat. Acad. Sci. USA* 42 (1956) 529–535; MR 18,326c.

[60] C. Domb, Graph theory and embeddings, *Phase Transitions and Critical Phenomena*, v. 3, ed. C. Domb and M. S. Green, Academic Press, 1974, pp. 33–37; MR 50 #6393.

[61] T. Fowler, I. Gessel, G. Labelle, and P. Leroux, Specifying 2-trees, *Formal Power Series and Algebraic Combinatorics (FPSAC)*, Proc. 2000 Moscow conf., ed. D. Krob, A. A. Mikhalev, and A. V. Mikhalev, Springer-Verlag, 2000, pp. 202–213; MR 2001m:05132.

[62] A. Meir and J. W. Moon, On random mapping patterns, *Combinatorica* 4 (1984) 61–70; MR 85g:05125.

[63] L. R. Mutafchiev, Large trees in a random mapping pattern, *Europ. J. Combin.* 14 (1993) 341–349; MR 94f:05072.

[64] L. R. Mutafchiev, Limit theorem concerning random mapping patterns, *Combinatorica* 8 (1988) 345–356; MR 90a:05170.

[65] N. J. A. Sloane, On-Line Encyclopedia of Integer Sequences, A001205, A003024, A003087, A005217, A006196, A008483, A015701, A014535, and A037026.

[66] P. Hanlon, Counting interval graphs, *Trans. Amer. Math. Soc.* 272 (1982) 383–426; MR 83h:05050.

[67] F. S. Roberts, *Discrete Mathematical Models*, Prentice-Hall, 1976, pp. 111–140.

[68] P. C. Fishburn, *Interval Orders and Interval Graphs: A Study of Partially Ordered Sets*, Wiley, 1985; MR 86m:06001.

[69] H. S. Wilf, *generatingfunctionology*, Academic Press, 1990, pp. 76–77, 151; MR 95a:05002.

[70] R. M. Robinson, A new absolute geometric constant, *Amer. Math. Monthly* 58 (1951) 462–469; addendum 59 (1952) 296–297; MR 13,200b.

[71] R. W. Robinson, Counting labeled acyclic digraphs, *New Directions in the Theory of Graphs*, Proc. 1971 Ann Arbor conf., ed. F. Harary, Academic Press, 1973, pp. 239–273; MR 51 #249.

[72] R. P. Stanley, Acyclic orientations of graphs, *Discrete Math.* 5 (1973) 171–178; MR 47 #6537.

[73] V. A. Liskovec, The number of maximal vertices of a random acyclic digraph (in Russian), *Teor. Veroyatnost. i Primenen.* 20 (1975) 412–421; Engl. transl. in *Theory Probab. Appl.* 20 (1975) 401–421; MR 52 #1822.

[74] E. A. Bender, L. B. Richmond, R. W. Robinson, and N. C. Wormald, The asymptotic number of acyclic digraphs. I, *Combinatorica* 6 (1986) 15–22; MR 87m:05102.

[75] K. Mahler, On a special functional equation, *J. London Math. Soc.* 15 (1940) 115–123; MR 2,133e.

[76] R. W. Robinson, Counting unlabeled acyclic digraphs, *Combinatorial Mathematics V*, Proc. 1976 Melbourne conf., ed. C. H. C. Little, Lect. Notes in Math. 622, Springer-Verlag, 1977, pp. 28–43; MR 57 #16129.

[77] E. A. Bender and R. W. Robinson, The asymptotic number of acyclic digraphs. II, *J. Combin. Theory Ser. B* 44 (1988) 363–369; MR 90a:05098.

[78] R. Kemp, A note on the number of leftist trees, *Inform. Process. Lett.* 25 (1987) 227–232.

[79] R. Kemp, Further results on leftist trees, *Random Graphs '87*, Proc. 1987 Poznan conf., ed. M. Karonski, J. Jaworski, and A. Rucinski, Wiley, 1990, pp. 103–130; MR 92e:05034.

[80] R. E. Miller, N. Pippenger, A. L. Rosenberg, and L. Snyder, Optimal 2,3-trees, *SIAM J. Comput.* 8 (1979) 42–59; MR 80c:68050.

[81] A. M. Odlyzko, Periodic oscillations of coefficients of power series that satisfy functional equations, *Adv. Math.* 44 (1982) 180–205; MR 84a:30042.

[82] A. M. Odlyzko, Some new methods and results in tree enumeration, *Proc. 13th Manitoba Conf. on Numerical Mathematics and Computing*, Winnipeg, 1983, ed. D. S. Meek and G. H. J. van Rees, Congr. Numer. 42, Utilitas Math., 1984, pp. 27–52; MR 85g:05061.

[83] H. Prodinger, Some recent results on the register function of a binary tree, *Random Graphs '85*, Proc. 1985 Poznan conf, ed. M. Karonski and Z. Palka, Annals of Discrete Math. 33, North-Holland, 1987, pp. 241–260; MR 89g:68058.

[84] H. Prodinger, On a problem of Yekutieli and Mandelbrot about the bifurcation ratio of binary trees, *Theoret. Comput. Sci.* 181 (1997) 181–194; also in *Proc. 1995 Latin American Theoretical Informatics Conf. (LATIN)*, Valparáiso, ed. R. A. Baeza-Yates, E. Goles Ch., and P. V. Poblete, Lect. Notes in Comp. Sci. 911, Springer-Verlag, 1995, pp. 461–468; MR 98i:68212.

[85] I. Yekutieli and B. B. Mandelbrot, Horton-Strahler ordering of random binary trees, *J. Phys. A* 27 (1994) 285–293; MR 94m:82022.

[86] T. E. Harris, *The Theory of Branching Processes*, Springer-Verlag, 1963; MR 29 #664.

[87] K. B. Athreya and P. Ney, *Branching Processes*, Springer-Verlag, 1972; MR 51 #9242.

[88] G. Sankaranarayanan, *Branching Processes and Its Estimation Theory*, Wiley, 1989; MR 91m:60156

[89] P. Erdös and A. Rényi, On random graphs. I, *Publ. Math. (Debrecen)* 6 (1959) 290–297; also in *Selected Papers of Alfréd Rényi*, v. 2, Akadémiai Kiadó, 1976, pp. 308–315; MR 22 #10924.

[90] B. Bollobás, The evolution of random graphs, *Trans. Amer. Math. Soc.* 286 (1984) 257–274; MR 85k:05090.

[91] B. Bollobás, *Random Graphs*, Academic Press, 1985; MR 87f:05152.

[92] S. Janson, T. Luczak, and A. Rucinski, *Random Graphs*, Wiley, 2000; MR 2001k:05180.

[93] S. Janson, D. E. Knuth, T. Luczak, and B. Pittel, The birth of the giant component, *Random Structures Algorithms* 4 (1993) 231–358; MR 94h:05070.

[94] M. A. Weiss, *Data Structures and Algorithm Analysis in C++*, 2nd ed., Addison-Wesley, 1999, pp. 320–322.

[95] A. C. C. Yao, On the average behavior of set merging algorithms, *8th ACM Symp. on Theory of Computing (STOC)*, Hershey, ACM, 1976, pp. 192–195; MR 55 #1819.

[96] D. E. Knuth and A. Schönhage, The expected linearity of a simple equivalence algorithm, *Theoret. Comput. Sci.* 6 (1978) 281–315; also in *Selected Papers on Analysis of Algorithms*, CSLI, 2000, pp. 341–389; MR 81a:68049.

[97] B. Bollobás and I. Simon, Probabilistic analysis of disjoint set union algorithms, *SIAM J. Comput.* 22 (1993) 1053–1074; also in *17th ACM Symp. on Theory of Computing (STOC)*, Providence, ACM, 1985, pp. 124–231; MR 94j:05110.

5.7 Lengyel's Constant

5.7.1 Stirling Partition Numbers

Let S be a set with n elements. The set of all subsets of S has 2^n elements. By a **partition** of S we mean a disjoint set of nonempty subsets (called **blocks**) whose union is S. The set of partitions of S that possess exactly k blocks has $S_{n,k}$ elements, where $S_{n,k}$ is a

Stirling number of the second kind. The set of *all* partitions of S has B_n elements, where B_n is a **Bell number**:

$$B_n = \sum_{k=1}^{n} S_{n,k} = \frac{1}{e} \sum_{j=0}^{\infty} \frac{j^n}{j!} = \frac{d^n}{dx^n} \exp(e^x - 1) \bigg|_{x=0}.$$

For example, $S_{4,1} = 1$, $S_{4,2} = 7$, $S_{4,3} = 6$, $S_{4,4} = 1$, and $B_4 = 15$. More generally, $S_{n,1} = 1$, $S_{n,2} = 2^{n-1} - 1$, and $S_{n,3} = \frac{1}{2}(3^{n-1} + 1) - 2^{n-1}$. The following recurrences are helpful [1–4]:

$$S_{n,0} = \begin{cases} 1 & \text{if } n = 0, \\ 0 & \text{if } n \geq 1, \end{cases} \quad S_{n,k} = k S_{n-1,k} + S_{n-1,k-1} \quad \text{if } n \geq k \geq 1,$$

$$B_0 = 1, \quad B_n = \sum_{k=0}^{n-1} \binom{n-1}{k} B_k,$$

and corresponding asymptotics are discussed in [5–9].

5.7.2 Chains in the Subset Lattice of S

If U and V are subsets of S, write $U \subset V$ if U is a proper subset of V. This endows the set of all subsets of S with a **partial ordering**; in fact, it is a **lattice** with maximum element S and minimum element $\emptyset$. The number of **chains** $\emptyset = U_0 \subset U_1 \subset \cdots \subset U_{k-1} \subset U_k = S$ of length k is $k! S_{n,k}$. Hence the number of all chains from $\emptyset$ to S is [1, 6, 10]

$$\sum_{k=0}^{n} k! S_{n,k} = \sum_{j=0}^{\infty} \frac{j^n}{2^{j+1}} = \frac{1}{2} \text{Li}_{-n}\left(\frac{1}{2}\right) = \frac{d^n}{dx^n} \frac{1}{2 - e^x} \bigg|_{x=0} \sim \frac{n!}{2} \left(\frac{1}{\ln(2)}\right)^{n+1},$$

where $\text{Li}_m(x)$ is the polylogarithm function. Wilf [10] marveled at how accurate this asymptotic approximation is.

If we further insist that the chains are **maximal**, equivalently, that additional proper insertions are impossible, then the number of such chains is $n!$ A general technique due to Doubilet, Rota & Stanley [11], involving what are called *incidence algebras*, can be used to obtain the two aforementioned results, as well as to enumerate chains within more complicated posets [12].

As an aside, we give a deeper application of incidence algebras: to enumerating chains of linear subspaces within finite vector spaces [6]. Define the q-**binomial coefficient** and q-**factorial** by

$$\binom{n}{k}_q = \frac{\prod_{j=1}^{n}(q^j - 1)}{\prod_{j=1}^{k}(q^j - 1) \cdot \prod_{j=1}^{n-k}(q^j - 1)},$$

$$[n!]_q = (1 + q)(1 + q + q^2) \cdots (1 + q + \cdots + q^{n-1}),$$

where $q > 1$. Note the special case in the limit as $q \to 1^+$. Consider the n-dimensional vector space $\mathbb{F}_q^n$ over the finite field $\mathbb{F}_q$, where q is a prime power [12–16]. The number of k-dimensional linear subspaces of $\mathbb{F}_q^n$ is $\binom{n}{k}_q$ and the total number of linear subspaces of $\mathbb{F}_q^n$ is asymptotically $c_e q^{n^2/4}$ if n is even and $c_o q^{n^2/4}$ if n is odd, where [17, 18]

$$c_e = \frac{\displaystyle\sum_{k=-\infty}^{\infty} q^{-k^2}}{\displaystyle\prod_{j=1}^{\infty}(1 - q^{-j})}, \quad c_o = \frac{\displaystyle\sum_{k=-\infty}^{\infty} q^{-(k+\frac{1}{2})^2}}{\displaystyle\prod_{j=1}^{\infty}(1 - q^{-j})}.$$

We give a recurrence for the number χ_n of chains of proper subspaces (again, ordered by inclusion):

$$\chi_1 = 1, \quad \chi_n = 1 + \sum_{k=1}^{n-1} \binom{n}{k}_q \chi_k \quad \text{for } n \geq 2.$$

For the asymptotics, it follows that [6, 17]

$$\chi_n \sim \frac{1}{\zeta_q'(r)r}\left(\frac{1}{r}\right)^n \prod_{j=1}^{n}(q^j - 1) = \frac{A}{r^n}(q - 1)(q^2 - 1)(q^3 - 1)\cdots(q^n - 1),$$

where $\zeta_q(x)$ is the zeta function for the poset of subspaces:

$$\zeta_q(x) = \sum_{k=1}^{\infty} \frac{x^k}{(q - 1)(q^2 - 1)(q^3 - 1)\cdots(q^k - 1)}$$

and $r > 0$ is the unique solution of the equation $\zeta_q(r) = 1$. In particular, when $q = 2$, we have $c_e = 7.3719688014\ldots$, $c_o = 7.3719494907\ldots$, and

$$\chi_n \sim \frac{A}{r^n} \cdot Q \cdot 2^{\frac{n(n+1)}{2}},$$

where $r = 0.7759021363\ldots$, $A = 0.8008134543\ldots$, and

$$Q = \prod_{k=1}^{\infty}\left(1 - \frac{1}{2^k}\right) = 0.2887880950\ldots$$

is one of the digital search tree constants [5.14]. If we further insist that the chains are maximal, then the number of such chains is $[n!]_q$.

5.7.3 Chains in the Partition Lattice of S

We have discussed chains in the poset of subsets of the set S. There is, however, another poset associated naturally with S that is less familiar and more difficult to study: the **poset of partitions** of S. Here is the partial ordering: Assuming P and Q are two partitions of S, then $P < Q$ if $P \neq Q$ and if $p \in P$ implies that p is a subset of q for some $q \in Q$. In other words, P is a *refinement* of Q in the sense that each of its blocks fits within a block of Q. For arbitrary n, the poset is, in fact, a lattice with minimum element $m = \{\{1\}, \{2\}, \ldots, \{n\}\}$ and maximum element $M = \{\{1, 2, \ldots, n\}\}$.

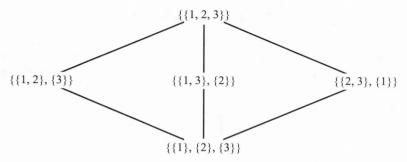

Figure 5.10. The number of chains $m < P_1 < M$ in the partition lattice of the set $\{1, 2, 3\}$ is three.

What is the number of chains $m = P_0 < P_1 < P_2 < \cdots < P_{k-1} < P_k = M$ of length k in the partition lattice of S? In the case $n = 3$, there is only one chain for $k = 1$, specifically, $m < M$. For $k = 2$, there are three such chains as pictured in Figure 5.10.

Let Z_n denote the number of all chains from m to M of any length; clearly $Z_1 = Z_2 = 1$ and, by the foregoing, $Z_3 = 4$. We have the recurrence

$$Z_n = \sum_{k=1}^{n-1} S_{n,k} Z_k$$

and exponential generating function

$$Z(x) = \sum_{n=1}^{\infty} \frac{Z_n}{n!} x^n, \quad 2Z(x) = x + Z(e^x - 1),$$

but techniques of Doubilet, Rota & Stanley and Bender do not apply here to give asymptotic estimates of Z_n. The partition lattice is the first natural lattice without the structure of a *binomial lattice*, which implies that well-known generating function techniques are no longer helpful.

Lengyel [19] formulated a different approach to prove that the quotient

$$r_n = \frac{Z_n}{(n!)^2 (2\ln(2))^{-n} n^{-1-\ln(2)/3}}$$

must be bounded between two positive constants as $n \to \infty$. He presented numerical evidence suggesting that r_n tends to a unique value. Babai & Lengyel [20] then proved a fairly general convergence criterion that enabled them to conclude that $\Lambda = \lim_{n \to \infty} r_n$ exists and $\Lambda = 1.09\ldots$. The analysis in [19] involves intricate estimates of the Stirling numbers; in [20], the focus is on nearly convex linear recurrences with finite retardation and active predecessors.

In an ambitious undertaking, Flajolet & Salvy [21] computed $\Lambda = 1.0986858055\ldots$. Their approach is based on (complex fractional) analytic iterates of $\exp(x) - 1$ and much more, but unfortunately their paper is presently incomplete. See [5.8] for related discussion of the Takeuchi-Prellberg constant.

By way of contrast, the number of *maximal* chains is given exactly by $n!(n-1)!/2^{n-1}$ and Lengyel [19] observed that Z_n exceeds this by an exponentially large factor.

5.7.4 Random Chains

Van Cutsem & Ycart [22] examined random chains in both the subset and partition lattices. It is remarkable that a common framework exists for studying these and that, in a certain sense, the limiting distributions of both types of chains are *identical*. We mention only one consequence: If $\kappa_n = k/n$ is the normalized length of the random chain, then

$$\lim_{n \to \infty} E(\kappa_n) = \frac{1}{2 \ln(2)} = 0.7213475204\ldots$$

and a corresponding Central Limit Theorem also holds.

[1] L. Lovász, *Combinatorial Problems and Exercises*, 2nd ed., North-Holland, 1993, pp. 16–18, 162–173; MR 94m:05001.

[2] L. Comtet, *Advanced Combinatorics: The Art of Finite and Infinite Expansions*, Reidel, 1974, pp. 59–60, 204–211; MR 57 #124.

[3] N. J. A. Sloane, On-Line Encyclopedia of Integer Sequences, A000110, A000670, A005121, and A006116.

[4] G.-C. Rota, The number of partitions of a set, *Amer. Math. Monthly* 71 (1964) 498–504; MR 28 #5009.

[5] N. G. de Bruijn, *Asymptotic Methods in Analysis*, Dover, 1958, pp. 102–109; MR 83m:41028.

[6] E. A. Bender, Asymptotic methods in enumeration, *SIAM Rev.* 16 (1974) 485–515; errata 18 (1976) 292; MR 51 #12545 and MR 55 #10276.

[7] A. M. Odlyzko, Asymptotic enumeration methods, *Handbook of Combinatorics*, v. I, ed. R. Graham, M. Grötschel, and L. Lovász, MIT Press, 1995, pp. 1063–1229; MR 97b:05012.

[8] B. Salvy and J. Shackell, Symbolic asymptotics: multiseries of inverse functions, *J. Symbolic Comput.* 27 (1999) 543–563; MR 2000h:41039.

[9] B. Salvy and J. Shackell, Asymptotics of the Stirling numbers of the second kind, *Studies in Automatic Combinatorics*, v. 2, Algorithms Project, INRIA, 1997.

[10] H. S. Wilf, *generatingfunctionology*, Academic Press, 1990, pp. 21–24, 146–147; MR 95a:05002.

[11] P. Doubilet, G.-C. Rota, and R. Stanley, On the foundations of combinatorial theory. VI: The idea of generating function, *Proc. Sixth Berkeley Symp. Math. Stat. Probab.*, v. 2, ed. L. M. Le Cam, J. Neyman, and E. L. Scott, Univ. of Calif. Press, 1972, pp. 267–318; MR 53 #7796.

[12] M. Aigner, *Combinatorial Theory*, Springer-Verlag, 1979, pp. 78–79, 142–143; MR 80h:05002.

[13] J. Goldman and G.-C. Rota, The number of subspaces of a vector space, *Recent Progress in Combinatorics*, Proc. 1968 Waterloo conf., ed. W. T. Tutte, Academic Press, 1969, pp. 75–83; MR 40 #5453.

[14] G. E. Andrews, *The Theory of Partitions*, Addison-Wesley, 1976; MR 99c:11126.

[15] H. Exton, *q-Hypergeometric Functions and Applications*, Ellis Horwood, 1983; MR 85g:33001.

[16] M. Sved, Gaussians and binomials, *Ars Combin.* 17 A (1984) 325–351; MR 85j:05002.

[17] T. Slivnik, Subspaces of $\mathbb{Z}_2^n$, unpublished note (1996).

[18] M. Wild, The asymptotic number of inequivalent binary codes and nonisomorphic binary matroids, *Finite Fields Appl.* 6 (2000) 192–202; MR 2001i:94077.

[19] T. Lengyel, On a recurrence involving Stirling numbers, *Europ. J. Combin.* 5 (1984) 313–321; MR 86c:11010.

[20] L. Babai and T. Lengyel, A convergence criterion for recurrent sequences with application to the partition lattice, *Analysis* 12 (1992) 109–119; MR 93f:05005.

[21] P. Flajolet and B. Salvy, Hierarchical set partitions and analytic iterates of the exponential function, unpublished note (1990).

[22] B. Van Cutsem and B. Ycart, Renewal-type behavior of absorption times in Markov chains, *Adv. Appl. Probab.* 26 (1994) 988–1005; MR 96f:60118.

5.8 Takeuchi–Prellberg Constant

In 1978, Takeuchi defined a triply recursive function [1,2]

$$t(x, y, z) = \begin{cases} y & \text{if } x \le y, \\ t(t(x-1, y, z), t(y-1, z, x), t(z-1, x, y)) & \text{otherwise} \end{cases}$$

that is useful for benchmark testing of programming languages. The value of $t(x, y, z)$ is of no practical significance; in fact, McCarthy [1,2] observed that the function can be described more simply as

$$t(x, y, z) = \begin{cases} y & \text{if } x \le y, \\ \begin{cases} z & \text{if } y \le z, \\ x & \text{otherwise,} \end{cases} & \text{otherwise.} \end{cases}$$

The interesting quantity is not $t(x, y, z)$, but rather $T(x, y, z)$, defined to be the number of times the *otherwise* clause is invoked in the recursion. We assume that the program is memoryless in the sense that previously computed results are not available at any time in the future. Knuth [1,3] studied the **Takeuchi numbers** $T_n = T(n, 0, n+1)$:

$$T_0 = 0, \ T_1 = 1, \ T_2 = 4, \ T_3 = 14, \ T_4 = 53, \ T_5 = 223, \ldots$$

and deduced that

$$e^{n \ln(n) - n \ln(\ln(n)) - n} < T_n < e^{n \ln(n) - n + \ln(n)}$$

for all sufficiently large n. He asked for more precise asymptotic information about the growth of T_n.

Starting with Knuth's recursive formula for the Takeuchi numbers

$$T_{n+1} = \sum_{k=0}^{n} \left[\binom{n+k}{n} - \binom{n+k}{n+1} \right] T_{n-k} + \sum_{k=1}^{n-1} \binom{2k}{k} \frac{1}{k+1}$$

and the somewhat related Bell numbers [5.7]

$$B_{n+1} = \sum_{k=0}^{n} \binom{n}{k} B_{n-k}, \quad B_0 = 1, \ B_1 = 1, \ B_2 = 2, \ B_3 = 5, \ B_4 = 15, \ B_5 = 52, \ldots,$$

Prellberg [4] observed that the following limit exists:

$$c = \lim_{n \to \infty} \frac{T_n}{B_n \exp\left(\frac{1}{2} W_n^2\right)} = 2.2394331040\ldots,$$

where $W_n \exp(W_n) = n$ are special values of the Lambert W function [6.11].

Since both the Bell numbers and the W function are well understood, this provides an answer to Knuth's question. The underlying theory is still under development, but

Prellberg's numerical evidence is persuasive. Recent theoretical work [5] relates the constant c to an associated functional equation,

$$T(z) = \sum_{n=0}^{\infty} T_n z^n, \quad T(z) = \frac{T(z - z^2)}{z} - \frac{1}{(1-z)(1-z+z^2)},$$

in a manner parallel to how Lengyel's constant [5.7] is obtained.

[1]   D. E. Knuth, Textbook examples of recursion, *Artificial Intelligence and Mathematical Theory of Computation*, ed. V. Lifschitz, Academic Press, 1991, pp. 207–229; also in *Selected Papers on Analysis of Algorithms*, CSLI, 2000, pp. 391–414; MR 93a:68093.
[2]   I. Vardi, *Computational Recreations in Mathematica*, Addison-Wesley, 1991, pp. 179–199; MR 93e:00002.
[3]   N. J. A. Sloane, On-Line Encyclopedia of Integer Sequences, A000651.
[4]   T. Prellberg, On the asymptotics of Takeuchi numbers, *Symbolic Computation, Number Theory, Special Functions, Physics and Combinatorics*, Proc. 1999 Gainesville conf., ed. F. G. Garvan and M. Ismail, Kluwer, 2001, pp. 231–242; math.CO/0005008.
[5]   T. Prellberg, On the asymptotic analysis of a class of linear recurrences, presentation at *Formal Power Series and Algebraic Combinatorics (FPSAC)* conf., Univ. of Melbourne, 2002.

5.9 Pólya's Random Walk Constants

Let L denote the d-dimensional cubic lattice whose vertices are precisely all integer points in d-dimensional space. A **walk** ω on L, beginning at the origin, is an infinite sequence of vertices $\omega_0, \omega_1, \omega_2, \omega_3, \ldots$ with $\omega_0 = 0$ and $|\omega_{j+1} - \omega_j| = 1$ for all j. Assume that the walk is random and symmetric in the sense that, at each time step, all $2d$ directions of possible travel have equal probability. What is the likelihood that $\omega_n = 0$ for some $n > 0$? That is, what is the **return probability** p_d?

Pólya [1–4] proved the remarkable fact that $p_1 = p_2 = 1$ but $p_d < 1$ for $d > 2$. Mc-Crea & Whipple [5], Watson [6], Domb [7] and Glasser & Zucker [8] each contributed facets of the following evaluations of $p_3 = 1 - 1/m_3 = 0.3405373295\ldots$, where the expected number m_3 of returns to the origin, plus one, is

$$
\begin{aligned}
m_3 &= \frac{3}{(2\pi)^3} \int_{-\pi}^{\pi}\int_{-\pi}^{\pi}\int_{-\pi}^{\pi} \frac{1}{3 - \cos(\theta) - \cos(\varphi) - \cos(\psi)}\, d\theta\, d\varphi\, d\psi \\
&= \frac{12}{\pi^2}\left(18 + 12\sqrt{2} - 10\sqrt{3} - 7\sqrt{6}\right) K\left[(2 - \sqrt{3})(\sqrt{3} - \sqrt{2})\right]^2 \\
&= 3\left(18 + 12\sqrt{2} - 10\sqrt{3} - 7\sqrt{6}\right)\left[1 + 2\sum_{k=1}^{\infty} \exp(-\sqrt{6}\pi k^2)\right]^4 \\
&= \frac{\sqrt{6}}{32\pi^3}\Gamma\left(\frac{1}{24}\right)\Gamma\left(\frac{5}{24}\right)\Gamma\left(\frac{7}{24}\right)\Gamma\left(\frac{11}{24}\right) = 1.5163860591\ldots.
\end{aligned}
$$

Hence the **escape probability** for a random walk on the three-dimensional cubic lattice is $1 - p_3 = 0.6594626704\ldots$. In these expressions, K denotes the complete elliptic integral of the first kind [1.4.6] and Γ denotes the gamma function [1.5.4]. Return and escape probabilities can also be computed for the body-centered or face-centered cubic

Table 5.1. *Expected Number of Returns and Return Probabilities*

d	m_d	p_d
4	1.2394671218...	0.1932016732...
5	1.1563081248...	0.1351786098...
6	1.1169633732...	0.1047154956...
7	1.0939063155...	0.0858449341...
8	1.0786470120...	0.0729126499...

lattices (as opposed to the simple cubic lattice), but we will not discuss these or other generalizations [9].

What can be said about p_d for $d > 3$? Closed-form expressions do not appear to exist here. Montroll [10–12] determined that $p_d = 1 - 1/m_d$, where

$$m_d = \frac{d}{(2\pi)^d} \int\limits_{-\pi}^{\pi} \int\limits_{-\pi}^{\pi} \cdots \int\limits_{-\pi}^{\pi} \left(d - \sum_{k=1}^{d} \cos(\theta_k) \right)^{-1} d\theta_1 \, d\theta_2 \cdots d\theta_d = \int\limits_{0}^{\infty} e^{-t} \left(I_0\left(\frac{t}{d}\right) \right)^d dt$$

and $I_0(x)$ denotes the zeroth modified Bessel function [3.6]. The corresponding numerical approximations, as functions of d, are listed in Table 5.1 [10, 13–17].

What is the length of travel required for a return? Let $U_{d,l,n}$ be the number of d-dimensional n-step walks that start from the origin and end at a lattice point l. Let $V_{d,l,n}$ be the number of d-dimensional n-step walks that start from the origin and reach the lattice point $l \neq 0$ for the *first time* at the end (second time if $l = 0$). Then the generating functions

$$U_{d,l}(x) = \sum_{n=0}^{\infty} \frac{U_{d,l,n}}{(2d)^n} x^n, \quad V_{d,l}(x) = \sum_{n=0}^{\infty} \frac{V_{d,l,n}}{(2d)^n} x^n$$

satisfy $V_{d,l}(x) = U_{d,l}(x)/U_{d,0}(x)$ if $l \neq 0$, $V_{d,l}(x) = 1 - 1/U_{d,0}(x)$ if $l = 0$, and $U_{d,0}(1) = m_d$, $V_{d,0}(1) = p_d$. For example,

$$U_{1,l}(x) = \sum_{n=0}^{\infty} \frac{1}{2^n} \binom{n}{\frac{l+n}{2}} x^n, \quad U_{2,l}(x) = \sum_{n=0}^{\infty} \frac{1}{4^n} \binom{n}{\frac{l_1+l_2+n}{2}} \binom{n}{\frac{l_1-l_2+n}{2}} x^n,$$

where we agree to set the binomial coefficients equal to 0 if $l + n$ is odd for $d = 1$ or $l_1 + l_2 + n$ is odd for $d = 2$. If $d = 3$, then $a_n = U_{3,0,2n}$ satisfies [18]

$$a_n = \binom{2n}{n} \sum_{k=0}^{n} \binom{n}{k}^2 \binom{2k}{k} = \sum_{k=0}^{n} \frac{(2n)!(2k)!}{(n-k)!^2 k!^4}, \quad \sum_{n=0}^{\infty} \frac{a_n}{(2n)!} y^{2n} = I_0(2y)^3,$$

$$(n+2)^3 a_{n+2} - 2(2n+3)(10n^2 + 30n + 23)a_{n+1} + 36(n+1)(2n+1)(2n+3)a_n = 0,$$

and if $d = 4$, then $b_n = U_{4,0,2n}$ satisfies [19]

$$(n+2)^4 b_{n+2} - 4(2n+3)^2(5n^2 + 15n + 12)b_{n+1}$$
$$+ 256(n+1)^2(2n+1)(2n+3)b_n = 0.$$

For any d, the mean **first-passage time** to arrive at any lattice point l is infinite (in spite of the fact that the associated probability $V_{d,l}(1) = 1$ for $d = 1$ or 2). There are several alternative ways of quantifying the length of required travel. Using our formulas for $V_{d,l}(x)$, the median first-passage times are 2-4, 1-3, 6-8, and 17-19 steps for $l = 0, 1,$ 2, and 3 when $d = 1$, and 2-4, 25-27, and 520-522 steps for $l = (0, 0), (1, 0),$ and $(1, 1)$ when $d = 2$. Hughes [3, 20] examined the conditional mean time to return to the origin (conditional upon return eventually occurring). Also, for $d = 1$, the mean time for the earliest of three independent random walkers to return to the origin is finite and has value [6, 21–23]

$$
2 \sum_{n=0}^{\infty} \frac{1}{2^{6n}} \binom{2n}{n}^3 = \frac{2}{\pi^3} \int_0^\pi \int_0^\pi \int_0^\pi \frac{1}{1 - \cos(\theta)\cos(\varphi)\cos(\psi)} \, d\theta \, d\varphi \, d\psi
$$

$$
= \frac{8}{\pi^2} K\left(\frac{1}{\sqrt{2}}\right)^2 = \frac{1}{2\pi^3} \Gamma\left(\frac{1}{4}\right)^4 = 2(1.3932039296\ldots),
$$

whereas for $d = 2$, the mean time for the earliest of an *arbitrary* number of independent random walkers is infinite. More on multiple random walkers, of both the friendly and vicious kinds, is found in [24].

It is known that

$$
U_{d,l}(x) = \frac{d}{(2\pi)^d} \int_{-\pi}^{\pi} \int_{-\pi}^{\pi} \cdots \int_{-\pi}^{\pi} \left(d - x \sum_{k=1}^{d} \cos(\theta_k)\right)^{-1}
$$

$$
\times \exp\left(i \sum_{k=1}^{d} \theta_k l_k\right) d\theta_1 \, d\theta_2 \cdots d\theta_d,
$$

which can be numerically evaluated for small d. Here are some sample probabilities [11, 16] that a three-dimensional walk reaches a point l:

$$
V_{3,l}(1) = \frac{U_{3,l}(1)}{m_3} = \begin{cases} 0.3405373295\ldots & \text{if } l = (1, 0, 0), \\ 0.2183801414\ldots & \text{if } l = (1, 1, 0), \\ 0.1724297877\ldots & \text{if } l = (1, 1, 1). \end{cases}
$$

An asymptotic expansion for these probabilities is [11, 12]

$$
V_{3,l}(1) = \frac{3}{2\pi m_3 |l|} \left[1 + \frac{1}{8|l|^2}\left(-3 + \frac{5(l_1^4 + l_2^4 + l_3^4)}{|l|^2} + \cdots\right)\right] \sim \frac{0.3148702313\ldots}{|l|}
$$

and is valid as $|l|^2 = l_1^2 + l_2^2 + l_3^2 \to \infty$.

Let $W_{d,n}$ be the average number of distinct vertices visited during a d-dimensional n-step walk. It can be shown that [25–28]

$$
W_d(x) = \sum_{n=0}^{\infty} W_{d,n} x^n = \frac{1}{(1-x)^2 U_{d,0}(x)}, \quad W_{d,n} \sim \begin{cases} \sqrt{\dfrac{8n}{\pi}} & \text{if } d = 1, \\ \dfrac{\pi n}{\ln(n)} & \text{if } d = 2, \\ (1 - p_3)n & \text{if } d = 3 \end{cases}
$$

as $n \to \infty$. Higher-order asymptotics for $W_{3,n}$ are possible using the expansion [11, 12, 29–31]

$$U_{3,0}(x) = m_3 - \frac{3\sqrt{3}}{2\pi}(1 - x^2)^{\frac{1}{2}} + c(1 - x^2) - \frac{3\sqrt{3}}{4\pi}(1 - x^2)^{\frac{3}{2}} + \cdots,$$

where $x \to 1^-$ and

$$c = \frac{9}{32}\left(m_3 + \frac{6}{\pi^2 m_3}\right) = 0.5392381750\ldots.$$

Other parameters, for example, the average growth of distance from the origin [32],

$$\lim_{n \to \infty} \frac{1}{\ln(n)} \sum_{j=1}^{n} \frac{j^{-1/2}}{1 + |\omega_j|} = \lambda_1 \quad \text{with probability 1, if } d = 1,$$

$$\lim_{n \to \infty} \frac{1}{\ln(n)^2} \sum_{j=1}^{n} \frac{1}{1 + |\omega_j|^2} = \lambda_2 \quad \text{with probability 1, if } d = 2,$$

$$\lim_{n \to \infty} \frac{1}{\ln(n)} \sum_{j=1}^{n} \frac{1}{1 + |\omega_j|^2} = \lambda_d \quad \text{with probability 1, if } d \geq 3,$$

are more difficult to analyze. The constants λ_d are known only to be finite and positive.

For a one-dimensional n-step walk ω, define M_n^+ to be the maximum value of ω_j and M_n^- to be the maximum value of $-\omega_j$. Then M_n^+ and M_n^- each follow the half-normal distribution [6.2] in the limit as $n \to \infty$, and [33, 34]

$$\lim_{n \to \infty} \mathrm{E}\left(n^{-\frac{1}{2}} M_n^+\right) = \sqrt{\frac{2}{\pi}} = \lim_{n \to \infty} \mathrm{E}\left(n^{-\frac{1}{2}} M_n^-\right).$$

Further, if T_n^+ is the smallest value of j for which $\omega_j = M_n^+$ and T_n^- is the smallest value of k for which $-\omega_k = M_n^-$, then the **arcsine law** applies:

$$\lim_{n \to \infty} \mathrm{P}\left(n^{-1} T_n^+ < x\right) = \frac{2}{\pi} \arcsin \sqrt{x} = \lim_{n \to \infty} \mathrm{P}\left(n^{-1} T_n^- < x\right),$$

which implies that a one-dimensional random walk tends to be either highly negative or highly positive (not both). Such detailed information about d-dimensional walks is not yet available. Define also $\tau_{d,r}$ to be the smallest value of j for which $|\omega_j| \geq r$, for any positive integer r. Then [35]

$$\tau_{1,r} = r^2, \quad \tau_{2,2} = \frac{9}{2}, \quad \tau_{2,3} = \frac{135}{13}, \quad \tau_{2,4} = \frac{11791}{668},$$

but a pattern is not evident. What precisely can be said about $\tau_{d,r}$ as $r \to \infty$?

As a computational aside, we mention a result of Odlyzko's [36–38]: Any algorithm that determines M_n^+ (or M_n^-) exactly must examine at least $(A + o(1))\sqrt{n}$ of the ω_j values on average, where $A = \sqrt{8/\pi} \ln(2) = 1.1061028674 \ldots$.

On the one hand, the waiting time N_n for a one-dimensional random walk to hit a new vertex, not visited in the first n steps, satisfies [39]

$$\limsup_{n \to \infty} \frac{N_n}{n \ln(\ln(n))^2} = \frac{1}{\pi^2} \quad \text{with probability 1.}$$

On the other hand, if F_n denotes the set of vertices that are maximally visited by the random walk up to step n, called **favorite sites**, then $|F_n| \geq 4$ only finitely often, with probability 1 [40].

For two-dimensional random walks, we may define F_n analogously. The number of visits to a selected point in F_n within the first n steps is $\sim \ln(n)^2/\pi$ with probability 1, as $n \to \infty$. This can be rephrased as the asymptotic number of times a drunkard drops by his favorite watering hole [41, 42]. Dually, the length of time C_r required to totally cover all vertices of the $r \times r$ torus (square with opposite sides identified) satisfies [43]

$$\lim_{r \to \infty} \mathrm{P} \left(\left| \frac{C_r}{r^2 \ln(r)^2} - \frac{4}{\pi} \right| < \varepsilon \right) = 1$$

for every $\varepsilon > 0$ (convergence in probability). This solves what is known as the "white screen problem" [44].

If a three-dimensional random walk ω is restricted to the region $x \geq y \geq z$, then the analogous series coefficients are

$$\bar{a}_n = \sum_{k=0}^{n} \frac{(2n)!(2k)!}{(n-k)!(n+1-k)!k!^2(k+1)!^2},$$

and from this we have [45]

$$\bar{m}_3 = \sum_{n=0}^{\infty} \frac{\bar{a}_n}{6^{2n}} = 1.0693411205 \ldots, \quad \bar{p}_3 = 1 - \frac{1}{\bar{m}_3} = 0.0648447153 \ldots$$

characterizing the return. What can be said concerning other regions, for example, a half-space, quarter-space, or octant?

Here is one variation. Let $X_1, X_2, X_3, \ldots$ be independent normally distributed random variables with mean μ and variance 1. Consider the partial sums $S_j = \sum_{k=1}^{j} X_k$, which constitute a random walk on the real line (rather than the one-dimensional lattice) with Gaussian increments (rather than Bernoulli increments). There is an enormous literature on $\{S_j\}$, but we shall mention only one result. Let H be the first positive value of S_j, called the **first ladder height** of the process; then the moments of H when $\mu = 0$ are [46]

$$\mathrm{E}_0(H) = \frac{1}{\sqrt{2}}, \quad \mathrm{E}_0(H^2) = -\frac{\zeta(\frac{1}{2})}{\sqrt{\pi}} = \sqrt{2}\rho = \sqrt{2}(0.5825971579 \ldots)$$

and, for arbitrary μ in a neighborhood of 0,

$$E_{\mu}(H) = \frac{1}{\sqrt{2}} \exp\left[-\frac{\mu}{\sqrt{2\pi}} \sum_{k=0}^{\infty} \frac{\zeta(\frac{1}{2}-k)}{k!(2k+1)} \left(-\frac{\mu^2}{2}\right)^k\right],$$

where $\zeta(x)$ is the Riemann zeta function [1.6]. Other occurrences of the interesting constant ρ in the statistical literature are in [47–50].

Here is another variation. Let Y_1, Y_2, Y_3, ... be independent Uniform $[-1, 1]$ random variables, $S_0 = 0$, and $S_j = \sum_{k=1}^{j} Y_k$. Then the expected maximum value of $\{S_0, S_1, \ldots, S_n\}$ is [51]

$$E\left(\max_{0 \le j \le n} S_j\right) = \sqrt{\frac{2}{3\pi}} n^{\frac{1}{2}} + \sigma + \frac{1}{5}\sqrt{\frac{2}{3\pi}} n^{-\frac{1}{2}} + O\left(n^{-\frac{3}{2}}\right)$$

as $n \to \infty$, where $\sigma = -0.2979521902\ldots$ is given by

$$\sigma = \frac{\zeta(\frac{1}{2})}{\sqrt{6\pi}} + \frac{\zeta(\frac{3}{2})}{20\sqrt{6\pi}} + \sum_{k=1}^{\infty}\left(\frac{t_k}{k} - \frac{k^{-\frac{1}{2}}}{\sqrt{6\pi}} - \frac{k^{-\frac{3}{2}}}{20\sqrt{6\pi}}\right)$$

and

$$t_k = \frac{2(-1)^k}{(k+1)!} \sum_{k/2 \le j \le k} (-1)^j \binom{k}{j} \left(j - \frac{k}{2}\right)^{k+1}.$$

A deeper connection between $\zeta(x)$ and random walks is discussed in [52].

5.9.1 Intersections and Trappings

A walk ω on the lattice L is **self-intersecting** if $\omega_i = \omega_j$ for some $i < j$, and the **self-intersection time** is the smallest value of j for which this happens. Computing self-intersection times is more difficult than first-passage times since the entire history of the walk requires memorization. If $d = 1$, then clearly the mean self-intersection time is 3. If $d = 2$, the mean self-intersection time is [53]

$$\frac{2 \cdot 4}{4^2} + \frac{3 \cdot 12}{4^3} + \frac{4 \cdot 44}{4^4} + \frac{5 \cdot 116}{4^5} + \cdots = \sum_{n=2}^{\infty} \frac{n(4c_{n-1} - c_n)}{4^n}$$

$$= \frac{c_1}{2} + \sum_{n=2}^{\infty} \frac{c_n}{4^n} = 4.5860790989\ldots,$$

where the sequence $\{c_n\}$ is defined in [5.10]. When n is large, no exact formula for evaluating c_n is known, unlike the sequences $\{a_n\}$, $\{\bar{a}_n\}$, and $\{b_n\}$ discussed earlier. We are, in this example, providing foreshadowing of difficulties to come later. See the generalization in [54, 55].

A walk ω is **self-trapping** if, for some k, $\omega_i \ne \omega_j$ for all $i < j \le k$ and ω_k is completely surrounded by previously visited vertices. If $d = 2$, there are eight self-trapping walks when $k = 7$ and sixteen such walks when $k = 8$. A Monte Carlo simulation in [56, 57] gave a mean self-trapping time of approximately $70.7\ldots$.

Two walks ω and ω' **intersect** if $\omega_i = \omega'_j$ for some nonzero i and j. The probability q_n that two n-step independent random walks never intersect satisfies [58–61]

$$\ln(q_n) \sim \begin{cases} -\frac{5}{8}\ln(n) & \text{if } d = 2, \\ -\xi \ln(n) & \text{if } d = 3, \\ -\frac{1}{2}\ln(\ln(n)) & \text{if } d = 4 \end{cases}$$

as $n \to \infty$, where the exponent ξ is approximately $0.29\ldots$ (again obtained by simulation). For each $d \geq 5$, it can be shown [62] that $\lim_{n\to\infty} q_n$ lies strictly between 0 and 1. Further simulation [63] yields $q_5 = 0.708\ldots$ and $q_6 = 0.822\ldots$, and we shall refer to these in [5.10].

5.9.2 Holonomicity

A **holonomic function** (in the sense of Zeilberger [45, 64, 65]) is a solution $f(z)$ of a linear homogeneous differential equation

$$f^{(n)}(z) + r_1(z)f^{(n-1)}(z) + \cdots + r_{n-1}(z)f'(z) + r_n(z)f(z) = 0,$$

where each $r_k(z)$ is a rational function with rational coefficients. **Regular holonomic constants** are values of f at algebraic points z_0 where each r_k is analytic; f can be proved to be analytic at z_0 as well. **Singular holonomic constants** are values of f at algebraic points z_0 where each r_k has, at worst, a pole of order k at z_0 (called Fuchsian or "regular" singularities [66–68]). The former include π, $\ln(2)$, and the tetralogarithm $\mathrm{Li}_4(1/2)$; the latter include Apéry's constant $\zeta(3)$, Catalan's constant G, and Pólya's constants p_d, $d > 2$. Holonomic constants of either type fall into the class of polynomial-time computable constants [69]. We merely mention a somewhat related theory of EL numbers due to Chow [70].

[1] G. Pólya, Über eine Aufgabe der Wahrscheinlichkeitsrechnung betreffend die Irrfahrt im Stassennetz, *Math. Annalen* 84 (1921) 149–160; also in *Collected Papers*, v. 4, ed. G.-C. Rota, MIT Press, 1984, pp. 69–80, 609.

[2] P. G. Doyle and J. L. Snell, *Random Walks and Electric Networks*, Math. Assoc. Amer., 1984; math.PR/0001057; MR 89a:94023.

[3] B. D. Hughes, *Random Walks and Random Environments*, v. 1, Oxford Univ. Press, 1995; MR 96i:60070.

[4] F. Spitzer, *Principles of Random Walks*, 2nd ed, Springer-Verlag, 1976, p. 103; MR 52 #9383.

[5] W. H. McCrea and F. J. W. Whipple, Random paths in two and three dimensions, *Proc. Royal Soc. Edinburgh* 60 (1940) 281–298; MR 2,107f.

[6] G. N. Watson, Three triple integrals, *Quart. J. Math.* 10 (1939) 266–276; MR 1,205b.

[7] C. Domb, On multiple returns in the random-walk problem, *Proc. Cambridge Philos. Soc.* 50 (1954) 586–591; MR 16,148f.

[8] M. L. Glasser and I. J. Zucker, Extended Watson integrals for the cubic lattices, *Proc. Nat. Acad. Sci. USA* 74 (1977) 1800–1801; MR 56 #686.

[9] D. J. Daley, Return probabilities for certain three-dimensional random walks, *J. Appl. Probab.* 16 (1979) 45–53; MR 80e:60083.

[10] E. W. Montroll, Random walks in multidimensional spaces, especially on periodic lattices, *J. SIAM* 4 (1956) 241–260; MR 19,470d.

[11] E. W. Montroll, Random walks on lattices, *Stochastic Processes in Mathematical Physics and Engineering*, ed. R. Bellman, Proc. Symp. Appl. Math. 16, Amer. Math. Soc., 1964, pp. 193–220; MR 28 #4585.

[12] E. W. Montroll and G. H. Weiss, Random walks on lattices. II, *J. Math. Phys.* 6 (1965) 167–181; MR 30 #2563.

[13] K. Kondo and T. Hara, Critical exponent of susceptibility for a class of general ferromagnets in $d > 4$ dimensions, *J. Math. Phys.* 28 (1987) 1206–1208; MR 88k:82052.

[14] D. I. Cartwright, Some examples of random walks on free products of discrete groups, *Annali Mat. Pura Appl.* 151 (1988) 1–15; MR 90f:60018.

[15] P. Griffin, Accelerating beyond the third dimension: Returning to the origin in simple random walk, *Math. Sci.* 15 (1990) 24–35; MR 91g:60083.

[16] T. Hara, G. Slade, and A. D. Sokal, New lower bounds on the self-avoiding-walk connective constant, *J. Stat. Phys.* 72 (1993) 479–517; erratum 78 (1995) 1187–1188; MR 94e:82053.

[17] J. Keane, Pólya's constants p_d to 80 digits for $3 \leq d \leq 64$, unpublished note (1998).

[18] N. J. A. Sloane, On-Line Encyclopedia of Integer Sequences, A002896, A039699, A049037, and A063888.

[19] M. L. Glasser and A. J. Guttmann, Lattice Green function (at 0) for the 4D hypercubic lattice, *J. Phys. A* 27 (1994) 7011–7014; MR 95i:82047.

[20] B. D. Hughes, On returns to the starting site in lattice random walks, *Physica* 134A (1986) 443–457; MR 87c:60057.

[21] K. Lindenberg, V. Seshadri, K. E. Shuler, and G. H. Weiss, Lattice random walks for sets of random walkers: First passage times, *J. Stat. Phys.* 23 (1980) 11–25; MR 83c:60100.

[22] W. D. Fryer and M. S. Klamkin, Comment on problem 612, *Math. Mag.* 40 (1967) 52–53.

[23] B. C. Berndt, *Ramanujan's Notebooks: Part II*, Springer-Verlag, 1989, p. 24; MR 90b:01039.

[24] M. E. Fisher, Walks, walls, wetting, and melting, *J. Stat. Phys.* 34 (1984) 667–729; MR 85j:82022.

[25] A. Dvoretzky and P. Erdös, Some problems on random walk in space, *Proc. Second Berkeley Symp. Math. Stat. Probab.*, ed. J. Neyman, Univ. of Calif. Press, 1951, pp. 353–367; MR 13,852b.

[26] G. H. Vineyard, The number of distinct sites visited in a random walk on a lattice, *J. Math. Phys.* 4 (1963) 1191–1193; MR 27 #4610.

[27] M. N. Barber and B. W. Ninham, *Random and Restricted Walks: Theory and Applications*, Gordon and Breach, 1970.

[28] E. W. Montroll and B. J. West, On an enriched collection of stochastic processes, *Studies in Statistical Mechanics*, v. 7, *Fluctuation Phenomena*, ed. E. W. Montroll and J. L. Lebowitz, North-Holland, 1979, pp. 61–175; MR 83g:82001.

[29] A. A. Maradudin, E. W. Montroll, G. H. Weiss, R. Herman, and H. W. Milnes, Green's functions for monatomic simple cubic lattices, *Acad. Royale Belgique Classe Sci. Mém. Coll. 4º, 2ᵉ Sér.*, v. 14 (1960) n. 7, 1–176; MR 22 #7440.

[30] G. S. Joyce, Lattice Green function for the simple cubic lattice, *J. Phys. A* (1972) L65–L68.

[31] G. S. Joyce, On the simple cubic lattice Green function, *Philos. Trans. Royal Soc. London Ser. A* 273 (1973) 583–610; MR 58 #28708.

[32] P. Erdös and S. J. Taylor, Some problems concerning the structure of random walk paths, *Acta Math. Acad. Sci. Hungar.* 11 (1960) 137–162; MR 22 #12599.

[33] P. Révész, *Random Walk in Random and Nonrandom Environments*, World Scientific, 1990; MR 92c:60096.

[34] W. Feller, *An Introduction to Probability Theory and Its Applications*, v. 1, 3ʳᵈ ed., Wiley, 1968; MR 37 #3604.

[35] I. Kastanas, Simple random walk barriers, unpublished note (1997).

[36] A. M. Odlyzko, Search for the maximum of a random walk, *Random Structures Algorithms* 6 (1995) 275–295; MR 97b:60117.

[37] H.-K. Hwang, A constant arising from the analysis of algorithms for determining the maximum of a random walk, *Random Structures Algorithms* 10 (1997) 333–335; MR 98i:05007.

[38] P. Chassaing, How many probes are needed to compute the maximum of a random walk?, *Stochastic Process. Appl.* 81 (1999) 129–153; MR 2000k:60087.

[39] E. Csáki, A note on: "Three problems on the random walk in Z^d" by P. Erdös and P. Révész, *Studia Sci. Math. Hungar.* 26 (1991) 201–205; MR 93k:60172.

[40] B. Tóth, No more than three favorite sites for simple random walk, *Annals of Probab.* 29 (2001) 484–503; MR 2002c:60076.

[41] A. Dembo, Y. Peres, J. Rosen, and O. Zeitouni, Thick points for planar Brownian motion and the Erdös-Taylor conjecture on random walk, *Acta Math.* 186 (2001) 239–270; math.PR/0105107.

[42] I. Stewart, Where drunkards hang out, *Nature* 413 (2001) 686–687.

[43] A. Dembo, Y. Peres, J. Rosen, and O. Zeitouni, Cover times for Brownian motion and random walks in two dimensions, math.PR/0107191.

[44] H. S. Wilf, The white screen problem, *Amer. Math. Monthly* 96 (1989) 704–707.

[45] J. Wimp and D. Zeilberger, How likely is Pólya's drunkard to stay in $x > y > z$?, *J. Stat. Phys.* 57 (1989) 1129–1135; MR 90m:82083.

[46] J. T. Chang and Y. Peres, Ladder heights, Gaussian random walks and the Riemann zeta function, *Annals of Probab.* 25 (1997) 787–802; MR 98c:60086.

[47] H. Chernoff, Sequential tests for the mean of a normal distribution. IV. (Discrete case), *Annals of Math. Statist.* 36 (1965) 55–68; MR 30 #681.

[48] T. L. Lai, Asymptotic moments of random walks with applications to ladder variables and renewal theory, *Annals of Probab.* 4 (1976) 51–66; MR 52 #12086.

[49] D. Siegmund, Corrected diffusion approximations in certain random walk problems, *Adv. Appl. Probab.* 11 (1979) 701–719; MR 80i:60096.

[50] S. Asmussen, P. Glynn, and J. Pitman, Discretization error in simulation of one-dimensional reflecting Brownian motion, *Annals of Appl. Probab.* 5 (1995) 875–896; MR 97e:65156.

[51] E. G. Coffman, P. Flajolet, L. Flatto, and M. Hofri, The maximum of a random walk and its application to rectangle packing, *Probab. Engin. Inform. Sci.* 12 (1998) 373–386; MR 99f:60127.

[52] P. Biane, J. Pitman, and M. Yor, Probability laws related to the Jacobi theta and Riemann zeta functions, and Brownian excursions, *Bull. Amer. Math. Soc.* 38 (2001) 435–465.

[53] A. J. Guttmann, Padé approximants and SAW generating functions, unpublished note (2001).

[54] D. J. Aldous, Self-intersections of random walks on discrete groups, *Math. Proc. Cambridge Philos. Soc.* 98 (1985) 155–177; MR 86j:60157.

[55] D. J. Aldous, Self-intersections of 1-dimensional random walks, *Probab. Theory Relat. Fields* 72 (1986) 559–587; MR 88a:60125.

[56] R. S. Lehman and G. H. Weiss, A study of the restricted random walk, *J. SIAM* 6 (1958) 257–278; MR 20 #4891.

[57] S. Hemmer and P. C. Hemmer, An average self-avoiding random walk on the square lattice lasts 71 steps, *J. Chem. Phys.* 81 (1984) 584–585; MR 85g:82099.

[58] K. Burdzy, G. F. Lawler, and T. Polaski, On the critical exponent for random walk intersections, *J. Stat. Phys.* 56 (1989) 1–12; MR 91h:60073.

[59] G. F. Lawler, *Intersections of Random Walks*, Birkhäuser, 1991; MR 92f:60122.

[60] G. Slade, Random walks, *Amer. Scientist*, v. 84 (1996) n. 2, 146–153.

[61] G. F. Lawler, O. Schramm, and W. Werner, Values of Brownian intersection exponents. II: Plane exponents, *Acta Math.* 187 (2001) 275–308; math.PR/0003156.

[62] G. F. Lawler, A self-avoiding random walk, *Duke Math. J.* 47 (1980) 655–693; MR 81j:60081.

[63] T. Prellberg, Intersection probabilities for high dimensional walks, unpublished note (2002).

[64] D. Zeilberger, A holonomic systems approach to special functions identities, *J. Comput. Appl. Math.* 32 (1990) 321–348; MR 92b:33014.

[65] H. S. Wilf and D. Zeilberger, Towards computerized proofs of identities, *Bull. Amer. Math. Soc.* 23 (1990) 77–83; MR 91a:33003.

[66] W. Wasow, *Asymptotic Expansions for Ordinary Differential Equations*, Wiley, 1965, pp. 1–29; MR 34 #3401.

[67] E. L. Ince, *Ordinary Differential Equations*, Dover, 1956, pp. 356–365; MR 6,65f.

[68] G. F. Simmons, *Differential Equations with Applications and Historical Notes*, McGraw-Hill, 1972, pp. 153–174; MR 58 #17258.

[69] P. Flajolet and B. Vallée, Continued fractions, comparison algorithms, and fine structure constants, *Constructive, Experimental, and Nonlinear Analysis*, Proc. 1999 Limoges conf., ed. M. Théra, Amer. Math. Soc., 2000, pp. 53–82; INRIA preprint RR4072; MR 2001h:11161.

[70] T. Y. Chow, What is a closed-form number?, *Amer. Math. Monthly* 106 (1999) 440–448; math.NT/9805045; MR 2000e:11156.

5.10 Self-Avoiding Walk Constants

Let L denote the d-dimensional cubic lattice whose vertices are precisely all integer points in d-dimensional space. An n-step **self-avoiding walk** ω on L, beginning at the origin, is a sequence of vertices $\omega_0, \omega_1, \omega_2, \ldots, \omega_n$ with $\omega_0 = 0$, $|\omega_{j+1} - \omega_j| = 1$ for all j and $\omega_i \neq \omega_j$ for all $i \neq j$. The number of such walks is denoted by c_n. For example, $c_0 = 1$, $c_1 = 2d$, $c_2 = 2d(2d - 1)$, $c_3 = 2d(2d - 1)^2$, and $c_4 = 2d(2d - 1)^3 - 2d(2d - 2)$. Self-avoiding walks are vastly more difficult to study than ordinary walks [1–6], and historically arose as a model for linear polymers in chemistry [7,8]. No exact combinatorial enumerations are possible for large n. The methods for analysis hence include finite series expansions and Monte Carlo simulations.

For simplicity's sake, we have suppressed the dependence of c_n on d; we will do this for associated constants too whenever possible.

What can be said about the asymptotics of c_n? Since $c_{n+m} \leq c_n c_m$, on the basis of Fekete's submultiplicativity theorem [9–12], it is known that the **connective constant**

$$\mu_d = \lim_{n \to \infty} c_n^{\frac{1}{n}} = \inf_n c_n^{\frac{1}{n}}$$

exists and is nonzero. Early attempts to estimate $\mu = \mu_d$ included [13–15]; see [2] for a detailed survey. The current best rigorous lower and upper bounds for μ, plus the best-known estimate, are given in Table 5.2 [16–24]. The extent of our ignorance is fairly surprising: Although we know that $\mu^2 = \lim_{n \to \infty} c_{n+2}/c_n$ and $c_{n+1} \geq c_n$ for all n and all d, proving that $\mu = \lim_{n \to \infty} c_{n+1}/c_n$ for $2 \leq d \leq 4$ remains an open problem [25, 26].

Table 5.2. *Estimates for Connective Constant μ*

d	Lower Bound	Best Estimate for μ	Upper Bound
2	2.6200	2.6381585303	2.6792
3	4.5721	4.68404	4.7114
4	6.7429	6.77404	6.8040
5	8.8285	8.83854	8.8602
6	10.8740	10.87809	10.8886

It is believed that there exists a positive constant $\gamma = \gamma_d$ such that the following limit exists and is nonzero:

$$A = \begin{cases} \displaystyle\lim_{n\to\infty} \frac{c_n}{\mu^n n^{\gamma-1}} & \text{if } d \neq 4, \\[2ex] \displaystyle\lim_{n\to\infty} \frac{c_n}{\mu^n n^{\gamma-1} \ln(n)^{1/4}} & \text{if } d = 4. \end{cases}$$

The **critical exponent** γ is conjectured to be [27–29]

$$\gamma_2 = \tfrac{43}{32} = 1.34375, \quad \gamma_3 = 1.1575\ldots, \quad \gamma_4 = 1$$

and has been proved [1, 30] to equal 1 for $d > 4$. For small d, we have bounds [1, 25, 31]

$$c_n \leq \begin{cases} \mu^n \exp\left(C n^{1/2}\right) & \text{if } d = 2, \\[1ex] \mu^n \exp\left(C n^{2/(d+2)} \ln(n)\right) & \text{if } 3 \leq d \leq 4, \end{cases}$$

which do not come close to proving the existence of A. It is known [32] that, for $d = 5$, $1 \leq A \leq 1.493$ and, for sufficiently large d, $A = 1 + (2d)^{-1} + d^{-2} + O(d^{-3})$.

Another interesting object of study is the **mean square end-to-end distance**

$$r_n = \mathrm{E}\left(|\omega_n|^2\right) = \frac{1}{c_n} \sum_\omega |\omega_n|^2,$$

where the summation is over all n-step self-avoiding walks ω on L. Like c_n, it is believed that there is a positive constant $\nu = \nu_d$ such that the following limit exists and is nonzero:

$$B = \begin{cases} \displaystyle\lim_{n\to\infty} \frac{r_n}{n^{2\nu}} & \text{if } d \neq 4, \\[2ex] \displaystyle\lim_{n\to\infty} \frac{r_n}{n^{2\nu} \ln(n)^{1/4}} & \text{if } d = 4. \end{cases}$$

As before, it is conjectured that [27, 33, 34]

$$\nu_2 = \tfrac{3}{4} = 0.75, \quad \nu_3 = 0.5877\ldots, \quad \nu_4 = \tfrac{1}{2} = 0.5$$

and has been proved [1, 30] that $\nu = 1/2$ for $d > 4$. This latter value is the same for Pólya walks, that is, the self-avoidance constraint has little effect in high dimensions. It is known [32] that, for $d = 5$, $1.098 \leq B \leq 1.803$ and, for sufficiently large d, $B = 1 + d^{-1} + 2d^{-2} + O(d^{-3})$. Hence a self-avoiding walk moves away from the origin faster than a Pólya walk, but only at the level of the amplitude and not at the level of the exponent.

If we accept the conjectured asymptotics $c_n \sim A\mu^n n^{\gamma-1}$ and $r_n \sim B n^{2\nu}$ as truth (for $d \neq 4$), then the calculations shown in Table 5.3 become possible [23, 24, 33, 35–37].

Table 5.3. *Estimates for Amplitudes A and B*

d	Estimate for A	Estimate for B	d	Estimate for A	Estimate for B
2	1.177043	0.77100	5	1.275	1.4767
3	1.205	1.21667	6	1.159	1.2940

(The logarithmic correction for $d = 4$ renders any reliable estimation of A or B very difficult.) Here is an application. Two walks ω and ω' **intersect** if $\omega_i = \omega'_j$ for some nonzero i and j. The probability that two n-step independent random self-avoiding walks never intersect is [1,38]

$$
\frac{c_{2n}}{c_n^2} \sim \begin{cases} A^{-1}2^{\gamma-1}n^{1-\gamma} \to 0 & \text{if } 2 \leq d \leq 3, \\ A^{-1}\ln(n)^{-1/4} \to 0 & \text{if } d = 4, \\ A^{-1} > 0 & \text{if } d \geq 5 \end{cases}
$$

as $n \to \infty$. This conjectured behavior is consistent with intuition: c_{2n}/c_n^2 is (slightly) larger than the corresponding probability q_n for ordinary walks [5.9.1] since self-avoiding walks tend to be more thinly dispersed in space.

Other interesting measures of the size of a walk include the **mean square radius of gyration**,

$$
s_n = \mathrm{E}\left(\left|\frac{1}{n+1}\sum_{i=0}^{n}\omega_i - \frac{1}{n+1}\sum_{j=0}^{n}\omega_j\right|^2\right) = \mathrm{E}\left(\frac{1}{2(n+1)^2}\sum_{i=0}^{n}\sum_{j=0}^{n}|\omega_i - \omega_j|^2\right),
$$

and the **mean square distance of a monomer from the endpoints**,

$$
t_n = \mathrm{E}\left(\frac{1}{n+1}\sum_{i=0}^{n}\frac{|\omega_i|^2 + |\omega_n - \omega_i|^2}{2}\right).
$$

The radius of gyration, for example, can be experimentally measured for polymers in a dilute solution via light scattering, but the end-to-end distance is preferred for theoretical simplicity [33, 39–41]. It is conjectured that $s_n \sim En^{2\nu}$ and $t_n \sim Fn^{2\nu}$, where ν is the same exponent as for r_n, and $E/B = 0.14026\ldots$, $F/B = 0.43961\ldots$ for $d = 2$ and $E/B = 0.1599\ldots$ for $d = 3$.

One can generalize this discussion to arbitrary lattices L in d-dimensional space. For example, in the case $d = 2$, there is a rigorous upper bound $\mu < 4.278$ and an estimate $\mu = 4.1507951\ldots$ for the equilateral triangular lattice [17, 35, 42–45], and it is conjectured that $\mu = \sqrt{2+\sqrt{2}} = 1.8477590650\ldots$ for the hexagonal (honeycomb) lattice [46–48]. The critical exponents γ, ν and amplitude ratios E/B, F/B, however, are thought to be *universal* in the sense that they are lattice-independent (although dimension-dependent). An important challenge, therefore, is to better understand the nature of such exponents and ratios, and certainly to prove their existence in low dimensions.

5.10.1 Polygons and Trails

The connective constant μ values given previously apply not only to the asymptotic growth of the number of self-avoiding walks, but also to the asymptotic growth of numbers of **self-avoiding polygons** and of self-avoiding walks with prescribed endpoints [2, 49]. See [5.19] for discussion of lattice animals or polyominoes, which are related to self-avoiding polygons.

No site or bond may be visited more than once in a self-avoiding walk. By way of contrast, a **self-avoiding trail** may revisit sites, but not bonds. Thus walks are a proper subset of trails [50–55]. The number h_n of trails is conjectured to satisfy $h_n \sim G\lambda^n n^{\gamma-1}$, where γ is the same exponent as for c_n. The connective constant λ provably exists as before and, in fact, satisfies $\lambda \geq \mu$. For the square lattice, there are rigorous bounds $2.634 < \lambda < 2.851$ and an estimate $\lambda = 2.72062\ldots$; the amplitude is approximately $G = 1.272\ldots$. For the cubic lattice, there is an upper bound $\lambda < 4.929$ and an estimate $\lambda = 4.8426\ldots$. Many related questions can be asked.

5.10.2 Rook Paths on a Chessboard

How many self-avoiding walks can a rook take from a fixed corner of an $m \times n$ chessboard to the opposite corner without ever leaving the chessboard? Denote the number of such **paths** by $p_{m-1,n-1}$; clearly $p_{k,1} = 2^k$, $p_{2,2} = 12$, and [56–58]

$$p_{k,2} \sim \frac{4+\sqrt{13}}{2\sqrt{13}} \left(\sqrt{\frac{3+\sqrt{13}}{2}} \right)^{2k} = 1.0547001962\ldots \cdot (1.8173540210\ldots)^{2k}$$

as $k \to \infty$. More broadly, the generating function for the sequence $\{p_{k,l}\}_{k=1}^{\infty}$ is rational for any integer $l \geq 1$ and thus relevant asymptotic coefficients are all algebraic numbers. What can be said about the asymptotics of $p_{k,k}$ as $k \to \infty$? Whittington & Guttmann [59] proved that

$$p_{k,k} \sim (1.756\ldots)^{k^2}$$

and conjectured the following [60,61]. If $\pi_{j,k}$ is the number of j-step paths with generating function

$$P_k(x) = \sum_{j=1}^{\infty} \pi_{j,k} x^j, \quad P_k(1) = p_{k,k}$$

then there is a *phase transition* in the sense that

$$0 < \lim_{k \to \infty} P_k(x)^{\frac{1}{k}} < 1 \quad \text{exists for } 0 < x < \mu^{-1} = 0.3790522777\ldots,$$
$$\lim_{k \to \infty} P_k(\mu^{-1})^{\frac{1}{k}} = 1,$$
$$1 < \lim_{k \to \infty} P_k(x)^{\frac{1}{k^2}} < \infty \text{ exists for } x > \mu^{-1}.$$

A proof was given by Madras [62]. This is an interesting occurrence of the connective constant $\mu = \mu_2$; an analogous theorem involving a d-dimensional chessboard also holds and naturally makes use of μ_d.

5.10.3 Meanders and Stamp Foldings

A **meander** of order n is a planar self-avoiding loop (road) crossing an infinite line (river) $2n$ times ($2n$ bridges). Define two meanders as equivalent if one may be deformed continuously into the other, keeping the bridges fixed. The number of inequivalent meanders M_n of order n satisfy $M_1 = 1$, $M_2 = 2$, $M_3 = 8$, $M_4 = 42$, $M_5 = 262, \ldots$.

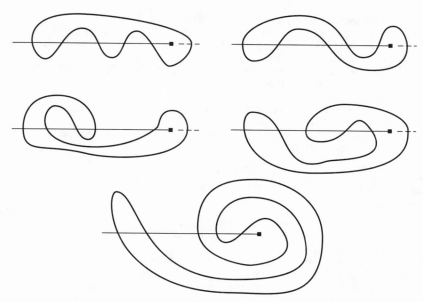

Figure 5.11. There are eight meanders of order 3 and ten semi-meanders of order 5; reflections across the river are omitted.

A **semi-meander** of order n is a planar self-avoiding loop (road) crossing a semi-infinite line (river with a source) n times (n bridges). Equivalence of semi-meanders is defined similarly. The number of inequivalent semi-meanders $\tilde{M}_n$ of order n satisfy $\tilde{M}_1 = 1$, $\tilde{M}_2 = 1$, $\tilde{M}_3 = 2$, $\tilde{M}_4 = 4$, $\tilde{M}_5 = 10$, ...

Counting meanders and semi-meanders has attracted much attention [63–73]. See Figure 5.11. As before, we expect asymptotic behavior

$$M_n \sim C\frac{R^{2n}}{n^\alpha}, \quad \tilde{M}_n \sim \tilde{C}\frac{R^n}{n^{\tilde\alpha}},$$

where $R = 3.501838\ldots$, that is, $R^2 = 12.262874\ldots$. No exact formula for the connective constant R is known. In contrast, there is a conjecture [74–76] that the critical exponents are given by

$$\alpha = \sqrt{29}\frac{\sqrt{29} + \sqrt{5}}{12} = 3.4201328816\ldots,$$

$$\tilde{\alpha} = 1 + \sqrt{11}\frac{\sqrt{29} + \sqrt{5}}{24} = 2.0531987328\ldots,$$

but doubt has been raised [77–79] about the semi-meander critical exponent value. The sequences $\tilde{M}_n$ and M_n are also related to enumerating the ways of folding a linear or circular row of stamps onto one stamp [80–87].

[1] N. Madras and G. Slade, *The Self-Avoiding Walk*, Birkhäuser, 1993; MR 94f:82002.
[2] B. D. Hughes, *Random Walks and Random Environments*, v. 1, Oxford Univ. Press, 1995; MR 96i:60070.
[3] G. Slade, Self-avoiding walks, *Math. Intellig.* 16 (1994) 29–35.

[4]   G. Slade, Random walks, *Amer. Scientist*, v. 84 (1996) n. 2, 146–153.

[5]   B. Hayes, How to avoid yourself, *Amer. Scientist*, v. 86 (1998) n. 4, 314–319.

[6]   N. J. A. Sloane, On-Line Encyclopedia of Integer Sequences, A001334, A001411, A001412, and A001668.

[7]   P. J. Flory, The configuration of real polymer chains, *J. Chem. Phys.* 17 (1949) 303–310.

[8]   K. F. Freed, Polymers as self-avoiding walks, *Annals of Probab.* 9 (1981) 537–556; MR 82j:60123.

[9]   M. Fekete, Über die Verteilung der Wurzeln bei gewissen algebraischen Gleichungen mit ganzzahligen Koeffizienten, *Math. Z.* 17 (1923) 228–249.

[10] G. Pólya and G. Szegö, *Problems and Theorems in Analysis*, v. 1, Springer-Verlag, 1972, ex. 98, pp. 23, 198; MR 81e:00002.

[11] J. M. Hammersley and K. W. Morton, Poor man's Monte Carlo, *J. Royal Statist. Soc. Ser. B.* 16 (1954) 23–38; discussion 61–75; MR 16,287i.

[12] J. M. Hammersley, Percolation processes. II: The connective constant, *Proc. Cambridge Philos. Soc.* 53 (1957) 642–645; MR 19,989f.

[13] M. E. Fisher and M. F. Sykes, Excluded-volume problem and the Ising model of ferromagnetism, *Phys. Rev.* 114 (1959) 45–58; MR 22 #10274.

[14] W. A. Beyer and M. B. Wells, Lower bound for the connective constant of a self-avoiding walk on a square lattice, *J. Combin. Theory Ser. A* 13 (1972) 176–182; MR 46 #1605.

[15] F. T. Wall and R. A. White, Macromolecular configurations simulated by random walks with limited orders of non-self-intersections, *J. Chem. Phys.* 65 (1976) 808–812.

[16] T. Hara, G. Slade, and A. D. Sokal, New lower bounds on the self-avoiding-walk connective constant, *J. Stat. Phys.* 72 (1993) 479–517; erratum 78 (1995) 1187–1188; MR 94e:82053.

[17] S. E. Alm, Upper bounds for the connective constant of self-avoiding walks, *Combin. Probab. Comput.* 2 (1993) 115–136; MR 94g:60126.

[18] A. R. Conway and A. J. Guttmann, Lower bound on the connective constant for square lattice self-avoiding walks, *J. Phys. A* 26 (1993) 3719–3724.

[19] J. Noonan, New upper bounds for the connective constants of self-avoiding walks, *J. Stat. Phys.* 91 (1998) 871–888; MR 99g:82030.

[20] J. Noonan and D. Zeilberger, The Goulden-Jackson cluster method: Extensions, applications and implementations, *J. Differ. Eq. Appl.* 5 (1999) 355–377; MR 2000f:05005.

[21] I. Jensen and A. J. Guttmann, Self-avoiding polygons on the square lattice, *J. Phys. A* 32 (1999) 4867–4876.

[22] A. Pönitz and P. Tittmann, Improved upper bounds for self-avoiding walks in $\mathbb{Z}^d$, *Elec. J. Combin.* 7 (2000) R21; MR 2000m:05015.

[23] D. MacDonald, S. Joseph, D. L. Hunter, L. L. Moseley, N. Jan, and A. J. Guttmann, Self-avoiding walks on the simple cubic lattice, *J. Phys. A* 33 (2000) 5973–5983; MR 2001g:82051.

[24] A. L. Owczarek and T. Prellberg, Scaling of self-avoiding walks in high dimensions, *J. Phys. A* 34 (2001) 5773–5780; cond-mat/0104135.

[25] H. Kesten, On the number of self-avoiding walks, *J. Math. Phys.* 4 (1963) 960–969; 5 (1964) 1128–1137; MR 27 #2006 and 29 #4118.

[26] G. L. O'Brien, Monotonicity of the number of self-avoiding walks, *J. Stat. Phys.* 59 (1990) 969–979; MR 91k:8007.

[27] P. Butera and M. Comi, N-vector spin models on the simple-cubic and the body-centered-cubic lattices: A study of the critical behavior of the susceptibility and of the correlation length by high-temperature series extended to order 21, *Phys. Rev. B* 56 (1997) 8212–8240; hep-lat/9703018.

[28] S. Caracciolo, M. S. Causo, and A. Pelissetto, Monte Carlo results for three-dimensional self-avoiding walks, *Nucl. Phys. Proc. Suppl.* 63 (1998) 652–654; hep-lat/9711051.

[29] S. Caracciolo, M. S. Causo, and A. Pelissetto, High-precision determination of the critical exponent gamma for self-avoiding walks, *Phys. Rev. E* 57 (1998) R1215–R1218; cond-mat/9703250.

[30] T. Hara and G. Slade, Self-avoiding walk in five or more dimensions. I: The critical behaviour, *Commun. Math. Phys.* 147 (1992) 101–136; MR 93j:82032.

[31] J. M. Hammersley and D. J. A. Welsh, Further results on the rate of convergence to the connective constant of the hypercubical lattice, *Quart. J. Math.* 13 (1962) 108–110; MR 25 #2967.

[32] T. Hara and G. Slade, The self-avoiding-walk and percolation critical points in high dimensions, *Combin. Probab. Comput.* 4 (1995) 197–215; MR 96i:82081.

[33] B. Li, N. Madras, and A. D. Sokal, Critical exponents, hyperscaling and universal amplitude ratios for two- and three-dimensional self-avoiding walks, *J. Stat. Phys.* 80 (1995) 661–754; hep-lat/9409003; MR 96e:82046.

[34] T. Prellberg, Scaling of self-avoiding walks and self-avoiding trails in three dimensions, *J. Phys. A* 34 (2001) L599–L602.

[35] I. G. Enting and A. J. Guttmann, Self-avoiding rings on the triangular lattice, *J. Phys. A* 25 (1992) 2791–2807; MR 93b:82030.

[36] A. R. Conway, I. G. Enting, and A. J. Guttmann, Algebraic techniques for enumerating self-avoiding walks on the square lattice, *J. Phys. A* 26 (1993) 1519–1534; MR 94f: 82040.

[37] A. R. Conway and A. J. Guttmann, Square lattice self-avoiding walks and corrections-to-scaling, *Phys. Rev. Lett.* 77 (1996) 5284–5287.

[38] G. F. Lawler, *Intersections of Random Walks*, Birkhäuser, 1991; MR 92f:60122.

[39] S. Caracciolo, A. Pelissetto, and A. D. Sokal, Universal distance ratios for two-dimensional self-avoiding walks: Corrected conformal-invariance predictions, *J. Phys. A* 23 (1990) L969–L974; MR 91g:81130.

[40] J. L. Cardy and A. J. Guttmann, Universal amplitude combinations for self-avoiding walks, polygons and trails, *J. Phys. A* 26 (1993) 2485–2494; MR 94f:82039.

[41] K. Y. Lin and J. X. Huang, Universal amplitude ratios for self-avoiding walks on the Kagomé lattice, *J. Phys. A* 28 (1995) 3641–3643.

[42] A. J. Guttmann, On two-dimensional self-avoiding random walks, *J. Phys. A* 17 (1984) 455–468; MR 85g:82096.

[43] T. Ishinabe, Critical exponents and corrections to scaling for the two-dimensional self-avoiding walk, *Phys. Rev. B* 37 (1988) 2376–2379.

[44] T. Ishinabe, Reassessment of critical exponents and corrections to scaling for self-avoiding walks, *Phys. Rev. B* 39 (1989) 9486–9495.

[45] A. J. Guttmann and J. Wang, The extension of self-avoiding random walk series in two dimensions, *J. Phys. A* 24 (1991) 3107–3109; MR 92b:82073.

[46] B. Nienhuis, Exact critical point and critical exponents of O(n) models in two dimensions, *Phys. Rev. Lett.* 49 (1982) 1062–1065.

[47] I. G. Enting and A. J. Guttmann, Polygons on the honeycomb lattice, *J. Phys. A* 22 (1989) 1371–1384; MR 90c:82050.

[48] D. MacDonald, D. L. Hunter, K. Kelly, and N. Jan, Self-avoiding walks in two to five dimensions: Exact enumerations and series study, *J. Phys. A* 25 (1992) 1429–1440.

[49] N. J. A. Sloane, On-Line Encyclopedia of Integer Sequences, A006817, A006818, A006819, and A006851.

[50] A. Malakis, The trail problem on the square lattice, *J. Phys. A* 9 (1976) 1283–1291.

[51] A. J. Guttmann and S. S. Manna, The geometric properties of planar lattice trails, *J. Phys. A* 22 (1989) 3613–3619.

[52] A. J. Guttmann, Lattice trails. I: Exact results, *J. Phys. A* 18 (1985) 567–573; MR 87f:82069.

[53] A. J. Guttmann, Lattice trails. II: Numerical results, *J. Phys. A* 18 (1985) 575–588; MR 87f:82070.

[54] A. R. Conway and A. J. Guttmann, Enumeration of self-avoiding trails on a square lattice using a transfer matrix technique, *J. Phys. A* 26 (1993) 1535–1552; MR 94f:82041.

[55] N. J. A. Sloane, On-Line Encyclopedia of Integer Sequences, A001335, A001413, A002931, and A036418.

[56] N. J. A. Sloane, On-Line Encyclopedia of Integer Sequences, A006192, A007764, A007786, and A007787.

[57] H. L. Abbott and D. Hanson, A lattice path problem, *Ars Combin.* 6 (1978) 163–178; MR 80m:05009.

[58] K. Edwards, Counting self-avoiding walks in a bounded region, *Ars Combin.* 20 *B* (1985) 271–281; MR 87h:05015.

[59] S. G. Whittington and A. J. Guttmann, Self-avoiding walks which cross a square, *J. Phys. A* 23 (1990) 5601–5609; MR 92e:82038.

[60] T. W. Burkhardt and I. Guim, Self-avoiding walks that cross a square, *J. Phys. A* 24 (1991) L1221–L1228.

[61] J. J. Prentis, Renormalization theory of self-avoiding walks which cross a square, *J. Phys. A* 24 (1991) 5097–5103.

[62] N. Madras, Critical behaviour of self-avoiding walks that cross a square, *J. Phys. A* 28 (1995) 1535–1547; MR 96d:82032.

[63] H. Poincaré, Sur un théorème de géométrie, *Rend. Circ. Mat. Palmero* 33 (1912) 375–407; also in *Oeuvres*, t. 6, Gauthier-Villars, 1953, pp. 499–538.

[64] J. Touchard, Contribution à l'étude du problème des timbres poste, *Canad. J. Math.* 2 (1950) 385–398; MR 12,312i.

[65] V. I. Arnold, The branched covering $CP^2 \rightarrow S^4$, hyperbolicity and projective topology (in Russian), *Sibirskii Mat. Zh.*, v. 29 (1988) n. 5, 36–47, 237; Engl. transl. in *Siberian Math. J.* 29 (1988) 717–726; MR 90a:57037.

[66] S. K. Lando and A. K. Zvonkin, Meanders, *Selecta Math. Soviet.* 11 (1992) 117–144; MR 93k:05013.

[67] S. K. Lando and A. K. Zvonkin, Plane and projective meanders, *Theoret. Comput. Sci.* 117 (1993) 227–241; MR 94i:05004.

[68] P. Di Francesco, O. Golinelli, and E. Guitter, Meanders: A direct enumeration approach, *Nucl. Phys. B* 482 (1996) 497–535; hep-th/9607039; MR 97j:82074.

[69] P. Di Francesco, O. Golinelli, and E. Guitter, Meander, folding and arch statistics, *Math. Comput. Modelling* 26 (1997) 97–147; hep-th/9506030; MR 99f:82029.

[70] P. Di Francesco, Meander determinants, *Commun. Math. Phys.* 191 (1998) 543–583; hep-th/9612026; MR 99e:05007.

[71] M. G. Harris, A diagrammatic approach to the meander problem, hep-th/9807193.

[72] J. Reeds and L. Shepp, An upper bound on the meander constant, unpublished note (1999).

[73] O. Golinelli, A Monte-Carlo study of meanders, *Europ. Phys. J. B* 14 (2000) 145–155; cond-mat/9906329.

[74] P. Di Francesco, O. Golinelli, and E. Guitter, Meanders: Exact asymptotics, *Nucl. Phys. B* 570 (2000) 699–712; cond-mat/9910453; MR 2001f:82032.

[75] P. Di Francesco, Folding and coloring problems in mathematics and physics, *Bull. Amer. Math. Soc.* 37 (2000) 251–307; MR 2001g:82004.

[76] P. Di Francesco, E. Guitter, and J. L. Jacobsen, Exact meander asymptotics: A numerical check, *Nucl. Phys. B* 580 (2000) 757–795; MR 2002b:82024.

[77] I. Jensen, Enumerations of plane meanders, cond-mat/9910313.

[78] I. Jensen, A transfer matrix approach to the enumeration of plane meanders, *J. Phys. A* 33 (2000) 5953–5963; cond-mat/0008178; MR 2001e:05008.

[79] I. Jensen and A. J. Guttmann, Critical exponents of plane meanders, *J. Phys. A* 33 (2000) L187–L192; MR 2001b:82024.

[80] W. F. Lunnon, A map-folding problem, *Math. Comp.* 22 (1968) 193–199; MR 36 #5009.

[81] J. E. Koehler, Folding a strip of stamps, *J. Combin. Theory* 5 (1968) 135–152; errata *J. Combin. Theory Ser. A* 19 (1975) 367; MR 37 #3945 and MR 52 #2910.

[82] W. F. Lunnon, Multi-dimensional map-folding, *Comput. J.* 14 (1971) 75–80; MR 44 #2627.

[83] W. F. Lunnon, Bounds for the map-folding function, unpublished note (1981).

[84] M. Gardner, The combinatorics of paper-folding, *Wheels, Life, and Other Mathematical Amusements*, W. H. Freeman, 1983, pp. 60–73.

[85] M. Gardner, *The Sixth Book of Mathematical Games from Scientific American*, Univ. of Chicago Press, 1984, pp. 21, 26–27.

[86] N. J. A. Sloane, My favorite integer sequences, *Sequences and Their Applications (SETA)*, Proc. 1998 Singapore conf., ed. C. Ding, T. Helleseth, and H. Niederreiter, Springer-Verlag, 1999, pp. 103–130; math.CO/0207175.

[87] N. J. A. Sloane, On-Line Encyclopedia of Integer Sequences, A000682, A001011, A005315, and A005316.

5.11 Feller's Coin Tossing Constants

Let w_n denote the probability that, in n independent tosses of an ideal coin, no run of three consecutive heads appears. Clearly $w_0 = w_1 = w_2 = 1$, $w_n = \frac{1}{2}w_{n-1} + \frac{1}{4}w_{n-2} + \frac{1}{8}w_{n-3}$ for $n \geq 3$, and $\lim_{n \to \infty} w_n = 0$. Feller [1] proved the following more precise asymptotic result:

$$\lim_{n \to \infty} w_n \alpha^{n+1} = \beta,$$

where

$$\alpha = \frac{\left(136 + 24\sqrt{33}\right)^{\frac{1}{3}} - 8\left(136 + 24\sqrt{33}\right)^{-\frac{1}{3}} - 2}{3} = 1.0873780254\ldots$$

and

$$\beta = \frac{2 - \alpha}{4 - 3\alpha} = 1.2368398446\ldots.$$

We first examine generalizations of these formulas. If runs of k consecutive heads, $k > 1$, are disallowed, then the analogous constants are [1,2]

$$\alpha \text{ is the smallest positive root of } 1 - x + \left(\frac{x}{2}\right)^{k+1} = 0$$

and

$$\beta = \frac{2 - \alpha}{k + 1 - k\alpha}.$$

Equivalently, the generating function that enumerates coin toss sequences with no runs of k consecutive heads is [3]

$$S_k(z) = \frac{1 - z^k}{1 - 2z + z^{k+1}}, \quad \frac{1}{n!}\frac{d^n}{dz^n}S_k(z)\Big|_{z=0} \sim \frac{\beta}{\alpha}\left(\frac{2}{\alpha}\right)^n.$$

See [4–8] for more material of a combinatorial nature.

If the coin is non-ideal, that is, if $P(H) = p$, $P(T) = q$, $p + q = 1$, but p and q are not equal, then the asymptotic behavior of w_n is governed by

$$\alpha \text{ is the smallest positive root of } 1 - x + qp^k x^{k+1} = 0$$

and

$$\beta = \frac{1 - p\alpha}{(k + 1 - k\alpha)q}.$$

A further generalization involves time-homogeneous two-state Markov chains. It makes little sense here to talk of coin tosses, so we turn attention to a different application. Imagine that a ground-based sensor determines once per hour whether a fixed line-of-sight through the atmosphere is cloud-obscured (0) or clear (1). Since meteorological events often display persistence through time, the sensor observations are not independent. A simple model for the time series $X_1, X_2, X_3, \ldots$ of observations might be a Markov chain with transition probability matrix

$$\begin{pmatrix} P(X_{j+1} = 0 | X_j = 0) & P(X_{j+1} = 1 | X_j = 0) \\ P(X_{j+1} = 0 | X_j = 1) & P(X_{j+1} = 1 | X_j = 1) \end{pmatrix} = \begin{pmatrix} \pi_{00} & \pi_{01} \\ \pi_{10} & \pi_{11} \end{pmatrix},$$

where conditional probability parameters satisfy $\pi_{00} + \pi_{01} = 1 = \pi_{10} + \pi_{11}$. The special case when $\pi_{00} = \pi_{10}$ and $\pi_{01} = \pi_{11}$ is equivalent to the Bernoulli trials scenario discussed in connection with coin tossing. Let $w_{n,k}$ denote the probability that no cloudy intervals of length $k > 1$ occur, and assume that initially $P(X_0 = 1) = \theta_1$. The asymptotic behavior is similar to before, where α is the smallest positive root of [9, 10]

$$1 - (\pi_{11} + \pi_{00})x + (\pi_{11} - \pi_{01})x^2 + \pi_{10}\pi_{01}\pi_{11}^{k-1}x^{k+1} = 0$$

and

$$\beta = \frac{[-1 + (2\pi_{11} - \pi_{01})\alpha - (\pi_{11} - \pi_{01})\pi_{11}\alpha^2][\theta_1 + (\pi_{01} - \theta_1)\alpha]}{\pi_{10}\pi_{01}[-1 - k + (\pi_{11} + \pi_{00})k\alpha + (\pi_{11} - \pi_{01})(1 - k)\alpha^2]}.$$

See [11] for a general technique for analysis of pattern statistics, with applications in molecular biology.

Of many possible variations on this problem, we discuss one. How many patterns of n children in a row are there if every girl is next to at least one other girl? If we denote the answer by Y_n, then $Y_1 = 1$, $Y_2 = 2$, $Y_3 = 4$, and $Y_n = 2Y_{n-1} - Y_{n-2} + Y_{n-3}$ for $n \geq 4$; hence

$$\lim_{n \to \infty} \frac{Y_{n+1}}{Y_n} = \frac{\left(100 + 12\sqrt{69}\right)^{\frac{1}{3}} + 4\left(100 + 12\sqrt{69}\right)^{-\frac{1}{3}} + 4}{6} = 1.7548776662\ldots.$$

A generalization of this, in which the girls must appear in groups of at least k, is given in [12, 13]. Similar cubic irrational numbers occur in [1.2.2].

Let us return to coin tossing. What is the expected length of the longest run of consecutive heads in a sequence of n ideal coin tosses? The answer is surprisingly complicated [14–21]:

$$\sum_{k=1}^{n}(1 - w_{n,k}) = \frac{\ln(n)}{\ln(2)} - \left(\frac{3}{2} - \frac{\gamma}{\ln(2)}\right) + \delta(n) + o(1)$$

as $n \to \infty$, where γ is the Euler-Mascheroni constant and

$$\delta(n) = \frac{1}{\ln(2)} \sum_{\substack{k=-\infty \\ k \neq 0}}^{\infty} \Gamma\left(\frac{2\pi i k}{\ln(2)}\right) \exp\left(-2\pi i k \frac{\ln(n)}{\ln(2)}\right).$$

That is, the expected length is $\ln(n)/\ln(2) - 0.6672538227\ldots$ plus an oscillatory, small-amplitude correction term. The function $\delta(n)$ is periodic ($\delta(n) = \delta(2n)$), has zero mean, and is "negligible" ($|\delta(n)| < 1.574 \times 10^{-6}$ for all n). The corresponding variance is $C + c + \varepsilon(n) + o(1)$, where $\varepsilon(n)$ is another small-amplitude function and

$$C = \frac{1}{12} + \frac{\pi^2}{6 \ln(2)^2} = 3.5070480758\ldots,$$

$$c = \frac{2}{\ln(2)} \sum_{k=0}^{\infty} \ln\left[1 - \exp\left(-\frac{2\pi^2}{\ln(2)}(2k+1)\right)\right] = (-1.237412\ldots) \times 10^{-12}.$$

Functions similar to $\delta(n)$ and $\varepsilon(n)$ appear in [2.3], [2.16], [5.6], and [5.14].

Also, if we toss n ideal coins, then toss those which show tails after the first toss, then toss those which show tails after the second toss, etc., what is the probability that the final toss involves exactly one coin? Again, the answer is complicated [22–25]:

$$\frac{n}{2} \sum_{j=0}^{\infty} 2^{-j}(1 - 2^{-j})^{n-1} \sim \frac{1}{2\ln(2)} + \rho(n) + o(1)$$

as $n \to \infty$, where

$$\rho(n) = \frac{1}{2\ln(2)} \sum_{\substack{k=-\infty \\ k \neq 0}}^{\infty} \Gamma\left(1 - \frac{2\pi i k}{\ln(2)}\right) \exp\left(2\pi i k \frac{\ln(n)}{\ln(2)}\right).$$

That is, the probability of a unique survivor (no ties) at the end is $1/(2\ln(2)) = 0.7213475204\ldots$ plus an oscillatory function satisfying $|\rho(n)| < 7.131 \times 10^{-6}$ for all n. The expected length of the longest of the n coin toss sequences is $\sum_{j=0}^{\infty}[1 - (1 - 2^{-j})^n]$ and can be analyzed similarly [26]. Related discussion is found in [27–31].

[1] W. Feller, *An Introduction to Probability Theory and Its Applications*, v. 1, 3rd ed., Wiley, 1968, pp. 278–279, 322–325; MR 37 #3604.
[2] W. Feller, Fluctuation theory of recurrent events, *Trans. Amer. Math. Soc.* 67 (1949) 98–119; MR 11,255c.
[3] R. Sedgewick and P. Flajolet, *Introduction to the Analysis of Algorithms*, Addison-Wesley, 1996, pp. 366–373.
[4] R. A. Howard, *Dynamic Probabilistic Systems: Markov Models*, v. 1, Wiley, 1971.
[5] A. N. Philippou and F. S. Makri, Successes, runs and longest runs, *Statist. Probab. Lett.* 4 (1986) 211–215; MR 88c:60035b.
[6] K. Hirano, Some properties of the distributions of order k, *Fibonacci Numbers and Their Applications*, Proc. 1984 Patras conf., ed. A. N. Philippou, G. E. Bergum, and A. F. Horadam, Reidel, 1986; MR 88b:62031.
[7] A. P. Godbole, Specific formulae for some success run distributions, *Statist. Probab. Lett.* 10 (1990) 119–124; MR 92e:60021.
[8] K. A. Suman, The longest run of any letter in a randomly generated word, *Runs and Patterns in Probability: Selected Papers,* ed. A. P. Godbole and S. G. Papastavnidis, Kluwer, 1994, pp. 119–130; MR 95k:60028.
[9] M. B. Rajarshi, Success runs in a two-state Markov chain, *J. Appl. Probab.* 11 (1974) 190–192; correction 14 (1977) 661; MR 51 #4402 and MR 57 #7777.
[10] C. Banderier and M. Vandenbogaert, A Markovian generalization of Feller's coin tossing constants, unpublished note (2000).
[11] P. Nicodème, B. Salvy, and P. Flajolet, Motif statistics, *Proc. 1999 European Symp. on Algorithms (ESA)*, Prague, ed. J. Nesetril, Lect. Notes in Comp. Sci. 1643, Springer-Verlag, 1999, pp. 194–211; INRIA research report RR-3606.

[12] J. H. Conway and R. K. Guy, *The Book of Numbers*, Springer-Verlag, 1996, pp. 205–206; MR 98g:00004.

[13] R. Austin and R. Guy, Binary sequences without isolated ones, *Fibonacci Quart.* 16 (1978) 84–86; MR 57 #5778.

[14] D. W. Boyd, Losing runs in Bernoulli trials, unpublished note (1972).

[15] P. Erdös and P. Révész, On the length of the longest head-run, *Topics in Information Theory*, Proc. 1975 Keszthely conf., ed. I. Csiszár and P. Elias, Colloq. Math. Soc. János Bolyai 16, North-Holland, 1977, pp. 219–228; MR 57 #17788.

[16] D. E. Knuth, The average time for carry propagation, *Proc. Konink. Nederl. Akad. Wetensch. Ser. A* 81 (1978) 238–242; *Indag. Math.* 40 (1978) 238–242; also in *Selected Papers on Analysis of Algorithms*, CSLI, 2000, pp. 467–471; MR 81b:68030.

[17] L. J. Guibas and A. M. Odlyzko, Long repetitive patterns in random sequences, *Z. Wahrsch. Verw. Gebiete* 53 (1980) 241–262; MR 81m:60047.

[18] L. Gordon, M. F. Schilling, and M. S. Waterman, An extreme value theory for long head runs, *Probab. Theory Relat. Fields* 72 (1986) 279–287; MR 87i:60023.

[19] H. Prodinger, Über längste 1-Teilfolgen in 0-1-Folgen, *Zahlentheoretische Analysis II*, Wien Seminar 1984-86, ed. E. Hlawka, Lect. Notes in Math. 1262, Springer-Verlag, 1987, pp. 124–133; MR 90g:11106.

[20] P. Hitczenko and G. Stengle, Expected number of distinct part sizes in a random integer composition, *Combin. Probab. Comput.* 9 (2000) 519–527; MR 2002d:05008.

[21] M. F. Schilling, The longest run of heads, *College Math J.* 21 (1990) 196–206.

[22] F. T. Bruss and C. A. O'Cinneide, On the maximum and its uniqueness for geometric random samples, *J. Appl. Probab.* 27 (1990) 598–610; MR 92a:60096.

[23] L. Räde, P. Griffin, and O. P. Lossers, Tossing coins until all show heads, *Amer. Math. Monthly* 101 (1994) 78–80.

[24] P. Kirschenhofer and H. Prodinger, The number of winners in a discrete geometrically distributed sample, *Annals of Appl. Probab.* 6 (1996) 687–694; MR 97g:60016.

[25] N. J. Calkin, E. R. Canfield, and H. S. Wilf, Averaging sequences, deranged mappings, and a problem of Lampert and Slater, *J. Combin. Theory Ser. A* 91 (2000) 171–190; MR 2002c:05019.

[26] C. F. Woodcock, On the asymptotic behaviour of a function arising from tossing coins, *Bull. London Math. Soc.* 28 (1996) 19–23; MR 96i:26001.

[27] B. Eisenberg, G. Stengle, and G. Strang, The asymptotic probability of a tie for first place, *Annals of Appl. Probab.* 3 (1993) 731–745; MR 95d:60044.

[28] J. J. A. M. Brands, F. W. Steutel, and R. J. G. Wilms, On the number of maxima in a discrete sample, *Statist. Probab. Lett.* 20 (1994) 209–217; MR 95e:60010.

[29] Y. Baryshnikov, B. Eisenberg, and G. Stengle, A necessary and sufficient condition for the existence of the limiting probability of a tie for first place, *Statist. Probab. Lett.* 23 (1995) 203–209; MR 96d:60015.

[30] Y. Qi, A note on the number of maxima in a discrete sample, *Statist. Probab. Lett.* 33 (1997) 373–377; MR 98f:60061.

[31] D. E. Lampert and P. J. Slater, Parallel knockouts in the complete graph, *Amer. Math. Monthly* 105 (1998) 556–558.

5.12 Hard Square Entropy Constant

Consider the set of all $n \times n$ binary matrices. What is the number $F(n)$ of such matrices with no pairs of adjacent 1s? Two 1s are said to be adjacent if they lie in positions (i, j) and $(i + 1, j)$, or if they lie in positions (i, j) and $(i, j + 1)$, for some i, j. Equivalently, $F(n)$ is the number of configurations of non-attacking Princes on an $n \times n$ chessboard, where a "Prince" attacks the four adjacent, non-diagonal places. Let $N = n^2$; then [1–3]

$$\kappa = \lim_{n \to \infty} F(n)^{\frac{1}{N}} = 1.5030480824\ldots = \exp(0.4074951009\ldots)$$

is the **hard square entropy constant**. Earlier estimates were obtained by both physicists [4–9] and mathematicians [10–13]. Some related combinatorial enumeration problems appear in [14–16].

Instead of an $n \times n$ binary matrix, consider an $n \times n$ binary array that looks like

$$\begin{pmatrix} a_{11} & & a_{23} & \\ & a_{22} & & a_{34} \\ a_{21} & & a_{33} & \\ & a_{32} & & a_{44} \\ a_{31} & & a_{43} & \\ & a_{42} & & a_{54} \\ a_{41} & & a_{53} & \\ & a_{52} & & a_{64} \end{pmatrix}$$

(here $n = 4$). What is the number $G(n)$ of such arrays with no pairs of adjacent 1s? Two 1s here are said to be adjacent if they lie in positions (i, j) and $(i + 1, j)$, or in (i, j) and $(i, j + 1)$, or in (i, j) and $(i + 1, j + 1)$, for some i, j. Equivalently, $G(n)$ is the number of configurations of non-attacking Kings on an $n \times n$ chessboard with regular hexagonal cells. It is surprising that the **hard hexagon entropy constant**

$$\kappa = \lim_{n \to \infty} G(n)^{\frac{1}{N}} = 1.3954859724 \ldots = \exp(0.3332427219 \ldots)$$

is *algebraic* (in fact, is solvable in radicals [17–22]) with minimal integer polynomial [23]

$$25937424601x^{24} + 2013290651222784x^{22} + 2505062311720673792x^{20}$$
$$+ 797726698866658379776x^{18} + 7449488310131083100160x^{16}$$
$$+ 2958015038376958230528x^{14} - 72405670285649161617408x^{12}$$
$$+ 10715544815044338804326 4x^{10} - 71220809441400405884928x^{8}$$
$$- 7334749118363010387148 8x^{6} + 9714313527737757519052 8x^{4}$$
$$- 3275169181047901598515 2.$$

This is a consequence of Baxter's exact solution of the hard hexagon model [24–27] via theta elliptic functions and the Rogers–Ramanujan identities from number theory [28–31]! The expression for κ, in fact, comes out of a more general expression for

$$\kappa(z) = \lim_{n \to \infty} Z_n(z)^{\frac{1}{N}},$$

where $Z_n(z)$ is known as the **partition function** for the model and $G(n) = Z_n(1)$, $\kappa = \kappa(1)$. More on the physics of phase transitions in lattice gas models is found in [5.12.1].

McKay and Calkin independently calculated that, if we replace Princes by Kings on the chessboard with square cells, then the corresponding constant κ is $1.3426439511 \ldots$; see also [32–34]. Note that the distinction between Princes and Kings on a chessboard with regular hexagonal cells is immaterial. (Clarification: If a Prince occupies cell c, then any cell sharing an edge with c is vulnerable to attack. If a King occupies cell c, by contrast, then any cell sharing *either* an edge or corner with c is vulnerable.)

If we examine instead a chessboard with equilateral triangular cells, then $\kappa = 1.5464407087\ldots$ for Princes [3]. This may be called the **hard triangle entropy constant**. The value of κ when replacing Princes by Kings here is not known.

What are the constants κ for non-attacking Knights or Queens on chessboards with square cells? The analysis for Knights should be similar to that for Princes and Kings, but for Queens everything is different since interactions are no longer local [35].

The hard square entropy constant also appears in the form $\ln(\kappa)/\ln(2) = 0.5878911617\ldots$ in several coding-theoretic papers [36–41], with applications including holographic data storage and retrieval.

5.12.1 Phase Transitions in Lattice Gas Models

Statistical mechanics is concerned with the average properties of a large system of particles. We consider here, for example, the phase transition from a disordered fluid state to an ordered solid state, as temperature falls or density increases.

A simple model for this phenomenon is a **lattice gas**, in which particles are placed on the sites of a regular lattice and only adjacent particles interact. This may appear to be hopelessly idealized, as rigid molecules could not possibly satisfy such strict symmetry requirements. The model is nevertheless useful in understanding the link between microscopic and macroscopic descriptions of matter.

Two types of lattice gas models that have been studied extensively are the **hard square** model and the **hard hexagon** model. Once a particle is placed on a lattice site, no other particle is allowed to occupy the same site or any next to it, as pictured in Figure 5.12. Equivalently, the indicated squares and hexagons cannot overlap, hence giving rise to the adjective "hard."

Given a (square or triangular) lattice of N sites, assign a variable $\sigma_i = 1$ if site i is occupied and $\sigma_i = 0$ if it is vacant, for each $1 \leq i \leq N$. We study the **partition function**

$$Z_n(z) = \sum_{\sigma} \left(z^{\sigma_1 + \sigma_2 + \sigma_3 + \cdots + \sigma_N} \cdot \prod_{(i,j)} (1 - \sigma_i \sigma_j) \right),$$

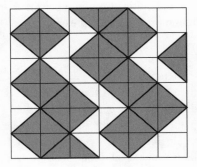 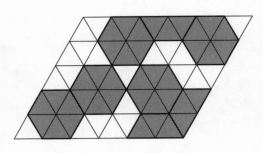

Figure 5.12. Hard squares and hard hexagons sit, respectively, on the square lattice and triangular lattice.

where the sum is over all 2^N possible values of the vector $\sigma = (\sigma_1, \sigma_2, \sigma_3, \ldots, \sigma_N)$ and the product is over all edges of the lattice (sites i and j are distinct and adjacent). Observe that the product enforces the nearest neighbor exclusion: If a configuration has two particles next to each other, then zero contribution is made to the partition function.

It is customary to deal with boundary effects by wrapping the lattice around to form a torus. More precisely, for the square lattice, $2n$ new edges are created to connect the n rightmost and n topmost points to corresponding n leftmost and n bottommost points. Hence there are a total of $2N$ edges in the square lattice, each site "looking like" every other. For the triangular lattice, $4n - 1$ new edges are created, implying a total of $3N$ edges. In both cases, the number of boundary sites, relative to N, is vanishingly small as $n \to \infty$, so this convention does not lead to any error.

Clearly the following combinatorial expressions are true [4, 42, 43]: For the square lattice,

$$Z_n = \sum_{k=0}^{\lfloor N/2 \rfloor} f_{k,n} z^k, \quad f_{0,n} = 1, \quad f_{1,n} = N, \quad f_{2,n} = \begin{cases} 2 & \text{if } n = 2, \\ \frac{1}{2} N(N - 5) & \text{if } n \geq 3, \end{cases}$$

$$f_{3,n} = \begin{cases} 6 & \text{if } n = 3, \\ \frac{1}{6} \left(N(N - 10)(N - 13) + 4N(N - 9) + 4N(N - 8) \right) & \text{if } n \geq 4, \end{cases}$$

where $f_{k,n}$ denotes the number of allowable tilings of the N-site lattice with k squares, and for the triangular lattice,

$$Z_n = \sum_{k=0}^{\lfloor N/3 \rfloor} g_{k,n} z^k, \quad g_{0,n} = 1, \quad g_{1,n} = N, \quad g_{2,n} = \frac{1}{2} N(N - 7),$$

$$g_{3,n} = \begin{cases} 0 & \text{if } n = 3, \\ \frac{1}{6} \left(N(N - 14)(N - 19) + 6N(N - 13) + 6N(N - 12) \right) & \text{if } n \geq 4, \end{cases}$$

where $g_{k,n}$ denotes the corresponding number of hexagonal tilings.

Returning to physics, we remark that the partition function is important since it acts as the "denominator" in probability calculations. For example, consider the two sublattices A and B of the square lattice with sites as shown in Figure 5.13. The probability that an arbitrary site α in the sublattice A is occupied is

$$\rho_A(z) = \lim_{n \to \infty} \frac{1}{Z_n} \sum_{\sigma} \left(\sigma_\alpha \cdot z^{\sigma_1 + \sigma_2 + \sigma_3 + \cdots + \sigma_N} \cdot \prod_{(i,j)} (1 - \sigma_i \sigma_j) \right),$$

which is also called the local density at α. We can define analogous probabilities for the three sublattices A, B, and C of the triangular lattice.

We are interested in the behavior of these models as a function of the positive variable z, known as the **activity**. Figure 5.14, for example, exhibits a graph of the mean density for the hard hexagon case:

$$\rho(z) = z \frac{d}{dz} (\ln(\kappa(z))) = \frac{\rho_A(z) + \rho_B(z) + \rho_C(z)}{3}$$

using the exact formulation given in [18].

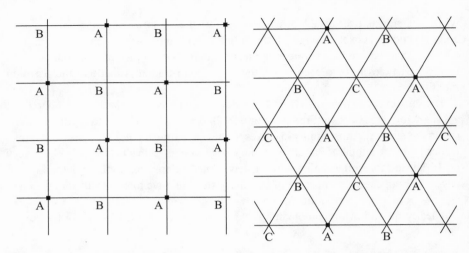

Figure 5.13. Two sublattices of the square lattice and three sublattices of the triangular lattice.

The existence of a phase transition is visually obvious. Let us look at the extreme cases: closely-packed configurations (large z) and sparsely-distributed configurations (small z). For infinite z, one of the possible sublattices is completely occupied, assumed to be the A sublattice, and the others are completely vacant; that is,

$$\rho_A = 1, \ \rho_B = 0 \quad \text{(for the square model)}$$

and

$$\rho_A = 1, \ \rho_B = \rho_C = 0 \quad \text{(for the hexagon model)}.$$

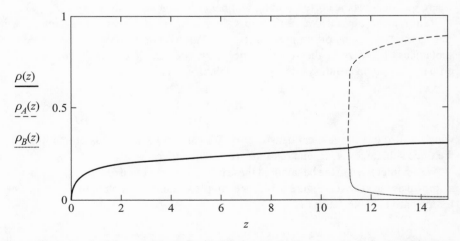

Figure 5.14. Graph of the mean density and sublattice densities, as functions of z, for the hexagon model.

For z close to zero, there is no preferential ordering on the sublattices; that is,

$\rho_A = \rho_B$ (for the square model) and $\rho_A = \rho_B = \rho_C$ (for the hexagon model).

Low activity corresponds to homogeneity and high activity corresponds to heterogeneity; thus there is a critical value, z_c, at which a phase transition occurs. Define the **order parameter**

$R = \rho_A - \rho_B$ (for squares) and $R = \rho_A - \rho_B = \rho_A - \rho_C$ (for hexagons);

then $R = 0$ for $z < z_c$ and $R > 0$ for $z > z_c$.

Elaborate numerical computations [7, 44, 45] have shown that, in the limit as $n \to \infty$,

$$z_c = 3.7962\ldots \text{ (for squares)} \text{ and } z_c = 11.09\ldots \text{ (for hexagons)},$$

assuming site α to be infinitely deep within the lattice. The computations involved highly-accurate series expansions for R and what are known as corner transfer matrices, which we cannot discuss here for reasons of space.

In a beautiful development, Baxter [24, 25] provided an exact solution of the hexagon model. The full breadth of this accomplishment cannot be conveyed here, but one of many corollaries is the exact formula

$$z_c = \frac{11 + 5\sqrt{5}}{2} = \left(\frac{1 + \sqrt{5}}{2}\right)^5 = 11.0901699437\ldots$$

for the hexagon model. No similar theoretical breakthrough has occurred for the square model and thus the identity of $3.7962\ldots$ remains masked from sight. The critical value $z_c = 7.92\ldots$ for the triangle model (on the hexagonal or honeycomb lattice) likewise is not exactly known [46].

For hard hexagons, the behavior of $\rho(z)$ and $R(z)$ at criticality is important [24, 26, 27]:

$$\rho \sim \rho_c - 5^{-3/2}\left(1 - \frac{z}{z_c}\right)^{2/3} \text{ as } z \to z_c^-, \ \rho_c = \frac{5 - \sqrt{5}}{10} = 0.2763932022\ldots,$$

$$R \sim \frac{3}{\sqrt{5}}\left[\frac{1}{5\sqrt{5}}\left(\frac{z}{z_c} - 1\right)\right]^{1/9} \text{ as } z \to z_c^+,$$

and it is conjectured that the exponents $1/3$ and $1/9$ are universal. For hard squares and hard triangles, we have only numerical estimates $\rho_c = 0.368\ldots$ and $0.422\ldots$, respectively. Far away from criticality, computations at $z = 1$ are less difficult [3, 47]:

$$\rho(1) = \begin{cases} 0.1624329213\ldots & \text{for hard hexagons,} \\ 0.2265708154\ldots & \text{for hard squares,} \\ 0.2424079763\ldots & \text{for hard triangles,} \end{cases}$$

and the first of these is algebraic of degree 12 [18, 22]. A generalization of $\rho(1)$ is the probability that an arbitrary point α and a specified configuration of neighboring points α' are all occupied; sample computations can be found in [3].

Needless to say, three-dimensional analogs of the models discussed here defy any attempt at exact solution [44].

[1]   N. J. Calkin and H. S. Wilf, The number of independent sets in a grid graph, *SIAM J. Discrete Math.* 11 (1998) 54–60; MR 99e:05010.

[2]   B. D. McKay, On Calkin and Wilf's limit theorem for grid graphs, unpublished note (1996).

[3]   R. J. Baxter, Planar lattice gases with nearest-neighbour exclusion, *Annals of Combin.* 3 (1999) 191–203; cond-mat/9811264; MR 2001h:82010.

[4]   D. S. Gaunt and M. E. Fisher, Hard-sphere lattice gases. I: Plane-square lattice, *J. Chem. Phys.* 43 (1965) 2840–2863; MR 32 #3716.

[5]   L. K. Runnels and L. L. Combs, Exact finite method of lattice statistics. I: Square and triangular lattice gases of hard molecules, *J. Chem. Phys.* 45 (1966) 2482–2492.

[6]   B. D. Metcalf and C. P. Yang, Degeneracy of antiferromagnetic Ising lattices at critical magnetic field and zero temperature, *Phys. Rev. B* 18 (1978) 2304–2307.

[7]   R. J. Baxter, I. G. Enting, and S. K. Tsang, Hard-square lattice gas, *J. Stat. Phys.* 22 (1980) 465–489; MR 81f:82037.

[8]   P. A. Pearce and K. A. Seaton, A classical theory of hard squares, *J. Stat. Phys.* 53 (1988) 1061–1072; MR 89j:82076.

[9]   S. Milosevic, B. Stosic, and T. Stosic, Towards finding exact residual entropies of the Ising antiferromagnets, *Physica A* 157 (1989) 899–906.

[10]   N. G. Markley and M. E. Paul, Maximal measures and entropy for $\mathbb{Z}^{\nu}$ subshifts of finite type, *Classical Mechanics and Dynamical Systems*, ed. R. L. Devaney and Z. H. Nitecki, Dekker, 1981, pp. 135–157; MR 83c:54059.

[11]   N. J. Calkin, *Sum-Free Sets and Measure Spaces*, Ph.D. thesis, Univ. of Waterloo, 1988.

[12]   K. Weber, On the number of stable sets in an $m \times n$ lattice, *Rostock. Math. Kolloq.* 34 (1988) 28–36; MR 89i:05172.

[13]   K. Engel, On the Fibonacci number of an $m \times n$ lattice, *Fibonacci Quart.* 28 (1990) 72–78; MR 90m:11033.

[14]   H. Prodinger and R. F. Tichy, Fibonacci numbers of graphs, *Fibonacci Quart.* 20 (1982) 16–21; MR 83m:05125.

[15]   Y. Kong, General recurrence theory of ligand binding on three-dimensional lattice, *J. Chem. Phys.* 111 (1999) 4790–4799.

[16]   N. J. A. Sloane, On-Line Encyclopedia of Integer Sequences, A000045, A001333, A006506, A051736, A051737, A050974, A066863, and A066864.

[17]   G. S. Joyce, Exact results for the activity and isothermal compressibility of the hard-hexagon model, *J. Phys. A* 21 (1988) L983–L988; MR 90a:82070.

[18]   G. S. Joyce, On the hard hexagon model and the theory of modular functions, *Philos. Trans. Royal Soc. London A* 325 (1988) 643–702; MR 90c:82055.

[19]   G. S. Joyce, On the icosahedral equation and the locus of zeros for the grand partition function of the hard hexagon model, *J. Phys. A* 22 (1989) L237–L242; MR 90e: 82101.

[20]   M. P. Richey and C. A. Tracy, Equation of state and isothermal compressibility for the hard hexagon model in the disordered regime, *J. Phys. A* 20 (1987) L1121–L1126; MR 89b:82121.

[21]   C. A. Tracy, L. Grove, and M. F. Newman, Modular properties of the hard hexagon model, *J. Stat. Phys.* 48 (1987) 477; MR 89b:82125.

[22]   M. P. Richey and C. A. Tracy, Algorithms for the computation of polynomial relationships for the hard hexagon model, *Nucl. Phys. B* 330 (1990) 681–704; MR 91c:82029.

[23]   P. Zimmermann, The hard hexagon entropy constant, unpublished note (1996).

[24]   R. J. Baxter, Hard hexagons: Exact solution, *J. Phys. A* 13 (1980) L61–L70; MR 80m:82052.

[25]   R. J. Baxter, Rogers-Ramanujan identities in the hard hexagon model, *J. Stat. Phys.* 26 (1981) 427–452; MR 84m:82104.

[26]   R. J. Baxter, *Exactly Solved Models in Statistical Mechanics*, Academic Press, 1982; MR 90b:82001.

[27] R. J. Baxter, Ramanujan's identities in statistical mechanics, *Ramanujan Revisited*, Proc. 1987 Urbana conf., ed. G. E. Andrews, R. A. Askey, B. C. Berndt, K. G. Ramanathan, and R. A. Rankin, Academic Press, 1988, pp. 69–84; MR 89h:82043.

[28] G. E. Andrews, The hard-hexagon model and Rogers-Ramanujan type identities, *Proc. Nat. Acad. Sci. USA* 78 (1981) 5290–5292; MR 82m:82005.

[29] G. E. Andrews, *q-Series: Their Development and Application in Analysis, Number Theory, Combinatorics, Physics and Computer Algebra*, Amer. Math. Soc., 1986; MR 88b:11063.

[30] G. E. Andrews, The reasonable and unreasonable effectiveness of number theory in statistical mechanics, *The Unreasonable Effectiveness of Number Theory*, Proc. 1991 Orono conf., ed. S. A. Burr, Amer. Math. Soc., 1992, pp. 21–34; MR 94c:82021.

[31] G. E. Andrews and R. J. Baxter, A motivated proof of the Rogers-Ramanujan identities, *Amer. Math. Monthly* 96 (1989) 401–409; 97 (1990) 214–215; MR 90e:11147 and MR 91j:11086.

[32] D. E. Knuth, Nonattacking kings on a chessboard, unpublished note (1994).

[33] H. S. Wilf, The problem of the kings, *Elec. J. Combin.* 2 (1995) R3; MR 96b:05012.

[34] M. Larsen, The problem of kings, *Elec. J. Combin.* 2 (1995) R18; MR 96m:05011.

[35] I. Rivin, I. Vardi, and P. Zimmermann, The n-queens problem, *Amer. Math. Monthly* 101 (1994) 629–638; MR 95d:05009.

[36] W. Weeks and R. E. Blahut, The capacity and coding gain of certain checkerboard codes, *IEEE Trans. Inform. Theory* 44 (1998) 1193–1203; MR 98m:94061.

[37] S. Forchhammer and J. Justesen, Entropy bounds for constrained two-dimensional random fields, *IEEE Trans. Inform. Theory* 45 (1999) 118–127; MR 99k:94023.

[38] A. Kato and K. Zeger, On the capacity of two-dimensional run-length constrained channels, *IEEE Trans. Inform. Theory* 45 (1999) 1527–1540; MR 2000c:94012.

[39] Z. Nagy and K. Zeger, Capacity bounds for the 3-dimensional (0, 1) runlength limited channel, *Applied Algebra, Algebraic Algorithms and Error-Correcting Codes (AAECC-13)*, Proc. 1999 Honolulu conf., ed. M. Fossorier, H. Imai, S. Lin, and A. Poli, Lect. Notes in Comp. Sci. 1719, Springer-Verlag, 1999, pp. 245–251.

[40] H. Ito, A. Kato, Z. Nagy, and K. Zeger, Zero capacity region of multidimensional run length constraints, *Elec. J. Combin.* 6 (1999) R33; MR 2000i:94036.

[41] R. M. Roth, P. H. Siegel, and J. K. Wolf, Efficient coding schemes for the hard-square model, *IEEE Trans. Inform. Theory* 47 (2001) 1166–1176; MR 2002b:94017.

[42] N. J. A. Sloane, On-Line Encyclopedia of Integer Sequences, A007197, A027683, A066866, and A067967.

[43] R. Hardin, Computation of $f_{k,n}$ and $g_{k,n}$, $1 \le n \le 9$, unpublished note (2002).

[44] D. S. Gaunt, Hard-sphere lattice gases. II: Plane-triangular and three-dimensional lattices, *J. Chem. Phys.* 46 (1967) 3237.

[45] R. J. Baxter and S. K. Tsang, Entropy of hard hexagons, *J. Phys. A* 13 (1980) 1023–1030.

[46] L. K. Runnels, L. L. Combs, and J. P. Salvant, Exact finite method of lattice statistics. II: Honeycomb lattice gas of hard molecules, *J. Chem. Phys.* 47 (1967) 4015–4020.

[47] C. Richard, M. Höffe, J. Hermisson, and M. Baake, Random tilings: Concepts and examples, *J. Phys. A* 31 (1998) 6385–6408; MR 99g:82033.

5.13 Binary Search Tree Constants

We first define a certain function f. The formulation may seem a little abstruse, but f has a natural interpretation as a path length along a type of weakly binary tree (an application of which we will discuss subsequently) [5.6].

Given a vector $V = (v_1, v_2, \ldots, v_k)$ of k distinct integers, define two subvectors V_L and V_R by

$$V_L = (v_j : v_j < v_1, \ 2 \le j \le k), \quad V_R = (v_j : v_j > v_1, \ 2 \le j \le k).$$

The subscripts L and R mean "left" and "right"; we emphasize that the sublists V_L and V_R preserve the ordering of the elements as listed in V.

Now, over all integers x, define the recursive function

$$f(x, V) = \begin{cases} 0 & \text{if } V = \emptyset \quad (\emptyset \text{ is the empty vector}), \\ \begin{cases} 1 & \text{if } x = v_1, \\ 1 + f(x, V_L) & \text{if } x < v_1, \\ 1 + f(x, V_R) & \text{if } x > v_1. \end{cases} & \text{otherwise} \quad (v_1 \text{ is the first vector component}), \end{cases}$$

Clearly $0 \leq f(x, V) \leq k$ always and the ordering of $v_1, v_2, \ldots, v_k$ is crucial in determining the value of $f(x, V)$. For example, $f(7, (3, 9, 5, 1, 7)) = 4$ and $f(4, (3, 9, 5, 1, 7)) = 3$.

Let V be a random permutation of $(1, 3, 5, \ldots, 2n - 1)$. We are interested in the probability distribution of $f(x, V)$ in two regimes:

- random odd x satisfying $1 \leq x \leq 2n - 1$ (successful search),
- random even x satisfying $0 \leq x \leq 2n$ (unsuccessful search).

Note that both V and x are random; it is assumed that they are drawn independently with uniform sampling. The expected value of $f(x, V)$ is, in the language of computer science [1–3],

- the average number of comparisons required to *find* an existing random record x in a data structure with n records,
- the average number of comparisons required to *insert* a new random record x into a data structure with n records,

where it is presumed the data structure follows that of a **binary search tree**. Figure 5.15 shows how such a tree is built starting with V as prescribed. Define also $g(l, V) = |\{x : f(x, V) = l, \ 1 \leq x \leq 2n - 1, \ x \text{ odd}\}|$, the number of vertices occupying the lth level of the tree ($l = 1$ is the root level). For example, $g(2, (3, 9, 5, 1, 7)) = 2$ and $g(3, (3, 9, 5, 1, 7)) = 1$.

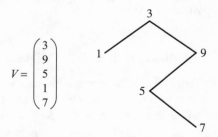

$$V = \begin{pmatrix} 3 \\ 9 \\ 5 \\ 1 \\ 7 \end{pmatrix}$$

Figure 5.15. Binary search tree constructed using V.

In addition to the two average-case parameters, we want the probability distribution of

$$h(V) = \max\{f(x, V) : 1 \leq x \leq 2n - 1, x \text{ odd}\} - 1,$$

the **height** of the tree (which captures the worst-case scenario for finding the record x, given V), and

$$s(V) = \max\{l : g(l, V) = 2^{l-1}\} - 1,$$

the **saturation level** of the tree (which provides the number of full levels of vertices in the tree, minus one). Thus $h(V)$ is the longest path length from the root of the tree to a leaf whereas $s(V)$ is the shortest such path. For example, $h(3, 9, 5, 1, 7) = 3$ and $s(3, 9, 5, 1, 7) = 1$.

Define, as is customary, the harmonic numbers

$$H_n = \sum_{k=1}^{n} \frac{1}{k} = \ln(n) + \gamma + \frac{1}{n} + O\left(\frac{1}{n^2}\right), \quad H_n^{(2)} = \sum_{k=1}^{n} \frac{1}{k^2} = \frac{\pi^2}{6} - \frac{1}{n} + O\left(\frac{1}{n^2}\right),$$

where γ is the Euler–Mascheroni constant [1.5]. Then the expected number of comparisons in a successful search (random, odd $1 \leq x \leq 2n - 1$) of a random tree is [2–4]

$$E(f(x, V)) = 2\left(1 + \frac{1}{n}\right) H_n - 3 = 2\ln(n) + 2\gamma - 3 + O\left(\frac{\ln(n)}{n}\right),$$

and in an unsuccessful search (random, even $0 \leq x \leq 2n$) the expected number is

$$E(f(x, V)) = 2(H_{n+1} - 1) = 2\ln(n) + 2\gamma - 2 + O\left(\frac{1}{n}\right).$$

The corresponding variances are, for odd x,

$$\text{Var}(f(x, V)) = \left(2 + \frac{10}{n}\right) H_n - 4\left(1 + \frac{1}{n}\right)\left(H_n^{(2)} + \frac{H_n^2}{4}\right) + 4$$
$$\sim 2\left(\ln(n) + \gamma - \frac{\pi^3}{3} + 2\right)$$

and, for even x,

$$\text{Var}(f(x, V)) = 2(H_{n+1} - 2H_{n+1}^{(2)} + 1) \sim 2\left(\ln(n) + \gamma - \frac{\pi^3}{3} + 1\right).$$

A complete analysis of $h(V)$ and $s(V)$ remained unresolved until 1985 when Devroye [3, 5–7], building upon work of Robson [8] and Pittel [9], proved that

$$\frac{h(V)}{\ln(n)} \to c, \quad \frac{s(V)}{\ln(n)} \to d,$$

almost surely as $n \to \infty$, where $c = 4.3110704070\ldots$ and $d = 0.3733646177\ldots$ are the only two real solutions of the equation

$$\frac{2}{x} \exp\left(1 - \frac{1}{x}\right) = 0.$$

Observe that the rate of convergence for $h(V)/\ln(n)$ and $s(V)/\ln(n)$ is slow; hence a numerical verification requires efficient simulation [10]. Considerable effort has been devoted to making these asymptotics more precise [11–14]. Reed [15, 16] and Drmota [17–19] recently proved that

$$E(h(V)) = c \ln(n) - \frac{3c}{2(c-1)} \ln(\ln(n)) + O(1),$$

$$E(s(V)) = d \ln(n) + O(\sqrt{\ln(n)} \ln(\ln(n)))$$

and $\mathrm{Var}(h(V)) = O(1)$ as $n \to \infty$. No numerical estimates of the latter are yet available. See also [20].

It is curious that for digital search trees [5.14], which are somewhat more complicated than binary search trees, the analogous limits

$$\frac{h(V)}{\ln(n)} \to \frac{1}{\ln(2)}, \quad \frac{s(V)}{\ln(n)} \to \frac{1}{\ln(2)}$$

do not involve new constants. The fact that limiting values for $h(V)/\ln(n)$ and $s(V)/\ln(n)$ are equal means that the trees are almost perfect (with only a small "fringe" around $\log_2(n)$). This is a hint that search/insertion algorithms on digital search trees are, on average, more efficient than on binary search trees.

Here is one related subject [21–23]. Break a stick of length r into two parts at random. Independently, break each of the two substicks into two parts at random as well. Continue inductively, so that at the end of the nth step, we have 2^n pieces. Let $P_n(r)$ denote the probability that all of the pieces have length < 1. For fixed r, clearly $P_n(r) \to 1$ as $n \to \infty$. More interestingly,

$$\lim_{n \to \infty} P_n(r^n) = \begin{cases} 0 & \text{if } r > e^{1/c}, \\ 1 & \text{if } 0 < r < e^{1/c}, \end{cases}$$

where $e^{1/c} = 1.2610704868\ldots$ and c is as defined earlier. The techniques for proving this are similar to those utilized in [5.3].

We merely mention a generalization of binary search trees called **quadtrees** [24–30], which also possess intriguing asymptotic constants. Quadtrees are useful for storing and retrieving multidimensional real data, for example, in cartography, computer graphics, and image processing [31–33].

[1]   R. Sedgewick and P. Flajolet, *Introduction to the Analysis of Algorithms*, Addison-Wesley, 1996, pp. 236–240, 246–250, 261.
[2]   D. E. Knuth, *The Art of Computer Programming*, v. 3, *Sorting and Searching*, Addison-Wesley, 1973, pp. 427, 448, 671–672; MR 56 #4281.
[3]   H. M. Mahmoud, *Evolution of Random Search Trees*, Wiley 1992, pp. 68–85, 92–95, 177–206; MR 93f:68045.

[4]   G. G. Brown and B. O. Shubert, On random binary trees, *Math. Oper. Res.* 9 (1984) 43–65; MR 86c:05099.

[5]   L. Devroye, A note on the height of binary search trees, *J. ACM* 33 (1986) 489–498; MR 87i:68009.

[6]   L. Devroye, Branching processes in the analysis of the heights of trees, *Acta Inform.* 24 (1987) 277–298; MR 88j:68022.

[7]   J. D. Biggins, How fast does a general branching random walk spread?, *Classical and Modern Branching Processes,* Proc. 1994 Minneapolis conf., ed. K. B. Athreya and P. Jagers, Springer-Verlag, 1997, pp. 19–39; MR 99c:60186.

[8]   J. M. Robson, The height of binary search trees, *Austral. Comput. J.* 11 (1979) 151–153; MR 81a:68071.

[9]   B. Pittel, On growing random binary trees, *J. Math. Anal. Appl.* 103 (1984) 461–480; MR 86c:05101.

[10] L. Devroye and J. M. Robson, On the generation of random binary search trees, *SIAM J. Comput.* 24 (1995) 1141–1156; MR 96j:68040.

[11] L. Devroye and B. Reed, On the variance of the height of random binary search trees, *SIAM J. Comput.* 24 (1995) 1157–1162; MR 96k:68033.

[12] J. M. Robson, On the concentration of the height of binary search trees, *Proc. 1997 Int. Colloq. on Automata, Languages and Programming (ICALP)*, Bologna, ed. P. Degano, R. Gorrieri, and A. Marchettio-Spaccamela, Lect. Notes in Comp. Sci. 1256, Springer-Verlag, pp. 441–448; MR 98m:68047.

[13] J. M. Robson, Constant bounds on the moments of the height of binary search trees, *Theoret. Comput. Sci.* 276 (2002) 435–444.

[14] M. Drmota, An analytic approach to the height of binary search trees, *Algorithmica* 29 (2001) 89–119.

[15] B. Reed, How tall is a tree?, *Proc. 32nd ACM Symp. on Theory of Computing (STOC)*, Portland, ACM, 2000, pp. 479–483.

[16] B. Reed, The height of a random binary search tree, *J. ACM*, to appear.

[17] M. Drmota, The variance of the height of binary search trees, *Theoret. Comput. Sci.* 270 (2002) 913–919.

[18] M. Drmota, An analytic approach to the height of binary search trees. II, *J. ACM*, to appear.

[19] M. Drmota, The saturation level in binary search trees, *Mathematics and Computer Science. Algorithms, Trees, Combinatorics and Probabilities*, Proc. 2000 Versailles conf., ed. D. Gardy and A. Mokkadem, Birkhäuser, 2000, pp. 41–51; MR 2001j:68026.

[20] C. Knessl and W. Szpankowski, The height of a binary search tree: The limiting distribution perspective, *Theoret. Comput. Sci.*, to appear.

[21] M. Sibuya and Y. Itoh, Random sequential bisection and its associated binary tree, *Annals Inst. Statist. Math.* 39 (1987) 69–84; MR 88e:60120.

[22] Y. Itoh, Binary search trees and 1-dimensional random packing, INRIA Project Algorithms Seminar 1997-1998, lecture summary.

[23] T. Hattori and H. Ochiai, A note on the height of binary search trees, random sequential bisection, and successive approximation for differential equation with moving singularity, unpublished note (1998).

[24] L. Laforest, *Étude des arbes hyperquaternaires*, LaCIM Tech. Report 3, Université du Québec à Montréal, 1990.

[25] L. Devroye and L. Laforest, An analysis of random d-dimensional quad trees, *SIAM J. Comput.* 19 (1990) 821–832; MR 91f:68018.

[26] P. Flajolet, G. Gonnet, C. Puech, and J. M. Robson, Analytic variations on quadtrees, *Algorithmica* 10 (1993) 473–500; MR 94i:68052.

[27] P. Flajolet, G. Labelle, L. Laforest, and B. Salvy, Hypergeometrics and the cost structure of quadtrees, *Random Structures Algorithms*, 7 (1995) 117–144; MR 96m:68034.

[28] G. Labelle and L. Laforest, Combinatorial variations on multidimensional quadtrees, *J. Combin. Theory Ser. A* 69 (1995) 1–16; MR 95m:05018.

[29] G. Labelle and L. Laforest, Sur la distribution de l'artié de la racine d'une arborescence hyperquaternaire à d dimensions, *Discrete Math.* 139 (1995) 287–302; MR 96f:05093.

[30] G. Labelle and L. Laforest, Etude de constantes universelles pour les arborescences hyper-quaternaires de recherche, *Discrete Math.* 153 (1996) 199–211; MR 97c:05003.
[31] H. Samet, The quadtree and related hierarchical structures, *ACM Comput. Surveys* 16 (1984) 187–206.
[32] H. Samet, *The Design and Analysis of Spatial Data Structures*, Addison-Wesley, 1990.
[33] H. Samet, *Applications of Spatial Data Structures*, Addison-Wesley, 1990.

5.14 Digital Search Tree Constants

Prior acquaintance with binary search trees [5.13] is recommended before reading this essay. Given a binary $k \times n$ matrix $M = (m_{i,j}) = (m_1, m_2, \ldots, m_k)$ of k distinct rows, define two submatrices $M_{L,p}$ and $M_{R,p}$ by

$$M_{L,p} = (m_i : m_{i,p} = 0, \ 2 \leq i \leq k), \quad M_{R,p} = (m_i : m_{i,p} = 1, \ 2 \leq i \leq k)$$

for any integer $1 \leq p \leq n$. That is, the pth column of $M_{L,p}$ is all zeros and the pth column of $M_{R,p}$ is all ones. The subscripts L and R mean "left" and "right"; we emphasize that the sublists $M_{L,p}$ and $M_{R,p}$ preserve the ordering of the rows as listed in M.

Now, over all binary n-vectors x, define the recursive function

$$f(x, M, p) = \begin{cases} 0 & \text{if } M = \emptyset, \\ \begin{cases} 1 & \text{if } x = m_1, \\ 1 + f(x, M_{L,p}, p+1) & \text{if } x \neq m_1 \text{ and } x_p = 0, \\ 1 + f(x, M_{R,p}, p+1) & \text{if } x \neq m_1 \text{ and } x_p = 1. \end{cases} & \text{otherwise,} \end{cases}$$

Clearly $0 \leq f(x, M, p) \leq k$ always and the ordering of $m_1, m_2, \ldots, m_k$, as well as the value of p, is crucial in determining the value of $f(x, M, p)$.

Let $M = (m_1, m_2, \ldots, m_k)$ be a random binary $n \times n$ matrix with n distinct rows, and let x denote a binary n-vector. We are interested in the probability distribution of $f(x, M, 1)$ in two regimes:

- random x satisfying $x = m_i$ for some i, $1 \leq i \leq n$ (successful search),
- random x satisfying $x \neq m_i$ for all i, $1 \leq i \leq n$ (unsuccessful search).

There is double randomness here as with binary search trees [5.13], but note that x depends on M more intricately than before. The expected value of $f(x, M, 1)$ is, in the language of computer science, [1–6]

- the average number of comparisons required to *find* an existing random record x in a data structure with n records,
- the average number of comparisons required to *insert* a new random record x into a data structure with n records,

where it is presumed the data structure follows that of a **digital search tree**. Figure 5.16 shows how such a tree is built starting with M as prescribed.

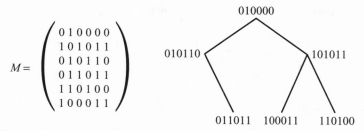

$$M = \begin{pmatrix} 0\,1\,0\,0\,0\,0 \\ 1\,0\,1\,0\,1\,1 \\ 0\,1\,0\,1\,1\,0 \\ 0\,1\,1\,0\,1\,1 \\ 1\,1\,0\,1\,0\,0 \\ 1\,0\,0\,0\,1\,1 \end{pmatrix}$$

Figure 5.16. Digital search tree constructed using M.

Another parameter of some interest is the number A_n of non-root vertices of degree 1, that is, nodes without children. For binary search trees [3, 7], it is known that $E(A_n) = (n + 1)/3$. For digital search trees, the corresponding result is more complicated, as we shall soon see. Because digital search trees are usually better "balanced" than binary search trees, one anticipates a linear coefficient closer to $1/2$ than $1/3$.

Let γ denote the Euler–Mascheroni constant [1.5] and define a new constant

$$\alpha = \sum_{k=1}^{\infty} \frac{1}{2^k - 1} = 1.6066951524\ldots.$$

Then the expected number of comparisons in a successful search (random, $x = m_i$ for some i) of a random tree is [3–6, 8, 9]

$$E(f(x, M, 1)) = \frac{1}{\ln(2)} \ln(n) + \frac{3}{2} + \frac{\gamma - 1}{\ln(2)} - \alpha + \delta(n) + O\left(\frac{\ln(n)}{n}\right)$$
$$\sim \log_2(n) - 0.716644\ldots + \delta(n),$$

and in an unsuccessful search (random $x \neq m_i$ for all i) the expected number is

$$E(f(x, M, 1)) = \frac{1}{\ln(2)} \ln(n) + \frac{1}{2} + \frac{\gamma}{\ln(2)} - \alpha + \delta(n) + O\left(\frac{\ln(n)}{n}\right)$$
$$\sim \log_2(n) - 0.273948\ldots + \delta(n),$$

where

$$\delta(n) = \frac{1}{\ln(2)} \sum_{\substack{k=-\infty \\ k \neq 0}}^{\infty} \Gamma\left(-1 - \frac{2\pi i k}{\ln(2)}\right) \exp\left(2\pi i k \frac{\ln(n)}{\ln(2)}\right).$$

The function $\delta(n)$ is oscillatory ($\delta(n) = \delta(2n)$), has zero mean, and is "negligible" ($|\delta(n)| < 1.726 \times 10^{-7}$ for all n). Similar functions $\varepsilon(n)$, $\rho(n)$, $\sigma(n)$ and $\tau(n)$ will be needed later. These arise in the analysis of many algorithms [3, 4, 6], as well as in problems discussed in [2.3], [2.16], [5.6], and [5.11]. Although such functions can be safely ignored for practical purposes, they need to be included in certain treatments for the sake of theoretical rigor.

The corresponding variances are, for searching,

$$\text{Var}(f(x, M, 1)) \sim \frac{1}{12} + \frac{\pi^2 + 6}{6 \ln(2)^2} - \alpha - \beta + \varepsilon(n) \sim 2.844383\ldots + \varepsilon(n)$$

and, for inserting,

$$\text{Var}(f(x, M, 1)) \sim \frac{1}{12} + \frac{\pi^2}{6 \ln(2)^2} - \alpha - \beta + \varepsilon(n) \sim 0.763014\ldots + \varepsilon(n),$$

where the new constant β is given by

$$\beta = \sum_{k=1}^{\infty} \frac{1}{(2^k - 1)^2} = 1.1373387363\ldots.$$

Flajolet & Sedgewick [3, 8, 10] answered an open question of Knuth's regarding the parameter A_n:

$$\text{E}(A_n) = \left[\theta + 1 - \frac{1}{Q}\left(\frac{1}{\ln(2)} + \alpha^2 - \alpha\right) + \rho(n)\right] n + O(n^{1/2}),$$

where the new constants Q and θ are given by

$$Q = \prod_{k=1}^{\infty}\left(1 - \frac{1}{2^k}\right) = 0.2887880950\ldots = (3.4627466194\ldots)^{-1},$$

$$\theta = \sum_{k=1}^{\infty} \frac{k 2^{k+1}}{1 \cdot 3 \cdot 7 \cdots (2^k - 1)} \sum_{j=1}^{k} \frac{1}{2^j - 1} = 7.7431319855\ldots.$$

The linear coefficient of $\text{E}(A_n)$ fluctuates around

$$c = \theta + 1 - \frac{1}{Q}\left(\frac{1}{\ln(2)} + \alpha^2 - \alpha\right) = 0.3720486812\ldots,$$

which is not as close to $1/2$ as one might have anticipated! Here also [11] is an integral representation for c:

$$c = \frac{1}{\ln(2)} \int_{0}^{\infty} \frac{x}{1+x}\left(1 + \frac{x}{1}\right)^{-1}\left(1 + \frac{x}{2}\right)^{-1}\left(1 + \frac{x}{4}\right)^{-1}\left(1 + \frac{x}{8}\right)^{-1} \cdots dx.$$

There are three main types of m-ary search trees: digital search trees, radix search tries (tries), and Patricia tries. We have assumed that $m = 2$ throughout. What, for example, is the variance for searching corresponding to Patricia tries? If we omit the fluctuation term, the remaining coefficient

$$\nu = \frac{1}{12} + \frac{\pi^2}{6 \ln(2)^2} + \frac{2}{\ln(2)} \sum_{k=1}^{\infty} \frac{(-1)^k}{k(2^k - 1)}$$

is interesting because, at first glance, it seems to be exactly 1! In fact, $\nu > 1 + 10^{-12}$ and this can be more carefully explained via the Dedekind eta function [12, 13].

5.14.1 Other Connections

In number theory, the divisor function $d(n)$ is the number of integers d, $1 \leq d \leq n$, that divide n. A special value of its generating function [4, 14, 15]

$$\sum_{n=1}^{\infty} d(n)q^n = \sum_{k=1}^{\infty} \frac{q^k}{1-q^k} = \sum_{k=1}^{\infty} \frac{q^{k^2}(1+q^k)}{1-q^k}$$

is α when $q = 1/2$. Erdös [16, 17] proved that α is irrational; forty years passed while people wondered about constants such as

$$\sum_{n=1}^{\infty} \frac{1}{2^n - 3} \text{ and } \sum_{n=1}^{\infty} \frac{1}{2^n + 1}$$

(the former appears in [18] whereas the latter is connected to tries [6] and mergesort asymptotics [19, 20]). Borwein [21, 22] proved that, if $|a| \geq 2$ is an integer, $b \neq 0$ is a rational number, and $b \neq -a^n$ for all n, then the series

$$\sum_{n=1}^{\infty} \frac{1}{a^n + b} \text{ and } \sum_{n=1}^{\infty} \frac{(-1)^n}{a^n + b}$$

are both irrational. Under the same conditions, the product

$$\prod_{n=1}^{\infty} \left(1 + \frac{b}{a^n}\right)$$

is irrational [23, 24], and hence so is Q. See [25] for recent computer-aided irrationality proofs.

On the one hand, from the combinatorics of integer partitions, we have Euler's pentagonal number theorem [14, 26–28]

$$\prod_{n=1}^{\infty}(1 - q^n) = \sum_{n=-\infty}^{\infty}(-1)^n q^{\frac{1}{2}(3n+1)n} = 1 + \sum_{n=1}^{\infty}(-1)^n \left(q^{\frac{1}{2}(3n-1)n} + q^{\frac{1}{2}(3n+1)n}\right)$$

and

$$\prod_{n=1}^{\infty}(1 - q^n)^{-1} = 1 + \sum_{n=1}^{\infty} \frac{q^n}{(1-q)(1-q^2)(1-q^3)\cdots(1-q^n)}$$

$$= 1 + \sum_{n=1}^{\infty} \frac{q^{n^2}}{(1-q)^2(1-q^2)^2(1-q^3)^2 \cdots (1-q^n)^2} = 1 + \sum_{n=1}^{\infty} p(n)q^n,$$

where $p(n)$ denotes the number of unrestricted partitions of n. If $q = 1/2$, these specialize to Q and $1/Q$. On the other hand, in the theory of finite vector spaces, Q appears in the asymptotic formula [5.7] for the number of linear subspaces of $\mathbb{F}_{q,n}$ when $q = 2$.

A substantial theory has emerged involving q-analogs of various classical mathematical objects. For example, the constant α is regarded as a $1/2$-analog of the Euler–Mascheroni constant [11]. Other constants (e.g., Apéry's constant $\zeta(3)$ or Catalan's constant G) can be similarly generalized.

Out of many more possible formulas, we mention three [4, 14, 26, 29]:

$$Q = \frac{1}{3} - \frac{1}{3 \cdot 7} + \frac{1}{3 \cdot 7 \cdot 15} - \frac{1}{3 \cdot 7 \cdot 15 \cdot 31} + - \cdots$$

$$= \exp\left(-\sum_{n=1}^{\infty} \frac{1}{n(2^n - 1)}\right)$$

$$= \sqrt{\frac{2\pi}{\ln(2)}} \exp\left(\frac{\ln(2)}{24} - \frac{\pi^2}{6\ln(2)}\right) \prod_{n=1}^{\infty}\left[1 - \exp\left(\frac{-4\pi^2 n}{\ln(2)}\right)\right].$$

The second makes one wonder if a simple relationship between Q and α exists. It can be shown that Q is the asymptotic probability that the determinant of a random $n \times n$ binary matrix is odd. A constant P similar to Q appears in [2.8]; exponents in P are constrained to be odd integers.

The reciprocal sum of repunits [30]

$$9\sum_{n=1}^{\infty} \frac{1}{10^n - 1} = \frac{1}{1} + \frac{1}{11} + \frac{1}{111} + \frac{1}{1111} + \cdots = 1.1009181908\ldots$$

is irrational by Borwein's theorem. The reciprocal series of Fibonacci numbers can be expressed as [31–33]

$$\sum_{k=1}^{\infty} \frac{1}{f_k} = \sqrt{5}\sum_{n=0}^{\infty} \frac{(-1)^n}{\varphi^{2n+1} - (-1)^n} = 3.3598856662\ldots,$$

where φ is the Golden mean, and this sum is known to be irrational [34–37]. Note that the subseries of terms with even subscripts can similarly be evaluated [26, 31]:

$$\sum_{k=1}^{\infty} \frac{1}{f_{2k}} = \sqrt{5}\left(\sum_{n=1}^{\infty} \frac{1}{\lambda^n - 1} - \sum_{n=1}^{\infty} \frac{1}{\mu^n - 1}\right) = 1.5353705088\ldots,$$

where $2\lambda = \sqrt{3} + 5$ and $2\mu = 7 + 3\sqrt{5}$. A completely different connection to the Fibonacci numbers (this time resembling the constant Q) is found in [1.2].

A certain normalizing constant [38–40]

$$K = \sqrt{\prod_{n=0}^{\infty}\left(1 + \frac{1}{2^{2n}}\right)} = 1.6467602581\ldots$$

occurs in efficient *binary cordic* implementations of two-dimensional vector rotation. Products such as Q and K, however, have no known closed-form expression except when $q = \exp(-\pi\xi)$, where $\xi > 0$ is an algebraic number [26, 41].

Observe that $2^{n+1} - 1$ is the smallest positive integer not representable as a sum of n integers of the form 2^i, $i \geq 0$. Define h_n to be the smallest positive integer not representable as a sum of n integers of the form $2^i 3^j$, $i \geq 0$, $j \geq 0$, that is, $h_0 = 1$, $h_1 = 5$, $h_2 = 23$, $h_3 = 431, \ldots$ [42, 43]. What is the precise growth rate of h_n as $n \to \infty$? What is the numerical value of the reciprocal sum of h_n (what might be

called the *2-3 analog* of the constant α)? This is vaguely related to our discussion in
[2.26] and [2.30.1].

5.14.2 Approximate Counting

Returning to computer science, we discuss **approximate counting**, an algorithm due
to Morris [44]. Approximate counting involves keeping track of a large number, N, of
events in only $\log_2(\log_2(N))$ bit storage, where accuracy is not paramount. Consider
the integer time series $X_0, X_1, \ldots, X_N$ defined recursively by

$$
X_n = \begin{cases} 1 & \text{if } n = 0, \\ \begin{cases} 1 + X_{n-1} & \text{with probability } 2^{-X_{n-1}}, \\ X_{n-1} & \text{with probability } 1 - 2^{-X_{n-1}}. \end{cases} & \text{otherwise,} \end{cases}
$$

It is not hard to prove that

$$
\mathrm{E}(2^{X_N} - 2) = N \text{ and } \mathrm{Var}(2^{X_N}) = \tfrac{1}{2} N(N + 1);
$$

hence probabilistic updates via this scheme give an unbiased estimator of N. Flajolet
[45–50] studied the distribution of X_N in much greater detail:

$$
\mathrm{E}(X_N) = \frac{1}{\ln(2)} \ln(N) + \frac{1}{2} + \frac{\gamma}{\ln(2)} - \alpha + \sigma(n) + O\left(\frac{\ln(N)}{N}\right)
$$
$$
\sim \log_2(N) - 0.273948\ldots + \sigma(N),
$$

$$
\mathrm{Var}(X_N) \sim \frac{1}{12} + \frac{\pi^2}{6\ln(2)^2} - \alpha - \beta - \chi + \tau(n) \sim 0.763014\ldots + \tau(N),
$$

where α and β are as before, the new constant χ is given by

$$
\chi = \frac{1}{\ln(2)} \sum_{n=1}^{\infty} \frac{1}{n} \operatorname{csch}\left(\frac{2\pi^2 n}{\ln(2)}\right) = (1.237412\ldots) \times 10^{-12},
$$

and $\sigma(n)$ and $\tau(n)$ are oscillatory "negligible" functions. In particular, since $\chi > 0$,
the constant coefficient for $\mathrm{Var}(X_N)$ is (slightly) smaller than that for $\mathrm{Var}(f(x, M, 1))$
given earlier. Similar ideas in probabilistic counting algorithms are found in [6.8].

[1] E. G. Coffman and J. Eve, File structures using hashing functions, *Commun. ACM* 13 (1970) 427–432.
[2] A. G. Konheim and D. J. Newman, A note on growing binary trees, *Discrete Math.* 4 (1973) 57–63; MR 47 #1650.
[3] P. Flajolet and R. Sedgewick, Digital search trees revisited, *SIAM Rev.* 15 (1986) 748–767; MR 87m:68014.
[4] D. E. Knuth, *The Art of Computer Programming*, v. 3, *Sorting and Searching*, Addison-Wesley, 1973, pp. 21, 134, 156, 493–502, 580, 685–686; MR 56 #4281.
[5] G. Louchard, Exact and asymptotic distributions in digital and binary search trees, *RAIRO Inform. Théor. Appl.* 21 (1987) 479–495; MR 89h:68031.
[6] H. M. Mahmoud, *Evolution of Random Search Trees*, Wiley, 1992, pp. 226–227, 260–291; MR 93f:68045.
[7] G. G. Brown and B. O. Shubert, On random binary trees, *Math. Oper. Res.* 9 (1984) 43–65; MR 86c:05099.

[8]   P. Kirschenhofer and H. Prodinger, Further results on digital search trees, *Theoret. Comput. Sci.* 58 (1988) 143–154; MR 89j:68022.

[9]   P. Kirschenhofer, H. Prodinger, and W. Szpankowski, Digital search trees again revisited: The internal path length perspective, *SIAM J. Comput.* 23 (1994) 598–616; MR 95i:68034.

[10] H. Prodinger, External internal nodes in digital search trees via Mellin transforms, *SIAM J. Comput.* 21 (1992) 1180–1183; MR 93i:68047.

[11] P. Flajolet and B. Richmond, Generalized digital trees and their difference-differential equations, *Random Structures Algorithms* 3 (1992) 305–320; MR 93f:05086.

[12] P. Kirschenhofer and H. Prodinger, Asymptotische Untersuchungen über charakteristische Parameter von Suchbäumen, *Zahlentheoretische Analysis II*, ed. E. Hlawka, Lect. Notes in Math. 1262, Springer-Verlag, 1987, pp. 93–107; MR 90h:68028.

[13] P. Kirschenhofer, H. Prodinger, and J. Schoissengeier, Zur Auswertung gewisser numerischer Reihen mit Hilfe modularer Funktionen, *Zahlentheoretische Analysis II*, ed. E. Hlawka, Lect. Notes in Math. 1262, Springer-Verlag, 1987, pp. 108–110; MR 90g:11057.

[14] G. H. Hardy and E. M. Wright, *An Introduction to the Theory of Numbers*, 5th ed., Oxford Univ. Press, 1985; Thms. 310, 350, 351, 353; MR 81i:10002.

[15] B. C. Berndt, *Ramanujan's Notebooks: Part I*, Springer-Verlag, 1985, p. 147; MR 86c:01062.

[16] P. Erdös, On arithmetical properties of Lambert series, *J. Indian Math. Soc.* 12 (1948) 63–66; MR 10,594c.

[17] D. H. Bailey and R. E. Crandall, Random generators and normal numbers, Perfectly Scientific Inc. preprint (2001).

[18] P. Erdös and R. L. Graham, *Old and New Problems and Results in Combinatorial Number Theory*, Enseignement Math. Monogr. 28, 1980, p. 62; MR 82j:10001.

[19] P. Flajolet and M. Golin, Exact asymptotics of divide-and-conquer recurrences, *Proc. 1993 Int. Colloq. on Automata, Languages and Programming (ICALP)*, Lund, ed. A. Lingas, R. Karlsson, and S. Carlsson, Lect. Notes in Comp. Sci. 700, Springer-Verlag, 1993, pp. 137–149.

[20] P. Flajolet and M. Golin, Mellin transforms and asymptotics: The mergesort recurrence, *Acta Inform.* 31 (1994) 673–696; MR 95h:68035.

[21] P. B. Borwein, On the irrationality of $\sum(1/(q^n + r))$, *J. Number Theory* 37 (1991) 253–259; MR 92b:11046.

[22] P. B. Borwein, On the irrationality of certain series, *Math. Proc. Cambridge Philos. Soc.* 112 (1992) 141–146; MR 93g:11074.

[23] J. Lynch, J. Mycielski, P. A. Vojta, and P. Bundschuh, Irrationality of an infinite product, *Amer. Math. Monthly* 87 (1980) 408–409.

[24] R. Wallisser, Rational approximation of the q-analogue of the exponential function and irrationality statements for this function, *Arch. Math. (Basel)* 44 (1985) 59–64; MR 86i:11036.

[25] T. Amdeberhan and D. Zeilberger, q-Apéry irrationality proofs by q-WZ pairs, *Adv. Appl. Math.* 20 (1998) 275–283; MR 99d:11074.

[26] J. M. Borwein and P. B. Borwein, *Pi and the AGM: A Study in Analytic Number Theory and Computational Complexity*, Wiley, 1987, pp. 62–75, 91–101; MR 99h:11147.

[27] G. Gasper and M. Rahman, *Basic Hypergeometric Series*, Cambridge Univ. Press, 1990; MR 91d:33034.

[28] G. E. Andrews, *q-Series: Their Development and Application in Analysis, Number Theory, Combinatorics, Physics and Computer Algebra*, CBMS, v. 66, Amer. Math. Soc., 1986; MR 88b:11063.

[29] R. J. McIntosh, Some asymptotic formulae for q-hypergeometric series, *J. London Math. Soc.* 51 (1995) 120–136; MR 95m:11112.

[30] A. H. Beiler, *Recreations in the Theory of Numbers*, Dover, 1966.

[31] A. F. Horadam, Elliptic functions and Lambert series in the summation of reciprocals in certain recurrence-generated sequences, *Fibonacci Quart.* 26 (1988) 98–114; MR 89e:11013.

[32] P. Griffin, Acceleration of the sum of Fibonacci reciprocals, *Fibonacci Quart.* 30 (1992) 179–181; MR 93d:11024.

[33] F.-Z. Zhao, Notes on reciprocal series related to Fibonacci and Lucas numbers, *Fibonacci Quart.* 37 (1999) 254–257; MR 2000d:11020.

[34] R. André-Jeannin, Irrationalité de la somme des inverses de certaines suites récurrentes, *C. R. Acad. Sci. Paris Sér. I Math.* 308 (1989) 539–541; MR 90b:11012.

[35] P. Bundschuh and K. Väänänen, Arithmetical investigations of a certain infinite product, *Compositio Math.* 91 (1994) 175–199; MR 95e:11081.

[36] D. Duverney, Irrationalité de la somme des inverses de la suite de Fibonacci, *Elem. Math.* 52 (1997) 31–36; MR 98c:11069.

[37] M. Prevost, On the irrationality of $\sum t^n/(A\alpha^n + B\beta^n)$, *J. Number Theory* 73 (1998) 139–161; MR 2000b:11085.

[38] J. E. Volder, The CORDIC trigonometric computing technique, *IRE Trans. Elec. Comput.* EC-8 (1959) 330–334; also in *Computer Arithmetic*, v. 1, ed. E. E. Swartzlander, IEEE Computer Soc. Press, 1990, pp. 226–230.

[39] J. S. Walther, A unified algorithm for elementary functions, *Spring Joint Computer Conf. Proc.* (1971) 379–385; also in *Computer Arithmetic*, v. 1, ed. E. E. Swartzlander, IEEE Computer Soc. Press, 1990, pp. 272–278.

[40] H. G. Baker, Complex Gaussian integers for 'Gaussian graphics,' *ACM Sigplan Notices*, v. 28 (1993) n. 11, 22–27.

[41] R. W. Gosper, Closed forms for $\prod_{n=1}^{\infty}(1 + \exp(-\pi \xi n))$, unpublished note (1998).

[42] V. S. Dimitrov, G. A. Jullien, and W. C. Miller, Theory and applications for a double-base number system, *IEEE Trans. Comput.* 48 (1999) 1098–1106; also in *Proc. 13th IEEE Symp. on Computer Arithmetic (ARITH)*, Asilomar, 1997, ed. T. Lang, J.-M. Muller, and N. Takagi, IEEE, 1997, pp. 44–51.

[43] N. J. A. Sloane, On-Line Encyclopedia of Integer Sequences, A018899.

[44] R. Morris, Counting large numbers of events in small registers, *Commun. ACM* 21 (1978) 840–842.

[45] P. Flajolet, Approximate counting: A detailed analysis, *BIT* 25 (1985) 113–134; MR 86j:68053.

[46] P. Kirschenhofer and H. Prodinger, Approximate counting: An alternative approach, *RAIRO Inform. Théor. Appl.* 25 (1991) 43–48; MR 92e:68070.

[47] H. Prodinger, Hypothetical analyses: Approximate counting in the style of Knuth, path length in the style of Flajolet, *Theoret. Comput. Sci.* 100 (1992) 243–251; MR 93j:68076.

[48] P. Kirschenhofer and H. Prodinger, A coin tossing algorithm for counting large numbers of events, *Math. Slovaca* 42 (1992) 531–545; MR 93j:68073.

[49] H. Prodinger, Approximate counting via Euler transform, *Math. Slovaca* 44 (1994) 569–574; MR 96h:11013.

[50] P. Kirschenhofer, A note on alternating sums, *Elec. J. Combin.* 3 (1996) R7; MR 97e:05025.

5.15 Optimal Stopping Constants

Consider the well-known **secretary problem**. An unordered sequence of **applicants** (distinct real numbers) $s_1, s_2, \ldots, s_n$ are interviewed by you one at a time. You have no prior information about the ss. You know the value of n, and as s_k is being interviewed, you must either accept s_k and end the process, or reject s_k and interview s_{k+1}. The decision to accept or reject s_k must be based solely on whether $s_k > s_j$ for all $1 \leq j < k$ (that is, on whether s_k is a **candidate**). An applicant once rejected cannot later be recalled.

If your objective is to select the most highly qualified applicant (the largest s_k), then the optimal strategy is to reject the first $m - 1$ applicants and accept the next candidate, where [1–4]

$$m = \min\left\{k \geq 1 : \sum_{j=k+1}^{n} \frac{1}{j-1} \leq 1\right\} \sim \frac{n}{e}$$

as $n \to \infty$. The asymptotic probability of obtaining the best applicant via this strategy is hence $1/e = 0.3678794411\ldots$, where e is the natural logarithmic base [1.3]. See a generalization of this in [5–7].

If your objective is instead to minimize the expected rank R_n of the chosen applicant (the largest s_k has rank 1, the second-largest has rank 2, etc.), then different formulation applies. Lindley [8] and Chow et al. [9] derived the optimal strategy in this case and proved that [10]

$$\lim_{n \to \infty} R_n = \prod_{k=1}^{\infty} \left(1 + \frac{2}{k}\right)^{\frac{1}{k+1}} = 3.8695192413\ldots = C.$$

A variation might include you knowing in advance that $s_1, s_2, \ldots, s_n$ are independent, uniformly distributed variables on the interval $[0, 1]$. This is known as a **full-information problem** (as opposed to the no-information problems just discussed). How does knowledge of the distribution improve your chances of success? For the "nothing but the best" objective, Gilbert & Mosteller [11] calculated the asymptotic probability of success to be [12, 13]

$$e^{-a} - (e^a - a - 1)\,\mathrm{Ei}(-a) = 0.5801642239\ldots,$$

where $a = 0.8043522628\ldots$ is the unique real solution of the equation $\mathrm{Ei}(a) - \gamma - \ln(a) = 1$, Ei is the exponential integral [6.2], and γ is the Euler-Mascheroni constant [1.5].

The full-information analog for $\lim_{n \to \infty} R_n$ appears to be an open problem [14–16]. Yet another objective, however, might be to maximize the hiree's expected quality Q_n itself (the kth applicant has quality s_k). Clearly

$$Q_0 = 0, \quad Q_n = \tfrac{1}{2}(1 + Q_{n-1}^2) \quad \text{if } n \geq 1,$$

and $Q_n \to 1$ as $n \to \infty$. Moser [11, 17–19] deduced that

$$Q_n \sim 1 - \frac{2}{n + \ln(n) + b},$$

where the constant b is estimated [10] to be $1.76799378\ldots$.

Here is a closely related problem. Assume $s_1, s_2, \ldots, s_n$ are independent, uniformly distributed variables on the interval $[0, N]$. Your objective is to minimize the number T_N of interviews necessary to select an applicant of expected quality $\geq N - 1$. Gum [20] sketched a proof that $T_N = 2N - O(\ln(N))$ as $N \to \infty$. Alternatively, assume everything as before except that $s_1', s_2', \ldots, s_n'$ are drawn with replacement from the set $\{1, 2, \ldots, N\}$. It can be proved here that $T_N' = c\,N + O(\sqrt{N})$, where [10]

$$c = 2 \sum_{k=3}^{\infty} \frac{\ln(k)}{k^2 - 1} - \frac{\ln(2)}{3} = 1.3531302722\ldots = \ln(C).$$

The secretary problem and its offshoots fall within the theory of **optimal stopping** [19]. Here is a sample exercise: We observe a fair coin being tossed repeatedly and can stop observing at any time. When we stop, the payoff is the average number of heads observed. What is the best strategy to maximize the expected payoff? Chow & Robbins [21, 22] described a strategy that achieves an expected payoff $> 0.79 = (0.59 + 1)/2$.

[1] T. S. Ferguson, Who solved the secretary problem?, *Statist. Sci.* 4 (1989) 282–296; MR 91k:01011.

[2] P. R. Freeman, The secretary problem and its extensions: A review, *Int. Statist. Rev.* 51 (1983) 189–206; MR 84k:62115.

[3] F. Mosteller, *Fifty Challenging Problems in Probability with Solutions*, Addison-Wesley, 1965, pp. 12, 74–79; MR 53 #1666.

[4] M. Gardner, *New Mathematical Diversions from Scientific American*, Simon and Schuster, 1966, pp. 35–36, 41–43.

[5] A. Q. Frank and S. M. Samuels, On an optimal stopping problem of Gusein-Zade, *Stochastic Process. Appl.* 10 (1980) 299–311; MR 83f:60067.

[6] M. P. Quine and J. S. Law, Exact results for a secretary problem, *J. Appl. Probab.* 33 (1996) 630–639; MR 97k:60127.

[7] G. F. Yeo, Duration of a secretary problem, *J. Appl. Probab.* 34 (1997) 556–558; MR 98a:60056.

[8] D. V. Lindley, Dynamic programming and decision theory, *Appl. Statist.* 10 (1961) 39–51; MR 23 #A740.

[9] Y. S. Chow, S. Moriguti, H. Robbins, and S. M. Samuels, Optimal selection based on relative rank (the "secretary problem"), *Israel J. Math.* 2 (1964) 81–90; MR 31 #855.

[10] P. Sebah, Computations of several optimal stopping constants, unpublished note (2001).

[11] J. P. Gilbert and F. Mosteller, Recognizing the maximum of a sequence, *J. Amer. Statist. Assoc.* 61 (1966) 35–73; MR 33 #6792.

[12] S. M. Samuels, Exact solutions for the full information best choice problem, Purdue Univ. Stat. Dept. report 82–17 (1982).

[13] S. M. Samuels, Secretary problems, in *Handbook of Sequential Analysis*, ed. B. K. Ghosh and P. K. Sen, Dekker, 1991, pp. 381–405; MR 93g:62102.

[14] F. T. Bruss and T. S. Ferguson, Minimizing the expected rank with full information, *J. Appl. Probab.* 30 (1993) 616–626; MR 94m:60090.

[15] F. T. Bruss and T. S. Ferguson, Half-prophets and Robbins' problem of minimizing the expected rank, *Proc. 1995 Athens Conf. on Applied Probability and Time Series Analysis*, v. 1, ed. C. C. Heyde, Yu. V. Prohorov, R. Pyke, and S. T. Rachev, Lect. Notes in Statist. 114, Springer-Verlag, 1996, pp. 1–17; MR 98k:60066.

[16] D. Assaf and E. Samuel-Cahn, The secretary problem: Minimizing the expected rank with i.i.d. random variables, *Adv. Appl. Probab.* 28 (1996) 828–852; MR 97f:60089.

[17] L. Moser, On a problem of Cayley, *Scripta Math.* 22 (1956) 289–292.

[18] I. Guttman, On a problem of L. Moser, *Canad. Math. Bull.* 3 (1960) 35–39; MR 23 #B2064.

[19] T. S. Ferguson, *Optimal Stopping and Applications*, unpublished manuscript (2000).

[20] B. Gum, The secretary problem with a uniform distribution, presentation at *Tenth SIAM Conf. on Discrete Math.*, Minneapolis, 2000.

[21] Y. S. Chow and H. Robbins, On optimal stopping rules for s_n/n, *Illinois J. Math.* 9 (1965) 444–454; MR 31 #4134.

[22] T. S. Ferguson, *Mathematical Statistics: A Decision Theoretic Approach*, Academic Press, 1967, p. 314; MR 35 #6231.

5.16 Extreme Value Constants

Let $X_1, X_2, \ldots, X_n$ denote a random sample from a population with continuous probability density function $f(x)$. Many interesting results exist concerning the distribution of the **order statistics**

$$X^{\langle 1 \rangle} < X^{\langle 2 \rangle} < \cdots < X^{\langle n \rangle},$$

where $X^{\langle 1 \rangle} = \min\{X_1, X_2, \ldots, X_n\} = m_n$ and $X^{\langle n \rangle} = \max\{X_1, X_2, \ldots, X_n\} = M_n$. We will focus only on the extreme values M_n for brevity's sake.

If $X_1, X_2, \ldots, X_n$ are taken from a Uniform $[0, 1]$ distribution (i.e., $f(x)$ is 1 for $0 \le x \le 1$ and is 0 otherwise), then the probability distribution of M_n is prescribed by

$$P(M_n < x) = \begin{cases} 0 & \text{if } x < 0, \\ x^n & \text{if } 0 \le x \le 1, \\ 1 & \text{if } x > 1 \end{cases}$$

and its moments are given by

$$\mu_n = E(M_n) = \frac{n}{n+1}, \quad \sigma_n^2 = \text{Var}(M_n) = \frac{n}{(n+1)^2(n+2)}.$$

These are all exact results [1–3]. Note that clearly

$$\lim_{n \to \infty} P\left(n\left(M_n - 1\right) < y\right) = \lim_{n \to \infty} P\left(M_n < 1 + \frac{1}{n}y\right) = \begin{cases} e^y & \text{if } y < 0, \\ 1 & \text{if } y \ge 0. \end{cases}$$

This asymptotic result is a special case of a far more general theorem due to Fisher & Tippett [4] and Gnedenko [5]. Under broad circumstances, the asymptotic distribution of M_n (suitably normalized) must belong to one of just three possible families. We see another, less trivial, example in the following.

If $X_1, X_2, \ldots, X_n$ are from a Normal $(0, 1)$ distribution, that is,

$$f(x) = \frac{1}{\sqrt{2\pi}} \exp\left(-\frac{x^2}{2}\right), \quad F(x) = \int\limits_{-\infty}^{x} f(\xi)\,d\xi = \frac{1}{2}\,\text{erf}\left(\frac{x}{\sqrt{2}}\right) + \frac{1}{2},$$

then the probability distribution of M_n is prescribed by

$$P(M_n < x) = F(x)^n = n \int\limits_{-\infty}^{x} F(\xi)^{n-1} f(\xi)\,d\xi$$

and its moments are given by

$$\mu_n = n \int\limits_{-\infty}^{\infty} x F(x)^{n-1} f(x)\,dx, \quad \sigma_n^2 = n \int\limits_{-\infty}^{\infty} x^2 F(x)^{n-1} f(x)\,dx - \mu_n^2.$$

For small n, exact expressions are possible [2, 3, 6–11]:

$$\mu_2 = \frac{1}{\sqrt{\pi}} = 0.564\ldots, \qquad\qquad \sigma_2^2 = 1 - \mu_2^2 = 0.681\ldots,$$

$$\mu_3 = \frac{3}{2\sqrt{\pi}} = 0.846\ldots, \qquad\qquad \sigma_3^2 = 1 + \frac{\sqrt{3}}{2\pi} - \mu_3^2 = 0.559\ldots,$$

$$\mu_4 = \frac{3}{\sqrt{\pi}}(1 - 2S_2) = 1.029\ldots, \qquad \sigma_4^2 = 1 + \frac{\sqrt{3}}{\pi} - \mu_4^2 = 0.491\ldots,$$

$$\mu_5 = \frac{5}{\sqrt{\pi}}(1 - 3S_2) = 1.162\ldots, \qquad \sigma_5^2 = 1 + \frac{5\sqrt{3}}{2\pi}(1 - 2S_3) - \mu_5^2 = 0.447\ldots,$$

$$\mu_6 = \frac{15}{2\sqrt{\pi}}(1 - 4S_2 + 2T_2) = 1.267\ldots, \quad \sigma_6^2 = 1 + \frac{5\sqrt{3}}{\pi}(1 - 3S_3) - \mu_6^2 = 0.415\ldots,$$

$$\mu_7 = \frac{21}{2\sqrt{\pi}}(1 - 5S_2 + 5T_2) = 1.352\ldots, \quad \sigma_7^2 = 1 + \frac{35\sqrt{3}}{4\pi}(1 - 4S_3 + 2T_3) - \mu_7^2$$
$$= 0.391\ldots,$$

where

$$S_k = \frac{\sqrt{k}}{\pi} \int\limits_0^{\frac{\pi}{4}} \frac{dx}{\sqrt{k + \sec(x)^2}} = \frac{1}{\pi} \arcsin\sqrt{\frac{k}{2(1+k)}},$$

$$T_k = \frac{\sqrt{k}}{\pi^2} \int\limits_0^{\frac{\pi}{4}} \int\limits_0^{\frac{\pi}{4}} \frac{dx\, dy}{\sqrt{k + \sec(x)^2 + \sec(y)^2}} = \frac{1}{\pi^2} \int\limits_0^{\pi S(k)} \arcsin\sqrt{\frac{1}{2}\frac{k(k+1)}{k(k+2) - \tan(z)^2}}\, dz.$$

Similar expressions for $\mu_8 = 1.423\ldots$ and $\sigma_8^2 = 0.372\ldots$ remain to be found. Ruben [12] demonstrated a connection between moments of order statistics and volumes of certain hyperspherical simplices (generalized spherical triangles). Calkin [13] discovered a binomial identity that, in a limiting case, yields the exact expression for μ_3.

We turn now to the asymptotic distribution of M_n. Let

$$a_n = \sqrt{2\ln(n)} - \frac{1}{2}\frac{\ln(\ln(n)) + \ln(4\pi)}{\sqrt{2\ln(n)}}.$$

It can be proved [14–18] that

$$\lim_{n\to\infty} P\left(\sqrt{2\ln(n)}(M_n - a_n) < y\right) = \exp(-e^{-y}),$$

and the resulting doubly exponential density function $g(y) = \exp(-y - e^{-y})$ is skewed to the right (called the Gumbel density or Fisher–Tippett Type I extreme values density). A random variable Y, distributed according to Gumbel's expression, satisfies [4]

$$E(Y) = \gamma = 0.577215\ldots, \qquad \text{Skew}(Y) = \frac{E\left[(Y - E(Y))^3\right]}{\text{Var}(Y)^{3/2}} = \frac{12\sqrt{6}}{\pi^3}\zeta(3)$$
$$= 1.139547\ldots,$$

$$\text{Var}(Y) = \frac{\pi^2}{6} = 1.644934\ldots, \quad \text{Kurt}(Y) = \frac{E\left[(Y - E(Y))^4\right]}{\text{Var}(Y)^2} - 3 = \frac{12}{5} = 2.4,$$

where γ is the Euler–Mascheroni constant [1.5] and $\zeta(3)$ is Apéry's constant [1.6]. (Some authors report the *square* of skewness; this explains the estimate 1.2986 in [2] and 1.3 in [19].) The constant $\zeta(3)$ also appears in [20]. Doubly exponential functions like $g(y)$ occur elsewhere (see [2.13], [5.7], and [6.10]).

The well-known Central Limit Theorem implies an asymptotic normal distribution for the *sum* of many independent, identically distributed random variables, whatever their common original distribution. A similar situation holds in extreme value theory. The asymptotic distribution of M_n (normalized) must belong to one of the following families [2, 14–17]:

$$G_{1,\alpha}(y) = \begin{cases} 0 & \text{if } y \leq 0, \\ \exp(-y^{-\alpha}) & \text{if } y > 0, \end{cases} \quad \text{``Fréchet'' or Type II,}$$

$$G_{2,\alpha}(y) = \begin{cases} \exp(-(-y)^{\alpha}) & \text{if } y \leq 0, \\ 1 & \text{if } y > 0, \end{cases} \quad \text{``Weibull'' or Type III,}$$

$$G_3(y) = \exp(-e^{-y}), \quad \text{``Gumbel'' or Type I,}$$

where $\alpha > 0$ is an arbitrary shape parameter. Note that $G_{2,1}(y)$ arose in our discussion of uniformly distributed X and $G_3(y)$ with regard to normally distributed X. It turns out to be unnecessary to know much about the distribution F of X to ascertain to which "domain of attraction" it belongs; the behavior of the tail of F is the crucial element. These three families can be further combined into a single one:

$$H_\beta(y) = \exp\left(-(1 + \beta y)^{-1/\beta}\right) \text{ if } 1 + \beta y > 0, \quad H_0(y) = \lim_{\beta \to 0} H_\beta(y),$$

which reduces to the three cases accordingly as $\beta > 0$, $\beta < 0$, or $\beta = 0$.

There is a fascinating connection between the preceding and random matrix theory (RMT). Consider first an $n \times n$ diagonal matrix with random diagonal elements X_1, X_2, ..., X_n; of course, its largest eigenvalue is equal to M_n. Consider now a random $n \times n$ complex Hermitian matrix. This means $X_{ij} = \bar{X}_{ij}$, so diagonal elements are real and off-diagonal elements satisfy a symmetry condition; further, all eigenvalues are real. A "natural" way of generating such matrices follows what is called the Gaussian Unitary Ensemble (GUE) probability distribution [21]. Exact moment formulas for the largest eigenvalue exist here for small n just as for the diagonal normally-distributed case discussed earlier [22]. The eigenvalues are independent in the diagonal case, but they are strongly dependent in the full Hermitian case. RMT is important in several ways: First, the spacing distribution between nontrivial zeros of the Riemann zeta function appears to be close to the eigenvalue distribution coming from GUE [2.15.3]. Second, RMT is pivotal in solving the longest increasing subsequence problem discussed in [5.20], and its tools are useful in understanding the two-dimensional Ising model [5.22]. Finally, RMT is associated with the physics of atomic energy levels, but elaboration on this is not possible here.

[1] J. D. Gibbons, *Nonparametric Statistical Inference*, McGraw-Hill, 1971; MR 86m:62067.

[2] H. A. David, *Order Statistics*, 2nd ed., Wiley, 1981; MR 82i:62073.

[3] N. Balakrishnan and A. Clifford Cohen, *Order Statistics and Inference*, Academic Press, 1991; MR 92k:62098.

[4] R. A. Fisher and L. H. C. Tippett, Limiting forms of the frequency distribution of the largest or smallest member of a sample, *Proc. Cambridge Philos. Soc.* 24 (1928) 180–190.

[5] B. Gnedenko, Sur la distribution limite du terme maximum d'une série aléatoire, *Annals of Math.* 44 (1943) 423–453; MR 5,41b.

[6] H. L. Jones, Exact lower moments of order statistics in small samples from a normal distribution, *Annals of Math. Statist.* 19 (1948) 270–273; MR 9,601d.

[7] H. J. Godwin, Some low moments of order statistics, *Annals of Math. Statist.* 20 (1949) 279–285; MR 10,722f.

[8] H. Ruben, On the moments of the range and product moments of extreme order statistics in normal samples, *Biometrika* 43 (1956) 458–460; MR 18,607d.

[9] J. K. Patel and C. B. Read, *Handbook of the Normal Distribution*, Dekker, 1982, pp. 238–241; MR 83j:62002.

[10] Y. Watanabe, M. Isida, S. Taga, Y. Ichijo, T. Kawase, G. Niside, Y. Takeda, A. Horisuzi, and I. Kuriyama, Some contributions to order statistics, *J. Gakugei, Tokushima Univ.* 8 (1957) 41–90; MR 20 #5545.

[11] Y. Watanabe, T. Yamamoto, T. Sato, T. Fujimoto, M. Inoue, T. Suzuki, and T. Uno, Some contributions to order statistics (continued), *J. Gakugei, Tokushima Univ.* 9 (1958) 31–86; MR 21 #2330.

[12] H. Ruben, On the moments of order statistics in samples from normal populations, *Biometrika* 41 (1954) 200–227; also in *Contributions to Order Statistics*, ed. A. E. Sarhan and B. G. Greenberg, Wiley, 1962, pp. 165–190; MR 16,153c.

[13] N. J. Calkin, A curious binomial identity, *Discrete Math.* 131 (1994) 335–337; MR 95i:05002.

[14] J. Galambos, *The Asymptotic Theory of Extreme Order Statistics*, 2nd ed., Krieger, 1987; MR 89a:60059.

[15] R.-D. Reiss, *Approximate Distributions of Order Statistics*, Springer-Verlag, 1989; MR 90e:62001.

[16] J. Galambos, Order statistics, *Handbook of Statistics*, v. 4, *Nonparametric Methods*, ed. P. R. Krishnaiah and P. K. Sens, Elsevier Science, 1984, pp. 359–382; MR 87g:62001.

[17] M. R. Leadbetter, G. Lindgren, and H. Rootzén, *Extremes and Related Properties of Random Sequences and Processes*, Springer-Verlag, 1983; MR 84h:60050.

[18] P. Hall, On the rate of convergence of normal extremes, *J. Appl. Probab.* 16 (1979) 433–439; MR 80d:60025.

[19] M. Abramowitz and I. A. Stegun, *Handbook of Mathematical Functions*, Dover, 1972, p. 930; MR 94b:00012.

[20] P. C. Joshi and S. Chakraborty, Moments of Cauchy order statistics via Riemann zeta functions, *Statistical Theory and Applications*, ed. H. N. Nagaraja, P. K. Sen, and D. F. Morrison, Springer-Verlag, 1996, pp. 117–127; MR 98f:62149.

[21] C. A. Tracy and H. Widom, Universality of the distribution functions of random matrix theory, *Integrable Systems: From Classical to Quantum*, Proc. 1999 Montréal conf., ed. J. Harnad, G. Sabidussi, and P. Winternitz, Amer. Math. Soc, 2000, pp. 251–264; math-ph/9909001; MR 2002f:15036.

[22] J. Gravner, C. A. Tracy, and H. Widom, Limit theorems for height fluctuations in a class of discrete space and time growth models, *J. Stat. Phys.* 102 (2001) 1085–1132; math.PR/0005133; MR 2002d:82065.

5.17 Pattern-Free Word Constants

Let a, b, c, ... denote the letters of a finite alphabet. A **word** is a finite sequence of letters; two examples are $abcacbacbc$ and $abcacbabcb$. A **square** is a word of the form xx, with x a nonempty word. A word is **square-free** if it contains no squares as factors. The first example contains the square $acbacb$ whereas the second is square-free. We ask the following question: How many square-free words of length n are there?

Over a two-letter alphabet, the only square-free words are a, b, ab, ba, aba, and bab; thus **binary** square-free words are not interesting. There do, however, exist arbitrarily long **ternary** square-free words, that is, over a three-letter alphabet. This fact was first proved by Thue [1, 2] using what is now called the Prouhet–Thue–Morse sequence [6.8]. Precise asymptotic enumeration of such words is complicated [3–7]. Brandenburg [8] proved that the number $s(n)$ of ternary square-free words of length $n > 24$ satisfies

$$6 \cdot 1.032^n < 6 \cdot 2^{\frac{n}{22}} \leq s(n) \leq 6 \cdot 1172^{\frac{n-2}{22}} < 3.157 \cdot 1.379^n,$$

and Brinkhuis [9] showed that $s(n) \leq A \cdot 1.316^n$ for some constant $A > 0$. Noonan & Zeilberger [10] improved the upper bound to $A' \cdot 1.302128^n$ for some constant $A' > 0$, and obtained a non-rigorous estimate of the limit

$$S = \lim_{n \to \infty} s(n)^{\frac{1}{n}} = 1.302 \ldots .$$

An independent computation [11] gave $S = \exp(0.263719 \ldots) = 1.301762 \ldots$, as well as estimates of S for k-letter alphabets, $k > 3$. Ekhad & Zeilberger [12] recently demonstrated that $1.041^n < 2^{n/17} \leq s(n)$, the first improvement in the lower bound in fifteen years. Note that S is a connective constant in the same manner as certain constants μ associated with self-avoiding walks [5.10]. In fact, Noonan & Zeilberger's computation of S is based on the same Goulden-Jackson technology used in bounding μ.

A **cube-free word** is a word that contains no factors of the form xxx, where x is a nonempty word. The Prouhet–Thue–Morse sequence gives examples of arbitrarily long binary cube-free words. Brandenburg [8] proved that the number $c(n)$ of binary cube-free words of length $n > 18$ satisfies

$$2 \cdot 1.080^n < 2 \cdot 2^{\frac{n}{9}} \leq c(n) \leq 2 \cdot 1251^{\frac{n-1}{17}} < 1.315 \cdot 1.522^n,$$

and Edlin [13] improved the upper bound to $B \cdot 1.45757921^n$ for some constant $B > 0$. Edlin also obtained a non-rigorous estimate of the limit:

$$C = \lim_{n \to \infty} c(n)^{\frac{1}{n}} = 1.457 \ldots .$$

A word is **overlap-free** if it contains no factor of the form $xyxyx$, with x nonempty. The Prouhet–Thue–Morse sequence, again, gives examples of arbitrarily long binary overlap-free words. Observe that a square-free word must be overlap-free, and that an overlap-free word must be cube-free. In fact, overlapping is the lowest pattern avoidable in arbitrarily long binary words. The number $t(n)$ of binary overlap-free words of length n satisfies [14, 15]

$$p \cdot n^{1.155} \leq t(n) \leq q \cdot n^{1.587}$$

for certain constants p and q. Therefore, $t(n)$ experiences only polynomial growth, unlike $s(n)$ and $c(n)$. Cassaigne [16] proved the interesting fact that $\lim_{n \to \infty} \ln(t(n)) / \ln(n)$ does not exist, but

$$1.155 < T_L = \liminf_{n \to \infty} \frac{\ln(t(n))}{\ln(n)} < 1.276 < 1.332 < T_U = \limsup_{n \to \infty} \frac{\ln(t(n))}{\ln(n)} < 1.587$$

(actually, he proved much more). We observed similar asymptotic misbehavior in [2.16].

An **abelian square** is a word xx', with x a nonempty word and x' a permutation of x. A word is **abelian square-free** if it contains no abelian squares as factors. The word *abcacbabcb* contains the abelian square *abcacb*. In fact, any ternary word of length at least 8 must contain an abelian square. Pleasants [17] proved that arbitrarily long abelian square-free words, based on five letters, exist. The four-letter case remained an open question until recently. Keränen [18] proved that arbitrarily long quaternary abelian square-free words also exist. Carpi [19] went farther to show that their number $h(n)$ must satisfy

$$\liminf_{n\to\infty} h(n)^{\frac{1}{n}} > 1.000021,$$

and he wrote, "... the closeness of this value to 1 leads us to think that, probably, it is far from optimal."

A ternary word w is a **partially abelian square** if $w = xx'$, with x a nonempty word and x' a permutation of x that leaves the letter b fixed, and that allows only adjacent letters a and c to commute. For example, the word *bacbca* is a partially abelian square. A word is **partially abelian square-free** if it contains no partially abelian squares as factors. Cori & Formisano [20] used Kobayashi's inequalities for $t(n)$ to derive bounds for the number of partially abelian square-free words.

Kolpakov & Kucherov [21, 22] asked: What is the minimal proportion of one letter in infinite square-free ternary words? Follow-on work by Tarannikov suggests [23] that the answer is $0.2746\ldots$.

A word over a k-letter alphabet is **primitive** if it is not a power of any subword [24]. The number of primitive words of length n is $\sum_{d|n} \mu(d) k^{n/d}$, where $\mu(d)$ is the Möbius mu function [2.2]. Hence, on the one hand, the proportion of words that are primitive is easily shown to approach 1 as $n \to \infty$. On the other hand, the problem of all counting words not *containing* a power is probably about as difficult as enumerating square-free words, cube-free words, etc.

A binary word $w_1 w_2 w_3 \ldots w_n$ of length n is said to be **unforgeable** if it never matches a left or right shift of itself, that is, it is never the same as any of $u_1 u_2 \ldots u_m w_1 w_2 \ldots w_{n-m}$ or $w_{m+1} w_{m+2} \ldots w_n v_1 v_2 \ldots v_m$ for any possible choice of u_is or v_js and any $1 \le m \le n - 1$. For example, we cannot have $w_1 = w_n$ because trouble would arise when $m = n - 1$. Let $f(n)$ denote the number of unforgeable words of length n. The example shows immediately that

$$0 \le \rho = \lim_{n\to\infty} \frac{f(n)}{2^n} \le \frac{1}{2}.$$

Further, via generating functions [7, 25–27],

$$\rho = \sum_{n=1}^{\infty} (-1)^{n-1} \frac{2}{2^{(2^{n+1}-1)} - 1} \prod_{m=2}^{n} \frac{2^{(2^m-1)}}{2^{(2^m-1)} - 1} = 0.2677868402\ldots$$
$$= 1 - 0.7322131597\ldots,$$

and this series is extremely rapidly convergent.

[1] A. Thue, Über die gegenseitige Lage gleicher Teile gewisser Zeichenreihen, *Videnskapssel-skapets Skrifter I, Matematisk-Naturvidenskapelig Klasse, Kristiania*, n. 1, Dybwad, 1912,

pp. 1–67; also in *Selected Mathematical Papers*, ed. T. Nagell, A. Selberg, S. Selberg, and K. Thalberg, Universitetsforlaget, 1977, pp. 413–478; MR 57 #46.

[2]   J.-P. Allouche and J. Shallit, The ubiquitous Prouhet-Thue-Morse sequence, *Sequences and Their Applications (SETA)*, Proc. 1998 Singapore conf., ed. C. Ding, T. Helleseth, and H. Niederreiter, Springer-Verlag, 1999, pp. 1–16; MR 2002e:11025.

[3]   M. Lothaire, *Combinatorics on Words*, Addison-Wesley, 1983; MR 98g:68134.

[4]   J. Berstel, Some recent results on squarefree words, *Proc. 1984 Symp. on Theoretical Aspects of Computer Science (STACS)*, Paris, ed. M. Fontet and K. Mehlhorn, Lect. Notes in Comp. Sci. 166, Springer-Verlag, 1984, pp. 14–25; MR 86e:68056.

[5]   J. Currie, Open problems in pattern avoidance, *Amer. Math. Monthly* 100 (1993) 790–793.

[6]   M. Lothaire, *Algebraic Combinatorics on Words*, Cambridge Univ. Press, 2002.

[7]   N. J. A. Sloane, On-Line Encyclopedia of Integer Sequences, A003000, A006156, A028445, and A007777.

[8]   F.-J. Brandenburg, Uniformly growing k^{th} power-free homomorphisms, *Theoret. Comput. Sci.* 23 (1983) 69–82; MR 84i:68148.

[9]   J. Brinkhuis, Non-repetitive sequences on three symbols, *Quart. J. Math.* 34 (1983) 145–149; MR 84e:05008.

[10] J. Noonan and D. Zeilberger, The Goulden-Jackson cluster method: Extensions, applications and implementations, *J. Differ. Eq. Appl.* 5 (1999) 355–377; MR 2000f:05005.

[11] M. Baake, V. Elser, and U. Grimm, The entropy of square-free words, *Math. Comput. Modelling* 26 (1997) 13–26; math-ph/9809010; MR 99d:68202.

[12] S. B. Ekhad and D. Zeilberger, There are more than $2^{n/17}$ n-letter ternary square-free words, *J. Integer Seq.* 1 (1998) 98.1.9.

[13] A. E. Edlin, The number of binary cube-free words of length up to 47 and their numerical analysis, *J. Differ. Eq. Appl.* 5 (1999) 353–354.

[14] A. Restivo and S. Salemi, Overlap-free words on two symbols, *Automata on Infinite Words*, ed. M. Nivat and D. Perrin, Lect. Notes in Comp. Sci. 192, Springer-Verlag, 1985, pp. 198–206; MR 87c:20101.

[15] Y. Kobayashi, Enumeration of irreducible binary words, *Discrete Appl. Math.* 20 (1988) 221–232; MR 89f:68036.

[16] J. Cassaigne, Counting overlap-free binary words, *Proc. 1993 Symp. on Theoretical Aspects of Computer Science (STACS)*, Würzburg, ed. P. Enjalbert, A. Finkel, and K. W. Wagner, Lect. Notes in Comp. Sci. 665, Springer-Verlag, 1993, pp. 216–225; MR 94j:68152.

[17] P. A. B. Pleasants, Non-repetitive sequences, *Proc. Cambridge Philos. Soc.* 68 (1970) 267–274; MR 42 #85.

[18] V. Keränen, Abelian squares are avoidable on 4 letters, *Proc. 1992 Int. Colloq. on Automata, Languages and Programming (ICALP)*, Vienna, ed. W. Kuich, Lect. Notes in Comp. Sci. 623, Springer-Verlag, 1992, pp. 41–52; MR 94j:68244.

[19] A. Carpi, On the number of abelian square-free words on four letters, *Discrete Appl. Math.* 81 (1998) 155–167; MR 98j:68139.

[20] R. Cori and M. R. Formisano, On the number of partially abelian square-free words on a three-letter alphabet, *Theoret. Comput. Sci.* 81 (1991) 147–153; MR 92i:68129.

[21] R. Kolpakov and G. Kucherov, Minimal letter frequency in n^{th} power-free binary words, *Mathematical Foundations of Computer Science (MFCS)*, Proc. 1997 Bratislava conf., ed. I. Prívara and P. Ruzicka, Lect. Notes in Comp. Sci. 1295, Springer-Verlag, pp. 347–357; MR 99d:68206.

[22] R. Kolpakov, G. Kucherov, and Y. Tarannikov, On repetition-free binary words of minimal density, *Theoret. Comput. Sci.* 218 (1999) 161–175; MR 2000b:68180.

[23] Y. Tarannikov, Minimal letter density in infinite ternary square-free word is 0.2746 . . . , *Proc. Two Joint French-Russian Seminars on Combinatorial and Algorithmical Properties of Discrete Structures*, Moscow State Univ., 2001, pp. 51–56.

[24] H. Petersen, On the language of primitive words, *Theoret. Comput. Sci.* 161 (1996) 141–156; MR 97e:68065.

[25] P. T. Nielsen, A note on bifix-free sequences, *IEEE Trans. Inform. Theory* 19 (1973) 704–706; MR 52 #2724.

[26] G. Blom and O. P. Lossers, Overlapping binary sequences, *SIAM Rev.* 37 (1995) 619–620.
[27] D. J. Greaves and S. J. Montgomery-Smith, Unforgeable marker sequences, unpublished
      note (2000).

5.18 Percolation Cluster Density Constants

Percolation theory is concerned with fluid flow in random media, for example, molecules penetrating a porus solid or wildfires consuming a forest. Broadbent & Hammersley [1–3] wondered about the probable number and structure of open channels in media for fluid passage. Answering their question has created an entirely new field of research [4–10]. Since the field is vast, we will attempt only to present a few constants.

Let $M = (m_{ij})$ be a random $n \times n$ binary matrix satisfying the following:

* $m_{ij} = 1$ with probability p, 0 with probability $1 - p$ for each i, j,
* m_{ij} and m_{kl} are independent for all $(i, j) \neq (k, l)$.

An *s*-**cluster** is an isolated grouping of s adjacent 1s in M, where adjacency means horizontal or vertical neighbors (not diagonal). For example, the 4×4 matrix

$$M = \begin{pmatrix} 1 & 0 & 1 & 1 \\ 1 & 1 & 0 & 0 \\ 0 & 1 & 0 & 1 \\ 1 & 0 & 0 & 1 \end{pmatrix}$$

has one 1-cluster, two 2-clusters, and one 4-cluster. The total number of clusters K_4 is 4 in this case. For arbitrary n, the total cluster count K_n is a random variable. The limit $\kappa_S(p)$ of the normalized expected value $\mathrm{E}(K_n)/n^2$ exists as $n \to \infty$, and $\kappa_S(p)$ is called the **mean cluster density** for the **site percolation model**. It is known that $\kappa_S(p)$ is twice continuously differentiable on [0, 1]; further, $\kappa_S(p)$ is analytic on [0, 1] except possibly at one point $p = p_c$. Monte Carlo simulation and numerical Padé approximants can be used to compute $\kappa_S(p)$. For example [11], it is known that $\kappa_S(1/2) = 0.065770\ldots$.

Instead of an $n \times n$ binary matrix M, consider a binary array A of $2n(n - 1)$ entries that looks like

$$A = \begin{pmatrix} & a_{12} & & a_{14} & & a_{16} & \\ a_{11} & & a_{13} & & a_{15} & & a_{17} \\ & a_{22} & & a_{24} & & a_{26} & \\ a_{21} & & a_{23} & & a_{25} & & a_{27} \\ & a_{32} & & a_{34} & & a_{36} & \\ a_{31} & & a_{33} & & a_{35} & & a_{37} \\ & a_{42} & & a_{44} & & a_{46} & \end{pmatrix}$$

(here $n = 4$). We associate a_{ij} not with a site of the $n \times n$ square lattice (as we do for m_{ij}) but with a bond. An *s*-cluster here is an isolated, connected subgraph of the graph of all bonds associated with 1s. For example, the array

$$A = \begin{pmatrix} & 1 & 0 & 0 & \\ 1 & 0 & 0 & 0 \\ & 0 & 1 & 0 & \\ 0 & 1 & 1 & 0 \\ & 0 & 1 & 0 & \\ 1 & 0 & 0 & 0 \\ & 0 & 0 & 0 & \end{pmatrix}$$

has one 1-cluster, one 2-cluster, and one 4-cluster. For **bond percolation models** such as this, we include 0-clusters in the total count as well, that is, isolated sites with no attached 1s bonds. In this case there are seven 0-clusters; hence the total number of clusters K_4 is 10. The mean cluster density $\kappa_B(p) = \lim_{n \to \infty} E(K_n)/n^2$ exists and similar smoothness properties hold. Remarkably, however, an exact integral expression can be found at $p = 1/2$ for the mean cluster density [13, 14]:

$$\kappa_B\left(\frac{1}{2}\right) = -\frac{1}{8}\cot(y) \cdot \frac{d}{dy}\left\{\frac{1}{y}\int_{-\infty}^{\infty} \text{sech}\left(\frac{\pi x}{2y}\right) \ln\left(\frac{\cosh(x) - \cos(2y)}{\cosh(x) - 1}\right) dx\right\}\Bigg|_{y=\frac{\pi}{3}},$$

which Adamchik [11, 12] recently simplified to

$$\kappa_B\left(\frac{1}{2}\right) = \frac{3\sqrt{3} - 5}{2} = 0.0980762113\ldots.$$

This constant is sometimes reported as $0.0355762113\ldots$, which is $\kappa_B(1/2) - 1/16$, if 0-clusters are not included in the total count. It may alternatively be reported as $0.0177881056\ldots$, which occurs if one normalizes not by the number of sites, n^2, but by the number of bonds, $2n(n - 1)$. Caution is needed when reviewing the literature. Other occurrences of this integral are in [15–18].

An expression for the limiting variance of bond cluster density is not known, but a Monte Carlo estimate $0.164\ldots$ and relevant discussion appear in [11]. The bond percolation model on the *triangular* lattice gives a limiting mean cluster density $0.111\ldots$ at a specific value $p = 0.347\ldots$ (see the next section for greater precision). The associated variance $0.183\ldots$, again, is not known.

5.18.1 Critical Probability

Let us turn attention away from mean cluster density $\kappa(p)$ and instead toward **mean cluster size** $\sigma(p)$. In the examples given earlier, $S_4 = (1 + 2 + 2 + 4)/4 = 9/4$ for the site case, $S_4 = (1 + 2 + 4)/3 = 7/3$ for the bond case, and $\sigma(p)$ is the limiting value of $E(S_n)$ as $n \to \infty$. The **critical probability** or **percolation threshold** p_c is defined to be [5, 6, 10]

$$p_c = \inf_{\substack{0 < p < 1 \\ \sigma(p) = \infty}} p,$$

that is, the concentration p at which an ∞-cluster appears in the infinite lattice. There are other possible definitions that turn out to be equivalent under most conditions. For example, if $\theta(p)$ denotes the **percolation probability**, that is, the probability that an ∞-cluster contains a prescribed site or bond, then p_c is the unique point for which $p < p_c$ implies $\theta(p) = 0$, and $p > p_c$ implies $\theta(p) > 0$. The critical probability indicates a phase transition in the system, analogous to that observed in [5.12] and [5.22].

For site percolation on the square lattice, there are rigorous bounds [19–24]

$$0.556 < p_c < 0.679492$$

and an estimate [25, 26] $p_c = 0.5927460\ldots$ based on extensive simulation. Ziff [11] additionally calculated that $\kappa_S(p_c) = 0.0275981\ldots$ via simulation. Parameter bounds for the cubic lattice and higher dimensions appear in [27–30].

In contrast, for bond percolation on the square and triangular lattices, there are exact results due to Sykes & Essam [31, 32]. Kesten [33] proved that $p_c = 1/2$ on the square lattice, corresponding to the expression $\kappa_B(1/2)$ in the previous section. On the triangular lattice, Wierman [34] proved that

$$p_c = 2 \sin\left(\frac{\pi}{18}\right) = 0.3472963553\ldots,$$

and this corresponds to another exact expression [11, 35–37],

$$\kappa_B(p_c) = -\frac{3}{8}\csc(2y) \cdot \frac{d}{dy}\left\{ \int_{-\infty}^{\infty} \frac{\sinh((\pi - y)x)\sinh(\frac{2}{3}yx)}{x\sinh(\pi x)\cosh(yx)}dx \right\}\Bigg|_{y=\frac{\pi}{3}} + \frac{3}{2} - \frac{2}{1+p_c}$$

$$= \frac{35}{4} - \frac{3}{p_c} = \frac{23}{4} - \frac{3}{2} \cdot \left\{ \sqrt[3]{4\left(1 + i\sqrt{3}\right)} + \sqrt[3]{4\left(1 - i\sqrt{3}\right)} \right\}$$

$$= 0.1118442752\ldots.$$

Similar results apply for the hexagonal (honeycomb) lattice by duality.

It is also known that $p_c = 1/2$ for site percolation on the triangular lattice [10] and, in this case, $\kappa_S(1/2) = 0.0176255\ldots$ via simulation [11, 38]. For site percolation on the hexagonal lattice, we have bounds [39]

$$0.6527 < 1 - 2\sin\left(\frac{\pi}{18}\right) \leq p_c \leq 0.8079$$

and an estimate $p_c = 0.6962\ldots$ [40, 41].

5.18.2 Series Expansions

Here are details on how the functions $\kappa_S(p)$ and $\kappa_B(p)$ may be computed [6, 42, 43]. We will work on the square lattice, focusing mostly on site percolation. Let g_{st} denote the number of lattice animals [5.19] with area s and perimeter t, and let $q = 1 - p$. The probability that a fixed site is a 1-cluster is clearly pq^4. Because a 2-cluster can be oriented either horizontally or vertically, the average 2-cluster count per site is $2p^2q^6$. A 3-cluster can be linear (two orientations) or L-shaped (four orientations); hence the

Table 5.4. *Mean s-Cluster Densities*

s	Mean s-Cluster Density for Site Model	Mean s-Cluster Density for Bond Model
0	0	q^4
1	pq^4	$2pq^6$
2	$2p^2q^6$	$6p^2q^8$
3	$p^3(2q^8 + 4q^7)$	$p^3(18q^{10} + 4q^9)$
4	$p^4(2q^{10} + 8q^9 + 9q^8)$	$p^4(55q^{12} + 32q^{11} + q^8)$

average 3-cluster count per site is $p^3(2q^8 + 4q^7)$. More generally, the mean s-cluster density is $\sum_t g_{st} p^s q^t$. Summing the left column entries in Table 5.4 [44, 45] gives $\kappa_S(p)$ as the number of entries $\to \infty$:

$$\kappa_S(p) = p - 2p^2 + p^4 + p^8 - p^9 + 2p^{10} - 4p^{11} + 11p^{12} + - \cdots$$
$$\sim \kappa_S(p_c) + a_S(p - p_c) + b_S(p - p_c)^2 + c_S |p - p_c|^{2-\alpha}.$$

Likewise, summing the right column entries in the table gives $\kappa_B(p)$:

$$\kappa_B(p) = q^4 + 2p - 6p^2 + 4p^3 + 2p^6 - 2p^7 + 7p^8 - 12p^9 + 28p^{10} + - \cdots$$
$$\sim \kappa_B(\tfrac{1}{2}) + a_B(p - \tfrac{1}{2}) + b_B(p - \tfrac{1}{2})^2 + c_B |p - \tfrac{1}{2}|^{2-\alpha},$$

where $a_B = -0.50\ldots$, $b_B = 2.8\ldots$, and $c_B = -8.48\ldots$ [46]. The exponent α is conjectured to be $-2/3$, that is, $2 - \alpha = 8/3$.

If instead of $\sum_{s,t} g_{st} p^s q^t$, we examine $\sum_{s,t} s^2 g_{st} p^{s-1} q^t$, then for the site model,

$$\sigma_S(p) = 1 + 4p + 12p^2 + 24p^3 + 52p^4 + 108p^5 + 224p^6 + 412p^7 + - \cdots$$
$$\sim C |p - p_c|^{-\gamma}$$

is the mean cluster size series (for low concentration $p < p_c$). The exponent γ is conjectured to be $43/18$.

The expression $1 - \sum_{s,t} s g_{st} p^{s-1} q^t$, when expanded in terms of q, gives

$$\theta_S(p) = 1 - q^4 - 4q^6 - 8q^7 - 23q^8 - 28q^9 - 186q^{10} + 48q^{11} - + \cdots$$
$$\sim D |p - p_c|^\beta,$$

which is the site percolation probability series (for high concentration $p > p_c$). The exponent β is conjectured to be $5/36$.

Smirnov & Werner [47] recently proved that α, β, and γ indeed exist and are equal to their conjectured values, for site percolation on the triangular lattice. A proof of universality would encompass both site and bond cases on the square lattice, but this has not yet been achieved.

5.18.3 Variations

Let the sites of an infinite lattice be independently labeled A with probability p and B with probability $1 - p$. Ordinary site percolation theory involves clusters of As. Let us instead connect adjacent sites that possess *opposite* labels and leave adjacent sites with the same labels disconnected. This is known as AB **percolation** or **antipercolation**. We wish to know what can be said of the probability $\theta(p)$ that an infinite AB cluster contains a prescribed site. It turns out that $\theta(p) = 0$ for all p for the infinite square lattice [48], but $\theta(p) > 0$ for all p lying in some nonempty subinterval containing $1/2$, for the infinite triangular lattice [49]. The exact extent of this interval is not known: Mai & Halley [50] gave $[0.2145, 0.7855]$ via Monte Carlo simulation whereas Wierman [51] gave $[0.4031, 0.5969]$. The function $\theta(p)$, for the triangular lattice, is nondecreasing on $[0, 1/2]$ and therefore was deemed unimodal on $[0, 1]$ by Appel [52].

Ordinary bond percolation theory is concerned with models in which any selected bond is either open (1) or closed (0). First-passage percolation [53] assigns not a binary random variable to each bond, but rather a nonnegative *real* random variable, thought of as length. Consider the square lattice in which each bond is independently assigned a length from the Uniform $[0, 1]$ probability distribution. Let T_n denote the shortest length of all lattice path lengths starting at the origin $(0, 0)$ and ending at $(n, 0)$; then it can be proved that the limit

$$\tau = \lim_{n \to \infty} \frac{E(T_n)}{n} = \inf_n \frac{E(T_n)}{n}$$

exists. Building upon earlier work [54–58], Alm & Parviainen [59] obtained rigorous bounds $0.243666 \leq \tau \leq 0.403141$ and an estimate $\tau = 0.312\ldots$ via simulation. If, instead, lengths are taken from the exponential distribution with unit mean, then we have bounds $0.300282 \leq \tau \leq 0.503425$ and an estimate $\tau = 0.402$. Godsil, Grötschel & Welsh [9] suggested the exact evaluation of τ to be a "hopelessly intractable problem."

We mention finally a constant $\lambda_c = 0.359072\ldots$ that arises in **continuum percolation** [5, 60]. Consider a homogeneous Poisson process of intensity λ on the plane, that is, points are uniformly distributed in the plane such that

- the probability of having exactly n points in a subset S of measure μ is $e^{-\lambda \mu} (\lambda \mu)^n / n!$ and
- the counts n_i of points in any collection of disjoint measurable subsets S_i are independent random variables.

Around each point, draw a disk of unit radius. The disks are allowed to overlap; that is, they are fully penetrable. There exists a unique critical intensity λ_c such that an unbounded connected cluster of disks develops with probability 1 if $\lambda > \lambda_c$ and with probability 0 if $\lambda < \lambda_c$. Hall [61] proved the best-known rigorous bounds $0.174 < \lambda_c < 0.843$, and the numerical estimate $0.359072\ldots$ is found in [62–64]. Among several alternative representations, we mention $\varphi_c = 1 - \exp(-\pi \lambda_c) = 0.676339\ldots$ [65] and $\pi \lambda_c = 1.128057\ldots$ [66]. The latter is simply the normalized total area of all the disks, disregarding whether they overlap or not, whereas φ_c takes overlapping portions into account. Continuum percolation shares many mathematical properties with lattice percolation, yet in many ways it is a more accurate model of physical disorder. Interestingly, it has also recently been applied in pure mathematics itself, to the study of gaps in the set of Gaussian primes [67].

[1] S. R. Broadbent and J. M. Hammersley, Percolation processes. I: Crystals and mazes, *Proc. Cambridge Philos. Soc.* 53 (1957) 629–641; MR 19,989e.

[2] J. M. Hammersley, Percolation processes. II: The connective constant, *Proc. Cambridge Philos. Soc.* 53 (1957) 642–645; MR 19,989f.

[3] J. M. Hammersley, Percolation processes: Lower bounds for the critical probability, *Annals of Math. Statist.* 28 (1957) 790–795; MR 21 #374.

[4] D. Stauffer, Scaling theory of percolation clusters, *Phys. Rep.* 54 (1979) 1–74.

[5] G. Grimmett, *Percolation*, Springer-Verlag, 1989; MR 90j:60109.

[6] D. Stauffer and A. Aharony, *Introduction to Percolation Theory*, 2nd ed., Taylor and Francis, 1992; MR 87k:82093.

[7] M. Sahimi, *Applications of Percolation Theory*, Taylor and Francis, 1994.

[8] S. Havlin and A. Bunde, Percolation, *Contemporary Problems in Statistical Physics*, ed. G. H. Weiss, SIAM, 1994, pp. 103–146.

[9] C. Godsil, M. Grötschel, and D. J. A. Welsh, Combinatorics in statistical physics, *Handbook of Combinatorics*, v. II, ed. R. Graham, M. Grötschel, and L. Lovász, MIT Press, 1995, pp. 1925–1954; MR 96h:05001.

[10] B. D. Hughes, *Random Walks and Random Environments*, v. 2, Oxford Univ. Press, 1996; MR 98d:60139.

[11] R. M. Ziff, S. R. Finch, and V. S. Adamchik, Universality of finite-size corrections to the number of critical percolation clusters, *Phys. Rev. Lett.* 79 (1997) 3447–3450.

[12] V. S. Adamchik, S. R. Finch, and R. M. Ziff, The Potts model on the square lattice, unpublished note (1996).

[13] H. N. V. Temperley and E. H. Lieb, Relations between the 'percolation' and 'colouring' problem and other graph-theoretical problems associated with regular planar lattices: Some exact results for the 'percolation' problem, *Proc. Royal Soc. London* A 322 (1971) 251–280; MR 58 #16425.

[14] J. W. Essam, Percolation and cluster size, *Phase Transitions and Critical Phenomena*, v. II, ed. C. Domb and M. S. Green, Academic Press, 1972, pp. 197–270; MR 50 #6392.

[15] M. L. Glasser, D. B. Abraham, and E. H. Lieb, Analytic properties of the free energy for the "ice" models, *J. Math. Phys.* 13 (1972) 887–900; MR 55 #7227.

[16] R. J. Baxter, Potts model at the critical temperature, *J. Phys.* C 6 (1973) L445–L448.

[17] H. N. V. Temperley, The shapes of domains occurring in the droplet model of phase transitions, *J. Phys.* A 9 (1976) L113–L117.

[18] R. J. Baxter, *Exactly Solved Models in Statistical Mechanics*, Academic Press, 1982, pp. 322–341; MR 90b:82001.

[19] B. Tóth, A lower bound for the critical probability of the square lattice site percolation, *Z. Wahr. Verw. Gebiete* 69 (1985) 19–22; MR 86f:60118.

[20] S. A. Zuev, Bounds for the percolation threshold for a square lattice (in Russian), *Teor. Veroyatnost. i Primenen.* 32 (1987) 606–609; Engl. transl. in *Theory Probab. Appl.* 32 (1987) 551–553; MR 89h:60171.

[21] S. A. Zuev, A lower bound for a percolation threshold for a square lattice (in Russian), *Vestnik Moskov. Univ. Ser. I Mat. Mekh.* (1988) n. 5, 59–61; Engl. transl. in *Moscow Univ. Math. Bull.*, v. 43 (1988) n. 5, 66–69; MR 91k:82035.

[22] M. V. Menshikov and K. D. Pelikh, Percolation with several defect types: An estimate of critical probability for a square lattice, *Math. Notes Acad. Sci. USSR* 46 (1989) 778–785; MR 91h:60116.

[23] J. C. Wierman, Substitution method critical probability bounds for the square lattice site percolation model, *Combin. Probab. Comput.* 4 (1995) 181–188; MR 97g:60136.

[24] J. van den Berg and A. Ermakov, A new lower bound for the critical probability of site percolation on the square lattice, *Random Structures Algorithms* 8 (1996) 199–212; MR 99b:60165.

[25] R. M. Ziff and B. Sapoval, The efficient determination of the percolation threshold by a frontier-generating walk in a gradient, *J. Phys.* A 19 (1986) L1169–L1172.

[26] R. M. Ziff, Spanning probability in 2D percolation, *Phys. Rev. Lett.* 69 (1992) 2670–2673.

[27] M. Campanino and L. Russo, An upper bound on the critical percolation probability for the three-dimensional cubic lattice, *Annals of Probab.* 13 (1985) 478–491; MR 86j: 60222.

[28] J. Adler, Y. Meir, A. Aharony, and A. B. Harris, Series study of percolation moments in general dimension, *Phys. Rev. B* 41 (1990) 9183–9206.

[29] B. Bollobás and Y. Kohayakawa, Percolation in high dimensions, *Europ. J. Combin.* 15 (1994) 113–125; MR 95c:60092.

[30] T. Hara and G. Slade, The self-avoiding-walk and percolation critical points in high dimensions, *Combin. Probab. Comput.* 4 (1995) 197–215; MR 96i:82081.

[31] M. F. Sykes and J. W. Essam, Exact critical percolation probabilities for site and bond problems in two dimensions, *J. Math. Phys.* 5 (1964) 1117–1121; MR 29 #1977.

[32] J. W. Essam and M. F. Sykes, Percolation processes. I: Low-density expansion for the mean number of clusters in a random mixture, *J. Math. Phys.* 7 (1966) 1573–1581; MR 34 #3952.

[33] H. Kesten, The critical probability of bond percolation on the square lattice equals 1/2, *Commun. Math. Phys.* 74 (1980) 41–59; MR 82c:60179.

[34] J. C. Wierman, Bond percolation on honeycomb and triangular lattices, *Adv. Appl. Probab.* 13 (1981) 298–313; MR 82k:60216.

[35] R. J. Baxter, H. N. V. Temperley, and S. E. Ashley, Triangular Potts model at its transition temperature, and related models, *Proc. Royal Soc. London A* 358 (1978) 535–559; MR 58 #20108.

[36] V. S. Adamchik, S. R. Finch, and R. M. Ziff, The Potts model on the triangular lattice, unpublished note (1996).

[37] V. S. Adamchik, A class of logarithmic integrals, *Proc. 1997 Int. Symp. on Symbolic and Algebraic Computation (ISSAC)*, ed. W. W. Küchlin, Maui, ACM, 1997, pp. 1–8; MR 2001k:33043.

[38] D. W. Erbach, Advanced Problem 6229, *Amer. Math. Monthly* 85 (1978) 686.

[39] T. Luczak and J. C. Wierman, Critical probability bounds for two-dimensional site percolation models, *J. Phys. A* 21 (1988) 3131–3138; MR 89i:82053.

[40] Z. V. Djordjevic, H. E. Stanley, and A. Margolina, Site percolation threshold for honeycomb and square lattices, *J. Phys. A* 15 (1982) L405–L412.

[41] R. P. Langlands, C. Pichet, P. Pouliot, and Y. Saint-Aubin, On the universality of crossing probabilities in two-dimensional percolation, *J. Stat. Phys.* 67 (1992) 553–574; MR 93e:82028.

[42] J. Adler, Series expansions, *Comput. in Phys.* 8 (1994) 287–295.

[43] A. R. Conway and A. J. Guttmann, On two-dimensional percolation, *J. Phys. A* 28 (1995) 891–904.

[44] M. F. Sykes and M. Glen, Percolation processes in two dimensions. I: Low-density series expansions, *J. Phys. A* 9 (1976) 87–95.

[45] M. F. Sykes, D. S. Gaunt, and M. Glen, Perimeter polynomials for bond percolation processes, *J. Phys. A* 14 (1981) 287–293; MR 81m:82045.

[46] C. Domb and C. J. Pearce, Mean number of clusters for percolation processes in two dimensions, *J. Phys. A* 9 (1976) L137–L140.

[47] S. Smirnov and W. Werner, Critical exponents for two-dimensional percolation, *Math. Res. Lett.* 8 (2001) 729–744; math.PR/0109120.

[48] M. J. Appel and J. C. Wierman, On the absence of infinite AB percolation clusters in bipartite graphs, *J. Phys. A* 20 (1987) 2527–2531; MR 89b:82061.

[49] J. C. Wierman and M. J. Appel, Infinite AB percolation clusters exist on the triangular lattice, *J. Phys. A* 20 (1987) 2533–2537; MR 89b:82062

[50] T. Mai and J. W. Halley, AB percolation on a triangular lattice, *Ordering in Two Dimensions*, ed. S. K. Sinha, North-Holland, 1980, pp. 369–371.

[51] J. C. Wierman, AB percolation on close-packed graphs, *J. Phys. A* 21 (1988) 1939–1944; MR 89m:60258.

[52] M. J. B. Appel, *AB* percolation on plane triangulations is unimodal, *J. Appl. Probab.* 31 (1994) 193–204; MR 95e:60101.

[53] R. T. Smythe and J. C. Wierman, *First-Passage Percolation on the Square Lattice*, Lect. Notes in Math. 671, Springer-Verlag, 1978; MR 80a:60135.

[54] J. M. Hammersley and D. J. A. Welsh, First-passage percolation, subadditive processes, stochastic networks, and generalized renewal theory, *Bernoulli, 1713; Bayes, 1763; Laplace, 1813. Anniversary Volume*, Proc. 1963 Berkeley seminar, ed. J. Neyman and L. M. Le Cam, Springer-Verlag, 1965, pp. 61–110; MR 33 #6731.

[55] S. Janson, An upper bound for the velocity of first-passage percolation, *J. Appl. Probab.* 18 (1981) 256–262; MR 82c:60178.

[56] D. J. A. Welsh, An upper bound for a percolation constant, *Z. Angew Math. Phys.* 16 (1965) 520–522.

[57] R. T. Smythe, Percolation models in two and three dimensions, *Biological Growth and Spread*, Proc. 1979 Heidelberg conf., ed. W. Jäger, H. Rost, and P. Tautu, Lect. Notes in Biomath. 38, Springer-Verlag, 1980, pp. 504–511; MR 82i:60183.

[58] R. Ahlberg and S. Janson, Upper bounds for the connectivity constant, unpublished note (1981).

[59] S. E. Alm and R. Parviainen, Lower and upper bounds for the time constant of first-passage percolation, *Combin. Probab. Comput*, to appear.

[60] R. Meester and R. Roy, *Continuum Percolation*, Cambridge Univ. Press, 1996; MR 98d:60193.

[61] P. Hall, On continuum percolation, *Annals of Probab.* 13 (1985) 1250–1266; MR 87f:60018.

[62] S. W. Haan and R. Zwanzig, Series expansions in a continuum percolation problem, *J. Phys. A* 10 (1977) 1547–1555.

[63] E. T. Gawlinski and H. E. Stanley, Continuum percolation in two dimensions: Monte Carlo tests of scaling and universality for noninteracting discs, *J. Phys. A* 14 (1981) L291–L299; MR 82m:82026.

[64] J. Quintanilla, S. Torquato, and R. M. Ziff, Efficient measurement of the percolation threshold for fully penetrable discs, *J. Phys. A* 33 (2000) L399–L407.

[65] C. D. Lorenz and R. M. Ziff, Precise determination of the critical percolation threshold for the three-dimensional "Swiss cheese" model using a growth algorithm, *J. Chem. Phys.* 114 (2001) 3659–3661.

[66] P. Hall, *Introduction to the Theory of Coverage Processes*, Wiley, 1988; MR 90f:60024.

[67] I. Vardi, Prime percolation, *Experim. Math.* 7 (1998) 275–289; MR 2000h:11081.

5.19 Klarner's Polyomino Constant

A **domino** is a pair of adjacent squares. Generalizing, we say that a **polyomino** or **lattice animal** of order n is a connected set of n adjacent squares [1–7]. See Figures 5.17 and 5.18.

Define $A(n)$ to be the number of polyominoes of order n, where it is agreed that two polyominoes are distinct if and only if they have different shapes *or* different

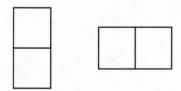

Figure 5.17. All dominoes (polyominoes of order 2); $A(2) = 2$.

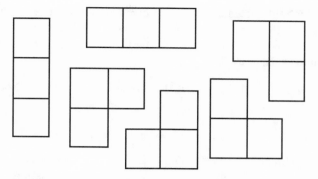

Figure 5.18. All polyominoes of order 3; $A(3) = 6$.

orientations:

$$A(1) = 1, \quad A(2) = 2, \quad A(3) = 6, \quad A(4) = 19, \quad A(5) = 63,$$
$$A(6) = 216, \quad A(7) = 760, \ldots.$$

There are different senses in which polyominoes are defined, for example, free versus fixed, bond versus site, simply-connected versus not necessarily so, and others. For brevity, we focus only on the fixed, site, possibly multiply-connected case.

Redelmeier [8] computed $A(n)$ up to $n = 24$, and Conway & Guttmann [9] found $A(25)$. In a recent flurry of activity, Oliveira e Silva [10] computed $A(n)$ up to $n = 28$, Jensen & Guttmann [11, 12] extended this to $A(46)$, and Knuth [13] found $A(47)$. Klarner [14, 15] proved that the limit

$$\alpha = \lim_{n \to \infty} A(n)^{\frac{1}{n}} = \sup_{n} A(n)^{\frac{1}{n}}$$

exists and is nonzero, although Eden [16] numerically investigated α several years earlier. The best-known bounds on α are $3.903184 \le \alpha \le 4.649551$, as discussed in [17–20]. Improvements are possible using the new value $A(47)$. The best-known estimate, obtained via series expansion analysis by differential approximants [11], is $\alpha = 4.062570\ldots$. A more precise asymptotic expression for $A(n)$ is

$$A(n) \sim \left(\frac{0.316915\ldots}{n} - \frac{0.276\ldots}{n^{3/2}} + \frac{0.335\ldots}{n^2} - \frac{0.25\ldots}{n^{5/2}} + O\left(\frac{1}{n^3}\right) \right) \alpha^n,$$

but such an empirical result is far from being rigorously proved.

Satterfield [5, 21] reported a lower bound of 3.91336 for α, using one of several algorithms he developed with Klarner and Shende. Details of their work unfortunately remain unpublished.

We mention that parallel analysis can be performed on the triangular and hexagonal lattices [7, 22].

Any self-avoiding polygon [5.10] determines a polyomino, but the converse is false since a polyomino can possess holes. A polyomino is **row-convex** if every (horizontal) row consists of a single strip of squares, and it is **convex** if this requirement is met for every column as well. Note that a convex polyomino does not generally determine a convex polygon in the usual sense. Counts of row-convex polyominoes obey a third-order linear recurrence [23–28], but counts $\tilde{A}(n)$ of convex polyominoes are somewhat more difficult to analyze [29, 30]:

$$\tilde{A}(1) = 1, \quad \tilde{A}(2) = 2, \quad \tilde{A}(3) = 6, \quad \tilde{A}(4) = 19, \quad \tilde{A}(5) = 59,$$

$$\tilde{A}(6) = 176, \quad \tilde{A}(7) = 502, \ldots,$$

$$\tilde{A}(n) \sim (2.67564\ldots)\tilde{\alpha}^n,$$

where $\tilde{\alpha} = 2.3091385933\ldots = (0.4330619231\ldots)^{-1}$. Exact generating function formulation for $\tilde{A}(n)$ was discovered only recently [31–33] but is too complicated to include here. Bender [30] further analyzed the expected shape of convex polyominoes, finding that, when viewed from a distance, most convex polyominoes resemble rods tilted $45°$ from the vertical with horizontal (and vertical) thickness roughly equal to $2.37597\ldots$. More results like this are found in [34–36].

It turns out that the growth constant $\tilde{\alpha}$ for convex polyominoes is the same as the growth constant α' for **parallelogram polyominoes**, that is, polyominoes whose left and right boundaries both climb in a northeasterly direction:

$$A'(1) = 1, \quad A'(2) = 2, \quad A'(3) = 4, \quad A'(4) = 9, \quad A'(5) = 20,$$

$$A'(6) = 46, \quad A'(7) = 105, \ldots.$$

These have the virtue of a simpler generating function $f(q)$. Let $(q)_0 = 1$ and $(q)_n = \prod_{j=1}^n (1 - q^j)$; then $f(q)$ is a ratio $J_1(q)/J_0(q)$ of q-analogs of Bessel functions:

$$J_0(q) = 1 + \sum_{n=1}^\infty \frac{(-1)^n q^{\binom{n+1}{2}}}{(q)_n (q)_n}, \quad J_1(q) = -\sum_{n=1}^\infty \frac{(-1)^n q^{\binom{n+1}{2}}}{(q)_{n-1}(q)_n},$$

which gives $\alpha' = \tilde{\alpha}$, but a different multiplicative constant $0.29745\ldots$.

There are many more counting problems of this sort than we can possibly summarize! Here is one more example, studied independently by Glasser, Privman & Svrakic [37] and Odlyzko & Wilf [38–40]. An **n-fountain** (Figure 5.19) is best pictured as a connected, self-supporting stacking of n coins in a triangular lattice array against a vertical wall.

Note that the bottom row cannot have gaps but the higher rows can; each coin in a higher row must touch two adjacent coins in the row below. Let $B(n)$ be the number of n-fountains. The generating function for $B(n)$ satisfies a beautiful identity involving

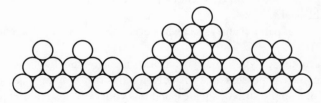

Figure 5.19. An example of an n-fountain.

Ramanujan's continued fraction:

$$1 + \sum_{n=1}^{\infty} B(n)x^n = 1 + x + x^2 + 2x^3 + 3x^4 + 5x^5 + 9x^6 + 15x^7 + 26x^8 + 45x^9 + \cdots$$

$$= \frac{1|}{|1} - \frac{x|}{|1} - \frac{x^2|}{|1} - \frac{x^3|}{|1} - \frac{x^4|}{|1} - \frac{x^5|}{|1} - \cdots,$$

and the following growth estimates arise:

$$\lim_{n \to \infty} B(n)^{\frac{1}{n}} = \beta = 1.7356628245\ldots = (0.5761487691\ldots)^{-1},$$

$$B(n) = (0.3123633245\ldots)\beta^n + O\left(\left(\frac{5}{3}\right)^n\right).$$

See [41] for other related counting problems.

[1] S. W. Golomb, *Polyominoes*, 2nd ed., Princeton Univ. Press, 1994; MR 95k:00006.

[2] A. J. Guttmann, Planar polygons: Regular, convex, almost convex, staircase and row convex, *Computer-Aided Statistical Physics*, Proc. 1991 Taipei symp., ed. C.-K. Hu, Amer. Inst. Phys., 1992, pp. 12–43.

[3] M. P. Delest, Polyominoes and animals: Some recent results, *J. Math. Chem.* 8 (1991) 3–18; MR 93e:05024.

[4] C. Godsil, M. Grötschel, and D. J. A. Welsh, Combinatorics in statistical physics, *Handbook of Combinatorics*, v. II, ed. R. Graham, M. Grötschel, and L. Lovász, MIT Press, 1995, pp. 1925–1954; MR 96h:05001.

[5] D. A. Klarner, Polyominoes, *Handbook of Discrete and Computational Geometry*, ed. J. E. Goodman and J. O'Rourke, CRC Press, 1997, pp. 225–240; MR 2000j:52001.

[6] D. Eppstein, Polyominoes and Other Animals (Geometry Junkyard).

[7] N. J. A. Sloane, On-Line Encyclopedia of Integer Sequences, A001168, A001169, A001207, A001420, A005169, A006958, and A067675.

[8] D. H. Redelmeier, Counting polyominoes: Yet another attack, *Discrete Math.* 36 (1981) 191–203; MR 84g:05049.

[9] A. R. Conway and A. J. Guttmann, On two-dimensional percolation, *J. Phys. A* 28 (1995) 891–904.

[10] T. Oliveira e Silva, Enumeration of animals on the (4^4) regular tiling of the Euclidean plane, unpublished note (1999).

[11] I. Jensen and A. J. Guttmann, Statistics of lattice animals (polyominoes) and polygons, *J. Phys. A* 33 (2000) L257–L263; MR 2001e:82025.

[12] I. Jensen, Enumerations of lattice animals and trees, *J. Stat. Phys.* 102 (2001) 865–881; MR 2002b:82026.

[13] D. E. Knuth, The number of 47-ominoes, unpublished note (2001).

[14] D. A. Klarner, Cell growth problems, *Canad. J. Math.* 19 (1967) 851–863; MR 35 #5339.

[15] D. A. Klarner, My life among the polyominoes, *Nieuw Arch. Wisk.* 29 (1981) 156–177; also in *The Mathematical Gardner*, ed. D. A. Klarner, Wadsworth, 1981, pp. 243–262; MR 83e:05038.

[16] M. Eden, A two-dimensional growth process, *Proc. Fourth Berkeley Symp. Math. Stat. Probab.*, v. 4, ed. J. Neyman, Univ. of Calif. Press, 1961, pp. 223–239; MR 24 #B2493.

[17] D. A. Klarner and R. L. Rivest, A procedure for improving the upper bound for the number of *n*-ominoes, *Canad. J. Math.* 25 (1973) 585–602; MR 48 #1943.

[18] B. M. I. Rands and D. J. A. Welsh, Animals, trees and renewal sequences, *IMA J. Appl. Math.* 27 (1981) 1–17; corrigendum 28 (1982) 107; MR 82j:05049 and MR 83c:05041.

[19] S. G. Whittington and C. E. Soteros, Lattice animals: Rigorous results and wild guesses, *Disorder in Physical Systems: A Volume in Honour of J. M. Hammersley*, ed. G. R. Grimmett and D. J. A. Welsh, Oxford Univ. Press, 1990, pp. 323–335; MR 91m:82061.

[20] A. J. Guttmann, On the number of lattice animals embeddable in the square lattice, *J. Phys. A* 15 (1982) 1987–1990.

[21] D. A. Klarner, S. Shende, and W. Satterfield, Lower-bounding techniques for lattice animals, unpublished work (2000).

[22] W. F. Lunnon, Counting hexagonal and triangular polyominoes, *Graph Theory and Computing*, ed. R. C. Read, Academic Press, 1972, pp. 87–100; MR 49 #2439.

[23] G. Pólya, On the number of certain lattice polygons, *J. Combin. Theory* 6 (1969) 102–105; also in *Collected Papers*, v. 4, ed. G.-C. Rota, MIT Press, 1984, pp. 441–444, 630; MR 38 #4329.

[24] H. N. V. Temperley, Combinatorial problems suggested by the statistical mechanics of domains and of rubber-like molecules, *Phys. Rev.* 103 (1956) 1–16; MR 17,1168f.

[25] D. A. Klarner, Some results concerning polyominoes, *Fibonacci Quart.* 3 (1965) 9–20; MR 32 #4028.

[26] M. P. Delest, Generating functions for column-convex polyominoes, *J. Combin. Theory Ser. A* 48 (1988) 12–31; MR 89e:05013.

[27] V. Domocos, A combinatorial method for the enumeration of column-convex polyominoes, *Discrete Math.* 152 (1996) 115–123; MR 97c:05005.

[28] D. Hickerson, Counting horizontally convex polyominoes, *J. Integer Seq.* 2 (1999) 99.1.8; MR 2000k:05023.

[29] D. A. Klarner and R. L. Rivest, Asymptotic bounds for the number of convex n-ominoes, *Discrete Math.* 8 (1974) 31–40; MR 49 #91.

[30] E. A. Bender, Convex n-ominoes, *Discrete Math.* 8 (1974) 219–226; MR 49 #67.

[31] M. Bousquet-Mélou and J.-M. Fédou, The generating function of convex polyominoes: The resolution of a q-differential system, *Discrete Math.* 137 (1995) 53–75; MR 95m:05009.

[32] M. Bousquet-Mélou and A. Rechnitzer, Lattice animals and heaps of dimers, *Discrete Math.*, to appear.

[33] K. Y. Lin, Exact solution of the convex polygon perimeter and area generating function, *J. Phys. A* 24 (1991) 2411–2417; MR 92f:82023.

[34] G. Louchard, Probabilistic analysis of some (un)directed animals, *Theoret. Comput. Sci.* 159 (1996) 65–79; MR 97b:68164.

[35] G. Louchard, Probabilistic analysis of column-convex and directed diagonally-convex animals, *Random Structures Algorithms* 11 (1997) 151–178; MR 99c:05047.

[36] G. Louchard, Probabilistic analysis of column-convex and directed diagonally-convex animals. II: Trajectories and shapes, *Random Structures Algorithms* 15 (1999) 1–23; MR 2000e:05042.

[37] M. L. Glasser, V. Privman, and N. M. Svrakic, Temperley's triangular lattice compact cluster model: Exact solution in terms of the q series, *J. Phys. A* 20 (1987) L1275–L1280; MR 89b:82107.

[38] R. K. Guy, The strong law of small numbers, *Amer. Math. Monthly* 95 (1988) 697–712; MR 90c:11002.

[39] A. M. Odlyzko and H. S. Wilf, The editor's corner: n coins in a fountain, *Amer. Math. Monthly* 95 (1988) 840–843.

[40] A. M. Odlyzko, Asymptotic enumeration methods, *Handbook of Combinatorics*, v. I, ed. R. Graham, M. Grötschel, and L. Lovász, MIT Press, 1995, pp. 1063–1229; MR 97b:05012.

[41] V. Privman and N. M. Svrakic, Difference equations in statistical mechanics. I: Cluster statistics models, *J. Stat. Phys.* 51 (1988) 1091–1110; MR 89i:82079.

5.20 Longest Subsequence Constants

5.20.1 Increasing Subsequences

Let π denote a random permutation on the symbols $1, 2, \ldots, N$. An **increasing subsequence** of π is a sequence $(\pi(j_1), \pi(j_2), \ldots, \pi(j_k))$ satisfying both $1 \leq j_1 < j_2 < \ldots < j_k \leq N$ and $\pi(j_1) < \pi(j_2) < \ldots < \pi(j_k)$. Define L_N to be the length of the longest increasing subsequence of π. For example, the permutation $\pi = (2, 7, 4, 1, 6, 3, 9, 5, 8)$ has longest increasing subsequences $(2, 4, 6, 9)$ and $(1, 3, 5, 8)$; hence $L_9 = 4$. What can be said about the probability distribution of L_N (e.g., its mean and variance) as $N \rightarrow \infty$?

This question has inspired an avalanche of research [1–4]. Vershik & Kerov [5] and Logan & Shepp [6] proved that

$$\lim_{N \to \infty} N^{-\frac{1}{2}} \, \mathrm{E}(L_N) = 2,$$

building upon earlier work in [7–10]. Odlyzko & Rains [11] conjectured in 1993 that both limits

$$\lim_{N \to \infty} N^{-\frac{1}{3}} \, \mathrm{Var}(L_N) = c_0, \quad \lim_{N \to \infty} N^{-\frac{1}{6}} (\mathrm{E}(L_N) - 2\sqrt{N}) = c_1$$

exist and are finite and nonzero; numerical approximations were computed via Monte Carlo simulation. In a showcase of analysis (using methods from mathematical physics), Baik, Deift & Johansson [12] obtained

$$c_0 = 0.81318\ldots \text{ (i.e., } \sqrt{c_0} = 0.90177\ldots), \quad c_1 = -1.77109\ldots,$$

confirming the predictions in [11]. These constants are defined exactly in terms of the solution to a Painlevé II equation. (Incidently, Painlevé III arises in [5.22] and Painlevé V arises in [2.15.3].) The derivation involves a relationship between random matrices and random permutations [13, 14]. More precisely, Tracy & Widom [15–17] derived a certain probability distribution function $F(x)$ characterizing the largest eigenvalue of a random Hermitian matrix, generated according to the Gaussian Unitary Ensemble (GUE) probability law. Baik, Deift & Johansson proved that the limiting distribution of L_N is Tracy & Widom's $F(x)$, and then obtained estimates of the constants c_0 and c_1 via moments quoted in [16].

Before presenting more details, we provide a generalization. A **2-increasing subsequence** of π is a union of two disjoint increasing subsequences of π. Define $\tilde{L}_N$ to be the length of the longest 2-increasing subsequence of π, minus L_N. For example, the permutation $\pi = (2, 4, 7, 9, 5, 1, 3, 6, 8)$ has longest increasing subsequence $(2, 4, 5, 6, 8)$ and longest 2-increasing subsequence $(2, 4, 7, 9) \cup (1, 3, 6, 8)$; hence $\tilde{L}_9 = 8 - 5 = 3$. As before, both

$$\lim_{N \to \infty} N^{-\frac{1}{3}} \, \mathrm{Var}(\tilde{L}_N) = \tilde{c}_0, \quad \lim_{N \to \infty} N^{-\frac{1}{6}} (\mathrm{E}(\tilde{L}_N) - 2\sqrt{N}) = \tilde{c}_1$$

exist and can be proved [18] to possess values

$$\tilde{c}_0 = 0.5405\ldots, \quad \tilde{c}_1 = -3.6754\ldots.$$

The corresponding distribution function $\tilde{F}(x)$ characterizes the second-largest eigenvalue of a random Hermitian matrix under GUE. Such proofs were extended to m-increasing subsequences, for arbitrary $m > 2$, and to the joint distribution of row lengths from random Young tableaux in [19–21].

Here are the promised details [12, 18]. Fix $0 < t \leq 1$. Let $q_t(x)$ be the solution of the Painlevé II differential equation

$$q_t''(x) = 2q_t(x)^3 + xq_t(x), \quad q_t(x) \sim \frac{1}{2}\left(\frac{t}{\pi}\right)^{\frac{1}{2}} x^{-\frac{1}{4}} \exp\left(-\frac{2}{3}x^{\frac{3}{2}}\right) \text{ as } x \to \infty,$$

and define

$$\Phi(x, t) = \exp\left[-\int_x^\infty (y - x)q_t(y)^2 dy\right].$$

The Tracy-Widom functions are

$$F(x) = \Phi(x, 1), \quad \tilde{F}(x) = \Phi(x, 1) - \frac{\partial\Phi}{\partial t}(x, t)\bigg|_{t=1}$$

and hence

$$c_0 = \int_{-\infty}^\infty x^2 F'(x)dx - \left(\int_{-\infty}^\infty xF'(x)dx\right)^2, \quad c_1 = \int_{-\infty}^\infty xF'(x)dx,$$

$$\tilde{c}_0 = \int_{-\infty}^\infty x^2 \tilde{F}'(x)dx - \left(\int_{-\infty}^\infty x\tilde{F}'(x)dx\right)^2, \quad \tilde{c}_1 = \int_{-\infty}^\infty x\tilde{F}'(x)dx$$

are the required formulas. Note that the values of c_0, c_1, $\tilde{c}_0$, and $\tilde{c}_1$ appear in the caption of Figure 2 of [16]. Hence these arguably should be called Odlyzko–Rains–Tracy–Widom constants.

What makes this work especially exciting [1, 22] is its connection with the common cardgame of solitaire (for which no successful analysis has yet been performed) and possibly with the unsolved Riemann hypothesis [1.6] from prime number theory. See [23, 24] for other applications.

5.20.2 Common Subsequences

Let a and b be random sequences of length n, with terms a_i and b_j taking values from the alphabet $\{0, 1, \ldots, k - 1\}$. A sequence c is a **common subsequence** of a and b if c is a subsequence of both a and b, meaning that c is obtained from a by deleting zero or more terms a_i and from b by deleting zero or more terms b_j. Define $\lambda_{n,k}$ to be the length of the longest common subsequence of a and b. For example, the sequences $a = (1, 0, 0, 2, 3, 2, 1, 1, 0, 2)$, $b = (0, 1, 1, 1, 3, 3, 3, 0, 2, 1)$ have longest common subsequence $c = (0, 1, 1, 0, 2)$ and $\lambda_{10,3} = 5$. What can be said about the mean of $\lambda_{n,k}$ as $n \to \infty$, as a function of k?

It can be proved that $E(\lambda_{n,k})$ is superadditive with respect to n, that is, $E(\lambda_{m,k}) + E(\lambda_{n,k}) \leq E(\lambda_{m+n,k})$. Hence, by Fekete's theorem [25, 26], the limit

$$\gamma_k = \lim_{n\to\infty} \frac{E(\lambda_{n,k})}{n} = \sup_n \frac{E(\lambda_{n,k})}{n}$$

Table 5.5. *Estimates for Ratios* γ_k

k	Lower Bound	Numerical Estimate	Upper Bound
2	0.77391	0.8118	0.83763
3	0.63376	0.7172	0.76581
4	0.55282	0.6537	0.70824
5	0.50952	0.6069	0.66443

exists. Beginning with Chvátal & Sankoff [27–30], a number of researchers [31–37] have investigated γ_k. Table 5.5 contains rigorous lower and upper bounds for γ_k, as well as the best numerical estimates of γ_k presently available [37].

It is known [27, 31] that $1 \leq \gamma_k \sqrt{k} \leq e$ for all k and conjectured [38] that $\lim_{k\to\infty} \gamma_k \sqrt{k} = 2$. There is interest in the rate of convergence of the limiting ratio [39–41]

$$\gamma_k \, n - O(\sqrt{n \ln(n)}) \leq E(\lambda_{n,k}) \leq \gamma_k \, n$$

as well as in $\text{Var}(\lambda_{n,k})$, which is conjectured [39, 41, 42] to grow linearly with n.

A sequence c is a **common supersequence** of a and b if c is a supersequence of both a and b, meaning that both a and b are subsequences of c. The shortest common subsequence length $\Lambda_{n,k}$ of a and b can be shown [34, 43, 44] to satisfy

$$\lim_{n\to\infty} \frac{E(\Lambda_{n,k})}{n} = 2 - \gamma_k.$$

Such nice duality as this fails, however, if we seek longest subsequences/shortest supersequences from a set of > 2 random sequences.

[1] D. Aldous and P. Diaconis, Longest increasing subsequences: From patience sorting to the Baik-Deift-Johansson theorem, *Bull. Amer. Math. Soc.* 36 (1999) 413–432; MR 2000g:60013.

[2] P. Deift, Integrable systems and combinatorial theory, *Notices Amer. Math. Soc.* 47 (2000) 631–640; MR 2001g:05012.

[3] C. A. Tracy and H. Widom, Universality of the distribution functions of random matrix theory, *Integrable Systems: From Classical to Quantum*, Proc. 1999 Montréal conf., ed. J. Harnad, G. Sabidussi, and P. Winternitz, Amer. Math. Soc, 2000, pp. 251–264; math-ph/9909001; MR 2002f:15036.

[4] R. P. Stanley, Recent progress in algebraic combinatorics, presentation at *Mathematical Challenges for the 21st Century* conf., Los Angeles, 2000; *Bull. Amer. Math. Soc.*, to appear; math.CO/0010218.

[5] A. M. Vershik and S. V. Kerov, Asymptotic behavior of the Plancherel measure of the symmetric group and the limit form of Young tableaux (in Russian), *Dokl. Akad. Nauk SSSR* 233 (1977) 1024–1027; Engl. transl. in *Soviet Math. Dokl.* 233 (1977) 527–531; MR 58 #562.

[6] B. F. Logan and L. A. Shepp, A variational problem for random Young tableaux, *Adv. Math.* 26 (1977) 206–222; MR 98e:05108.

[7] S. M. Ulam, Monte Carlo calculations in problems of mathematical physics, *Modern Mathematics for the Engineer: Second Series*, ed. E. F. Beckenbach, McGraw-Hill, 1961, pp. 261–281; MR 23 #B2202.

[8] R. M. Baer and P. Brock, Natural sorting over permutation spaces, *Math. Comp.* 22 (1968) 385–410; MR 37 #3800.

[9] J. M. Hammersley, A few seedlings of research, *Proc. Sixth Berkeley Symp. Math. Stat. Probab.*, v. 1, ed. L. M. Le Cam, J. Neyman, and E. L. Scott, Univ. of Calif. Press, 1972, pp. 345–394; MR 53 #9457.

[10] J. F. C. Kingman, Subadditive ergodic theory, *Annals of Probab.* 1 (1973) 883–909; MR 50 #8663.

[11] A. M. Odlyzko and E. M. Rains, On longest increasing subsequences in random permutations, *Analysis, Geometry, Number Theory: The Mathematics of Leon Ehrenpreis*, Proc. 1998 Temple Univ. conf., ed. E. L. Grinberg, S. Berhanu, M. Knopp, G. Mendoza, and E. T. Quinto, Amer. Math. Soc., 2000, pp. 439–451; MR 2001d:05003.

[12] J. Baik, P. Deift, and K. Johansson, On the distribution of the length of the longest increasing subsequence of random permutations, *J. Amer. Math. Soc.* 12 (1999) 1119–1178; math.CO/9810105; MR 2000e:05006.

[13] C. A. Tracy and H. Widom, Random unitary matrices, permutations and Painlevé, *Commun. Math. Phys.* 207 (1999) 665–685; math.CO/9811154; MR 2001h:15019.

[14] E. M. Rains, Increasing subsequences and the classical groups, *Elec. J. Combin.* 5 (1998) R12; MR 98k:05146.

[15] C. A. Tracy and H. Widom, Level-spacing distributions and the Airy kernel, *Phys. Lett. B* 305 (1993) 115–118; hep-th/9210074; MR 94f:82046.

[16] C. A. Tracy and H. Widom, Level-spacing distributions and the Airy kernel, *Commun. Math. Phys.* 159 (1994) 151–174; hep-th/9211141; MR 95e:82003.

[17] C. A. Tracy and H. Widom, The distribution of the largest eigenvalue in the Gaussian ensembles: $\beta = 1, 2, 4$, *Calogero-Moser-Sutherland Models*, Proc. 1997 Montréal conf., ed. J. F. van Diejen and L. Vinet, Springer-Verlag, 2000, pp. 461–472; solv-int/9707001; MR 2002g:82021.

[18] J. Baik, P. Deift, and K. Johansson, On the distribution of the length of the second row of a Young diagram under Plancherel measure, *Geom. Func. Anal.* 10 (2000) 702–731; addendum 10 (2000) 1606–1607; math.CO/9901118; MR 2001m:05258.

[19] A. Okounkov, Random matrices and random permutations, *Int. Math. Res. Notices* (2000) 1043–1095; math.CO/9903176; MR 2002c:15045.

[20] A. Borodin, A. Okounkov, and G. Olshanski, Asymptotics of Plancherel measures for symmetric groups. *J. Amer. Math. Soc.* 13 (2000) 481–515; math.CO/9905032; MR 2001g:05103

[21] K. Johansson, Discrete orthogonal polynomial ensembles and the Plancherel measure, *Annals of Math.* 153 (2001) 259–296; math.CO/9906120; MR 2002g:05188.

[22] D. Mackenzie, From solitaire, a clue to the world of prime numbers, *Science* 282 (1998) 1631–1632; 283 (1999) 794–795.

[23] I. M. Johnstone, On the distribution of the largest principal component, *Annals of Statist.* 29 (2001) 295–327; Stanford Univ. Dept. of Statistics TR 2000-27.

[24] C. A. Tracy and H. Widom, A distribution function arising in computational biology, *MathPhys Odyssey 2001: Integrable Models and Beyond*, Proc. 2001 Okayama/Kyoto conf., ed. M. Kashiwara and T. Miwa, Birkhäuser, 2002, pp. 467–474; math.CO/0011146.

[25] M. Fekete, Über die Verteilung der Wurzeln bei gewissen algebraischen Gleichungen mit ganzzahligen Koeffizienten, *Math. Z.* 17 (1923) 228–249.

[26] G. Pólya and G. Szegö, *Problems and Theorems in Analysis*, v. 1, Springer-Verlag, 1972, ex. 98, pp. 23, 198; MR 81e:00002.

[27] V. Chvátal and D. Sankoff, Longest common subsequences of two random sequences, *J. Appl. Probab.* 12 (1975) 306–315; MR 53 #9324.

[28] V. Chvátal and D. Sankoff, An upper-bound technique for lengths of common subsequences, *Time Warps, String Edits, and Macromolecules: The Theory and Practice of Sequence Comparison*, ed. D. Sankoff and J. B. Kruskal, Addison-Wesley, 1983, pp. 353–357; MR 85h:68073.

[29] R. Durrett, *Probability: Theory and Examples*, Wadsworth, 1991, pp. 361–373; MR 91m:60002.

[30] I. Simon, Sequence comparison: Some theory and some practice, *Electronic Dictionaries and Automata in Computational Linguistics*, Proc. 1987 St. Pierre d'Oléron conf., ed. M. Gross and D. Perrin, Lect. Notes in Comp. Sci. 377, Springer-Verlag, 1987, pp. 79–92.

[31] J. G. Deken, Some limit results for longest common subsequences, *Discrete Math.* 26 (1979) 17–31; MR 80e:68100.

[32] J. G. Deken, Probabilistic behavior of longest-common-subsequence length, *Time Warps, String Edits, and Macromolecules*, ed. D. Sankoff and J. B. Kruskal, Addison-Wesley, 1983, pp. 359–362; MR 85h:68073.

[33] V. Dancik and M. S. Paterson, Upper bounds for the expected length of a longest common subsequence of two binary sequences, *Random Structures Algorithms* 6 (1995) 449–458; also in *Proc. 1994 Symp. on Theoretical Aspects of Computer Science (STACS)*, Caen, ed. P. Enjalbert, E. W. Mayr, and K. W. Wagner, Lect. Notes in Comp. Sci. 775, Springer-Verlag, 1994, pp. 669–678; MR 95g:68040 and MR 96h:05016.

[34] V. Dancik, *Expected Length of Longest Common Subsequences*, Ph.D. thesis, Univ. of Warwick, 1994.

[35] M. Paterson and V. Dancík, Longest common subsequences, *Mathematical Foundations of Computer Science (MFCS)*, Proc. 1994 Kosice conf., ed. I. Privara, B. Rovan, and P. Ruzicka, Lect. Notes in Comp. Sci. 841, Springer–Verlag, Berlin, 1994, pp. 127–142; MR 95k:68180.

[36] V. Dancík, Upper bounds for the expected length of longest common subsequences, unpublished note (1996); abstract in *Bull. EATCS* 54 (1994) 248.

[37] R. A. Baeza-Yates, R. Gavaldà, G. Navarro, and R. Scheihing, Bounding the expected length of longest common subsequences and forests, *Theory Comput. Sys.* 32 (1999) 435–452; also in *Proc. Third South American Workshop on String Processing (WSP)*, Recife, ed. R. Baeza-Yates, N. Ziviani, and K. Guimarães, Carleton Univ. Press, 1996, pp. 1–15; MR 2000k:68076.

[38] D. Sankoff and S. Mainville, Common subsequences and monotone subsequences, *Time Warps, String Edits, and Macromolecules*, ed. D. Sankoff and J. B. Kruskal, Addison-Wesley, 1983, pp. 363–365; MR 85h:68073.

[39] K. S. Alexander, The rate of convergence of the mean length of the longest common subsequence, *Annals of Appl. Probab.* 4 (1994) 1074–1082; MR 95k:60020.

[40] W. T. Rhee, On rates of convergence for common subsequences and first passage time, *Annals of Appl. Probab.* 5 (1995) 44–48; MR 96e:60023.

[41] J. Boutet de Monvel, Extensive simulations for longest common subsequences: Finite size scaling, a cavity solution, and configuration space properties, *Europ. Phys. J. B* 7 (1999) 293–308; cond-mat/9809280.

[42] M. S. Waterman, Estimating statistical significance of sequence alignments, *Philos. Trans. Royal Soc. London Ser. B* 344 (1994) 383–390.

[43] V. Dancik, Common subsequences and supersequences and their expected length, *Combin. Probab. Comput.* 7 (1998) 365–373; also in *Sixth Combinatorial Pattern Matching Symp. (CPM)*, Proc. 1995 Espoo conf., ed. Z. Galil and E. Ukkonen, Lect. Notes in Comp. Sci. 937, Springer-Verlag, 1995, pp. 55–63; MR 98e:68100 and MR 99m:05007.

[44] T. Jiang and M. Li, On the approximation of shortest common supersequences and longest common subsequences, *SIAM J. Comput.* 24 (1995) 1122–1139; also in *Proc. 1994 Int. Colloq. on Automata, Languages and Programming (ICALP)*, Jerusalem, ed. S. Abiteboul and E. Shamir, Lect. Notes in Comp. Sci. 820, Springer-Verlag, 1994, pp. 191–202; MR 97a:68081.

5.21 *k*-Satisfiability Constants

Let $x_1, x_2, \ldots, x_n$ be Boolean variables. Choose k elements randomly from the set $\{x_1, \neg x_1, x_2, \neg x_2, \ldots, x_n, \neg x_n\}$ under the restriction that x_j and $\neg x_j$ cannot both be selected. These k **literals** determine a **clause**, which is the disjunction ($\bigvee$, that is, "inclusive or") of the literals.

Perform this selection process m times. The m independent clauses determine a **formula**, which is the conjunction ($\bigwedge$, that is, "and") of the clauses. A sample formula, in the special case $n = 5$, $k = 3$, and $m = 4$, is

$$[x_1 \vee (\neg x_5) \vee (\neg x_2)] \wedge [(\neg x_3) \vee x_2 \vee (\neg x_1)] \wedge [x_5 \vee x_2 \vee x_4] \wedge [x_4 \vee (\neg x_3) \vee x_1].$$

A formula is **satisfiable** if there exists an assignment of 0s and 1s to the xs so that the formula is true (that is, has value 1). The design of efficient algorithms for discovering such an assignment, given a large formula, or for proving that the formula is **unsatisfiable**, is an important topic in theoretical computer science [1–3].

The k-satisfiability problem, or k-SAT, behaves differently for $k = 2$ and $k \geq 3$. For $k = 2$, the problem can be solved by a linear time algorithm, whereas for $k \geq 3$, the problem is NP-complete.

There is another distinction involving ideas from percolation theory [5.18]. As $m \to \infty$ and $n \to \infty$ with limiting ratio $m/n \to r$, empirical evidence suggests that the random k-SAT problem undergoes a phase transition at a critical value $r_c(k)$ of the parameter r. For $r < r_c$, a random formula is satisfiable with probability $\to 1$ as $m, n \to \infty$. For $r > r_c$, a random formula is likewise unsatisfiable almost surely. Away from the boundary, k-SAT is relatively easy to solve; computational difficulties appear to be maximized at the threshold $r = r_c$ itself. This observation may ultimately help in improving algorithms for solving the traveling salesman problem [8.5] and other combinatorial nightmares.

In the case of 2-SAT, it has been proved [4–6] that $r_c(2) = 1$. A rigorous understanding of 2-SAT from a statistical mechanical point-of-view was achieved in [7].

In the case of k-SAT, $k \geq 3$, comparatively little has been proved. Here is an inequality [4] valid for all $k \geq 3$:

$$\frac{3}{8} \frac{2^k}{k} \leq r_c(k) \leq \ln(2) \cdot \ln\left(\frac{2^k}{2^k - 1}\right)^{-1} \sim \ln(2) \cdot 2^k.$$

Many researchers have contributed to placing tight upper bounds [8–16] and lower bounds [17–20] on the 3-SAT threshold:

$$3.26 \leq r_c(3) \leq 4.506.$$

Large-scale computations [21–23] give an estimate $r_c(3) = 4.25\ldots$. Estimates for larger k [1] include $r_c(4) = 9.7\ldots$, $r_c(5) = 20.9\ldots$, and $r_c(6) = 43.2\ldots$, but these can be improved. Unlike 2-SAT, we do not yet possess a proof that $r_c(k)$ exists, for $k \geq 3$, but Friedgut [24] took an important step in this direction. Sharp phase transitions, corresponding to certain properties of random graphs, play an essential role in his paper. The possibility that $r_c(k)$ oscillates between the bounds $O(2^k/k)$ and $O(2^k)$ has not been completely ruled out, but this would be unexpected.

We mention a similar instance of threshold phenomena for random graphs. When $m \to \infty$ and $n \to \infty$ with limiting ratio $m/n \to s$, then in a random graph G on n vertices and with m edges, it appears that G is k-colorable with probability $\to 1$ for $s < s_c(k)$ and G is not k-colorable with probability $\to 1$ for $s > s_c(k)$. As before, the existence of $s_c(k)$ is only conjectured if $k \geq 3$, but we have bounds [25–33]

$$1.923 \leq s_c(3) \leq 2.495, \quad 2.879 \leq s_c(4) \leq 4.587,$$
$$3.974 \leq s_c(5) \leq 6.948, \quad 5.190 \leq s_c(6) \leq 9.539$$

and an estimate [34] $s_c(3) = 2.3$.

Consider also the discrete n-cube Q of vectors of the form $(\pm 1, \pm 1, \pm 1, \ldots, \pm 1)$. The **half cube** H_v generated by any $v \in Q$ is the set of all vectors $w \in Q$ having negative inner product with v. If a vector $u \in H_v$, it is natural to say that H_v **covers** u. Let $v_1, v_2, \ldots, v_m$ be drawn randomly from Q. When $m \to \infty$ and $n \to \infty$ with limiting ratio $m/n \to t$, it appears that $\bigcup_{k=1}^{m} H_{v_k}$ covers all of Q with probability $\to 1$ for $t > t_c$ but fails to do so with probability $\to 1$ for $t < t_c$. The existence of t_c was conjectured in [35] but a proof is not known. We have bounds [36, 37]

$$0.005 \leq t_c \leq 0.9963 = 1 - 0.0037$$

and an estimate [38, 39] $t_c = 0.82$. The motivation for studying this problem arises in binary neural networks.

Here is an interesting variation that encompasses both 2-SAT and 3-SAT. Fix a number $0 \leq p \leq 1$. When selecting m clauses at random, choose a 3-clause with probability p and a 2-clause with probability $1 - p$. This is known as $(2 + p)$-SAT and is useful in understanding the onset of complexity when moving from 2-SAT to 3-SAT [3, 40–42]. Clearly the critical value for this model satisfies

$$r_c(2 + p) \leq \min \left\{ \frac{1}{1 - p}, \frac{1}{p} r_c(3) \right\}$$

for all p. Further [43], if $p \leq 2/5$, then with probability $\to 1$, a random $(2 + p)$-SAT formula is satisfiable if and only if its 2-SAT subformula is satisfiable. This is a remarkable result: A random mixture containing 60% 2-clauses and 40% 3-clauses behaves like 2-SAT! Evidence for a conjecture that the critical threshold $p_c = 2/5$ appears in [44]. See also [45].

Another variation involves replacing "inclusive or" when forming clauses by "exclusive or." By way of contrast with k-SAT, $k \geq 3$, the XOR-SAT problem can be solved in polynomial time, and its transition from satisfiability to unsatisfiability is completely understood [46].

[1] S. Kirkpatrick and B. Selman, Critical behavior in the satisfiability of random Boolean expressions, *Science* 264 (1994) 1297–1301; MR 96e:68063.

[2] B. Hayes, Can't get no satisfaction, *Amer. Scientist*, v. 85 (1997) n. 2, 108–112.

[3] R. Monasson, R. Zecchina, S. Kirkpatrick, B. Selman, and L. Troyansky, Determining computational complexity from characteristic phase transitions, *Nature* 400 (1999) 133–137; MR 2000f:68055.

[4] V. Chvátal and B. Reed, Mick gets some (the odds are on his side), *Proc. 33rd Symp. on Foundations of Computer Science (FOCS)*, Pittsburgh, IEEE, 1992, pp. 620–627.

[5] A. Goerdt, A threshold for unsatisfiability, *J. Comput. Sys. Sci.* 53 (1996) 469–486; also in *Mathematical Foundations of Computer Science (MFCS)*, Proc. 1992 Prague conf., ed. I. M. Havel and V. Koubek, Lect. Notes in Comp. Sci. 629, Springer-Verlag, 1992, pp. 264–274; MR 94j:03011 and MR 98i:03012.

[6]   W. Fernandez de la Vega, On random 2-SAT, unpublished note (1992).

[7]   B. Bollobás, C. Borgs, J. T. Chayes, J. H. Kim, and D. B. Wilson, The scaling window of the 2-SAT transition, *Random Structures Algorithms* 18 (2001) 201–256; MR 2002a:68052.

[8]   J. Franco and M. Paull, Probabilistic analysis of the Davis-Putnam procedure for solving the satisfiability problem, *Discrete Appl. Math.* 5 (1983) 77–87; correction 17 (1987) 295–299; MR 84e:68038 and MR 88e:68050.

[9]   A. Z. Broder, A. M. Frieze, and E. Upfal, On the satisfiability and maximum satisfiability of random 3-CNF formulas, *Proc. 4th ACM-SIAM Symp. on Discrete Algorithms (SODA)*, Austin, ACM, 1993, pp. 322–330; MR 94b:03023.

[10] A. El Maftouhi and W. Fernandez de la Vega, On random 3-SAT, *Combin. Probab. Comput.* 4 (1995) 189–195; MR 96f:03007.

[11] A. Kamath, R. Motwani, K. Palem, and P. Spirakis, Tail bounds for occupancy and the satisfiability threshold conjecture, *Random Structures Algorithms* 7 (1995) 59–80; MR 97b:68091.

[12] L. M. Kirousis, E. Kranakis, D. Krizanc, and Y. C. Stamatiou, Approximating the unsatisfiability threshold of random formulas, *Random Structures Algorithms* 12 (1998) 253–269; MR 2000c:68069.

[13] O. Dubois and Y. Boufkhad, A general upper bound for the satisfiability threshold of random r-SAT formulae, *J. Algorithms* 24 (1997) 395–420; MR 98e:68103.

[14] S. Janson, Y. C. Stamatiou, and M. Vamvakari, Bounding the unsatisfiability threshold of random 3-SAT, *Random Structures Algorithms* 17 (2000) 103–116; erratum 18 (2001) 99–100; MR 2001c:68065 and MR 2001m:68064.

[15] A. C. Kaporis, L. M. Kirousis, Y. C. Stamatiou, M. Vamvakari, and M. Zito, Coupon collectors, q-binomial coefficients and the unsatisfiability threshold, *Seventh Italian Conf. on Theoretical Computer Science (ICTCS)*, Proc. 2001 Torino conf., ed. A. Restivo, S. Ronchi Della Rocca, and L. Roversi, Lect. Notes in Comp. Sci. 2202, Springer-Verlag, 2001, pp. 328–338.

[16] O. Dubois, Y. Boufkhad, and J. Mandler, Typical random 3-SAT formulae and the satisfiability threshold, *Proc. 11th ACM-SIAM Symp. on Discrete Algorithms (SODA)*, San Francisco, ACM, 2000, pp. 126–127.

[17] M.-T. Chao and J. Franco, Probabilistic analysis of two heuristics for the 3-satisfiability problem, *SIAM J. Comput.* 15 (1986) 1106–1118; MR 88b:68079.

[18] A. Frieze and S. Suen, Analysis of two simple heuristics on a random instance of k-SAT, *J. Algorithms* 20 (1996) 312–355; MR 97c:68062.

[19] D. Achlioptas, Setting 2 variables at a time yields a new lower bound for random 3-SAT, *Proc. 32nd ACM Symp. on Theory of Computing (STOC)*, Portland, ACM, 2000, pp. 28–37.

[20] D. Achlioptas and G. B Sorkin, Optimal myopic algorithms for random 3-SAT, *Proc. 41st Symp. on Foundations of Computer Science (FOCS)*, Redondo Beach, IEEE, 2000, pp. 590–600.

[21] T. Larrabee and Y. Tsuji, Evidence for a satisfiability threshold for random 3CNF formulas, presentation at *AAAI Spring Symp. on AI and NP-Hard Problems*, Palo Alto, 1993; Univ. of Calif. at Santa Cruz Tech. Report UCSC-CRL-92-42.

[22] B. Selman, D. G. Mitchell, and H. J. Levesque, Generating hard satisfiability problems, *Artificial Intellig.* 81 (1996) 17–29; Hard and easy distributions of SAT problems, *Proc. Tenth Nat. Conf. on Artificial Intelligence*, San Jose, AAAI Press, 1992, pp. 459–465; MR 98b:03013.

[23] J. M. Crawford and L. D. Auton, Experimental results on the crossover point in random 3-SAT, *Artificial Intellig.* 81 (1996) 31–57; also in *Proc. Eleventh Nat. Conf. on Artificial Intelligence,* Washington DC, AAAI Press, 1993, pp. 21–27; MR 97d:03055.

[24] E. Friedgut, Sharp thresholds of graph properties, and the k-SAT problem (appendix by J. Bourgain), *J. Amer. Math. Soc.* 12 (1999) 1017–1054; MR 2000a:05183.

[25] T. Luczak, Size and connectivity of the k-core of a random graph, *Discrete Math.* 91 (1991) 61–68; MR 92m:05171.

[26] V. Chvátal, Almost all graphs with $1.44n$ edges are 3-colorable, *Random Structures Algorithms* 2 (1991) 11–28; MR 92c:05056.

[27] M. Molloy and B. Reed, A critical point for random graphs with a given degree sequence, *Random Structures Algorithms* 6 (1995) 161–179; MR 97a:05191.

[28] B. Pittel, J. Spencer, and N. Wormald, Sudden emergence of a giant k-core in a random graph, *J. Combin. Theory Ser. B* 67 (1996) 111–151; MR 97e:05176.

[29] M. Molloy, A gap between the appearances of a k-core and a $(k + 1)$-chromatic graph, *Random Structures Algorithms* 8 (1996) 159–160.

[30] D. Achlioptas and M. Molloy, The analysis of a list-coloring algorithm on a random graph, *Proc. 38th Symp. on Foundations of Computer Science (FOCS)*, Miami Beach, IEEE, 1997, pp. 204–212.

[31] P. E. Dunne and M. Zito, An improved upper bound on the non-3-colourability threshold, *Inform. Process. Lett.* 65 (1998) 17–23; MR 98i:05073.

[32] D. Achlioptas and M. Molloy, Almost all graphs with $2.522n$ edges are not 3-colorable, *Elec. J. Combin.* 6 (1999) R29; MR 2000e:05140.

[33] A. C. Kaporis, L. M. Kirousis, and Y. C. Stamatiou, A note on the non-colorability threshold of a random graph, *Elec. J. Combin.* 7 (2000) R29; MR 2001e:05116.

[34] T. Hogg and C. P. Williams, The hardest constraint problems: A double phase transition, *Artificial Intellig.* 69 (1994) 359–377.

[35] E. Gardner, Maximum storage capacity in neural networks, *Europhys. Lett.* 4 (1987) 481–485.

[36] J. H. Kim and J. R. Roche, Covering cubes by random half cubes, with applications to binary neural networks, *J. Comput. Sys. Sci.* 56 (1998) 223–252; MR 2000g:68129.

[37] M. Talagrand, Intersecting random half cubes, *Random Structures Algorithms* 15 (1999) 436–449; MR 2000i:60011.

[38] W. Krauth and M. Opper, Critical storage capacity of the $J = \pm 1$ neural network, *J. Phys. A* 22 (1989) L519–L523.

[39] W. Krauth and M. Mézard, Storage capacity of memory networks with binary couplings, *J. Physique* 50 (1989) 3057–3066.

[40] R. Monasson and R. Zecchina, The entropy of the k-satisfiability problem, *Phys. Rev. Lett.* 76 (1996) 3881–3885; cond-mat/9603014; MR 97a:82053.

[41] R. Monasson and R. Zecchina, Statistical mechanics of the random k-satisfiability model, *Phys. Rev. E* 56 (1997) 1357–1370; MR 98g:82022.

[42] R. Monasson, R. Zecchina, S. Kirkpatrick, B. Selman, and L. Troyansky, $(2 + p)$-SAT: Relation of typical-case complexity to the nature of the phase transition, *Random Structures Algorithms* 15 (1999) 414–435; cond-mat/9910080; MR 2000i:68076.

[43] D. Achlioptas, L. M. Kirousis, E. Kranakis, and D. Krizanc, Rigorous results for $(2 + p)$-SAT, *Theoret. Comput. Sci.* 265 (2001) 109–129; MR 2002g:68047.

[44] G. Biroli, R. Monasson, and M. Weigt, A variational description of the ground state structure in random satisfiability problems, *Europ. Phys. J. B* 14 (2000) 551–568; cond-mat/9907343.

[45] I. Gent and T. Walsh, The SAT phase transition, *Proc. 11th European Conf. on Artificial Intelligence (ECAI)*, Amsterdam, Wiley, 1994, pp. 105–109.

[46] C. Creignou and H. Daudé, Satisfiability threshold for random XOR-CNF formulas, *Discrete Appl. Math.* 96–97 (1999) 41–53; MR 2000i:68072.

5.22 Lenz–Ising Constants

The Ising model is concerned with the physics of phase transitions, for example, the tendency of a magnet to lose strength as it is heated, with total loss occurring above a certain finite critical temperature. This essay can barely introduce the subject. Unlike hard squares [5.12] and percolation clusters [5.18], a concise complete problem statement here is not possible. We are concerned with large arrays of 1s and -1s whose joint distribution passes through a singularity as a parameter T increases. The definition and characterization of the joint distribution is elaborate; our treatment is combinatorial and focuses on series expansions. See [1–10] for background.

Let L denote the regular d-dimensional cubic lattice with $N = n^d$ sites. For example, in two dimensions, L is the $n \times n$ square lattice with $N = n^2$. To eliminate boundary effects, L is wrapped around to form a d-dimensional torus so that, without exception, every site has $2d$ nearest neighbors. This convention leads to negligible error for large N.

5.22.1 Low-Temperature Series Expansions

Suppose that the N sites of L are colored black or white at random. The dN edges of L fall into three categories: black-black, black-white, and white-white. What can be said jointly about the relative numbers of these? Over all possible such colorings, let $A(p, q)$ be the number of colorings for which there are exactly p black sites and exactly q black-white edges. (See Figure 5.20.)

Then, for large enough N [11–14],

$$
\begin{array}{ll}
A(0, 0) = 1 & \text{(all white),} \\
A(1, 2d) = N & \text{(one black),} \\
A(2, 4d - 2) = dN & \text{(two black, adjacent),} \\
A(2, 4d) = \frac{1}{2}(N - 2d - 1)N & \text{(two black, not adjacent),} \\
A(3, 6d - 4) = (2d - 1)dN & \text{(three black, adjacent).}
\end{array}
$$

Properties of this sequence can be studied via the bivariate generating function

$$
a(x, y) = \sum_{p,q} A(p, q)x^p y^q
$$

and the formal power series

$$
\alpha(x, y) = \lim_{n \to \infty} \frac{1}{N} \ln(a(x, y))
$$

$$
= xy^{2d} + dx^2 y^{4d-2} - \frac{2d + 1}{2}x^2 y^{4d} + (2d - 1)dx^3 y^{6d-4} + \cdots
$$

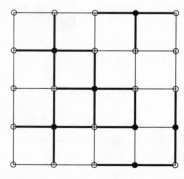

Figure 5.20. Sample coloring with $d = 2$, $N = 25$, $p = 7$, and $q = 21$ (ignoring wraparound).

obtained by merely collecting the coefficients that are linear in N. The latter is sometimes written as [15]

$$\exp(\alpha(x, y)) = 1 + xy^{2d} + dx^2y^{4d-2} - dx^2y^{4d} + (2d-1)dx^3y^{6d-4} + \cdots,$$

a series whose coefficients are integers only. This is what physicists call the **low-
temperature series** for the **Ising free energy per site**. The letters x and y are not
dummy variables but are related to temperature and magnetic field; the series $\alpha(x, y)$ is
not merely a mathematical construct but is a thermodynamic function with properties
that can be measured against physical experiment [16]. In the special case when $x = 1$,
known as the **zero magnetic field case**, we write $\alpha(y) = \alpha(1, y)$ for convenience.

When $d = 2$, we have [11, 17]

$$\exp(\alpha(y)) = 1 + y^4 + 2y^6 + 5y^8 + 14y^{10} + 44y^{12} + 152y^{14} + 566y^{16} + \cdots.$$

Onsager [18–23] discovered an astonishing closed-form expression:

$$\alpha(y) = \frac{1}{2} \int\limits_0^1 \int\limits_0^1 \ln\left[(1 + y^2)^2 - 2y(1 - y^2)(\cos(2\pi u) + \cos(2\pi v))\right] du\, dv$$

that permits computation of series coefficients to arbitrary order [24] and much more.

When $d = 3$, we have [11, 25–30]

$$\exp(\alpha(y)) = 1 + y^6 + 3y^{10} - 3y^{12} + 15y^{14} - 30y^{16} + 101y^{18} - 261y^{16} + - \cdots$$

No closed-form expression for this series has been found, and the required computations
are much more involved than those for $d = 2$.

5.22.2 High-Temperature Series Expansions

The associated high-temperature series arises via a seemingly unrelated combinatorial
problem. Let us assume that a nonempty *subgraph* of L is connected and contains at
least one edge. Suppose that several subgraphs are drawn on L with the property that

- each edge of L is used at most once, and
- each site of L is used an *even* number of times (possibly zero).

Call such a configuration on L an **even polygonal drawing**. (See Figure 5.21.) An even
polygonal drawing is the union of simple, closed, edge-disjoint polygons that need not
be connected.

Let $B(r)$ be the number of even polygonal drawings for which there are exactly r
edges. Then, for large enough N [4, 11, 31],

$$B(4) = \tfrac{1}{2}d(d-1)N \qquad\qquad \text{(square)},$$
$$B(6) = \tfrac{1}{3}d(d-1)(8d-13)N \qquad\qquad \text{(two squares, adjacent)},$$
$$B(8) = \tfrac{1}{8}d(d-1)\left(d(d-1)N + 216d^2 - 848d + 850\right)N \quad \text{(many possibilities)}.$$

On the one hand, for $d \geq 3$, the drawings can intertwine and be knotted [32], so computing $B(r)$ for larger r is quite complicated! On the other hand, for $d = 2$, clearly

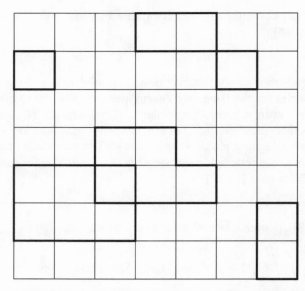

Figure 5.21. An even polygonal drawing for $d = 2$; other names include closed or Eulerian subgraph.

$B(q) = \sum_p A(p, q)$ always. As before, we define a (univariate) generating function

$$b(z) = 1 + \sum_r B(r)z^r$$

and a formal power series

$$\beta(z) = \lim_{n \to \infty} \frac{1}{N} \ln(b(z))$$
$$= \frac{1}{2}d(d - 1)z^4 + \frac{1}{3}d(d - 1)(8d - 13)z^6 + \frac{1}{4}d(d - 1)(108d^2 - 424d + 425)z^8$$
$$+ \frac{2}{15}d(d - 1)(2976d^3 - 19814d^2 + 44956d - 34419)z^{10} + \cdots$$

called the **high-temperature zero-field series** for the **Ising free energy**. When $d = 3$ [11, 25, 29, 33–36],

$$\exp(\beta(z)) = 1 + 3z^4 + 22z^6 + 192z^8 + 2046z^{10} + 24853z^{12} + 329334z^{14} + \cdots,$$

but again our knowledge of the series coefficients is limited.

5.22.3 Phase Transitions in Ferromagnetic Models

The two major unsolved problems connected to the Ising model are [4, 31, 37]:

- Find a closed-form expression for $\alpha(x, y)$ when $d = 2$.
- Find a closed-form expression for $\beta(z)$ when $d = 3$.

Why are these so important? We discuss now the underlying physics, as well its relationship to the aforementioned combinatorial problems.

Place a bar of iron in an external magnetic field at constant absolute temperature T. The field will induce a certain amount of magnetization into the bar. If the external field is then slowly turned off, we empirically observe that, for small T, the bar retains some of its internal magnetization, but for large T, the bar's internal magnetization disappears completely.

There is a unique **critical temperature**, T_c, also called the **Curie point**, where this qualitative change in behavior occurs. The Ising model is a simple means for explaining the physical phenomena from a microscopic point of view.

At each site of the lattice L, define a "spin variable" $\sigma_i = 1$ if site i is "up" and $\sigma_i = -1$ if site i is "down." This is known as the **spin-1/2 model**. We study the **partition function**

$$Z(T) = \sum_{\sigma} \exp\left[\frac{1}{\kappa T} \left(\sum_{(i,j)} \xi \sigma_i \sigma_j + \sum_k \eta \sigma_k \right) \right],$$

where ξ is the coupling (or interaction) constant between nearest neighbor spin variables, $\eta \geq 0$ is the intensity constant of the external magnetic field, and $\kappa > 0$ is Boltzmann's constant.

The function $Z(T)$ captures all of the thermodynamic features of the physical system and acts as a kind of "denominator" when calculating state probabilities. Observe that the first summation is over all 2^N possible values of the vector $\sigma = (\sigma_1, \sigma_2, \ldots, \sigma_N)$ and the second summation is over all edges of the lattice (sites i and j are distinct and adjacent). Henceforth we will assume $\xi > 0$, which corresponds to the **ferromagnetic case**. A somewhat different theory emerges in the antiferromagnetic case ($\xi < 0$), which we will not discuss.

How is Z connected to the combinatorial problems discussed earlier? If we assign a spin 1 to the color white and a spin -1 to the color black, then

$$\sum_{(i,j)} \sigma_i \sigma_j = (dN - q) \cdot 1 + q \cdot (-1) = dN - 2q,$$

$$\sum_k \sigma_k = (N - p) \cdot 1 + p \cdot (-1) = N - 2p,$$

and therefore

$$Z = x^{-\frac{1}{2}N} y^{-\frac{d}{2}N} a(x, y),$$

where

$$x = \exp\left(-\frac{2\eta}{\kappa T} \right), \quad y = \exp\left(-\frac{2\xi}{\kappa T} \right).$$

Since small T gives small values of x and y, the phrase low-temperature series for $\alpha(x, y)$ is justified. (Observe that $T = \infty$ corresponds to the case when lattice site colorings are assigned equal probability, which is precisely the combinatorial problem described earlier. The range $0 < T < \infty$ corresponds to unequal weighting, accentuating the states with small p and q. The point $T = 0$ corresponds to an ideal case when all spins are aligned; heat introduces disorder into the system.)

For the high-temperature case, rewrite Z as

$$Z = \left(\frac{4}{(1-z^2)^d(1-w^2)}\right)^{\frac{N}{2}} \frac{1}{2^N} \sum_\sigma \left(\prod_{(i,j)}(1 + \sigma_i\sigma_j z) \cdot \prod_k (1 + \sigma_k w)\right),$$

where

$$z = \tanh\left(\frac{\xi}{\kappa T}\right), \quad w = \tanh\left(\frac{\eta}{\kappa T}\right).$$

In the zero-field scenario ($\eta = 0$), this expression simplifies to

$$Z = \left(\frac{4}{(1-z^2)^d}\right)^{\frac{N}{2}} b(z),$$

and since large T gives small z, the phraseology again makes sense.

5.22.4 Critical Temperature

We turn attention to some interesting constants. The radius of convergence y_c in the complex plane of the low-temperature series $\alpha(y) = \sum_{k=0}^\infty \alpha_k y^k$ is given by [29]

$$y_c = \lim_{k\to\infty} |\alpha_{2k}|^{-\frac{1}{2k}} = \begin{cases} \sqrt{2} - 1 = 0.4142135623\ldots & \text{if } d = 2, \\ \sqrt{0.2853\ldots} = 0.5341\ldots & \text{if } d = 3; \end{cases}$$

hence, if $d = 2$, the ferromagnetic critical temperature T_c satisfies

$$K_c = \frac{\xi}{\kappa T_c} = \frac{1}{2}\ln\left(\frac{1}{y_c}\right) = \frac{1}{2}\ln(\sqrt{2} + 1) = 0.4406867935\ldots.$$

The two-dimensional result is a famous outcome of work by Kramers & Wannier [38] and Onsager [18]. For $d = 3$, the singularity at $y^2 = -0.2853\ldots$ is nonphysical and thus is not relevant to ferromagnetism; a second singularity at $y^2 = 0.412048\ldots$ is what we want but it is difficult to compute directly [29, 39]. To accurately obtain the critical temperature here, we examine instead the high-temperature series $\beta(z) = \sum_{k=0}^\infty \beta_k z^k$ and compute

$$z_c = \lim_{k\to\infty} \beta_{2k}^{-\frac{1}{2k}} = 0.218094\ldots, \quad K_c = \frac{1}{2}\ln\left(\frac{1+z_c}{1-z_c}\right) = 0.221654\ldots.$$

There is a huge literature of series and Monte Carlo analyses leading to this estimate [40–53]. (A conjectured exact expression for z_c in [54] appears to be false [55].) For $d > 3$, the following estimates are known [56–65]:

$$z_c = \begin{cases} 0.14855\ldots & \text{if } d = 4, \\ 0.1134\ldots & \text{if } d = 5, \\ 0.0920\ldots & \text{if } d = 6, \\ 0.0775\ldots & \text{if } d = 7, \end{cases} \quad K_c = \begin{cases} 0.14966\ldots & \text{if } d = 4, \\ 0.1139\ldots & \text{if } d = 5, \\ 0.0923\ldots & \text{if } d = 6, \\ 0.0777\ldots & \text{if } d = 7. \end{cases}$$

An associated critical exponent γ will be discussed shortly.

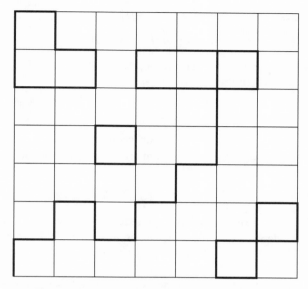

Figure 5.22. An odd polygonal drawing for $d = 2$.

5.22.5 Magnetic Susceptibility

Here is another combinatorial problem. Suppose that several subgraphs are drawn on L with the property that

- each edge of L is used at most once,
- all sites of L, except two, are even, and
- the two remaining sites are odd and must lie in the same (connected) subgraph.

Call this configuration an **odd polygonal drawing**. (See Figure 5.22.) Note that an odd polygonal drawing is the edge-disjoint union of an even polygonal drawing and an (undirected) self-avoiding walk [5.10] linking the two odd sites.

Let $C(r)$ be twice the number of odd polygonal drawings for which there are exactly r edges. Then, for large enough N [12, 66],

$$
\begin{aligned}
C(1) &= 2dN & \text{(SAW)}, \\
C(2) &= 2d(2d-1)N & \text{(SAW)}, \\
C(3) &= 2d(2d-1)^2N & \text{(SAW)}, \\
C(4) &= 2d\left(2d(2d-1)^3 - 2d(2d-2)\right)N & \text{(SAW)}, \\
C(5) &= d^2(d-1)N^2 + 2d\left(16d^4 - 32d^3 + 16d^2 + 4d - 3\right)N & \text{(square and/or SAW)}.
\end{aligned}
$$

As before, we may define a generating function and a formal power series

$$
c(z) = N + \sum_r C(r)z^r, \quad \chi(z) = \lim_{n \to \infty} \frac{1}{N} \ln(c(z)) = \sum_{k=0}^{\infty} \chi_k z^k,
$$

which is what physicists call the **high-temperature zero-field series** for the **Ising magnetic susceptibility per site**. The radius of convergence z_c of $\chi(z)$ is the same as that for $\beta(z)$ for $d > 1$. For example, when $d = 3$, analyzing the series [67–73]

$$\chi(z) = 1 + 6z + 30z^2 + 150z^3 + 726z^4 + 3510z^5 + 16710z^6 + \cdots$$

is the preferred way to obtain critical parameter estimates (being the best behaved of several available series). Further, the limit

$$\lim_{k \to \infty} \frac{\chi_k}{z_c^{-k} k^{\gamma - 1}}$$

appears to exist and is nonzero for a certain positive constant γ depending on dimensionality. As an example, if $d = 2$, numerical evidence surrounding the series [67, 74, 75]

$$\chi(z) = 1 + 4z + 12z^2 + 36z^3 + 100z^4 + 276z^5 + 740z^6 + 1972z^7 + 5172z^8 + \cdots$$

suggests that the **critical susceptibility exponent** γ is $7/4$ and that γ is *universal* (in the sense that it is independent of the choice of lattice). No analogous exact expressions appear to be valid for γ when $d \geq 3$; for $d = 3$, the consensus is that $\gamma = 1.238\ldots$ [40, 44, 46, 49–52, 71, 73].

We finally make explicit the association of $\chi(z)$ with the Ising model [76]:

$$\lim_{n \to \infty} \frac{1}{N} \ln(Z(z, w)) = \ln(2) - \frac{d}{2} \ln(1 - z^2) - \frac{1}{2} \ln(1 - w^2) + \beta(z)$$

$$+ \frac{1}{2} (\chi(z) - 1) w^2 + O(w^4),$$

where the big O depends on z. Therefore $\chi(z)$ occurs when evaluating a second derivative with respect to w, specifically, when computing the variance of P (defined momentarily).

5.22.6 Q and P Moments

Let us return to the random coloring problem, suitably generalized to incorporate temperature. Let

$$Q = d - \frac{2}{N} q = \frac{1}{N} \sum_{(i,j)} \sigma_i \sigma_j, \quad P = 1 - \frac{2}{N} p = \frac{1}{N} \sum_k \sigma_k$$

for convenience and assume henceforth that $d = 2$. To study the asymptotic distribution of Q, define

$$F(z) = \lim_{n \to \infty} \frac{1}{N} \ln(Z(z)).$$

Then clearly

$$\lim_{n \to \infty} \mathrm{E}(Q) = (\kappa T) \frac{dF}{d\xi}, \quad \lim_{n \to \infty} N \, \mathrm{Var}(Q) = (\kappa T)^2 \frac{d^2 F}{d\xi^2}$$

via term-by-term differentiation of $\ln(Z)$. Exact expressions for both moments are possible using Onsager's formula:

$$F(z) = \ln\left(\frac{2}{1-z^2}\right)$$

$$+ \frac{1}{2} \int_0^1 \int_0^1 \ln\left[(1+z^2)^2 - 2z(1-z^2)(\cos(2\pi u) + \cos(2\pi v))\right] du\, dv,$$

but we give results at only two special temperatures. In the case $T = \infty$, for which states are assigned equal weighting, $E(Q) \to 0$ and $N \operatorname{Var}(Q) \to 2$, confirming reasoning in [77]. In the case $T = T_c$, note that the singularity is fairly subtle since F and its first derivative are both well defined [11]:

$$F(z_c) = \frac{\ln(2)}{2} + \frac{2G}{\pi} = 0.9296953983\ldots = \frac{1}{2}\left(\ln(2) + 1.1662436161\ldots\right),$$

$$\lim_{n\to\infty} E(Q) = \sqrt{2},$$

where G is Catalan's constant [1.7]. The second derivative of F, however, is unbounded in the vicinity of $z = z_c$ and, in fact [5],

$$\lim_{n\to\infty} N \operatorname{Var}(Q) \approx -\frac{8}{\pi}\left(\ln\left|\frac{T}{T_c} - 1\right| + g\right),$$

where g is the constant

$$g = 1 + \frac{\pi}{4} + \ln\left(\frac{\sqrt{2}}{4}\ln(\sqrt{2}+1)\right) = 0.6194036984\ldots.$$

This is related to what physicists call the **logarithmic divergence** of the **Ising specific heat**. (See Figure 5.23.)

As an aside, we mention that corresponding values of $F(z_c)$ on the triangular and hexagonal planar lattices are, respectively [11],

$$\ln(2) + \frac{\ln(3)}{4} + \frac{H}{2} = 0.8795853862\ldots,$$

$$\frac{3\ln(2)}{4} + \frac{\ln(3)}{2} + \frac{H}{4} = 1.0250590965\ldots.$$

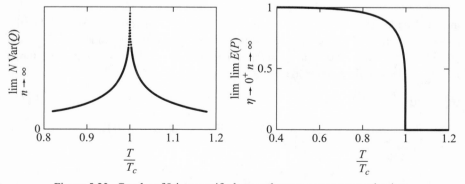

Figure 5.23. Graphs of Ising specific heat and spontaneous magnetization.

Both results feature a new constant [78, 79]:

$$H = \frac{5\sqrt{3}}{6\pi}\psi'\left(\frac{1}{3}\right) - \frac{5\sqrt{3}}{9}\pi - \ln(6) = \frac{\sqrt{3}}{6\pi}\psi'\left(\frac{1}{6}\right) - \frac{\sqrt{3}}{3}\pi - \ln(6)$$
$$= -0.1764297331\ldots,$$

where $\psi'(x)$ is the trigamma function (derivative of the digamma function $\psi(x)$ [1.5.4]). See [80–82] for other occurrences of H; note that the formula

$$\ln(2) + \ln(3) + H = \frac{1}{4\pi^2} \int\limits_{-\pi}^{\pi}\int\limits_{-\pi}^{\pi} \ln\left[6 - 2\cos(\theta) - 2\cos(\varphi) - 2\cos(\theta + \varphi)\right] d\theta\, d\varphi$$

$$= \frac{3\sqrt{3}}{\pi}\left(1 - \frac{1}{5^2} + \frac{1}{7^2} - \frac{1}{11^2} + \frac{1}{13^2} - \frac{1}{17^2} + - \cdots\right)$$

$$= 1.6153297360\ldots$$

parallels nicely similar results in [3.10] and [5.23].

A more difficult analysis allows us to compute the corresponding two moments of P and also to see more vividly the significance of magnetic susceptibility and critical exponents. Let

$$F(z, w) = \lim_{n\to\infty} \frac{1}{N}\ln(Z(z, w));$$

then clearly

$$\lim_{\eta\to 0^+}\lim_{n\to\infty} E(P) = (\kappa T)\frac{\partial F}{\partial \eta}\bigg|_{\eta=0}, \quad \lim_{\eta\to 0^+}\lim_{n\to\infty} N\,\text{Var}(P) = (\kappa T)^2\frac{\partial^2 F}{\partial \eta^2}\bigg|_{\eta=0}$$

as before. Of course, we do not know $F(z, w)$ exactly when $w \neq 0$. Its derivative at $w = 0$, however, has a simple expression valid for all z:

$$\lim_{\eta\to 0^+}\lim_{n\to\infty} E(P) = \begin{cases} \left[1 - \sinh\left(\dfrac{2\xi}{\kappa T}\right)^{-4}\right]^{\frac{1}{8}} & \text{if } T < T_c, \\ 0 & \text{if } T > T_c, \end{cases}$$

$$= \begin{cases} (1 + y^2)^{\frac{1}{4}}(1 - 6y^2 + y^4)^{\frac{1}{8}}(1 - y^2)^{-\frac{1}{2}} & \text{if } T < T_c, \\ 0 & \text{if } T > T_c \end{cases}$$

due to Onsager and Yang [83–85]. A rigorous justification is found in [86–88]. For the special temperature $T = \infty$, we have $E(P) \to 0$ and $N\,\text{Var}(P) \to 1$ since p is Binomial $(N, 1/2)$ distributed. At criticality, $E(P) \to 0$ as well, but the second derivative exhibits fascinatingly complicated behavior:

$$\lim_{\eta\to 0^+}\lim_{n\to\infty} N\,\text{Var}(P) = \chi(z) \approx c_0^+ t^{-\frac{7}{4}} + c_1^+ t^{-\frac{3}{4}} + d_0 + c_2^+ t^{\frac{1}{4}} + e_0\, t\ln(t) + d_1 t + c_3^+ t^{\frac{5}{4}},$$

where $0 < t = 1 - T_c/T$, $c_0^+ = 0.9625817323\ldots$, $d_0 = -0.1041332451\ldots$, $e_0 = 0.0403255003\ldots$, $d_1 = -0.14869\ldots$, and

$$c_1^+ = \frac{\sqrt{2}}{8}K_c c_0^+, \quad c_2^+ = \frac{151}{192}K_c^2 c_0^+, \quad c_3^+ = \frac{615\sqrt{2}}{512}K_c^3 c_0^+.$$

Wu, McCoy, Tracy & Barouch [89–99] determined exact expressions for these series coefficients in terms of the solution to a Painlevé III differential equation (described in the next section). Different numerical values of the coefficients apply for $T < T_c$, as well as for the antiferromagnetic case [100, 101]. For example, when $t < 0$, the corresponding leading coefficient is $c_0^- = 0.0255369745\ldots$. The study of magnetic susceptibility $\chi(z)$ is far more involved than the other thermodynamic functions mentioned in this essay, and there are still gaps in the rigorous line of thought [102]. Also, in a recent breakthrough [103, 104], the entire asymptotic structure of $\chi(z)$ has now largely been determined.

5.22.7 Painlevé III Equation

Let $f(x)$ be the solution of the Painlevé III differential equation [105]

$$\frac{f''(x)}{f(x)} = \left(\frac{f'(x)}{f(x)}\right)^2 - \frac{1}{x}\frac{f'(x)}{f(x)} + f(x)^2 - \frac{1}{f(x)^2}$$

satisfying the boundary conditions

$$f(x) \sim 1 - \frac{e^{-2x}}{\sqrt{\pi x}} \text{ as } x \to \infty, \quad f(x) \sim x\,(2\ln(2) - \gamma - \ln(x)) \text{ as } x \to 0^+,$$

where γ is Euler's constant [1.5]. Define

$$g(x) = \left[\frac{xf'(x)}{2f(x)} + \frac{x^2}{4f(x)^2}\left((1 - f(x)^2)^2 - f'(x)^2\right)\right]\ln(x).$$

Then exact expressions for c_0^+ and c_0^- are

$$c_0^+ = 2^{\frac{5}{8}}\pi\ln(\sqrt{2} + 1)^{-\frac{7}{4}}\int_0^\infty y(1 - f(y))$$

$$\times \exp\left[\int_y^\infty x\ln(x)\left(1 - f(x)^2\right)dx - g(y)\right]dy,$$

$$c_0^- = 2^{\frac{5}{8}}\pi\ln(\sqrt{2} + 1)^{-\frac{7}{4}}\int_0^\infty y$$

$$\times \left\{(1 + f(y))\exp\left[\int_y^\infty x\ln(x)\left(1 - f(x)^2\right)dx - g(y)\right] - 2\right\}dy.$$

Painlevé II arises in our discussion of the longest increasing subsequence problem [5.20], and Painlevé V arises in connection with the GUE hypothesis [2.15.3].

Here is a slight variation of these results. Define

$$h(x) = -\ln\left(f\left(\frac{x}{c}\right)\right)$$

for any constant $c > 0$; then the function $h(x)$ satisfies what is known as the sinh-Gordon differential equation:

$$h''(x) + \frac{1}{x}h'(x) = \frac{2}{c^2}\sinh(2h(x)),$$

$$h(x) \sim \sqrt{\frac{c}{\pi x}}\exp\left(-\frac{2x}{c}\right) \text{ as } x \to \infty.$$

Finally, we mention a beautiful formula:

$$\int\limits_0^\infty x\ln(x)\left(1 - f(x)^2\right)dx = \frac{1}{4} + \frac{7}{12}\ln(2) - 3\ln(A),$$

where A is Glaisher's constant [2.15]. Conceivably, c_0^+ and c_0^- may someday be related to A as well.

[1] G. F. Newell and E. W. Montroll, On the theory of the Ising model of ferromagnetism, *Rev. Mod. Phys.* 25 (1953) 353–389; MR 15,88b.
[2] M. E. Fisher, The theory of cooperative phenomena, *Rep. Prog. Phys.* 30 (1967) 615–730.
[3] S. G. Brush, History of the Lenz-Ising model, *Rev. Mod. Phys.* 39 (1967) 883–893.
[4] C. Thompson, *Mathematical Statistical Mechanics*, Princeton Univ. Press, 1972; MR 80h:82001.
[5] B. M. McCoy and T. T. Wu, *The Two-Dimensional Ising Model*, Harvard Univ. Press, 1973.
[6] R. J. Baxter, *Exactly Solved Models in Statistical Mechanics*, Academic Press, 1982; MR 90b:82001.
[7] G. A. Baker, *Quantitative Theory of Critical Phenomena*, Academic Press, 1990; MR 92d:82039.
[8] C. Domb, *The Critical Point: A Historical Introduction to the Modern Theory of Critical Phenomena*, Taylor and Francis, 1996.
[9] G. M. Bell and D. A. Lavis, *Statistical Mechanics of Lattice Systems*, v. 1-2, Springer-Verlag, 1999.
[10] D. S. Gaunt and A. J. Guttmann, Asymptotic analysis of coefficients, *Phase Transitions and Critical Phenomena*, v. 3, ed. C. Domb and M. S. Green, Academic Press, 1974, pp. 181–243; A. J. Guttmann, Asymptotic analysis of power-series expansions, *Phase Transitions and Critical Phenomena,* v. 13, ed. C. Domb and J. L. Lebowitz, Academic Press, 1989, pp. 1–234; MR 50 #6393 and MR 94i:82003.
[11] C. Domb, On the theory of cooperative phenomena in crystals, *Adv. Phys.* 9 (1960) 149–361.
[12] T. Oguchi, Statistics of the three-dimensional ferromagnet. II and III, *J. Phys. Soc. Japan* 6 (1951) 27–35; MR 15,188h.
[13] A. J. Wakefield, Statistics of the simple cubic lattice, *Proc. Cambridge Philos. Soc.* 47 (1951) 419–429, 719–810; MR 13,308a and MR 13,417c.
[14] A. Rosengren and B. Lindström, A combinatorial series expansion for the Ising model, *Europ. J. Combin.* 8 (1987) 317–323; MR 89c:82062.
[15] R. J. Baxter and I. G. Enting, Series expansions for corner transfer matrices: The square lattice Ising model, *J. Stat. Phys.* 21 (1979) 103–123.
[16] C. Domb, Some statistical problems connected with crystal lattices, *J. Royal Statist. Soc.* B 26 (1964) 367–397.
[17] N. J. A. Sloane, On-Line Encyclopedia of Integer Sequences, A001393, A002891, A001408, and A002916.
[18] L. Onsager, Crystal physics. I: A two-dimensional model with an order-disorder transition, *Phys. Rev.* 65 (1944) 117–149.

[19] M. Kac and J. C. Ward, A combinatorial solution of the two-dimensional Ising model, *Phys. Rev.* 88 (1952) 1332–1337.

[20] S. Sherman, Combinatorial aspects of the Ising model for ferromagnetism. I: A conjecture of Feynman on paths and graphs, *J. Math. Phys.* 1 (1960) 202–217, addendum 4 (1963) 1213–1214; MR 22 #10273 and MR 27 #6560.

[21] N. V. Vdovichenko, A calculation of the partition function for a plane dipole lattice (in Russian), *Z. Èksper. Teoret. Fiz.* 47 (1965) 715–719; Engl. transl. in *Soviet Physics JETP* 20 (1965) 477–488; MR 31 #5622.

[22] M. L. Glasser, Exact partition function for the two-dimensional Ising model, *Amer. J. Phys.* 38 (1970) 1033–1036.

[23] F. Harary, A graphical exposition of the Ising problem, *J. Austral. Math. Soc.* 12 (1971) 365–377; MR 45 #5032.

[24] P. D. Beale, Exact distribution of energies in the two-dimensional Ising model, *Phys. Rev. Lett.* 76 (1996) 78–81.

[25] N. J. A. Sloane, On-Line Encyclopedia of Integer Sequences, A002890, A029872, A029873, and A029874.

[26] M. Creutz, State counting and low-temperature series, *Phys. Rev. B* 43 (1991) 10659–10662.

[27] G. Bhanot, M. Creutz, and J. Lacki, Low temperature expansion for the 3-d Ising model, *Phys. Rev. Lett.* 69 (1992) 1841–1844; hep-lat/9206020.

[28] G. Bhanot, M. Creutz, I. Horvath, J. Lacki, and J. Weckel, Series expansions without diagrams, *Phys. Rev. E* 49 (1994) 2445–2453; hep-lat/9303002.

[29] A. J. Guttmann and I. G. Enting, Series studies of the Potts model. I: The simple cubic Ising model, *J. Phys. A* 26 (1993) 807–821; MR 94a:82009.

[30] C. Vohwinkel, Yet another way to obtain low temperature expansions for discrete spin systems, *Phys. Lett. B* 301 (1993) 208–212.

[31] B. A. Cipra, An introduction to the Ising model, *Amer. Math. Monthly* 94 (1987) 937–959; MR 89g:82001.

[32] M. E. Fisher, The nature of critical points, *Statistical Physics, Weak Interactions, Field Theory – Lectures in Theoretical Physics*, v. 7C, ed. W. E. Brittin, Univ. of Colorado Press, 1964, pp. 1–159.

[33] G. S. Rushbrooke and J. Eve, High-temperature Ising partition function and related non-crossing polygons for the simple cubic lattice, *J. Math. Phys.* 3 (1962) 185–189; MR 25 #1907.

[34] S. McKenzie, Derivation of high temperature series expansions: Ising model, *Phase Transitions – Cargèse 1980*, ed. M. Lévy, J.-C. Le Guillou, and J. Zinn-Justin, Plenum Press, 1982, pp. 247–270.

[35] G. Bhanot, M. Creutz, U. Glässner, and K. Schilling, Specific heat exponent for the 3-d Ising model from a 24-th order high temperature series, *Phys. Rev. B* 49 (1994) 12909–12914; *Nucl. Phys. B (Proc. Suppl.)* 42 (1995) 758–760; hep-lat/9312048.

[36] A. J. Guttmann and I. G. Enting, The high-temperature specific heat exponent of the 3D Ising model, *J. Phys. A* 27 (1994) 8007–8010.

[37] F. Harary and E. M. Palmer, *Graphical Enumeration*, Academic Press, 1973, pp. 11–16, 113–117, 236–237; MR 50 #9682.

[38] H. A. Kramers and G. H. Wannier, Statistics of the two-dimensional ferromagnet. I and II, *Phys. Rev.* 60 (1941) 252–276; MR 3,63i and MR 3,64a.

[39] C. Domb and A. J. Guttmann, Low-temperature series for the Ising model, *J. Phys. C* 3 (1970) 1652–1660.

[40] J. Zinn-Justin, Analysis of Ising model critical exponents from high temperature series expansions, *J. Physique* 40 (1979) 969–975.

[41] J. Adler, Critical temperatures of the $d = 3, s = 1/2$ Ising model: The effect of confluent corrections to scaling, *J. Phys. A* 16 (1983) 3585–3599.

[42] A. J. Liu and M. E. Fisher, The three-dimensional Ising model revisited numerically, *Physica A* 156 (1989) 35–76; MR 90c:82059.

[43] A. M. Ferrenberg and D. P. Landau, Critical behavior of the three-dimensional Ising model: A high-resolution Monte Carlo study, *Phys. Rev. B* 44 (1991) 5081–5091.

[44] B. G. Nickel, Confluent singularities in 3D continuum ϕ^4 theory: Resolving critical point discrepancies, *Physica A* 177 (1991) 189–196.

[45] N. Ito and M. Suzuki, Monte Carlo study of the spontaneous magnetization of the three-dimensional Ising model, *J. Phys. Soc. Japan* 60 (1991) 1978–1987.

[46] Y. Kinosita, N. Kawahima, and M. Suzuki, Coherent-anomaly analysis of series expansions and its application to the Ising model, *J. Phys. Soc. Japan* 61 (1992) 3887–3901; MR 93j:82037.

[47] C. F. Baillie, R. Gupta, K. A. Hawick, and G. S. Pawley, Monte Carlo renomalization-group study of the three-dimensional Ising model, *Phys. Rev. B* 45 (1992) 10438–10453.

[48] H. W. J. Blöte and G. Kamieniarz, Finite-size calculations on the three-dimensional Ising model, *Physica A* 196 (1993) 455–460.

[49] D. P. Landau, Computer simulation studies of critical phenomena, *Physica A* 205 (1994) 41–64.

[50] M. Kolesik and M. Suzuki, Accurate estimates of 3D Ising critical exponents using the coherent-anomaly method, *Physica A* 215 (1995) 138–151.

[51] H. W. J. Blöte, E. Luijten, and J. R. Heringa, Ising universality in three dimensions: A Monte Carlo study, *J. Phys. Math. A* 28 (1995) 6289–6313.

[52] R. Gupta and P. Tamayo, Critical exponents of the 3D Ising model, *Int. J. Mod. Phys. C* 7 (1996) 305–319.

[53] A. L. Talapov and H. W. J. Blöte, The magnetization of the 3D Ising model, *J. Phys. A* 29 (1996) 5727–5733.

[54] A. Rosengren, On the combinatorial solution of the Ising model, *J. Phys. A* 19 (1986) 1709–1714; MR 87k:82149.

[55] M. E. Fisher, On the critical polynomial of the simple cubic Ising model, *J. Phys. A.* 28 (1995) 6323–6333; corrigenda 29 (1996) 1145; MR 97b:82018a and MR 97b:82018b.

[56] N. J. A. Sloane, On-Line Encyclopedia of Integer Sequences, A010556, A010579, A010580, A030008, A030044, A030045, A030046, A030047, A030048, and A030049.

[57] M. E. Fisher and D. S. Gaunt, Ising model and self-avoiding walks on hypercubical lattices and high density expansions, *Phys. Rev.* 133 (1964) A224–A239.

[58] M. A. Moore, Critical behavior of the four-dimensional Ising ferromagnet and the breakdown of scaling, *Phys. Rev. B* 1 (1970) 2238–2240.

[59] D. S. Gaunt, M. F. Sykes, and S. McKenzie, Susceptibility and fourth-field derivative of the spin-1/2 Ising model for $T > T_c$ and $d = 4$, *J. Phys. A* 12 (1979) 871–877.

[60] M. F. Sykes, Derivation of low-temperature expansions for Ising model. X: The four-dimensional simple hypercubic lattice, *J. Phys. A* 12 (1979) 879–892.

[61] C. Vohwinkel and P. Weisz, Low-temperature expansion in the $d = 4$ Ising model, *Nucl. Phys. B* 374 (1992) 647–666; MR 93a:82015.

[62] A. J. Guttmann, Correction to scaling exponents and critical properties of the n-vector model with dimensionality > 4, *J. Phys. A* 14 (1981) 233–239.

[63] A. B. Harris and Y. Meir, Recursive enumeration of clusters in general dimension on hypercubic lattices, *Phys. Rev. A* 36 (1987) 1840–1848; MR 88m:82037.

[64] C. Münkel, D. W. Heermann, J. Adler, M. Gofman, and D. Stauffer, The dynamical critical exponent of the two-, three- and five-dimensional kinetic Ising model, *Physica A* 193 (1993) 540–552.

[65] M. Gofman, J. Adler, A. Aharony, A. B. Harris, and D. Stauffer, Series and Monte Carlo study of high-dimensional Ising models, *J. Stat. Phys.* 71 (1993) 1221–1230.

[66] M. F. Sykes, Some counting theorems in the theory of the Ising model and the excluded volume problem, *J. Math. Phys.* 2 (1961) 52–59; MR 22 #8749.

[67] N. J. A. Sloane, On-Line Encyclopedia of Integer Sequences, A002906, A002913, A002926, and A002927.

[68] D. S. Gaunt and M. F. Sykes, The critical exponent γ for the three-dimensional Ising model, *J. Phys. A* 12 (1979) L25–L28.

[69] D. S. Gaunt, High temperature series analysis for the three-dimensional Ising model: A review of some recent work, *Phase Transitions – Cargèse 1980*, ed. M. Lévy, J.-C. Le Guillou, and J. Zinn-Justin, Plenum Press, 1982, pp. 217–246.

[70] A. J. Guttmann, The high temperature susceptibility and spin-spin correlation function of the three-dimensional Ising model, *J. Phys. A* 20 (1987) 1855–1863; MR 88h:82075.

[71] P. Butera and M. Comi, N-vector spin models on the simple-cubic and the body-centered-cubic lattices: A study of the critical behavior of the susceptibility and of the correlation length by high-temperature series extended to order 21, *Phys. Rev. B* 56 (1997) 8212–8240; hep-lat/9703018.

[72] M. Campostrini, Linked-cluster expansion of the Ising model, *J. Stat. Phys.* 103 (2001) 369–394; cond-mat/0005130.

[73] P. Butera and M. Comi, Extension to order β^{23} of the high-temperature expansions for the spin-1/2 Ising model on the simple-cubic and the body-centered-cubic lattices, *Phys. Rev. B* 62 (2000) 14837–14843; hep-lat/0006009.

[74] M. F. Sykes, D. S. Gaunt, P. D. Roberts, and J. A. Wyles, High temperature series for the susceptibility of the Ising model. I: Two dimensional lattices, *J. Phys. A* 5 (1972) 624–639.

[75] B. G. Nickel, On the singularity structure of the 2D Ising model, *J. Phys. A* 32 (1999) 3889–3906; addendum 33 (2000) 1693–1711; MR 2000d:82013 and MR 2001a: 82022.

[76] C. Domb, Ising model, *Phase Transitions and Critical Phenomena*, v. 3, ed. C. Domb and M. S. Green, Academic Press, 1974, pp. 357–484; MR 50 #6393.

[77] P. A. P. Moran, Random associations on a lattice, *Proc. Cambridge Philos. Soc.* 34 (1947) 321–328; 45 (1949) 488; MR 8,592b.

[78] R. M. F. Houtappel, Order-disorder in hexagonal lattices, *Physica* 16 (1950) 425–455; MR 12,576j.

[79] V. S. Adamchik, Exact formulas for some Ising-related constants, unpublished note (1997).

[80] R. Burton and R. Pemantle, Local characteristics, entropy and limit theorems for spanning trees and domino tilings via transfer-impedances, *Annals of Probab.* 21 (1993) 1329–1371; MR 94m:60019.

[81] F. Y. Wu, Number of spanning trees on a lattice, *J. Phys. A* 10 (1977) L113–L115; MR 58 #8974.

[82] R. Shrock and F. Y. Wu, Spanning trees on graphs and lattices in d dimensions, *J. Phys. A* 33 (2000) 3881–3902; MR 2001b:05111.

[83] L. Onsager, Statistical hydrodynamics, *Nuovo Cimento Suppl.* 6 (1949) 279–287.

[84] C. N. Yang, The spontaneous magnetization of a two-dimensional Ising model, *Phys. Rev.* 85 (1952) 808–817; MR 14,522e.

[85] E. W. Montroll and R. B. Potts, Correlations and spontaneous magnetization of the two-dimensional Ising model, *J. Math. Phys.* 4 (1963) 308–319; MR 26 #5913.

[86] G. Benettin, G. Gallavotti, G. Jona-Lasinio, and A. L. Stella, On the Onsager-Yang value of the spontaneous magnetization, *Commun. Math. Phys.* 30 (1973) 45–54.

[87] D. B. Abraham and A. Martin-Löf, The transfer matrix for a pure phase in the two-dimensional Ising model, *Commun. Math. Phys.* 32 (1973) 245–268; MR 49 #6851.

[88] G. Gallavotti, *Statistical Mechanics: A Short Treatise*, Springer-Verlag, 1999.

[89] M. E. Fisher, The susceptibility of the plane Ising model, *Physica* 25 (1959) 521–524.

[90] E. Barouch, B. M. McCoy, and T. T. Wu, Zero-field susceptibility of the two-dimensional Ising model near T_c, *Phys. Rev. Lett.* 31 (1973) 1409–1411.

[91] C. A. Tracy and B. M. McCoy, Neutron scattering and the correlation functions of the Ising model near T_c, *Phys. Rev. Lett.* 31 (1973) 1500–1504.

[92] T. T. Wu, B. M. McCoy, C. A. Tracy, and E. Barouch, Spin-spin correlation functions for the two-dimensional Ising model: Exact theory in the scaling region, *Phys. Rev. B* 13 (1976) 316–374.

[93] B. M. McCoy, C. A. Tracy, and T. T. Wu, Painlevé functions of the third kind, *J. Math. Phys.* 18 (1977) 1058–1092; MR 57 #12993.

[94] C. A. Tracy, Painlevé transcendents and scaling functions of the two-dimensional Ising model, *Nonlinear Equations in Physics and Mathematics*, ed. A. O. Barut, Reidel, 1978, pp. 221–237; MR 84k:35001.

[95] X.-P. Kong, H. Au-Yang, and J. H. H. Perk, New results for the susceptibility of the two-dimensional Ising model at criticality, *Phys. Lett. A* 116 (1986) 54–56.

[96] X.-P. Kong, *Wave-Vector Dependent Susceptibility of the Two-Dimensional Ising Model*, Ph.D. thesis, State Univ. of New York at Stony Brook, 1987.

[97] S. Gartenhaus and W. S. McCullough, Higher order corrections for the quadratic Ising lattice susceptibility at criticality, *Phys. Rev. B* 38 (1988) 11688–11703; *Phys. Lett. A* 127 (1988) 315–318; MR 89b:82105.

[98] C. A. Tracy, Asymptotics of a tau-function arising in the two-dimensional Ising model, *Commun. Math. Phys.* 142 (1991) 298–311; MR 93c:82014.

[99] O. Babelon and D. Bernard, From form factors to correlation functions; the Ising model, *Phys. Lett. B* 288 (1992) 113–120; MR 94e:82015.

[100] X.-P. Kong, H. Au-Yang, and J. H. H. Perk, Comment on a paper by Yamadi and Suzuki, *Prog. Theor. Phys.* 77 (1987) 514–516.

[101] S. S. C. Burnett and S. Gartenhaus, Zero-field susceptibility of an antiferromagnetic square Ising lattice, *Phys. Rev. B* 47 (1993) 7944–7956.

[102] J. Palmer and C. A. Tracy, Two-dimensional Ising correlations: Convergence of the scaling limit, *Adv. Appl. Math* 2 (1981) 329–388; MR 84m:82024.

[103] W. P. Orrick, B. G. Nickel, A. J. Guttmann, and J. H. H. Perk, Critical behaviour of the two-dimensional Ising susceptibility, *Phys. Rev. Lett.* 86 (2001) 4120–4123.

[104] W. P. Orrick, B. G. Nickel, A. J. Guttmann, and J. H. H. Perk, The susceptibility of the square lattice Ising model: New developments, *J. Stat. Phys.* 102 (2001) 795–841; MR 2002e:82013.

[105] C. A. Tracy and H. Widom, Universality of the distribution functions of random matrix theory, *Integrable Systems: From Classical to Quantum*, Proc. 1999 Montréal conf., ed. J. Harnad, G. Sabidussi, and P. Winternitz, Amer. Math. Soc, 2000, pp. 251–264; math-ph/9909001; MR 2002f:15036.

5.23 Monomer-Dimer Constants

Let L be a graph [5.6]. A **dimer** consists of two adjacent vertices of L and the (non-oriented) bond connecting them. A **dimer arrangement** is a collection of disjoint dimers on L. Uncovered vertices are called **monomers**, so dimer arrangements are also known as **monomer-dimer coverings**. We will discuss such coverings only briefly at the beginning of the next section.

A **dimer covering** is a dimer arrangement whose union contains all the vertices of L. Dimer coverings and the closely-related topic of tilings will occupy the remainder of this essay.

5.23.1 2D Domino Tilings

Let a_n denote the number of distinct monomer-dimer coverings of an $n \times n$ square lattice L and $N = n^2$; then $a_1 = 1$, $a_2 = 7$, $a_3 = 131$, $a_4 = 10012$ [1,2], and asymptotically [3–6]

$$A = \lim_{n \to \infty} a_n^{\frac{1}{N}} = 1.940215351\ldots = (3.764435608\ldots)^{\frac{1}{2}}.$$

No exact expression for the constant A is known. Baxter's approach for estimating A was based on the corner transfer matrix variational approach, which also played a role in [5.12]. A natural way for physicists to discuss the monomer-dimer problem is to associate an activity z with each dimer; A thus corresponds to the case $z = 1$. The mean number ρ of dimers per vertex is 0 if $z = 0$ and $1/2$ if $z = \infty$; when $z = 1$, ρ is $0.3190615546\ldots$, for which again there is no closed-form expression [3]. Unlike other lattice models (see [5.12], [5.18], and [5.22]), monomer-dimer systems do not have a phase transition [7].

Computing a_n is equivalent to counting (not necessarily perfect) **matchings** in L, that is, to counting independent sets of edges in L. This is related to the difficult problem of computing permanents of certain binary incidence matrices [8–14]. Kenyon, Randall & Sinclair [15] gave a randomized polynomial-time approximation algorithm for computing the number of monomer-dimer coverings of L, assuming ρ to be given.

Let us turn our attention henceforth to the zero monomer density case, that is, $z = \infty$. If b_n is the number of distinct dimer coverings of L, then $b_n = 0$ if n is odd and

$$b_n = 2^{N/2} \prod_{j=1}^{n/2} \prod_{k=1}^{n/2} \left(\cos^2 \frac{j\pi}{n+1} + \cos^2 \frac{k\pi}{n+1} \right)$$

if n is even. This exact expression is due to Kastelyn [16] and Fisher & Temperley [17, 18]. Further,

$$\lim_{\substack{n\to\infty \\ n \text{ even}}} \frac{1}{N} \ln(b_n) = \frac{1}{16\pi^2} \int_{-\pi}^{\pi} \int_{-\pi}^{\pi} \ln\left[4 + 2\cos(\theta) + 2\cos(\varphi)\right] d\theta\, d\varphi$$

$$= \frac{G}{\pi} = 0.2915609040\ldots;$$

that is,

$$B = \lim_{\substack{n\to\infty \\ n \text{ even}}} b_n^{\frac{1}{N}} = \exp\left(\frac{G}{\pi}\right) = 1.3385151519\ldots = (1.7916228120\ldots)^{\frac{1}{2}},$$

where G is Catalan's constant [1.7]. This is a remarkable solution, in graph theoretic terms, of the problem of counting **perfect matchings** on the square lattice. It is also an answer to the following question: What is the number of ways of tiling an $n \times n$ chessboard with 2×1 or 1×2 **dominoes**? See [19–26] for more details. The constant B^2 is called δ in [3.10] and appears in [1.8] too; the expression $4G/\pi$ arises in [5.22], $G/(\pi \ln(2))$ in [5.6], and $8G/\pi^2$ in [7.7].

If we wrap the square lattice around to form a torus, the counts b_n differ somewhat, but the limiting constant B remains the same [16, 27]. If, instead, we assume the chessboard to be shaped like an Aztec diamond [28], then the associated constant $B = 2^{1/4} = 1.189\ldots < 1.338\ldots = e^{G/\pi}$. Hence, even though the square chessboard has slightly less area than the diamond chessboard, the former possesses many more domino tilings [29]. Lattice boundary effects are thus seen to be nontrivial.

5.23.2 Lozenges and Bibones

The analog of $\exp(2G/\pi)$ for dimers on a hexagonal (honeycomb) lattice with wraparound is [30–32]

$$C^2 = \lim_{n\to\infty} c_n^{\frac{2}{N}} = \exp\left(\frac{1}{8\pi^2} \int\limits_{-\pi}^{\pi}\int\limits_{-\pi}^{\pi} \ln\left[3 + 2\cos(\theta) + 2\cos(\varphi) + 2\cos(\theta+\varphi)\right]\, d\theta\, d\varphi\right)$$

$$= 1.3813564445\ldots.$$

This constant is called β in [3.10] and can be expressed by other formulas too. It characterizes lozenge tilings on a chessboard with triangular cells satisfying periodic boundary conditions. See [33–38] as well.

If there is no wraparound, then the sequence [39]

$$c_n = \prod_{j=1}^{n}\prod_{k=1}^{n} \frac{n+j+k-1}{j+k-1}$$

emerges, and a different growth constant $3\sqrt{3}/4$ applies. We have assumed that the hexagonal grid is center-symmetric with sides n, n, and n (i.e., the simplest possible boundary conditions). The sequence further enumerates plane partitions contained within an $n \times n \times n$ box [40,41].

The corresponding analog for dimers on a triangular lattice with wraparound is [30,42,43]

$$D^2 = \lim_{n\to\infty} d_n^{\frac{2}{N}} = \exp\left(\frac{1}{8\pi^2} \int\limits_{-\pi}^{\pi}\int\limits_{-\pi}^{\pi} \ln\left[6 + 2\cos(\theta) + 2\cos(\varphi) + 2\cos(\theta+\varphi)\right]\, d\theta\, d\varphi\right)$$

$$= 2.3565273533\ldots.$$

The expression $4\ln(D)$ bears close similarity to a constant $\ln(6) + H$ described in [5.22]. It also characterizes bibone tilings on a chessboard with hexagonal cells satisfying periodic boundary conditions. The case of no wraparound [1,44,45] apparently remains open.

5.23.3 3D Domino Tilings

Let h_n denote the number of distinct dimer coverings of an $n \times n \times n$ cubic lattice L and $N = n^3$. Then $h_n = 0$ if n is odd, $h_2 = 9$, and $h_4 = 5051532105$ [46,47]. An important unsolved problem in solid-state chemistry is the estimation of

$$\lim_{\substack{n\to\infty\\ n \text{ even}}} h_n^{\frac{1}{N}} = \exp(\lambda)$$

or, equivalently,

$$\lambda = \lim_{\substack{n\to\infty\\ n \text{ even}}} \frac{1}{N} \ln(h_n).$$

Hammersley [48] proved that λ exists and $\lambda \geq 0.29156$. Lower bounds were improved by Fisher [49] to 0.30187, Hammersley [50, 51] to 0.418347, and Priezzhev [52, 53] to 0.419989. In a review of [54], Minc pointed out that a conjecture due to Schrijver & Valiant on lower bounds for permanents of certain binary matrices would imply that $\lambda \geq 0.44007584$. Schrijver [55] proved this conjecture, and this is the best-known result.

Fowler & Rushbrooke [56] gave an upper bound of 0.54931 for λ over sixty years ago (assuming λ exists). Upper bounds have been improved by Minc [8, 57, 58] to 0.5482709, Ciucu [59] to 0.463107, and Lundow [60] to 0.457547.

A sequence of nonrigorous numerical estimates by Nagle [30], Gaunt [31], and Beichl & Sullivan [61] has culminated with $\lambda = 0.4466\ldots$. As with a_n, computing h_n for even small values of n is hard and matrix permanent approximation schemes offer the only hope. The field is treacherously difficult: Conjectured exact asymptotic formulas for h_n in [62, 63] are incorrect.

A related topic is the number, k_n, of dimer coverings of the n-dimensional unit cube, whose 2^n vertices consist of all n-tuples drawn from $\{0, 1\}$ [47, 64]. The term $k_6 = 16332454526976$ was computed independently by Lundow [46] and Weidemann [65]. In this case, we know the asymptotic behavior of k_n rather precisely [44, 65, 66]:

$$\lim_{n \to \infty} \frac{1}{n} k_n^{2^{1-n}} = \frac{1}{e} = 0.3678794411\ldots,$$

where e is the natural logarithmic base [1.3].

[1] N. J. A. Sloane, On-Line Encyclopedia of Integer Sequences, A004003, A006125, A008793, A028420, and A039907.

[2] J. J. Henry, Monomer-dimer counts, $1 \leq n \leq 21$, unpublished note (1997).

[3] R. J. Baxter, Dimers on a rectangular lattice, *J. Math. Phys.* 9 (1968) 650–654.

[4] L. K. Runnels, Exact finite method of lattice statistics. III: Dimers on the square lattice, *J. Math. Phys.* 11 (1970) 842–850.

[5] M. Heise, Upper and lower bounds for the partition function of lattice models, *Physica A* 157 (1989) 983–999; MR 91c:82014.

[6] F. Cazals, Monomer-dimer tilings, *Studies in Automatic Combinatorics*, v. 2, Algorithms Project, INRIA, 1997.

[7] O. J. Heilmann and E. H. Lieb, Theory of monomer-dimer systems, *Commun. Math. Phys.* 25 (1972) 190–232; MR 45 #6337.

[8] H. Minc, *Permanents*, Addision-Wesley, 1978; MR 80d:15009.

[9] R. A. Brualdi and H. J. Ryser, *Combinatorial Matrix Theory*, Cambridge Univ. Press, 1991; MR 93a:05087.

[10] J. M. Hammersley, A. Feuerverger, A. Izenman, and K. Makani, Negative finding for the three-dimensional dimer problem, *J. Math. Phys.* 10 (1969) 443–446.

[11] M. Jerrum, Two-dimensional monomer-dimer systems are computationally intractable, *J. Stat. Phys.* 48 (1987) 121–134; erratum 59 (1990) 1087–1088; MR 89d:82008 and MR 91h:82002.

[12] M. Luby, A survey of approximation algorithms for the permanent, *Sequences: Combinatorics, Compression, Security and Transmission*, Proc. 1988 Naples workshop, ed. R. M. Capocelli, Springer-Verlag, 1990, pp. 75–91; MR 90m:68059.

[13] M. Jerrum and A. Sinclair, Approximating the permanent, *SIAM J. Comput.* 18 (1989) 1149–1178; MR 91a:05075.

[14] A. Frieze and M. Jerrum, An analysis of a Monte-Carlo algorithm for estimating the permanent, *Combinatorica* 15 (1995) 67–83; MR 96g:68052.

[15] C. Kenyon, D. Randall, and A. Sinclair, Approximating the number of monomer-dimer coverings of a lattice, *J. Stat. Phys.* 83 (1996) 637–659; MR 97g:82003.

[16] P. W. Kasteleyn, The statistics of dimers on a lattice. I: The number of dimer arrangements on a quadratic lattice, *Physica* 27 (1961) 1209–1225.

[17] M. E. Fisher, Statistical mechanics of dimers on a plane lattice, *Phys. Rev.* 124 (1961) 1664–1672; MR 24 #B2437.

[18] H. N. V. Temperley and M. E. Fisher, Dimer problem in statistical mechanics – An exact result, *Philos. Mag.* 6 (1961) 1061–1063; MR 24 #B2436.

[19] E. W. Montroll, Lattice statistics, *Applied Combinatorial Mathematics*, ed. E. F. Beckenbach, Wiley, 1964, pp. 96–143; MR 30 #4687.

[20] P. W. Kasteleyn, Graph theory and crystal physics, *Graph Theory and Theoretical Physics*, ed. F. Harary, Academic Press, 1967, pp. 43–110; MR 40 #6903.

[21] J. K. Percus, *Combinatorial Methods*, Springer-Verlag, 1971; MR 49 #10555.

[22] L. Lovász and M. D. Plummer, *Matching Theory*, North-Holland, 1986; MR 88b:90087.

[23] P. John, H. Sachs, and H. Zernitz, Counting perfect matchings in polyminoes with an application to the dimer problem, *Zastos. Mat.* 19 (1987) 465–477; MR 89e: 05158.

[24] H. Sachs and H. Zernitz, Remark on the dimer problem, *Discrete Appl. Math.* 51 (1994) 171–179; MR 97e:05067.

[25] D. M. Cvetkovic, M. Doob, and H. Sachs, *Spectra of Graphs: Theory and Applications*, 3rd ed., Johann Ambrosius Barth Verlag, 1995, pp. 245–251; MR 96b:05108.

[26] D. A. Lavis and G. M. Bell, *Statistical Mechanics of Lattice Systems*, v. 2, Springer-Verlag, 1999; MR 2001g:82002.

[27] J. Propp, Dimers and dominoes, unpublished note (1992).

[28] N. Elkies, G. Kuperberg, M. Larsen, and J. Propp, Alternating-sign matrices and domino tilings. I, *J. Algebraic Combin.* 1 (1992) 111–132; MR 94f:52035.

[29] H. Cohn, R. Kenyon, and J. Propp, A variational principle for domino tilings, *J. Amer. Math. Soc.* 14 (2001) 297–346; math.CO/0008220.

[30] J. F. Nagle, New series-expansion method for the dimer problem, *Phys. Rev.* 152 (1966) 190–197.

[31] D. S. Gaunt, Exact series-expansion study of the monomer-dimer problem, *Phys. Rev.* 179 (1969) 174–186.

[32] A. J. Phares and F. J. Wunderlich, Thermodynamics and molecular freedom of dimers on plane honeycomb and Kagomé lattices, *Nuovo Cimento B* 101 (1988) 653–686; MR 89m:82067.

[33] G. H. Wannier, Antiferromagnetism: The triangular Ising net, *Phys. Rev.* 79 (1950) 357–364; MR 12,576e.

[34] P. W. Kasteleyn, Dimer statistics and phase transitions, *J. Math. Phys.* 4 (1963) 287–293; MR 27 #3394.

[35] F. Y. Wu, Remarks on the modified potassium dihydrogen phosphate model of a ferroelectric, *Phys. Rev.* 168 (1968) 539–543.

[36] J. F. Nagle, Critical points for dimer models with 3/2-order transitions, *Phys. Rev. Lett.* 34 (1975) 1150–1153.

[37] H. W. J. Blöte and H. J. Hilhorst, Roughening transitions and the zero-temperature triangular Ising antiferromagnet, *J. Phys. A* 15 (1982) L631–L637; MR 83k:82046.

[38] C. Richard, M. Höffe, J. Hermisson, and M. Baake, Random tilings: Concepts and examples, *J. Phys. A* 31 (1998) 6385–6408; MR 99g:82033.

[39] V. Elser, Solution of the dimer problem on a hexagonal lattice with boundary, *J. Phys. A* 17 (1984) 1509–1513.

[40] G. David and C. Tomei, The problem of the calissons, *Amer. Math. Monthly* 96 (1989) 429–431; MR 90c:51024.

[41] P. A. MacMahon, *Combinatory Analysis*, Chelsea, 1960, pp. 182–183, 239–242; MR 25 #5003.

[42] A. J. Phares and F. J. Wunderlich, Thermodynamics and molecular freedom of dimers on plane triangular lattices, *J. Math. Phys.* 27 (1986) 1099–1109; MR 87c:82071.

[43] R. Kenyon, The planar dimer model with boundary: A survey, *Directions in Mathematical Quasicrystals*, ed. M. Baake and R. V. Moody, CRM Monogr. 13, Amer. Math. Soc., 2000, pp. 307–328; MR 2002e:82011.

[44] J. Propp, Enumeration of matchings: Problems and progress, *New Perspectives in Algebraic Combinatorics*, Proc. 1996-1997 MSRI Berkeley Program on Combinatorics, ed. L. J. Billera, A. Björner, C. Greene, R. E. Simion, and R. P. Stanley, Cambridge Univ. Press, 1999, pp. 255–291; math.CO/9904150; MR 2001c:05008.

[45] H. Sachs, A contribution to problem 18 in "Twenty open problems in enumeration of matchings," unpublished note (1997).

[46] P. H. Lundow, Computation of matching polynomials and the number of 1-factors in polygraphs, research report 12-1996, Umeå Universitet.

[47] N. J. A. Sloane, On-Line Encyclopedia of Integer Sequences, A005271, A028446, A033535, and A045310.

[48] J. M. Hammersley, Existence theorems and Monte Carlo methods for the monomer-dimer problem, *Research Papers in Statistics: Festschrift for J. Neyman*, ed. F. N. David, Wiley, 1966, pp. 125–146; MR 35 #2595.

[49] J. A. Bondy and D. J. A. Welsh, A note on the monomer-dimer problem, *Proc. Cambridge Philos. Soc.* 62 (1966) 503–505; MR 34 #3958.

[50] J. M. Hammersley, An improved lower bound for the multidimensional dimer problem, *Proc. Cambridge Philos. Soc.* 64 (1968) 455–463; MR 38 #5639.

[51] J. M. Hammersley and V. V. Menon, A lower bound for the monomer-dimer problem, *J. Inst. Math. Appl.* 6 (1970) 341–364; MR 44 #3886.

[52] V. B. Priezzhev, The statistics of dimers on a three-dimensional lattice. I: An exactly solved model, *J. Stat. Phys.* 26 (1981) 817–828; MR 84h:82059a.

[53] V. B. Priezzhev, The statistics of dimers on a three-dimensional lattice. II: An improved lower bound, *J. Stat. Phys.* 26 (1981) 829–837; MR 84h:82059b.

[54] A. Schrijver and W. G. Valiant, On lower bounds for permanents, *Proc. Konink. Nederl. Akad. Wetensch. Ser. A* 83 (1980) 425–427; *Indag. Math.* 42 (1980) 425–427; MR 82a:15004.

[55] A. Schrijver, Counting 1-factors in regular bipartite graphs, *J. Combin. Theory B* 72 (1998) 122–135; MR 99b:05117.

[56] R. H. Fowler and G. S. Rushbrooke, An attempt to extend the statistical theory of perfect solutions, *Trans. Faraday Soc.* 33 (1937) 1272–1294.

[57] H. Minc, An upper bound for the multidimensional dimer problem, *Math. Proc. Cambridge Philos. Soc.* 83 (1978) 461–462; MR 58 #289.

[58] H. Minc, An asymptotic solution of the multidimensional dimer problem, *Linear Multilinear Algebra* 8 (1980) 235–239; MR 81e:82063.

[59] M. Ciucu, An improved upper bound for the 3-dimensional dimer problem, *Duke Math. J.* 94 (1998) 1–11; MR 99f:05026.

[60] P. H. Lundow, Compression of transfer matrices, *Discrete Math.* 231 (2001) 321–329; MR 2002a:05200.

[61] I. Beichl and F. Sullivan, Approximating the permanent via importance sampling with application to the dimer covering problem, *J. Comput. Phys.* 149 (1999) 128–147; MR 99m:82021.

[62] A. J. Phares and F. J. Wunderlich, Thermodynamics of dimers on a rectangular $L \times M \times N$ lattice, *J. Math. Phys.* 26 (1985) 2491–2499; comment by J. C. Wheeler, 28 (1987) 2739–2740; MR 86m:82050 and MR 88m:82038.

[63] H. Narumi, H. Kita, and H. Hosoya, Expressions for the perfect matching numbers of cubic $l \times m \times n$ lattices and their asymptotic values, *J. Math. Chem.* 20 (1996) 67–77; MR 98c:82030.

[64] N. Graham and F. Harary, The number of perfect matchings in a hypercube, *Appl. Math. Lett.* 1 (1988) 45–48.

[65] L. H. Clark, J. C. George, and T. D. Porter, On the number of 1-factors in the n-cube, *Proc. 28th Southeastern Conf. on Combinatorics, Graph Theory and Computing*, Boca Raton, 1997, Congr. Numer. 127, Utilitas Math., 1997, pp. 67–69; MR 98i:05127.

[66]   H. Sachs, Problem 298, How many perfect matchings does the graph of the n-cube have?, *Discrete Math.* 191 (1998) 251.

5.24 Lieb's Square Ice Constant

Let L denote the $n \times n$ planar square lattice with wraparound and let $N = n^2$. An **orientation** of L is an assignment of a direction (or arrow) to each edge of L. What is the number, f_n, of orientations of L such that at each vertex there are exactly two inward and two outward pointing edges? Such orientations are said to obey the **ice rule** and are also called **Eulerian orientations**. The sequence $\{f_n\}$ starts with the terms $f_1 = 4$, $f_2 = 18$, $f_3 = 148$, and $f_4 = 2970$ [1,2]. After intricate analysis, Lieb [3–5] proved that

$$\lim_{n \to \infty} f_n^{\frac{1}{N}} = \left(\frac{4}{3}\right)^{\frac{3}{2}} = \sqrt{\frac{64}{27}} = 1.5396007178\ldots.$$

This constant is known as the **residual entropy for square ice**. A brief discussion of the underlying physics appears in [5.24.3]. The model is also called a **six-vertex model** since, at each vertex, there are six possible configurations of arrows [6–9]. See Figure 5.24.

We turn to several related results. Let $\tilde{f}_n$ denote the number of orientations of L such that at each vertex there are an even number of edges pointing in and an even number pointing out. Clearly $\tilde{f}_n \geq f_n$ and the model is called an **eight-vertex model**. In this case, however, the analysis is not quite so intricate and we have $\tilde{f}_n = 2^{N+1}$ via elementary linear algebra. The corresponding expression for the **sixteen-vertex model** (with no restrictions on the arrows) is obviously 2^{2N}.

Let us focus instead on the planar triangular lattice L with N vertices. What is the number, g_n, of orientations of L such that at each vertex there are exactly three inward and three outward pointing edges? (The phrase *Eulerian orientation* applies here, but not *ice rule*.) Baxter [10] proved that this **twenty-vertex model** satisfies

$$\lim_{n \to \infty} g_n^{\frac{1}{N}} = \sqrt{\frac{27}{4}} = 2.5980762113\ldots.$$

The problem of computing f_n and g_n is the same as counting nowhere-zero flows modulo

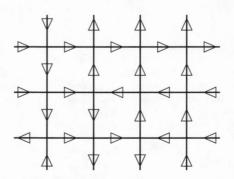

Figure 5.24. A sample planar configuration of arrows satisfying the ice rule.

3 on L [9, 11, 12]. Mihail & Winkler [13] studied related computational complexity issues.

One of several solutions of the famous alternating sign matrix conjecture [1, 14–16] is closely related to the square ice model. This achievement serves to underscore (once again) the commonality of combinatorial theory and statistical physics.

5.24.1 Coloring

Here is a fascinating topic that anticipates the next essay [5.25]. Let u_n denote the number of ways of coloring the vertices of the square lattice with three colors so that no two adjacent vertices are colored alike. Lenard [5] pointed out that $u_n = 3 f_n$. In words, the number of 3-colorings of a square map is thrice the number of square ice configurations. We will return to u_n momentarily, with generalization in mind.

Replace the square lattice by the triangular lattice L and fix an integer $q \geq 4$. Let v_n denote the number of ways of coloring the vertices of L with q colors so that no two adjacent vertices are colored alike. Baxter [17, 18] proved that, if a parameter $-1 < x < 0$ is defined for $q > 4$ by $q = 2 - x - x^{-1}$, then

$$\lim_{n \to \infty} v_n^{\frac{1}{N}} = -\frac{1}{x} \prod_{j=1}^{\infty} \frac{(1 - x^{6j-3})(1 - x^{6j-2})^2(1 - x^{6j-1})}{(1 - x^{6j-5})(1 - x^{6j-4})(1 - x^{6j})(1 - x^{6j+1})}.$$

In particular, letting $q \to 4^+$ (note that the formula makes sense for real q), we obtain

$$C^2 = \lim_{n \to \infty} v_n^{\frac{1}{N}} = \prod_{j=1}^{\infty} \frac{(3j - 1)^2}{(3j - 2)(3j)} = \frac{3}{4\pi^2} \Gamma\left(\tfrac{1}{3}\right)^3$$

$$= 1.4609984862\ldots = (1.2087177032\ldots)^2,$$

which we call **Baxter's 4-coloring constant** for a triangular lattice.

Define likewise u_n and w_n for the number of q-colorings of the square lattice and the hexagonal (honeycomb) lattice with N vertices, respectively. Analytical expressions for the corresponding limiting values are not available, but numerical assessment of certain series expansions provide the list in Table 5.6 [19–21]. The only known quantity in this table is Lieb's constant in the upper left corner. See [5.25] for related discussion on chromatic polynomials.

Table 5.6. *Limiting Values of Roots* $u_n^{1/N}$ *and* $w_n^{1/N}$

q	$\lim_{n \to \infty} u_n^{1/N}$	$\lim_{n \to \infty} w_n^{1/N}$
3	1.5396...	1.6600...
4	2.3360...	2.6034...
5	3.2504...	3.5795...
6	4.2001...	4.5651...
7	5.1667...	5.5553...

5.24.2 Folding

The *square-diagonal folding* problem may be translated into the following coloring problem. Cover the faces of the square lattice with either of the two following square tiles.

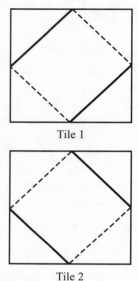

Tile 1

Tile 2

Tile 1: Alternating black and white segments join the centers of the consecutive edges around the square; west-to-north segment is black, north-to-east is white, east-to-south is black, and south-to-west is white. Tile 2: The opposite convention is adopted; west-to-north segment is white, north-to-east is black, east-to-south is white, and south-to-west is black.

There are $2N$ such coverings for a lattice made of N squares. Now, surrounding each vertex of the original lattice, there is a square *loop* formed from the four neighboring tiles. Count the number K_w of purely white loops and the number K_b of purely black loops, assuming wraparound. In the sample covering of Figure 5.25, both K_w and K_b are zero. Define

$$s = \lim_{n \to \infty} \frac{1}{4N} \ln \left(\sum_{\text{coverings}} 2^{K_w + K_b} \right)$$

to be the **entropy of folding** of the **square-diagonal lattice**, where the sum is over all 2^N tiling configurations. (This entropy is per triangle rather than per tile, which explains the additional factor of $1/4$.)

An obvious lower bound for s is

$$s \geq \lim_{n \to \infty} \frac{1}{4N} \ln(2^N + 2^N) = \lim_{n \to \infty} \frac{N+1}{4N} \ln(2) = \frac{1}{4} \ln(2) = 0.1732\ldots,$$

which is obtained by allowing the tiling configurations to alternate like a chessboard. There are two such possibilities (by simple exchanging of all tile 1s by tile 2s and all tile 2s by tile 1s). A more elaborate argument [22, 23] gives $s = 0.2299\ldots$.

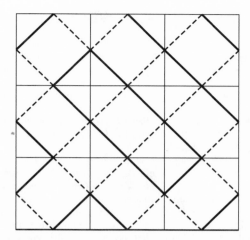

Figure 5.25. Sample covering of a lattice by tiles of both types.

The corresponding **entropy of folding** of the **triangular lattice** is $\ln(C) = 0.1895600483\ldots$ due to Baxter [17, 18] and possesses a simpler coloring interpretation, as already mentioned.

5.24.3 Atomic Arrangement in an Ice Crystal

Square ice is a two-dimensional idealization of water (H_2O) in its solid phase. The oxygen (O) atoms are pictured as the vertices of the square lattice, with outward pointing edges interpreted as the hydrogen (H) atoms. In actuality, however, there are several kinds of three-dimensional ice, depending on temperature and pressure [24, 25]. The residual entropies W for *ordinary hexagonal ice* Ice-Ih and for *cubic ice* Ice-Ic satisfy [3, 26–30]

$$1.5067 < W < 1.5070$$

and are equal within the limits of Nagle's estimation error. These complicated three-dimensional lattices are not the same as the simple models mathematicians tend to focus on.

It would be interesting to see the value of W for the customary $n \times n \times n$ cubic lattice, either with the ice rule in effect (two arrows point out, two arrows point in, and two null arrows) or with Eulerian orientation (three arrows point out and three arrows point in). No one appears to have done this.

[1] N. J. A. Sloane, On-Line Encyclopedia of Integer Sequences, A005130, A050204, and A054759.
[2] J. J. Henry, Ice configuration counts, $1 \leq n \leq 13$, unpublished note (1998).
[3] E. H. Lieb and F. Y. Wu, Two-dimensional ferroelectric models, *Phase Transitions and Critical Phenomena*, v. 1, ed. C. Domb and M. S. Green, Academic Press, 1972, pp. 331–490; MR 50 #6391.

[4]   E. H. Lieb, Exact solution of the problem of the entropy of two-dimensional ice, *Phys. Rev. Lett.* 18 (1967) 692–694.

[5]   E. H. Lieb, Residual entropy of square ice, *Phys. Rev.* 162 (1967) 162–172.

[6]   J. K. Percus, *Combinatorial Methods*, Springer-Verlag, 1971; MR 49 #10555.

[7]   R. J. Baxter, *Exactly Solved Models in Statistical Mechanics*, Academic Press, 1982; MR 90b:82001.

[8]   G. M. Bell and D. A. Lavis, *Statistical Mechanics of Lattice Systems*, v. 1-2, Springer-Verlag, 1999.

[9]   C. Godsil, M. Grötschel, and D. J. A. Welsh, Combinatorics in Statistical Physics, *Handbook of Combinatorics*, v. II, ed. R. Graham, M. Grötschel, and L. Lovász, MIT Press, 1995, pp. 1925–1954; MR 96h:05001.

[10] R. J. Baxter, *F* model on a triangular lattice, *J. Math. Phys.* 10 (1969) 1211–1216.

[11] D. H. Younger, Integer flows, *J. Graph Theory* 7 (1983) 349–357; MR 85d:05223.

[12] C.-Q. Zhang, *Integer Flows and Cycle Covers of Graphs*, Dekker, 1997; MR 98a:05002.

[13] M. Mihail and P. Winkler, On the number of Eulerian orientations of a graph, *Algorithmica* 16 (1996) 402–414; also in *Proc. 3rd ACM-SIAM Symp. on Discrete Algorithms (SODA)*, Orlando, ACM, 1992, pp. 138–145; MR 93f:05059 and MR 97i:68096.

[14] D. Bressoud and J. Propp, How the Alternating Sign Matrix conjecture was solved, *Notices Amer. Math. Soc.* 46 (1999) 637–646; corrections 1353–1354, 1419; MR 2000k:15002.

[15] D. Bressoud, *Proofs and Confirmations: The Story of the Alternating Sign Matrix Conjecture*, Math. Assoc. Amer. and Cambridge Univ. Press, 1999; MR 2000i:15002.

[16] A. Lascoux, Square-ice enumeration, *Sémin. Lothar. Combin.* 42 (1999) B42p; MR 2000f:05086.

[17] R. J. Baxter, Colorings of a hexagonal lattice, *J. Math. Phys.* 11 (1970) 784–789; MR 42 #1457.

[18] R. J. Baxter, *q* colourings of the triangular lattice, *J. Phys. A* 19 (1986) 2821–2839; MR 87k:82123.

[19] J. F. Nagle, A new subgraph expansion for obtaining coloring polynomials for graphs, *J. Combin. Theory* 10 (1971) 42–59; MR 44 #2663.

[20] A. V. Bakaev and V. I. Kabanovich, Series expansions for the q-colour problem on the square and cubic lattices, *J. Phys. A.* 27 (1994) 6731–6739; MR 95i:82014.

[21] R. Shrock and S.-H. Tsai, Asymptotic limits and zeros of chromatic polynomials and ground state entropy of Potts antiferromagnets, *Phys. Rev. E* 55 (1997) 5165; cond-mat/9612249.

[22] P. Di Francesco, Folding the square-diagonal lattice, *Nucl. Phys. B* 525 (1998) 507–548; cond-mat/9803051; MR 99k:82033.

[23] P. Di Francesco, Folding and coloring problems in mathematics and physics, *Bull. Amer. Math. Soc.* 37 (2000) 251–307; MR 2001g:82004.

[24] L. Pauling, *The Nature of the Chemical Bond*, 3rd ed., Cornell Univ. Press, 1960.

[25] *Advances in Physics* 7 (1958) 171–297 (entire issue devoted to the physics of water and ice).

[26] H. Takahasi, Zur Slaterschen Theorie der Umwandlung von KH2PO4 (Teil 1), *Proc. Physico-Math. Soc. Japan* 23 (1941) 1069–1079.

[27] E. A. DiMarzio and F. H. Stillinger, Residual entropy of ice, *J. Chem. Phys.* 40 (1964) 1577–1581.

[28] J. F. Nagle, Lattice statistics of hydrogen bonded crystals. I: The residual entropy of ice, *J. Math. Phys.* 7 (1966) 1484–1491.

[29] J. F. Nagle, Ferroelectric models, *Phase Transitions and Critical Phenomena*, v. 3, ed. C. Domb and M. S. Green, Academic Press, 1974, pp. 653–666; MR 50 #6393.

[30] L. K. Runnels, Ice, *Sci. Amer.*, v. 215 (1966) n. 6, 118–126.

5.25 Tutte–Beraha Constants

Let G be a graph with n vertices v_j [5.6] and let λ be a positive integer. A λ-**coloring** of G is a function $\{v_1, v_2, \ldots, v_n\} \to \{1, 2, \ldots, \lambda\}$ with the property that adjacent vertices must be colored differently. Define $P(\lambda)$ to be the number of λ-colorings of G. Then $P(\lambda)$ is a polynomial of degree n, called the **chromatic polynomial** (or **chromial**) of G. For example, if G is a triangle (three vertices with each pair connected), then $P(\lambda) = \lambda(\lambda - 1)(\lambda - 2)$. Chromatic polynomials were first extensively studied by Birkhoff & Lewis [1]; see [2–6] for introductory material.

A graph G is **planar** if it can be drawn in the plane in such a way that no two edges cross except at a common vertex. The famous Four Color Theorem for geographic maps can be restated as follows: If G is a planar graph, then $P(4) > 0$. Among several restatements of the theorem, we mention Kauffman's combinatorial three-dimensional vector cross product result [7–9].

We can ask about the behavior of $P(\lambda)$ at other real values. Clearly $P(0) = 0$ and, if G is connected, then $P(1) = 0$ and $P(\lambda) \neq 0$ for $\lambda < 0$ or $0 < \lambda < 1$. Further, $P(\varphi + 1) \neq 0$, where φ is the Golden mean [1.2]; more concerning φ will be said shortly.

A connected planar graph G determines a subdivision of the 2-sphere (under stereographic projection) into simply connected regions (faces). If each such region is bounded by a simple closed curve made up of exactly three edges of G, then G is called a **spherical triangulation**. We henceforth assume that this condition is always met.

Clearly $P(2) = 0$ for any spherical triangulation G. Empirical studies of typical G suggest that $P(\lambda) \neq 0$ for $1 < \lambda < 2$, but a single zero is expected in the interval $2 < \lambda < 3$. Tutte [10, 11] proved that

$$0 < |P(\varphi + 1)| \leq \varphi^{5-n};$$

hence $\varphi + 1$, although not itself a zero of $P(\lambda)$, is arbitrarily close to being a zero for large enough n. For this reason, the constant $\varphi + 1$ is called the **golden root**.

It is known that $P(3) > 0$ if and only if G is Eulerian; that is, the number of edges incident with each vertex is even [5]. Hence for non-Eulerian triangulations, we have $P(3) = 0$.

Tutte [12–14] subsequently proved a remarkable identity:

$$P(\varphi + 2) = (\varphi + 2)\varphi^{3n-10} \left(P(\varphi + 1) \right)^2,$$

which implies that $P(\varphi + 2) > 0$. Note that $\varphi + 2 = \sqrt{5}\varphi = 3.6180339887\ldots$. As stated earlier, $P(4) > 0$, and $P(\lambda) > 0$ for $\lambda \geq 5$ [1]. It is natural to ask about the possible whereabouts of the next accumulation point for zeros (after $2.618\ldots$).

Rigorous theory fails us here, so numerical evidence must suffice [15–18]. In the following, fix a family $\{G_k\}$ of spherical triangulations, where n_k is the order of G_k and $n_k \to \infty$ as $k \to \infty$. Typically, the graph G_k is recursively constructed from G_{k-1} for each k, but this is not essential. Experimental results indicate that the next batch of chromatic zeros might cluster around the point

$$\psi = 2 + 2\cos\left(\frac{2\pi}{7}\right) = 4\cos\left(\frac{\pi}{7}\right)^2 = 3.2469796037\ldots,$$

that is, a solution of the cubic equation $\psi^3 - 5\psi^2 + 6\psi - 1 = 0$. The constant ψ is called the **silver root** by analogy with the golden root $\varphi + 1$.

Or the zeros might cluster around some other point $> \psi$, but ≤ 4. Beraha [19] observed a pattern in the potential accumulation points, independent of the choice of $\{G_k\}$. He conjectured that, for arbitrary $\{G_k\}$, if chromatic zeros z_k cluster around a real number x, then $x = B_N$ for some $N \geq 1$, where

$$B_N = 2 + 2\cos\left(\frac{2\pi}{N}\right) = 4\cos\left(\frac{\pi}{N}\right)^2.$$

In words, the limiting values x cannot fall outside of a certain countably infinite set. Note that the **Tutte–Beraha constants** B_N include all the roots already discussed:

$$B_2 = 0, \quad B_3 = 1, \qquad B_4 = 2, \qquad B_5 = \varphi + 1,$$
$$B_6 = 3, \quad B_7 = \psi, \quad B_{10} = \varphi + 2, \quad \lim_{N\to\infty} B_N = 4.$$

Specific families $\{G_k\}$ have been constructed that can be proved to possess B_5, B_7, or B_{10} as accumulation points [20–23]. The marvel of Beraha's conjecture rests in its generality: It applies regardless of the configuration of G_k.

Beraha & Kahane also built a family $\{G_k\}$ possessing $B_1 = 4$ as an accumulation point. This is surprising since we know $P(4) > 0$ always, but $P_k(z_k) = 0$ for all k and $\lim_{k\to\infty} z_k = 4$. Hence the Four Color Theorem, although true, is nearly false [24].

The Tutte–Beraha constants also arise in mathematical physics [25–28] since evaluating $P(\lambda)$ over a lattice is equivalent to solving the λ-state zero-temperature anti-ferromagnetic Potts model. A heuristic explanation of the Beraha conjecture in [27] is insightful but is not a rigorous proof [8]. See [5.24] for related discussion on coloring and ice models. Other expressions containing $\cos(\pi/7)$ are mentioned in [2.23] and [8.2].

[1]   G. D. Birkhoff and D. C. Lewis, Chromatic polynomials, *Trans. Amer. Math. Soc.* 60 (1946) 355–451; MR 8,284f.

[2]   T. L. Saaty and P. C. Kainen, *The Four-Color Problem: Assaults and Conquest*, McGraw-Hill, 1977; MR 87k:05084.

[3]   R. C. Read and W. T. Tutte, Chromatic polynomials, *Selected Topics in Graph Theory. 3*, ed. L. W. Beineke and R. J. Wilson, Academic Press, 1988, pp. 15–42; MR 93h:05003.

[4]   W. T. Tutte, Chromials, *Hypergraph Seminar*, Proc. 1972 Ohio State Univ. conf., ed. C. Berge and D. Ray-Chaudhuri, Lect. Notes in Math. 411, Springer-Verlag, 1974, pp. 243–266; MR 51 #5370.

[5]   W. T. Tutte, The graph of the chromial of a graph, *Combinatorial Mathematics III*, Proc. 1974 Univ. of Queensland conf., ed. A. P. Street and W. D. Wallis, Lect. Notes in Math. 452, Springer-Verlag, 1975, pp. 55–61; MR 51 #10152.

[6]   W. T. Tutte, Chromials, *Studies in Graph Theory. Part II*, ed. D. R. Fulkerson, Math. Assoc. Amer., 1975, pp. 361–377; MR 53 #10637.

[7]   L. H. Kauffman, Map coloring and the vector cross product, *J. Combin. Theory Ser. B* 48 (1990) 145–154; MR 91b:05078.

[8]   L. H. Kauffman and H. Saluer, An algebraic approach to the planar coloring problem, *Commun. Math. Phys.* 152 (1993) 565–590; MR 94f:05056.

[9]   R. Thomas, An update on the four-color theorem, *Notices Amer. Math. Soc.* 45 (1998) 848–859; MR 99g:05082.

[10] G. Berman and W. T. Tutte, The golden root of a chromatic polynomial, *J. Combin. Theory* 6 (1969) 301–302; MR 39 #98.

[11] W. T. Tutte, On chromatic polynomials and the golden ratio, *J. Combin. Theory* 9 (1970) 289–296; MR 42 #7557.

[12] W. T. Tutte, More about chromatic polynomials and the golden ratio, *Combinatorial Structures and Their Applications*, Proc. 1969 Univ. of Calgary conf., ed. R. K. Guy, H. Hanani, N. Sauer, and J. Schönheim, Gordon and Breach, 1970, pp. 439–453; MR 41 #8299.

[13] W. T. Tutte, The golden ratio in the theory of chromatic polynomials, *Annals New York Acad. Sci.* 175 (1970) 391–402; MR 42 #130.

[14] D. W. Hall, On golden identities for constrained chromials, *J. Combin. Theory Ser. B* 11 (1971) 287–298; MR 44 #6510.

[15] D. W. Hall and D. C. Lewis, Coloring six-rings, *Trans. Amer. Math. Soc.* 64 (1948) 184–191; MR 10,136g.

[16] D. W. Hall, J. W. Siry, and B. R. Vanderslice, The chromatic polynomial of the truncated icosahedron, *Proc. Amer. Math. Soc.* 16 (1965) 620–628; MR 31 #3361.

[17] D. W. Hall, Coloring seven-circuits, *Graphs and Combinatorics*, Proc. 1973 George Washington Univ. conf., ed. R. A. Bari and F. Harary, Lect. Notes in Math. 406, Springer-Verlag, 1974, pp. 273–290; MR 51 #5366.

[18] W. T. Tutte, Chromatic sums for rooted planar triangulations. V: Special equations, *Canad. J. Math.* 26 (1974) 893–907; MR 50 #167.

[19] S. Beraha, *Infinite Non-trivial Families of Maps and Chromials*, Ph.D. thesis, Johns Hopkins Univ., 1974.

[20] S. Beraha, J. Kahane, and R. Reid, B_7 and B_{10} are limit points of chromatic zeroes, *Notices Amer. Math. Soc.* 20 (1973) A-5.

[21] S. Beraha, J. Kahane, and N. J. Weiss, Limits of zeroes of recursively defined polynomials, *Proc. Nat. Acad. Sci. USA* 72 (1975) 4209; MR 52 #5946.

[22] S. Beraha, J. Kahane, and N. J. Weiss, Limits of zeros of recursively defined families of polynomials, *Studies in Foundations and Combinatorics*, ed. G.-C. Rota, Academic Press, 1978, pp. 213–232; MR 80c:30005.

[23] S. Beraha, J. Kahane, and N. J. Weiss, Limits of chromatic zeros of some families of maps, *J. Combin. Theory Ser. B* 28 (1980) 52–65; MR 81f:05076.

[24] S. Beraha and J. Kahane, Is the four-color conjecture almost false?, *J. Combin. Theory Ser. B* 27 (1979) 1–12; MR 80j:05061.

[25] R. J. Baxter, *Exactly Solved Models in Statistical Mechanics*, Academic Press, 1982; MR 90b:82001.

[26] R. J. Baxter, Chromatic polynomials of large triangular lattices, *J. Phys. A.* 20 (1987) 5241–5261; MR 89a:82033.

[27] H. Saleur, Zeroes of chromatic polynomials: A new approach to Beraha conjecture using quantum groups, *Commun. Math. Phys.* 132 (1990) 657–679; MR 91k:17014.

[28] H. Saleur, The antiferromagnetic Potts model in two dimensions: Berker Kadanoff phases, antiferromagnetic transition and the role of Beraha numbers, *Nucl. Phys. B* 360 (1991) 219–263; MR 92j:82016.

6

Constants Associated with Functional Iteration

6.1 Gauss' Lemniscate Constant

In 1799, Gauss observed that the limiting value, M, of the following sequence:

$$a_0 = 1, \quad b_0 = \sqrt{2}, \quad a_n = \frac{a_{n-1} + b_{n-1}}{2}, \quad b_n = \sqrt{a_{n-1}b_{n-1}} \text{ for } n \geq 1$$

must satisfy

$$\frac{1}{M} = \lim_{n \to \infty} \frac{1}{a_n} = \lim_{n \to \infty} \frac{1}{b_n} = \frac{2}{\pi} \int_0^1 \frac{dx}{\sqrt{1-x^4}} = 0.8346268416\ldots$$

$$= \frac{1}{1.1981402347\ldots}.$$

The recursive formulation is based on what is called the **arithmetic-geometric-mean (AGM) algorithm**. Gauss recognized this limit to be an extraordinary result and pointed out an interesting connection to geometry as well. The total arclength of the lemniscate $r^2 = \cos(2\theta)$ is given by $2L$, where

$$L = \int_0^\pi \frac{d\theta}{\sqrt{1 + \sin(\theta)^2}} = 2 \int_0^1 \frac{dx}{\sqrt{1-x^4}} = 2.6220575542\ldots$$

and thus $L = \pi/M$. The **lemniscate constant** L plays a role for the lemniscate analogous to what π plays for the circle, and the AGM algorithm provides a quadratically convergent method of computing it [1–5].

Other representations of L are

$$L = \sqrt{2}K\left(\frac{1}{\sqrt{2}}\right) = \frac{1}{2\sqrt{2\pi}}\Gamma\left(\frac{1}{4}\right)^2 = \frac{\pi}{\sqrt{2}}\exp\left(\frac{1}{2}\left[\gamma - \frac{\beta'(1)}{\beta(1)}\right]\right),$$

where K denotes the complete elliptic integral of the first kind [1.4.6], $\Gamma(x)$ is the Euler gamma function [1.5.4], γ is the Euler–Mascheroni constant [1.5], and $\beta(x)$ is Dirichlet's beta function [1.7]. As stated in [2.10], clearly this is a meeting place for many ideas! Two rapidly convergent series are [4, 6]

$$\frac{1}{M} = \left[\sum_{n=-\infty}^{\infty} (-1)^n e^{-\pi n^2}\right]^2 = 2^{\frac{5}{4}} e^{\frac{-\pi}{3}} \left[\sum_{n=-\infty}^{\infty} (-1)^n e^{-2\pi(3n+1)n}\right]^2.$$

A third series involving central binomial coefficients appears in [1.5.4].

Several authors [7, 8] identify $M/\sqrt{2} = 0.8472130848\ldots$ as the so-called "ubiquitous constant," and the value $L/\sqrt{2} = 1.8540746773\ldots$ is also given in [9]. The definite integrals

$$\int_0^1 \frac{dx}{\sqrt{1-x^4}} = \frac{L}{2} = 1.3110287771\ldots, \quad \int_0^1 \frac{x^2 dx}{\sqrt{1-x^4}} = \frac{M}{2} = 0.5990701173\ldots$$

are sometimes called, respectively, the first and second lemniscate constants [4, 10, 11].

Gauss correctly anticipated that his limiting result and others like it would ignite research for many years to come. The massive field of *elliptic modular functions*, associated with names such as Abel, Jacobi, Cayley, Klein, and Fricke, can be said to have started with Gauss' observation [1, 4]. Although the theory slipped into obscurity by the 1900s, it has recently enjoyed a renaissance. Two contributing factors in this renaissance are the widespread awakening to Ramanujan's achievements and the discovery of fast algorithms for computing π, based on AGM-like recursions.

The constant L was proved in 1937 to be transcendental by Schneider [12]. Let us now consider something slightly more complicated. The infinite product over all nonzero Gaussian integers

$$\sigma(z) = z \prod_{\omega \neq 0} \left(1 - \frac{z}{\omega}\right) \exp\left(\frac{z}{\omega} + \frac{z^2}{2\omega^2}\right)$$

is called the **Weierstrass sigma function** [13, 14]. One has [15–17]

$$\sigma\left(\tfrac{1}{2}\right) = 2^{\frac{5}{4}} \pi^{\frac{1}{2}} e^{\frac{\pi}{8}} \Gamma\left(\tfrac{1}{4}\right)^{-2} = 2^{-\frac{1}{4}} e^{\frac{\pi}{8}} L^{-1} = 0.4749493799\ldots,$$

and this is transcendental, thanks to work by Nesterenko in 1996. Hence it took nearly sixty years for sufficient progress to be made to deal with the extra $\exp(\pi/8)$ factor in $\sigma(1/2)$! More results of this nature appear in [1.5.4].

Instead of the Gaussian integers ω, examine the lattice of points

$$\left\{\tilde{\omega} = j \cdot \left(\tfrac{1}{2} - i\tfrac{\sqrt{3}}{2}\right) + k \cdot \left(\tfrac{1}{2} + i\tfrac{\sqrt{3}}{2}\right) : -\infty < j, k < \infty \text{ are integers}\right\},$$

and define $\tilde{\sigma}(z)$ analogously over all such nonzero $\tilde{\omega}$. We will need this function shortly [6.1.1].

Starting with work of Erdös, Herzog & Piranian [18], Borwein [19] studied an interesting question. Let $p(z)$ denote a monic polynomial of degree n. Consider the curve in the complex plane given by $|p(z)| = 1$. Is the total arclength of this curve no greater than that for $p(z) = z^n - 1$? In the special case when $n = 2$, this reduces to the lemniscate $r^2 = 2\cos(2\theta)$, which has arclength $2\sqrt{2}L$. See [20] for recent progress on answering this question.

The integral

$$\int\limits_0^1 \sqrt{1 - x^4}\,dx = \frac{L}{3} = 0.8740191847\ldots$$

occurs in our discussion of the Landau–Ramanujan constant [2.3], in connection with recent number theoretic work by Friedlander & Iwaniec. Also, from geometric probability, M arises in an expression for the expected perimeter of the convex hull of N random points in the unit square, as discussed in [8.1].

6.1.1 Weierstrass Pe Function

Given $\sigma(z)$ and $\tilde{\sigma}(z)$ as defined in the previous section, let

$$\wp(z) = -\frac{d^2}{dz^2}\ln(\sigma(z)), \quad \tilde{\wp}(z) = -\frac{d^2}{dz^2}\ln(\tilde{\sigma}(z)).$$

Like the Jacobi elliptic functions [1.4.6], both $\wp(z)$ and $\tilde{\wp}(z)$ are doubly periodic meromorphic functions. The real half-period r of $\wp(x)$ is $L/\sqrt{2} = 1.8540746773\ldots$, whereas the real half-period $\tilde{r}$ of $\tilde{\wp}(x)$ is [1, 9, 21]

$$\frac{\sqrt[3]{2}}{\sqrt[4]{3}} K\left(\frac{\sqrt{2 - \sqrt{3}}}{2}\right) = \frac{1}{4\pi}\Gamma\left(\frac{1}{3}\right)^3 = 1.5299540370.\ldots$$

Further, for all $0 < x \le r$ and $0 < y \le \tilde{r}$, we have

$$x = \int\limits_{\wp(x)}^{\infty} \frac{1}{\sqrt{(4t^2 - 1)t}}\,dt, \quad y = \int\limits_{\tilde{\wp}(y)}^{\infty} \frac{1}{\sqrt{4t^3 - 1}}\,dt,$$

which suggest why $\wp(z)$ and $\tilde{\wp}(z)$ are important in elliptic curve theory [22]. The **Weierstrass pe function** is, in fact, a two-parameter family of functions and encompasses the two examples provided here.

[1] J. M. Borwein and P. B. Borwein, *Pi and the AGM: A Study in Analytic Number Theory and Computational Complexity*, Wiley, 1987, pp. 1–15, 27–32; MR 99h:11147.
[2] D. A. Cox, The arithmetic-geometric mean of Gauss, *Enseign. Math.* 30 (1984) 275–330; MR 86a:01027.
[3] G. Miel, Of calculations past and present: The Archimedean algorithm, *Amer. Math. Monthly* 90 (1983) 17–35; MR 85a:01006.
[4] J. Todd, The lemniscate constants, *Commun. ACM* 18 (1975) 14–19, 462; MR 51 #11935.
[5] D. Shanks, The second-order term in the asymptotic expansion of $B(x)$, *Math. Comp.* 18 (1964) 75–86; MR 28 #2391.
[6] D. H. Lehmer, The lemniscate constant, *Math. Tables Other Aids Comput.* 3 (1948-49) 550–551.
[7] J. Spanier and K. B. Oldham, *An Atlas of Functions*, Hemisphere, 1987.
[8] M. Schroeder, How probable is Fermat's last theorem?, *Math. Intellig.* 16 (1994) 19–20; MR 95e:11040.
[9] M. Abramowitz and I. A. Stegun, *Handbook of Mathematical Functions*, Dover, 1972, pp. 652, 658; MR 94b:00012.

[10] R. W. Gosper, A calculus of series rearrangements, *Algorithms and Complexity: New Directions and Recent Results*, Proc. 1976 Carnegie-Mellon conf., ed. J. F. Traub, Academic Press, 1976, pp. 121–151; MR 56 #9899.

[11] S. Lewanowicz and S. Paszkowski, An analytic method for convergence acceleration of certain hypergeometric series, *Math. Comp.* 64 (1995) 691–713; MR 95h:33006.

[12] C. L. Siegel, *Transcendental Numbers*, Princeton Univ. Press, 1949, pp. 95–100; MR 11,330c.

[13] S. Lang, *Complex Analysis*, 3rd ed., Springer-Verlag, 1993; MR 99i:30001.

[14] K. Chandrasekharan, *Elliptic Functions*, Springer-Verlag, 1985; MR 87e:11058.

[15] M. Waldschmidt, Nombres transcendants et fonctions sigma de Weierstrass, *C. R. Math. Rep. Acad. Sci. Canada* 1 (1978/79) 111–114; MR 80f:10044.

[16] F. Le Lionnais, *Les Nombres Remarquables*, Hermann, 1983.

[17] S. Plouffe, Weierstrass constant (Plouffe's Tables).

[18] P. Erdős, F. Herzog, and G. Piranian, Metric properties of polynomials, *J. d'Analyse Math.* 6 (1958) 125–148; MR 21 #123.

[19] P. Borwein, The arc length of the lemniscate $|p(z)| = 1$, *Proc. Amer. Math. Soc.* 123 (1995) 797–799; MR 95d:31001.

[20] A. Eremenko and W. Hayman, On the length of lemniscates, *Michigan Math. J.* 46 (1999) 409–415; MR 2000k:30001.

[21] T. H. Southard, Approximation and table of the Weierstrass $\wp$ function in the equianharmonic case for real argument, *Math. Tables Aids Comput.* 11 (1957) 99–100; MR 19,182c.

[22] J. H. Silverman, *The Arithmetic of Elliptic Curves*, Springer-Verlag, 1986, pp. 150–159; MR 87g:11070.

6.2 Euler–Gompertz Constant

The regular continued fraction

$$c_1 = 0 + \frac{1|}{|1} + \frac{1|}{|2} + \frac{1|}{|3} + \frac{1|}{|4} + \frac{1|}{|5} + \cdots$$

is convergent (hence it differs from the harmonic series in this regard). Its limiting value is [1–3]

$$\frac{I_1(2)}{I_0(2)} = c_1 = 0.6977746579\ldots,$$

where $I_0(x)$, $I_1(x)$ denote modified Bessel functions [3.6]. Using this formula, Siegel [4, 5] proved that c_1 is transcendental.

What happens if we reverse the patterns of the numerators and denominators prescribed in c_1? We obtain [6, 7]

$$C_1 = 0 + \frac{1|}{|1} + \frac{1|}{|1} + \frac{2|}{|1} + \frac{3|}{|1} + \frac{4|}{|1} + \frac{5|}{|1} + \cdots = \sqrt{\frac{\pi e}{2}} \operatorname{erfc}\left(\frac{1}{\sqrt{2}}\right)$$

$$= \int_1^\infty \exp\left[\tfrac{1}{2}(1 - x^2)\right] dx = \sqrt{\frac{\pi e}{2}} - \tilde{C}_1 = 0.6556795424\ldots,$$

where erfc is the complementary error function [4.6] and

$$\tilde{C}_1 = \sum_{n=1}^{\infty} \frac{1}{1 \cdot 3 \cdot 5 \cdots (2n-1)} = \sqrt{\frac{\pi e}{2}} \operatorname{erf}\left(\frac{1}{\sqrt{2}}\right) = 1.4106861346\ldots.$$

What happens if we additionally repeat each numerator? In this case, we obtain [6, 8]

$$C_2 = 0 + \frac{1|}{|1} + \frac{1|}{|1} + \frac{1|}{|1} + \frac{2|}{|1} + \frac{2|}{|1} + \frac{3|}{|1} + \frac{3|}{|1} + \frac{4|}{|1} + \frac{4|}{|1} + \frac{5|}{|1} + \frac{5|}{|1} + \cdots$$

$$= -e\,\mathrm{Ei}(-1) = \int\limits_{1}^{\infty} \frac{\exp(1-x)}{x}dx = 0.5963473623\ldots,$$

where Ei is the exponential integral [6.2.1]. More about the **Euler–Gompertz constant** C_2 appears shortly.

No one knows the exact outcome if we instead repeat each denominator in c_1, although numerically we find $c_2 = 0.5851972651\ldots$.

Euler [9–11] discovered that

$$0 + \frac{1|}{|1} + \frac{1^2|}{|1} + \frac{2^2|}{|1} + \frac{3^2|}{|1} + \frac{4^2|}{|1} + \frac{5^2|}{|1} + \cdots = \ln(2) = 0.6931471805\ldots$$

and Ramanujan [12, 13] discovered that

$$0 + \frac{1|}{|1} + \frac{1^2|}{|1} + \frac{1^2|}{|1} + \frac{2^2|}{|1} + \frac{2^2|}{|1} + \frac{3^2|}{|1} + \frac{3^2|}{|1} + \frac{4^2|}{|1} + \frac{4^2|}{|1} + \frac{5^2|}{|1} + \frac{5^2|}{|1} + \cdots$$

$$= 4\int\limits_{1}^{\infty} \frac{x\exp(-\sqrt{5}x)}{\cosh(x)}dx = 0.5683000031\ldots.$$

Again, however, no one knows the exact outcome if we reverse the patterns of the numerators and denominators, or if the exponents are chosen to be ≥ 3.

6.2.1 Exponential Integral

Let γ be the Euler–Mascheroni constant [1.5]. The **exponential integral** $\mathrm{Ei}(x)$ is defined by

$$\mathrm{Ei}(x) = \gamma + \ln|x| + \sum_{k=1}^{\infty} \frac{x^k}{k \cdot k!} = \begin{cases} \displaystyle\lim_{\varepsilon \to 0^+} \left(\int\limits_{-\infty}^{-\varepsilon} \frac{e^t}{t}dt + \int\limits_{\varepsilon}^{x} \frac{e^t}{t}dt \right) & \text{if } x > 0, \\[4mm] \displaystyle\int\limits_{-\infty}^{x} \frac{e^t}{t}dt & \text{if } x < 0; \end{cases}$$

that is, $\mathrm{Ei}(x)$ is the Cauchy principal value of the improper integral. Sample applications of $\mathrm{Ei}(x)$ include evaluating the Raabe integrals [14–16]

$$A = \int\limits_{0}^{\infty} \frac{\sin(x)}{1+x^2}dx = \tfrac{1}{2}\left(e^{-1}\,\mathrm{Ei}(1) - e\,\mathrm{Ei}(-1)\right),$$

$$B = \int\limits_{0}^{\infty} \frac{x\cos(x)}{1+x^2}dx = -\tfrac{1}{2}\left(e^{-1}\,\mathrm{Ei}(1) + e\,\mathrm{Ei}(-1)\right),$$

which provide closure to an issue raised in [1.4.3].

6.2.2 Logarithmic Integral

Define the **logarithmic integral** for $0 < x \neq 1$ by the formula $\text{Li}(x) = \text{Ei}(\ln(x))$. There exists a unique number $\mu > 1$ satisfying $\text{Li}(\mu) = 0$, and Ramanujan and Soldner [17–22] numerically calculated $\mu = 1.4513692348\ldots$ For example [23],

$$\text{Li}(2) = \lim_{\varepsilon \to 0^+} \left(\int_0^{1-\varepsilon} \frac{1}{\ln(t)} dt + \int_{1+\varepsilon}^{2} \frac{1}{\ln(t)} dt \right) = \int_\mu^2 \frac{1}{\ln(t)} dt = 1.0451637801\ldots.$$

The famous Prime Number Theorem [2.1] is usually stated in terms of $\text{Li}(x)$ or $\text{li}(x) = \text{Li}(x) - \text{Li}(2)$. Since these are both $O(x/\ln(x))$ as $x \to \infty$, the difference $\text{Li}(2)$ is regarded by analytic number theorists as (asymptotically) insignificant.

6.2.3 Divergent Series

What meaning can be given to the divergent alternating factorial series $0! - 1! + 2! - 3! + - \cdots$? Euler formally deduced that [24–28]

$$\sum_{n=0}^{\infty} (-1)^n \, n! = \sum_{n=0}^{\infty} \left((-1)^n \int_0^\infty x^n e^{-x} dx \right) = \int_0^\infty \frac{e^{-x}}{1+x} dx = C_2.$$

The even and odd parts of the series can be evaluated separately [29–31]:

$$\sum_{n=0}^{\infty} (2n)! = A = 0.6467611227\ldots, \quad \sum_{n=0}^{\infty} (2n+1)! = -B = 0.0504137604\ldots,$$

where A and B are the definite integrals defined earlier. Also, in the same extended sense [32,33],

$$\sum_{n=1}^{\infty} (-1)^{n+1} (2n+1)!! = 1 \cdot 3 - 1 \cdot 3 \cdot 5 + 1 \cdot 3 \cdot 5 \cdot 7 - 1 \cdot 3 \cdot 5 \cdot 7 \cdot 9 + - \cdots = C_1.$$

6.2.4 Survival Analysis

Le Lionnais [34] called C_2 Gompertz's constant; it is interesting to attempt an explanation. Let the lifetime X of an individual be a random variable with cumulative distribution function $F(x) = \text{P}(X \leq x)$ and probability density function $f(x) = F'(x)$. Then the probability that an individual, having survived to time x, will survive at most an additional time t, is

$$\text{P}(X - x \leq t \mid X > x) = \frac{\text{P}(x < X \leq x + t)}{\text{P}(X > x)} = \frac{F(x+t) - F(x)}{1 - F(x)}.$$

This is related to what is known in actuarial science as the **force of mortality** or the **hazard function** [35,36]. The conditional expectation of $X - x$, given $X > x$, is hence

$$\text{E}(X - x \mid X > x) = \int_0^\infty \frac{t \cdot f(x+t)}{1 - F(x)} \, dt.$$

Consider the well-known Gompertz distribution [37]

$$F(x) = 1 - \exp\left[\frac{b}{a}(1 - e^{ax})\right], \quad x > 0, \ a > 0, \ b > 0,$$

and let $x = m$ be the mode of f, that is, the unique point at which $f'(m) = 0$. Then it is easily shown that [38], for all a and b,

$$E(X - m \mid X > m) = \frac{C_2}{a},$$

which is a curious occurrence of Euler's original constant.

Similarly, if $\Phi(x) = \text{erf}(x/\sqrt{2})$ and $\varphi(x) = \Phi'(x)$, that is, if X follows the half-normal (folded) distribution, then at the point of inflection $x = 1$,

$$E(X - 1 \mid X > 1) = \sqrt{\frac{\pi}{2}}\left(\frac{1}{C_1} - 1\right), \quad \frac{1 - \Phi(1)}{\varphi(1)} = C_1.$$

In closing, here are two additional continued fraction expansions [6, 10, 39–41]:

$$\tilde{C}_1 = 0 + \frac{1|}{|1} - \frac{1|}{|3} + \frac{2|}{|5} - \frac{3|}{|7} + \frac{4|}{|9} - + \cdots,$$

$$C_2 = 0 + \frac{1|}{|2} - \frac{1^2|}{|4} - \frac{2^2|}{|6} - \frac{3^2|}{|8} - \frac{4^2|}{|10} - \cdots.$$

Note that $(1 - C_2)/e = 0.1484955067\ldots$ is connected with two-sided generalized Fibonacci sequences [42]. The Euler–Gompertz constant also appears in [5.6.2] with regard to increasing mobile trees.

[1] D. H. Lehmer, Continued fractions containing arithmetic progressions, *Scripta Math.* 29 (1973) 17–24; MR 48 #5979.

[2] S. Rabinowitz, Asymptotic estimates for convergents of a continued fraction, *Amer. Math. Monthly* 97 (1990) 157.

[3] N. Robbins, A note regarding continued fractions, *Fibonacci Quart.* 33 (1995) 311–312; MR 96d:11010.

[4] C. L. Siegel, Über einige Anwendungen diophantischer Approximationen, *Abh. Preuss. Akad. Wiss., Phys.-Math. Klasse* (1929) n. 1, 1–70; also in *Gesammelte Abhandlungen*, v. 1, ed. K. Chandrasekharan and H. Maass, Springer-Verlag, 1966, pp. 209–266.

[5] C. L. Siegel, *Transcendental Numbers*, Chelsea 1965, pp. 59, 71–72; MR 11,330c.

[6] H. S. Wall, *Analytic Theory of Continued Fractions*, Van Nostrand, 1948, pp. 356–358, 367; MR 10,32d

[7] B. C. Berndt, Y.-S. Choi, and S.-Y. Kang, The problems submitted by Ramanujan to the Journal of the Indian Mathematical Society, *Continued Fractions: From Analytic Number Theory to Constructive Approximation*, Proc. 1998 Univ. of Missouri conf., ed. B. C. Berndt and F. Gesztesy, Amer. Math. Soc., 1999, pp. 15–56; MR 2000i:11003.

[8] L. Lorentzen and H. Waadeland, *Continued Fractions with Applications*, North-Holland 1992, pp. 576–577; MR 93g:30007.

[9] L. Euler, *Introduction to Analysis of the Infinite. Book I*, 1748, transl. J. D. Blanton, Springer-Verlag, 1988, pp. 311–312; MR 89g:01067.

[10] B. C. Berndt, *Ramanujan's Notebooks: Part II*, Springer-Verlag, 1989, pp. 147–149, 167–172; MR 90b:01039.

[11] B. C. Berndt, *Ramanujan's Notebooks: Part V*, Springer-Verlag, 1998, p. 56; MR 99f:11024.

[12] G. H. Hardy, Srinivasa Ramanujan obituary notice, *Proc. London Math. Soc.* 19 (1921) xl–lviii.

[13] C. T. Preece, Theorems stated by Ramanujan. X, *J. London Math. Soc.* 6 (1931) 22–32.

[14] A. Erdélyi, W. Magnus, F. Oberhettinger, and F. G. Tricomi, *Higher Transcendental Functions*, v. 2, McGraw-Hill, 1953, pp. 143–147; MR 15, 419.

[15] I. S. Gradshteyn and I. M. Ryzhik, *Table of Integrals, Series and Products*, 6th ed., Academic Press, 2000, pp. 417–418; MR 2001c:00002.

[16] M. Abramowitz and I. A. Stegun, *Handbook of Mathematical Functions*, Dover, 1972, pp. 78, 230–233, 302; MR 94b:00012.

[17] G. H. Hardy, P. V. Seshu Aiyar, and B. M. Wilson (eds.), Further extracts from Ramanujan's letters, *Collected Papers of Srinivasa Ramanujan*, Cambridge Univ. Press, 1927, pp. 349–355.

[18] G. H. Hardy, *Ramanujan: Twelve Lectures on Subjects Suggested by His Life and Work*, Chelsea, 1959, p. 45; MR 21 #4881.

[19] N. Nielsen, *Theorie des Integrallogarithmus und verwandter Transzendenten*, Chelsea, 1965, p. 88; MR 32 #2622.

[20] B. C. Berndt and R. J. Evans, Some elegant approximations and asymptotic formulas for Ramanujan, *J. Comput. Appl. Math.* 37 (1991) 35–41; MR 93a:41055.

[21] B. C. Berndt, *Ramanujan's Notebooks: Part IV*, Springer-Verlag, 1994, pp. 123–124; MR 95e:11028.

[22] P. Sebah, 75500 digits of the Ramanujan-Soldner constant via fast quartic Newton iteration, unpublished note (2001).

[23] A. E. Ingham, *The Distribution of Prime Numbers*, Cambridge Univ. Press, 1932, p. 3.

[24] G. N. Watson, Theorems stated by Ramanujan. VIII: Theorems on divergent series, *J. London Math. Soc.* 4 (1929) 82–86.

[25] T. J. I'A. Bromwich, *An Introduction to the Theory of Infinite Series*, 2nd ed., MacMillan, 1942, pp. 323–324, 336.

[26] G. H. Hardy, *Divergent Series*, Oxford Univ. Press, 1949, pp. 26–29; MR 11,25a.

[27] E. J. Barbeau, Euler subdues a very obstreperous series, *Amer. Math. Monthly* 86 (1979) 356–372; MR 80i:01007.

[28] B. C. Berndt, *Ramanujan's Notebooks: Part I*, Springer-Verlag, 1985, pp. 101–103, 143–145; MR 86c:01062.

[29] J. Keane, Subseries of the alternating factorial series, unpublished note (2001).

[30] R. B. Dingle, Asymptotic expansions and converging factors. I: General theory and basic converging factors, *Proc. Royal Soc. London. Ser. A* 244 (1958) 456–475; MR 21 #2145.

[31] R. B. Dingle, *Asymptotic Expansions: Their Derivation and Interpretation*, Academic Press, 1973, pp. 447–448; MR 58 #17673.

[32] L. Euler, De seriebus divergentibus, 1754, *Opera Omnia Ser. I*, v. 14, Lipsiae, 1911, pp. 585–617.

[33] E. J. Barbeau and P. J. Leah, Euler's 1760 paper on divergent series, *Historia Math.* 3 (1976) 141–160; 5 (1978) 332; MR 58 #21162a-b.

[34] F. Le Lionnais, *Les Nombres Remarquables*, Hermann 1983.

[35] R. C. Elandt-Johnson and N. L. Johnson, *Survival Models and Data Analysis*, Wiley, 1980; MR 81j:62195.

[36] M. L. Garg, B. Raja Rao, and C. K. Redmond, Maximum-likelihood estimation of the parameters of the Gompertz survival function, *J. Royal Statist. Soc. Ser. C Appl. Statist.* 19 (1970) 152–159; MR 42 #2581.

[37] B. Gompertz, On the nature of the function expressive of the law of human mortality, and on the new mode of determining the value of life contingencies, *Philos. Trans. Royal Soc. London* 115 (1825) 513–585.

[38] J. H. Pollard, Expectation of life and Gompertz's distribution, unpublished note (2001).

[39] L. R. Shenton, Inequalities for the normal integral including a new continued fraction, *Biometrika* 41 (1954) 177–189; MR 15,884e.

[40] N. L. Johnson and S. Kotz, *Distributions in Statistics: Continuous Univariate Distributions*, v. 2. Houghton Mifflin, 1970; MR 42 #5364.

[41] T. J. Stieltjes, Recherches sur les fractions continues, *Annales Faculté Sciences Toulouse*
8 (1894) J1-J122; 9 (1895) A1-A47; also in *Oeuvres Complètes*, t. 2, ed. W. Kapteyn and
J. C. Kluyver, Noordhoff, 1918, pp. 402–566; Engl. transl. in *Collected Papers*, v. 2, ed.
G. van Dijk, Springer-Verlag, 1993, pp. 406–570, 609–745; MR 95g:01033.

[42] P. C. Fishburn, A. M. Odlyzko, and F. S. Roberts, Two-sided generalized Fibonacci sequences, *Fibonacci Quart.* 27 (1989) 352–361; MR 90k:11019.

6.3 Kepler–Bouwkamp Constant

Draw a circle C_1 of unit radius and inscribe it with an equilateral triangle. Inscribe the
triangle with another circle C_2 and inscribe C_2 with a square. Continue with a third
circle C_3 inscribing the square and inscribe C_3 with a regular pentagon. Repeat this
procedure indefinitely, each time increasing the number of sides of the regular polygon
by one. The radius of the limiting circle C_∞ is given by [1–3]

$$\rho = \prod_{j=3}^{\infty} \cos\left(\frac{\pi}{j}\right) = 0.1149420448\ldots = (8.7000366252\ldots)^{-1}.$$

This construction originated with Kepler [4, 5], who at one point believed that the orbits
of Jupiter and Saturn around the sun might be approximated by the circumscribed and
inscribed circles of an equilateral triangle, that is, by suitably scaled C_1 and C_2. Since
the equilateral triangle is the first regular polygon, he thought that the orbit of Mars
would thus correspond to C_3, the orbit of Earth would correspond to C_4, etc. (This
model, however, could not explain the fact that there were only six known planets.
Kepler subsequently replaced two-dimensional regular polygons by three-dimensional
regular polyhedra, of which there are precisely five, and also obtained better agreement
with astronomical data.)

Consider the same construction with the word "inscribe" replaced everywhere by
"circumscribe." The limiting radius is not a new constant, but simply ρ^{-1} [6]. Consider
as well the infinite product

$$\sigma = \prod_{j=2}^{\infty} \frac{j}{\pi} \sin\left(\frac{\pi}{j}\right) = 0.3287096916\ldots = \frac{2}{\pi}(0.5163359762\ldots),$$

which has no apparent link with ρ. By way of contrast, the product

$$\prod_{j=3}^{\infty} \left(1 - \sin\left(\frac{\pi}{j}\right)\right)$$

diverges to zero.

Bouwkamp apparently was the first mathematician to exploit the more rapidly convergent formulas [7, 8]

$$\rho = \frac{2}{\pi} \prod_{m=1}^{\infty} \prod_{n=1}^{\infty} \left(1 - \frac{1}{m^2\left(n + \frac{1}{2}\right)^2}\right) = \frac{2}{\pi} \exp\left[-\sum_{k=1}^{\infty} \frac{\zeta(2k)2^{2k}(\lambda(2k) - 1)}{k}\right],$$

$$\sigma = \prod_{m=1}^{\infty} \prod_{n=2}^{\infty} \left(1 - \frac{1}{m^2 n^2}\right) = \exp\left[-\sum_{k=1}^{\infty} \frac{\zeta(2k)(\zeta(2k) - 1)}{k}\right]$$

for computation's sake. Here $\zeta(x)$ is defined in [1.6] and $\lambda(x)$ is defined in [1.7].

A recent result involves the function

$$f(x) = \prod_{j=1}^{\infty} \cos\left(\frac{x}{j}\right), \quad \lim_{x \to \pi} \frac{f(x)}{x - \pi} = \frac{\rho}{2},$$

for which it is known that [9]

$$\int_0^{\infty} f(x)\,dx = 0.7853805572\ldots < \frac{\pi}{4} = 0.7853981633\ldots.$$

The function

$$g(x) = \prod_{j=1}^{\infty} \frac{j}{x} \sin\left(\frac{x}{j}\right), \quad \lim_{x \to \pi} \frac{g(x)}{x - \pi} = -\frac{\sigma}{\pi},$$

can be similarly analyzed. See also [10–12] for an intriguing connection between $f(x)$, $g(x)$ and the divisor problem from number theory.

[1] R. W. Hamming, *Numerical Methods for Scientists and Engineers*, 2nd ed., McGraw-Hill, 1973, pp. 193–194.

[2] T. Curnow, Falling down a polygonal well, *Math. Spectrum* 26 (1993/94) 110–118.

[3] R. S. Pinkham, Mathematics and modern technology, *Amer. Math. Monthly* 103 (1996) 539–545.

[4] J. Kepler, *Mysterium Cosmographicum*, transl. by A. M. Duncan, Abaris Books, 1981.

[5] O. Lodge, Johann Kepler, *The World of Mathematics*, v. 1, ed. J. R. Newman, Simon and Schuster, 1956, pp. 220–234.

[6] E. Kasner and J. Newman, *Mathematics and the Imagination*, Simon and Schuster, 1940, pp. 310–312.

[7] C. J. Bouwkamp, An infinite product, *Proc. Konink. Nederl. Akad. Wetensch. Ser. A* 68 (1965) 40–46; *Indag. Math.* 27 (1965) 40–46; MR 30 #5468.

[8] P. T. Wahl and S. Robins, Evaluating Kepler's concentric circles product, unpublished note (1993).

[9] D. Borwein and J. M. Borwein, Some remarkable properties of sinc and related integrals, *Ramanujan J.* 5 (2001) 73–89; CECM preprint 99:142.

[10] G. af Hällström, Zwei Beispiele ganzer Funktionen mit algebraischen Höchstindex einer Stellensorte, *Math. Z.* 47 (1941) 161–174; MR 4,7a.

[11] D. J. Newman and N. J. Fine, A trigonometric limit, *Amer. Math. Monthly* 63 (1956) 128–129.

[12] N. A. Bowen and A. J. Macintyre, Entire functions related to the Dirichlet divisor problem, *Entire Functions and Related Parts of Analysis*, ed. J. Korevaar, S. S. Chern, L. Ehrenpreis, W. H. J. Fuchs, and L. A. Rubel, Proc. Symp. Pure Math., 11, Amer. Math. Soc., pp. 66–78; MR 38 #3434.

6.4 Grossman's Constant

Grossman [1] defined a sequence of real numbers via the nonlinear recurrence

$$a_0 = 1, \qquad a_1 = y, \qquad a_{n+2} = \frac{a_n}{1 + a_{n+1}} \quad \text{for } n \geq 0.$$

On the basis of compelling numerical evidence, he conjectured that there is precisely one real value of $y = \eta$ for which this sequence converges, namely, $\eta = 0.7373383033\ldots.$

Janssen & Tjaden [2] succeeded in proving Grossman's conjecture. Nyerges [3] further demonstrated that existence and uniqueness of $y = F(x)$ holds, given an *arbitrary* starting point $a_0 = x \geq 0$. This gives rise to the functional equation

$$x = (1 + F(x)) F(F(x)), \quad F : [0, \infty) \to [0, \infty) \text{ continuous,}$$

and Grossman's constant is the special value $\eta = F(1)$. Other than this, there is no easily available description of η in terms of well-known constants or functions.

Ewing & Foias [4] examined the recurrence

$$b_1 = x > 0, \quad b_{n+1} = \left(1 + \frac{1}{b_n}\right)^n \text{ for } n \geq 1$$

and determined that there is exactly one value $x = \xi$ for which $b_n \to \infty$. In this case, $\xi = 1.1874523511\ldots$ thanks to a computation by Ross [4]. Again, there is a shortage of representations of ξ, as with η.

In [3.5] and [6.10], we observe other constants reminiscent of Grossman's constant.

[1]   J. W. Grossman, Problem 86-2, *Math. Intellig.* 8 (1986) 31.
[2]   A. J. E. M. Janssen and D. L. A. Tjaden, Solution to Problem 86-2, *Math. Intellig.* 9 (1987) 40–43.
[3]   G. Nyerges, The solution of the functional equation $x = (1 + F(x)) F^2(x)$, unpublished note (2000).
[4]   J. Ewing and C. Foias, An interesting serendiptous real number, *Finite Versus Infinite: Contributions to an Eternal Dilemma*, ed. C. S. Calude and G. Paun, Springer-Verlag, 2000, pp. 119–126; MR 2001k:11267.

6.5 Plouffe's Constant

We start with a formula that is surprising at first glance:

$$\sum_{n=0}^{\infty} \frac{\rho(a_n)}{2^{n+1}} = \frac{1}{2\pi},$$

where

$$a_n = \sin(2^n) = \begin{cases} \sin(1) & \text{if } n = 0, \\ 2a_0\sqrt{1 - a_0^2} & \text{if } n = 1, \\ 2a_{n-1}\left(1 - 2a_{n-2}^2\right) & \text{if } n \geq 2, \end{cases}$$

and $\rho(x) = 1$ if $x < 0$ and $\rho(x) = 0$ if $x \geq 0$. In words, the binary expansion of $1/(2\pi)$ is completely determined by the sign pattern of the second-order recurrence $\{a_n\}$. The trivial proof uses the double-angle formulas for sine and cosine. One might believe that we have uncovered here a fast way of computing the binary expansion of $1/(2\pi)$, but this would be a mistake. The reason is that we would need $\sin(1)$ to high accuracy for initialization, but computing $\sin(1)$ is no easier than computing $1/(2\pi)$.

The double-angle formula for cosine gives rise to a simpler, first-order recurrence

$$b_n = \cos(2^n) = \begin{cases} \cos(1) & \text{if } n = 0, \\ 2b_{n-1}^2 - 1 & \text{if } n \geq 1, \end{cases}$$

but the sum

$$K = \sum_{n=0}^{\infty} \frac{\rho(b_n)}{2^{n+1}} = 0.4756260767\ldots$$

does not appear to have a closed-form expression. (We will revisit this question later.) The double-angle formula for tangent, however, gives rise to both a first-order recursion

$$c_n = \tan(2^n) = \begin{cases} \tan(1) & \text{if } n = 0, \\ \dfrac{2c_{n-1}}{1 - c_{n-1}^2} & \text{if } n \geq 1 \end{cases}$$

and a closed-form expression for the sum

$$\sum_{n=0}^{\infty} \frac{\rho(c_n)}{2^{n+1}} = \frac{1}{\pi}$$

by a trivial proof like before. Again, computing $\tan(1)$ is no easier than computing $1/\pi$.

We have observed so far that, for sine and tangent, certain irrational inputs yield recognizable irrational outputs. Plouffe [1–3] wondered if this process could be adjusted somewhat. He asked whether it was possible to initialize any of these three recurrences with *rational* values, such as $1/2$, and still obtain recognizable irrational binary expansions. Define

$$\alpha_n = \sin\left(2^n \arcsin\left(\tfrac{1}{2}\right)\right) = \begin{cases} 1/2 & \text{if } n = 0, \\ \sqrt{3}/2 & \text{if } n = 1, \\ 2\alpha_{n-1}\left(1 - 2\alpha_{n-2}^2\right) & \text{if } n \geq 2, \end{cases}$$

$$\beta_n = \cos\left(2^n \arccos\left(\tfrac{1}{2}\right)\right) = \begin{cases} 1/2 & \text{if } n = 0, \\ 2\beta_{n-1}^2 - 1 & \text{if } n \geq 1, \end{cases}$$

$$\gamma_n = \tan\left(2^n \arctan\left(\tfrac{1}{2}\right)\right) = \begin{cases} 1/2 & \text{if } n = 0, \\ \dfrac{2\gamma_{n-1}}{1 - \gamma_{n-1}^2} & \text{if } n \geq 1; \end{cases}$$

then the first two sums

$$\sum_{n=0}^{\infty} \frac{\rho(\alpha_n)}{2^{n+1}} = \frac{1}{12}, \quad \sum_{n=0}^{\infty} \frac{\rho(\beta_n)}{2^{n+1}} = \frac{1}{2}$$

are rational, but the third sum

$$C = \sum_{n=0}^{\infty} \frac{\rho(\gamma_n)}{2^{n+1}} = 0.1475836176\ldots$$

is more mysterious. Plouffe numerically determined that

$$C = \frac{1}{\pi} \arctan\left(\tfrac{1}{2}\right),$$

but rigorous justification remained an open problem.

Borwein & Girgensohn [4] succeeded in proving Plouffe's formula for C and much more. They demonstrated that, given an arbitrary real value x, if

$$\xi_n = \tan\left(2^n \arctan(x)\right) = \begin{cases} x & \text{if } n = 0, \\ \dfrac{2\xi_{n-1}}{1 - \xi_{n-1}^2} & \text{if } n \geq 1 \text{ and } |\xi_{n-1}| \neq 1, \\ -\infty & \text{if } n \geq 1 \text{ and } |\xi_{n-1}| = 1, \end{cases}$$

then

$$\sum_{n=0}^{\infty} \frac{\rho(\xi_n)}{2^{n+1}} = \begin{cases} \dfrac{\arctan(x)}{\pi} & \text{if } x \geq 0, \\ 1 + \dfrac{\arctan(x)}{\pi} & \text{if } x < 0, \end{cases}$$

which we call **Plouffe's recursion**.

This, however, was only one facet of their paper. It turns out to be crucial that the aforementioned sum, call it $f(x)$, satisfies the functional equation

$$2f(x) = f\left(\frac{2x}{1 - x^2}\right) \text{ if } x \geq 0, \quad 2f(x) - 1 = f\left(\frac{2x}{1 - x^2}\right) \text{ if } x < 0.$$

A vastly more general functional equation gives rise to other interesting recurrences and binary expansions. We will not attempt to summarize these results except to remark that Plouffe's recursion appears to be the simplest example in the theory. Other examples, associated with logarithmic, hyperbolic, and elliptic integrals of the first kind, are presented in [4] as well.

A well-known theorem of Lehmer [5] gives that C is irrational. In fact, C is transcendental [6].

Chowdhury [7] recently observed that the constant K defined earlier can be expressed in binary as the bitwise XOR sum of $1/(2\pi)$ and $1/\pi$. That is,

$$\begin{aligned} & 0.00101000101111100110\ldots \\ \oplus\ & 0.01010001011111001100\ldots \\ =\ & 0.01111001110000101010\ldots \end{aligned}$$

and "addition exclusive or" is identical to addition modulo two without carries. Since $1/(2\pi)$ is simply a shifted version of $1/\pi$, the constant K is truly quite interesting! More generally, if $-1 \leq x \leq 1$, the bitwise XOR sum of $\arccos(x)/(2\pi)$ and $\arccos(x)/\pi$ is $\sum_{n=0}^{\infty} \rho(\eta_n) 2^{-n-1}$, where

$$\eta_n = \cos\left(2^n \arccos(x)\right) = \begin{cases} x & \text{if } n = 0, \\ 2\eta_{n-1}^2 - 1 & \text{if } n \geq 1. \end{cases}$$

This is a well-studied object: The sequence $\{1 - 2\eta_n\}$ is equal to iterates of the chaotic logistic map $y \mapsto 4y(1 - y)$ defined in [1.9] with seed value $1 - 2x$. Unfortunately, this insight does not help us in more clearly identifying the constant K.

[1] S. Plouffe, Why build the Inverse Symbolic Calculator?, unpublished note (1995).
[2] S. Plouffe, The computation of certain numbers using a ruler and compass, *J. Integer Seq.* 1 (1998) 98.1.3; MR 2000c:11211.
[3] N. J. A. Sloane, On-Line Encyclopedia of Integer Sequences, A004715, A004716, and A004717.
[4] J. M. Borwein and R. Girgensohn, Addition theorems and binary expansions, *Canad. J. Math.* 47 (1995) 262–273; MR 96i:39037.
[5] I. Niven, *Irrational Numbers*, Math. Assoc. Amer., 1956, pp. 36–41; MR 18,195c.
[6] B. H. Margolius, Plouffe's constant is transcendental, unpublished note (2002).
[7] M. Chowdhury, A formula for 0.4756260767 . . . , unpublished note (2001).

6.6 Lehmer's Constant

Every irrational number x has a unique infinite continued fraction representation of the form

$$x = a_0 + \frac{1|}{|a_1|} + \frac{1|}{|a_2|} + \frac{1|}{|a_3|} + \cdots,$$

where each a_k is a positive integer for $k \geq 1$ and a_0 is an integer [1]. Conversely, every such expression is convergent. The Golden mean

$$\frac{1 + \sqrt{5}}{2} = 1 + \frac{1|}{|1|} + \frac{1|}{|1|} + \frac{1|}{|1|} + \cdots$$

can be said to be the case for which the convergence rate is slowest.

Lehmer [2, 3] discovered an interesting analog of continued fractions. Every positive irrational x has a unique infinite **continued cotangent representation** of the form

$$x = \cot\left(\sum_{k=0}^{\infty}(-1)^k \operatorname{arccot}(b_k)\right),$$

where each b_k is a nonnegative integer for $k \geq 0$ and $b_k \geq b_{k-1}^2 + b_{k-1} + 1$ for $k \geq 1$. Conversely, every such expression is convergent. Lehmer's constant, ξ, corresponds to the Golden mean under the analogy and

$$\xi = \cot\left(\operatorname{arccot}(0) - \operatorname{arccot}(1) + \operatorname{arccot}(3) - \operatorname{arccot}(13) + - \cdots + (-1)^k c_k + \cdots\right)$$
$$= 0.5926327182\ldots$$

can be said to be the case for which the convergence rate is slowest. Here the kth arccotangent argument is defined via the quadratic recurrence [4]

$$c_0 = 0, \quad c_k = c_{k-1}^2 + c_{k-1} + 1 \text{ for } k \geq 1,$$

which is itself an interesting object of study. Lehmer proved that ξ is not an algebraic number of degree < 4. When coupled with Roth's theorem [2.22], which Lehmer did not have available back in 1938, the argument implies the transcendence of ξ [5].

What inspired Lehmer to even begin examining continued cotangents? He observed that the iteration of simple two-variable functions such as

$$f(x, y) = x + y, \qquad g(x, y) = x + \frac{1}{y},$$

$$h(x, y) = \frac{xy + 1}{y - x} = \cot(\text{arccot}(x) - \text{arccot}(y))$$

give rise to

$$f(x_1, f(x_2, f(x_3, \dots))) = \sum_{j=1}^{\infty} x_j,$$

$$g(x_1, g(x_2, g(x_3, \dots))) = x_1 + \frac{1|}{|x_2} + \frac{1|}{|x_3} + \cdots,$$

$$h(x_1, h(x_2, h(x_3, \dots))) = \cot\left(\sum_{j=1}^{\infty} (-1)^{j+1} \text{arccot}(x_j)\right).$$

The first two results, infinite sums and infinite continued fractions, occur throughout mathematics. Lehmer's result and conceivably others might find applications in the future.

[1] G. H. Hardy and E. M. Wright, *An Introduction to the Theory of Numbers*, 5th ed., Oxford Univ. Press, 1985; MR 81i:10002.
[2] D. H. Lehmer, A cotangent analogue of continued fractions, *Duke Math. J.* 4 (1938) 323–340.
[3] J. Shallit, Predictable regular continued cotangent expansions, *J. Res. Nat. Bur. Standards B.* 80 (1976) 285–290; MR 55 #2734.
[4] N. J. A. Sloane, On-Line Encyclopedia of Integer Sequences, A002065.
[5] P. Borwein, Lehmer's constant is transcendental, unpublished note (1999).

6.7 Cahen's Constant

Here is a little known example of a **self-generating continued fraction**. Start with

$$\frac{0}{1} = 0, \quad \frac{1}{1} = 0 + \frac{1}{1}$$

and define $q_0 = 1$ and $q_1 = 1$, the denominators on the left-hand side. Continue with

$$\frac{p_2}{q_2} = 0 + \frac{1}{1 + \dfrac{1}{q_0}} = 0 + \frac{1|}{|1} + \frac{1|}{|q_0},$$

where $\gcd(p_2, q_2) = 1$, obtaining $q_2 = 2$. (Henceforth, whenever we write a fraction p/q, it is assumed, for simplicity, to be in lowest terms.) Continue with

$$\frac{p_3}{q_3} = 0 + \frac{1|}{|1} + \frac{1|}{|q_0} + \frac{1|}{|q_1},$$

obtaining $q_3 = 3$. Continue with

$$\frac{p_4}{q_4} = 0 + \frac{1|}{|1} + \frac{1|}{|q_0} + \frac{1|}{|q_1} + \frac{1|}{|q_2},$$

obtaining $q_4 = 8$. At each step in the process, the nth partial denominator q_n is defined in terms of the finite continued fraction with partial quotients up to q_{n-2}. Maintaining this indefinitely, one finds that the sequence of qs

$$1, 1, 2, 3, 8, 27, 224, 6075, 1361024, 8268226875, 11253255215681024, \ldots$$

satisfies the quadratic recurrence $q_{n+2} = q_n(q_{n+1} + 1)$ and that the limiting value of the continued fraction coincides with the sum of a certain alternating infinite series:

$$\lim_{n \to \infty} \frac{p_n}{q_n} = \sum_{j=0}^{\infty} \frac{(-1)^j}{q_j q_{j+1}} = 0.6294650204\ldots.$$

This constant was apparently first discussed by Davison & Shallit [1], who proved it is transcendental.

Let us now start over, but proceeding more generally. Let $w_0, w_1, w_2, \ldots$ be an infinite sequence of positive integers. From

$$\frac{0}{1} = 0, \quad \frac{1}{w_0} = 0 + \frac{1}{w_0}$$

define $q_0 = 1$ and $q_1 = w_0$. From

$$\frac{p_2}{q_2} = 0 + \frac{1|}{|w_0} + \frac{1|}{|w_1 q_0}$$

obtain $q_2 = q_0(w_1 q_1 + 1)$. From

$$\frac{p_3}{q_3} = 0 + \frac{1|}{|w_0} + \frac{1|}{|w_1 q_0} + \frac{1|}{|w_2 q_1}$$

obtain $q_3 = q_1(w_2 q_2 + 1)$. Maintaining this indefinitely, one finds that the sequence of qs satisfies the recurrence $q_{n+2} = q_n(w_{n+1}q_{n+1} + 1)$ and that the limiting value of the continued fraction coincides with the series

$$\xi(w) = \lim_{n \to \infty} \frac{p_n}{q_n} = \sum_{j=0}^{\infty} \frac{(-1)^j}{q_j q_{j+1}}.$$

It can be proved [1] that the number $\xi(w)$ is always transcendental, regardless of the choice of ws.

Let k be a positive integer. As a special case of the preceding, define $w_0 = 1$ and $w_{j+1} = q_j^{k-1}$ for all $j \geq 0$. Then the sequence of qs satisfies the recurrence $q_{n+2} = q_n(q_n^{k-1}q_{n+1} + 1)$ and the corresponding limiting value $\xi(w)$ is

$$0 + \frac{1|}{|1} + \frac{1|}{|q_0^k} + \frac{1|}{|q_1^k} + \frac{1|}{|q_2^k} + \cdots = \xi_k = \sum_{j=0}^{\infty} \frac{(-1)^j}{q_j q_{j+1}}.$$

The Davison–Shallit constant arises from the instance for which $k = 1$. The case $k = 2$ is often rewritten as $s_n = q_n q_{n+1} + 1$; hence

$$\xi_2 = c = \sum_{j=0}^{\infty} \frac{(-1)^j}{s_j - 1} = 0.6434105462\ldots,$$

where $s_0 = 2$, $s_{n+1} = s_n^2 - s_n + 1$ is **Sylvester's sequence**. This sequence is also discussed in [6.10]. Cahen [2] was the first to examine the constant c. Subsequent references include [3–6]. In the 1930s, Mahler partitioned the set of all transcendental numbers into three classes: S, T, and U, the classification being determined by how small a polynomial with bounded degree and height can be when evaluated at the point in question. Töpfner [7] succeeded in proving that c must fall in the class S. The case $k \geq 3$ has not been examined, as far as is known: $\xi_3 = 0.6539007091\ldots$, $\xi_4 = 0.6600049346\ldots$, and $\xi_5 = 0.6632657345\ldots$.

Some variations on Cahen's constant c are worth pointing out. The number $c' = \sum_{j=0}^{\infty} (-1)^j / s_j$ satisfies $2c = c' + 1$, and thus c' is also transcendental, whereas $\sum_{j=0}^{\infty} 1/s_j = 1$. What can be said about $\sum_{j=0}^{\infty} 1/(s_j - 1) = 1.6910302067\ldots$? Finally, what other kinds of self-generating continued fractions have appeared in the literature?

[1] J. L. Davison and J. O. Shallit, Continued fractions for some alternating series, *Monatsh. Math.* 111 (1991) 119–126; MR 92f:11094.

[2] M. E. Cahen, Note sur un développement des quantites numériques, qui présente quelque analogie avec celui des fractions continues, *Nouvelles Annales de Mathematiques* 10 (1891) 508–514.

[3] E. Ya. Remez, On series with alternating signs which may be connected with two algorithms of M. V. Ostrogadskii for the approximation of irrational numbers (in Russian), *Uspekhi Mat. Nauk*, v. 6 (1951) n. 5, 33–42; MR 13,444d.

[4] P.-G. Becker, Algebraic independence of the values of certain series by Mahler's method, *Monatsh. Math.* 114 (1992) 183–198; MR 94b:11066.

[5] T. Töpfer, On the transcendence and algebraic independence of certain continued fractions, *Monatsh. Math.* 117 (1994) 255–262; MR 95e:11079.

[6] C. Baxa, Fast growing sequences of partial denominators, *Acta Math. Inform. Univ. Ostraviensis* 2 (1994) 81–84; MR 95k:11091.

[7] T. Töpfer, Algebraic independence of the values of generalized Mahler functions, *Acta Arith.* 70 (1995) 161–181; MR 96a:11070.

6.8 Prouhet–Thue–Morse Constant

The Prouhet–Thue–Morse binary sequence $\{t_n\} = \{0, 1, 1, 0, 1, 0, 0, 1, 1, 0, \ldots\}$ has several equivalent definitions: [1]

- $t_0 = 0$, $t_{2n} = t_n$, and $t_{2n+1} = 1 - t_n$ for all $n \geq 0$;
- t_n is the number of ones, modulo two, in the binary expansion of n [2.16];
- $(-1)^{t_n}$ is the coefficient of x^n in the power series expansion of $\prod_{k=0}^{\infty}(1 - x^{2^k})$;
- $\{0, 0, 1, 0, 0, 1, 1, 1 - t_0, 1 - t_1, 1 - t_2, 1 - t_3, \ldots\}$ is the lexicographically smallest overlap-free infinite binary word [5.17].

We begin with the constant

$$\tau = \sum_{n=0}^{\infty} \frac{t_n}{2^{n+1}} = 0.4124540336\ldots = \frac{1}{2}(0.8249080672\ldots),$$

sometimes called the **parity constant**, which is known to be transcendental [2–6]. Less "artificial" formulas include the infinite product [7, 8]

$$\prod_{k=0}^{\infty} \left(1 - \frac{1}{2^{2^k}}\right) = 2(1 - 2\tau)$$

and the continued fraction

$$2 - \frac{1|}{|4} - \frac{3|}{|16} - \frac{15|}{|256} - \frac{255|}{|65536} - \frac{65535|}{|4294967296} - \cdots = \frac{\tau}{3\tau - 1},$$

where the pattern is generated by 2^{2^n} and $2^{2^n} - 1$.

6.8.1 Probabilistic Counting

Woods & Robbins [9] proved that

$$\prod_{m=0}^{\infty} \left(\frac{2m + 1}{2m + 2}\right)^{(-1)^{t_m}} = \frac{1}{\sqrt{2}}.$$

Shallit [10] generalized this result and wrote a base-3 version. Other generalizations include [11–14]

$$\prod_{m=0}^{\infty} \left(\frac{(2m + 1)^2}{(m + 1)(4m + 1)}\right)^{(-1)^{u_m}} = \frac{1}{\sqrt{2}},$$

where u_m is the Golay–Rudin–Shapiro sequence, which counts the number of (possibly overlapping) elevens in the binary expansion of m, modulo two.

Here is a problem involving n coins. For each $1 \leq k \leq n$, let X_k be the number of independent tosses of the kth coin required for heads to appear, minus one. Define R_n to be the smallest nonnegative integer $\neq X_k$ for all k; then clearly $0 \leq R_n \leq n$. Flajolet & Martin [15] proved that

$$E(R_n) = \frac{1}{\ln(2)} \ln(\psi n) + \delta(n) + o(1),$$

where

$$\psi = \frac{e^\gamma}{\sqrt{2}} \prod_{m=1}^{\infty} \left(\frac{2m + 1}{2m}\right)^{(-1)^{t_m}} = 0.7735162909\ldots,$$

γ is the Euler–Mascheroni constant [1.5], and $\delta(n)$ is a "negligible" periodic function of small amplitude ($|\delta(n)| < 10^{-5}$) of the type mentioned in [5.14]. A more complicated expression for $\text{Var}(R_n) \sim 1.257\ldots + \varepsilon(n)$ appears in [15–17]. The proof involves the analytic continuation of a function

$$F(z) = \sum_{k=1}^{\infty} \frac{(-1)^{t_k}}{k^z}, \quad \mathrm{Re}(z) > 1,$$

to the entire complex plane. This is useful in assessing **probabilistic counting algorithms** for data mining, and it is interesting how the sequence $\{t_n\}$ persists throughout. Plouffe [18] gave the following products:

$$\prod_{m=1}^{\infty} \left(\frac{m}{m+1} \right)^{(-1)^{t_{m-1}}} = 0.8116869215\ldots,$$

$$\prod_{m=1}^{\infty} \left(\frac{2m}{2m+1} \right)^{(-1)^{t_{m-1}}} = 0.8711570464\ldots,$$

$$\prod_{m=1}^{\infty} \left(\frac{2m}{2m+1} \right)^{(-1)^{t_m}} = 1.6281601297\ldots,$$

$$\prod_{m=1}^{\infty} \left(\frac{m}{m+1} \right)^{(-1)^{t_m}} = 2.3025661371\ldots,$$

due to Flajolet; the third is $2^{-1/2} e^{\gamma} \psi^{-1}$ of course. A finite expression for these in terms of more familiar constants is not known. This situation makes the Woods–Robbins formula and others all the more remarkable!

6.8.2 Non-Integer Bases

Fix q to be a real number satisfying $1 < q \le 2$. Define a q-**development** to be a series

$$\sum_{n=1}^{\infty} \varepsilon_n q^{-n} = 1,$$

where $\varepsilon_n = 0$ or 1 for every n. The greedy algorithm shows that q-developments exist. If $q = 2$, then $\varepsilon_n = 1$ for all n and this is the unique 2-development. Do there exist other values of q, $1 < q < 2$, for which there is a unique q-development?

Intuitively, one would expect the answer to be no. Indeed, if we fix $1 < q < \varphi$, where φ is the Golden mean [1.2], then there exist uncountably many q-developments. Also, if $q = \varphi$, then there exist a countably infinite number of q-developments [19–21].

If we fix $\varphi < q < 2$, however, intuition fails. There is an uncountable, measure-zero subset of exceptional q-values, each with only one q-development. Moreover, the exceptional subset possesses a minimum element that can be characterized exactly [22]. This special q-value is the unique positive solution of the equation

$$\prod_{k=0}^{\infty} \left(1 - \frac{1}{q^{2^k}} \right) = \left(1 - \frac{1}{q} \right)^{-1} - 2;$$

hence $q = 1.7872316501\ldots$. The corresponding q-development satisfies $\varepsilon_n = t_n$ for all $n \geq 1$, an unexpected occurrence of the Prouhet–Thue–Morse sequence. Also, the **Komornik–Loreti constant** q is transcendental, as shown by Allouche & Cosnard [23].

6.8.3 External Arguments

Here is a connection between τ and the Myrberg constant $c_\infty = 1.4011551890\ldots$ from fractal geometry [1.9]. Imagine the Mandelbrot set M [6.10] to be electrically charged; thus it determines in the plane **equipotential curves** (which encircle M) and **field trajectories** (which are orthogonal to the equipotential curves). Seen from far away, M resembles a point charge and the field trajectories approach rays of the form $r \exp(2\pi i \theta)$ as $r \to \infty$. The **external arguments** θ_k corresponding to the bifurcation points c_k of $1 - cx^2$, given by [1.9]

$$c_2 = \tfrac{5}{4} = 1.25, \quad c_3 = 1.3680\ldots, \quad c_4 = 1.3940\ldots,$$

are (in binary)

$$\theta_2 = 0.\overline{01} = \tfrac{1}{3}, \quad \theta_3 = 0.\overline{0110} = \tfrac{2}{5}, \quad \theta_4 = 0.\overline{01101001} = \tfrac{7}{17},$$

with limiting value $\theta_\infty = \tau$. Unfortunately the details are too elaborate to explain further [24–26].

6.8.4 Fibonacci Word

Another "self-generating" constant is the so-called **rabbit constant**, which can be defined via recursive bit substitutions $0 \mapsto 1$, $1 \mapsto 10$ leading to the infinite binary Fibonacci word [27–32]. (The analogous substitution map for the Thue–Morse word is $0 \mapsto 01$, $1 \mapsto 10$.) A simpler definition is

$$\rho = \sum_{k=1}^{\infty} \frac{1}{2^{\lfloor k\varphi \rfloor}} = 0.7098034428\ldots,$$

where φ is the Golden mean [1.2]. It is known that [33–37]

$$\rho = 0 + \frac{1|}{|2^0} + \frac{1|}{|2^1} + \frac{1|}{|2^1} + \frac{1|}{|2^2} + \frac{1|}{|2^3} + \frac{1|}{|2^5} + \frac{1|}{|2^8} + \cdots,$$

where the exponents form none other than the classical Fibonacci sequence, and hence ρ is transcendental.

6.8.5 Paper Folding

Consider the act of folding a strip of paper in half, right over left [38]. Iterating this process gives a sequence of creases in the strip, appearing when unfolded as either valleys (1) or peaks (0). The **paper folding sequence** $\{s_n\} = \{1, 1, 0, 1, 1, 0, 0, 1, 1, 1, 1, \ldots\}$ is defined by $s_{4n-3} = 1$, $s_{4n-1} = 0$, and $s_{2n} = s_n$ for all $n \geq 1$, or alternatively, by the word transformation $w \mapsto w1\tilde{w}$, where $\tilde{w}$ is the mirror image of w with 0s replaced by 1s and 1s by 0s. It can be shown that

$$\sigma = \sum_{n=1}^{\infty} \frac{s_n}{2^n} = 0.8507361882\ldots = \sum_{k=0}^{\infty} \frac{1}{2^{2^k}} \left(1 - \frac{1}{2^{2^{k+2}}}\right)^{-1}$$

and transcendentality of σ follows [5, 39].

[1] J.-P. Allouche and J. Shallit, The ubiquitous Prouhet-Thue-Morse sequence, *Sequences and Their Applications (SETA)*, Proc. 1998 Singapore conf., ed. C. Ding, T. Helleseth, and H. Niederreiter, Springer-Verlag, 1999, pp. 1–16; MR 2002e:11025.

[2] K. Mahler, Arithmetische Eigenschaften der Lösungen einer Klasse von Funktionalgleichungen, *Math. Annalen* 101 (1929) 342–366; corrigendum 103 (1930) 532.

[3] A. Cobham, *A Proof of Transcendence Based on Functional Equations*, IBM Tech. Report RC-2041, 1968.

[4] M. Dekking, Transcendance du nombre de Thue-Morse, *C. R. Acad. Sci. Paris Sér. A-B* 285 (1977) A157–A160; MR 56 #15571.

[5] J. H. Loxton and A. J. van der Poorten, Arithmetic properties of the solutions of a class of functional equations, *J. Reine Angew. Math.* 330 (1982) 159–172; MR 83i: 10046.

[6] J. Shallit, Number theory and formal languages, *Emerging Applications of Number Theory*, Proc. 1996 Minneapolis conf., ed. D. A. Hejhal, J. Friedman, M. C. Gutzwiller, and A. M. Odlyzko, Springer-Verlag, 1999, pp. 547–570; MR 2000d:68123.

[7] M. Beeler, R. W. Gosper, and R. Schroeppel, Parity number, HAKMEM, MIT AI Memo 239, item 122.

[8] R. W. Gosper, Some identities for your amusement, *Ramanujan Revisited*, Proc. 1987 Urbana conf., ed. G. E. Andrews, R. A. Askey, B. C. Berndt, K. G. Ramanathan, and R. A. Rankin, Academic Press, 1987, pp. 607–609; MR 89d:05016.

[9] D. R. Woods and D. Robbins, Solution to problem E2692, *Amer. Math. Monthly* 86 (1979) 394–395.

[10] J. O. Shallit, On infinite products associated with sums of digits, *J. Number Theory* 21 (1985) 128–134; MR 86m:11007.

[11] J.-P. Allouche and H. Cohen, Dirichlet series and curious infinite products, *Bull. London Math. Soc.* 17 (1985) 531–538; MR 87b:11085.

[12] J.-P. Allouche, H. Cohen, M. Mendès France, and J. O. Shallit, De nouveaux curieux produits infinis, *Acta Arith.* 49 (1987) 141–153; MR 89f:11022.

[13] J.-P. Allouche and J. O. Shallit, Infinite products associated with counting blocks in binary strings, *J. London Math. Soc.* 39 (1989) 193–204; MR 90g:11013.

[14] J.-P. Allouche, P. Hajnal, and J. O. Shallit, Analysis of an infinite product algorithm, *SIAM J. Discrete Math.* 2 (1989) 1–15; MR 90f:68073.

[15] P. Flajolet and G. N. Martin, Probabilistic counting algorithms for data base applications, *J. Comput. Sys. Sci.* 31 (1985) 182–209; MR 87h:68023.

[16] P. Kirschenhofer and H. Prodinger, On the analysis of probabilistic counting, *Number-Theoretic Analysis: Vienna 1988-89*, ed. E. Hlawka and R. F. Tichy, Lect. Notes in Math. 1452, Springer-Verlag, 1990, pp. 117–120; MR 92a:11087.

[17] P. Kirschenhofer, H. Prodinger, and W. Szpankowski, How to count quickly and accurately, *Proc. 1992 Int. Colloq. on Automata, Languages and Programming (ICALP)*, Vienna, ed. W. Kuich, Lect. Notes in Comp. Sci. 623, Springer-Verlag, 1992, pp. 211–222; MR 94j:68099.

[18] S. Plouffe, Flajolet constants (Plouffe's Tables).

[19] P. Erdős, I. Joó, and V. Komornik, Characterization of the unique expansions $1 = \sum_{i=1}^{\infty} q^{-n_i}$ and related problems, *Bull. Soc. Math. France* 118 (1990) 377–390; MR 91j:11006.

[20] P. Erdős and I. Joó, On the expansion $1 = \sum q^{-n_i}$, *Period. Math. Hungar.* 23 (1991) 27–30; corrigendum 25 (1992) 113; MR 92i:11030 and MR 93k:11017.

[21] P. Erdős, M. Horváth, and I. Joó, On the uniqueness of the expansions $1 = \sum q^{-n_i}$, *Acta Math. Hungar.* 58 (1991) 333–342; MR 93e:11012.

[22] V. Komornik and P. Loreti, Unique developments in non-integer bases, *Amer. Math. Monthly* 105 (1998) 636–639; MR 99k:11017.

[23] J.-P. Allouche and M. Cosnard, The Komornik-Loreti constant is transcendental, *Amer. Math. Monthly* 107 (2000) 448–449.

[24] H.-O. Peitgen and P. H. Richter, *The Beauty of Fractals. Images of Complex Dynamical Systems*, Springer-Verlag, 1986; MR 88e:00019.

[25] A. Douady, Algorithms for computing angles in the Mandelbrot set, *Chaotic Dynamics and Fractals*, Proc. 1985 Atlanta conf., ed. M. F. Barnsley and S. G. Demko, Academic Press, 1986, pp. 155–168; MR 88a:58142.

[26] S. Bullett and P. Sentenac, Ordered orbits of the shift, square roots, and the devil's staircase, *Math. Proc. Cambridge Philos. Soc.* 115 (1994) 451–481; MR 95j: 58043.

[27] M. R. Schroeder, *Number Theory in Science and Communication: With Applications in Cryptography, Physics, Digital Information, Computing and Self-Similarity*, 2nd ed., Springer-Verlag, 1986; MR 99c:11165.

[28] M. Gardner, *Penrose Tiles and Trapdoor Ciphers*, W. H. Freeman, 1989, pp. 21–22; MR 97m:00004.

[29] M. Schroeder, *Fractals, Chaos, Power Laws: Minutes from an Infinite Paradise*, W. H. Freeman, 1991, pp. 53–57, 306–310; MR 92m:00018.

[30] J. C. Lagarias, Number theory and dynamical systems, *The Unreasonable Effectiveness of Number Theory*, Proc. 1991 Orono conf., ed. S. A. Burr, Amer. Math. Soc., 1992, pp. 35–72; MR 93m:11143.

[31] T. Gramss, Entropy of the symbolic sequence for critical circle maps, *Phys. Rev. E* 50 (1994) 2616–2620; MR 96m:58072.

[32] J. Grytczuk, Infinite self-similar words, *Discrete Math.* 161 (1996) 133–141; MR 98a:68154.

[33] P. E. Böhmer, Über die Transzendenz gewisser dyadischer Brüche, *Math. Annalen* 96 (1927) 367–377, 735.

[34] D. E. Knuth, Transcendental numbers based on the Fibonacci sequence, *Fibonacci Quart.* 2 (1964) 43–44.

[35] J. L. Davison, A series and its associated continued fraction, *Proc. Amer. Math. Soc.* 63 (1977) 29–32; MR 55 #2788.

[36] W. W. Adams and J. L. Davison, A remarkable class of continued fractions, *Proc. Amer. Math. Soc.* 65 (1977) 194–198; MR 56 #270.

[37] D. Bowman, A new generalization of Davison's theorem, *Fibonacci Quart.* 26 (1988) 40–45; MR 89c:11016.

[38] M. Dekking, M. Mendès France, and A. van der Poorten, Folds, *Math. Intellig.* 4 (1982) 130–138, 173–181, 190–195; MR 84f:10016.

[39] J. H. Loxton, A method of Mahler in transcendence theory and some of its applications, *Bull. Austral. Math. Soc.* 29 (1984) 127–136; MR 85i:11059.

6.9 Minkowski–Bower Constant

Define a function $? : [0, 1] \to [0, 1]$ by

$$? \left(0 + \frac{1|}{|a} + \frac{1|}{|b} + \frac{1|}{|c} + \frac{1|}{|d} + \cdots \right) = 0.\overbrace{00\ldots0}^{a-1}\underbrace{11\ldots1}_{b}\overbrace{00\ldots0}^{c}\underbrace{11\ldots1}_{d}00\ldots,$$

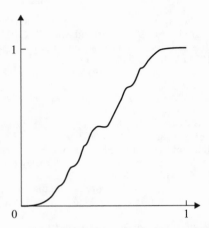

Figure 6.1. A graph of Minkowski's question mark function.

where the input is a regular continued fraction and the output is written in binary [1–3]. This is known as **Minkowski's question mark function** (see Figure 6.1). It is continuous, strictly increasing, but fractal-like. In fact, it is *singular* in the sense that its derivative is zero almost everywhere (except on a set of Lebesgue measure zero). Special values include

$$? \left(\tfrac{-1+\sqrt{5}}{2} \right) = \tfrac{2}{3}, \quad ? \left(-1 + \sqrt{2} \right) = \tfrac{2}{5}, \quad ? \left(\tfrac{-1+\sqrt{3}}{2} \right) = \tfrac{2}{7}.$$

Bower [4, 5] asked about the fixed points of ? other than 0, 1/2, and 1. There appear to be at least two more, arranged symmetrically around the center point. Are there exactly two? He computed the lesser value to be 0.4203723394 . . . (in decimal). Does this constant have a closed-form expression? Is it algebraic? A definition of ? in terms of Farey fractions is also possible.

While on the subject of artificial constants, let us mention the **Champernowne number** [6]

$$C = 0.12345678910111213141516171819202122232425 \ldots,$$

which is constructed by concatenating the digits of all positive integers, and the **Copeland–Erdös number** [7]

$$0.235711131719232931374143475359616771737379 \ldots,$$

which is likewise constructed by concatenating the digits of all primes. Both are known to be irrational; see [8–10] for recent proofs. Mahler [11] was the first to prove that C is transcendental. His theorem is consistent with the observation that relatively "short" rational numbers (e.g., 10/81 or 60499999499/490050000000) yield excellent approximations of C. This observation, in turn, implies the existence of extraordinarily large partial denominators in the regular continued fraction expansion for C (e.g., the 1709th partial denominator is $\approx 10^{4911098}$, due to Sofroniou & Spaletta [12]).

We also mention **Trott's constant** E, defined to be the (apparently unique) number with decimal digits $\{\varepsilon_k\}$ that coincide with its partial fraction denominators [12]:

$$E = 0.\varepsilon_1\varepsilon_2\varepsilon_3\varepsilon_4\ldots = 0 + \frac{1|}{|\varepsilon_1} + \frac{1|}{|\varepsilon_2} + \frac{1|}{|\varepsilon_3} + \frac{1|}{|\varepsilon_4} + \cdots, \quad 0 \le \varepsilon_k \le 9 \text{ for all } k,$$

and this turns out to be $0.1084101512\ldots$ Is E transcendental? Are alternative expressions for E possible?

[1] R. Salem, On some singular monotonic functions which are strictly increasing, *Trans. Amer. Math. Soc.* 53 (1943) 427–439; MR 4,217b.

[2] J. H. Conway, *On Numbers and Games*, Academic Press, 1976, pp. 82–86; MR 56 #8365.

[3] P. Viader and J. Paradis, A new light on Minkowski's ?(x) function, *J. Number Theory* 73 (1998) 212–227; MR 2000a:11104.

[4] N. J. A. Sloane, On-Line Encyclopedia of Integer Sequences, A048817, A048818, A048819, A048820, A048821, and A048822.

[5] C. Bower, Fixed points of Minkowski's ?(x) function, unpublished note (1999).

[6] D. G. Champernowne, The construction of decimals normal in the scale of ten, *J. London Math. Soc.* 8 (1933) 254–260.

[7] A. H. Copeland and P. Erdös, Note on normal numbers, *Bull. Amer. Math. Soc.* 52 (1946) 857–860; MR 8,194b.

[8] N. Hegyvári, On some irrational decimal fractions, *Amer. Math. Monthly* 100 (1993) 779–780; MR 94e:11080.

[9] A. M. Mercer, A note on some irrational decimal fractions, *Amer. Math. Monthly* 101 (1994) 567–568; MR 95d:11088.

[10] P. Martinez, Some new irrational decimal fractions, *Amer. Math. Monthly* 108 (2001) 250–253; MR 2002b:11096.

[11] K. Mahler, Arithmetische Eigenschaften einer Klasse von Dezimalbrüchen, *Konink. Akad. Wetensch. Proc. Sci. Sect.* 40 (1937) 421–428; Zbl. 17,56.

[12] N. J. A. Sloane, On-Line Encyclopedia of Integer Sequences, A030167, A030168, A033307, A033308, A039662, and A039663.

6.10 Quadratic Recurrence Constants

Linear recurrences include the Fibonacci sequence, which is discussed in [1.2]. Quadratic recurrences are far less understood and far more mysterious than linear recurrences. The simplest example is

$$a_0 = 2, \qquad a_n = a_{n-1}^2 \quad \text{for } n \ge 1,$$

with solution $a_n = 2^{2^n}$. A more challenging example is the total number of strongly binary trees [5.6] of height at most n:

$$b_0 = 1, \qquad b_n = b_{n-1}^2 + 1 \quad \text{for } n \ge 1.$$

(See Figure 6.2.) Aho & Sloane [1, 2] showed that this quadratic recurrence likewise has a doubly exponential solution $b_n = \lfloor \beta^{2^n} \rfloor$, but β is not precisely known and, in fact,

$$\beta = \exp\left[\sum_{j=0}^{\infty} 2^{-j-1} \ln\left(1 + b_j^{-2}\right)\right] = 1.5028368010\ldots.$$

If one could find an expression for β independent of $\{b_n\}$, this would be very surprising.

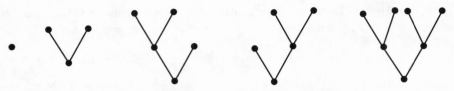

Figure 6.2. There are five strongly binary trees of height at most 2.

Another example is the closest strict under-approximation $C_n = \sum_{i=1}^{n} 1/c_i$ of the number 1, where $1 < c_1 < c_2 < \ldots < c_n$ are integers. This is given by the quadratic recurrence [6.7]

$$c_1 = 2, \qquad c_n = c_{n-1}^2 - c_{n-1} + 1 \quad \text{for } n \geq 2,$$

known as **Sylvester's sequence**. Further, $C_n = 1 - 1/(c_{n+1} - 1)$, which implies that C_n is formed by the greedy algorithm, equivalently, by choosing for the next term the largest feasible unit fraction [3–13]. Here, Aho & Sloane determined $c_n = \lfloor \chi^{2^n} + 1/2 \rfloor$, where

$$\chi = \frac{\sqrt{6}}{2} \exp\left[\sum_{j=1}^{\infty} 2^{-j-1} \ln\left(1 + (2c_j - 1)^{-2}\right) \right] = 1.2640847353\ldots.$$

Again, an independent expression for χ would be very surprising. We have encountered such doubly exponential functions elsewhere in [2.13], [5.7], and [5.16].

A well-known example is the Lucas recurrence [14–21]

$$u_n = u_{n-1}^2 - 2,$$

which has been studied extensively because of its connection with Mersenne prime theory when $|u_0| > 2$. In this case we have

$$u_n = \left(\frac{1}{2}u_0 + \frac{1}{2}\sqrt{u_0^2 - 4} \right)^{2^n} + \left(\frac{1}{2}u_0 - \frac{1}{2}\sqrt{u_0^2 - 4} \right)^{2^n},$$

so divergence always occurs in this regime. For $|u_0| < 2$ the long-term behavior is more intricate and interesting to dynamical system theorists. See [1.9] for a related discussion of the recurrence

$$0 \leq x_0 \leq 1, \quad x_n = a\, x_{n-1}(1 - x_{n-1}) \quad \text{for } n \geq 1, \quad 0 \leq a \leq 4,$$

with its cycle structure and period-doubling bifurcations.

Another well-known example is the Lehmer recurrence

$$v_0 = 1, \qquad v_n = v_{n-1}^2 + v_{n-1} + 1 \quad \text{for } n \geq 1,$$

which generates the coefficients of the least rapidly convergent continued cotangent [6.6].

Quadratic recurrences arise in tree-related contexts in other ways [5.6]: in the extinction probabilities associated with Galton–Watson branching processes,

$$y_0 = 0, \quad y_n = (1 - p) + p\, y_{n-1}^2 \quad \text{for } n \geq 1, \quad 0 < p < 1,$$

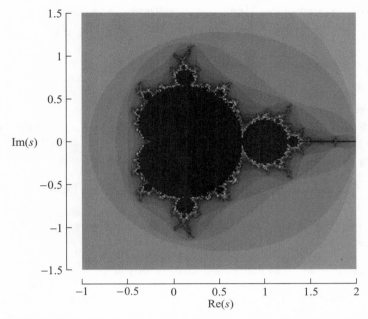

Figure 6.3. The Mandelbrot set is the black cardiod-shaped region and is entirely contained within the indicated rectangle. Its intersection with the real line is the interval $[-1/4, 2]$.

and in the asymptotics of non-isomorphic binary trees,

$$w_0 = 2, \qquad w_n = w_{n-1}^2 + 2 \quad \text{for } n \geq 1.$$

In the study of 1-additive sequences, the ternary quadratic recurrence

$$t_n = 2\left(t_{n-2}(t_{n-2} + 1) + t_{n-4k-3}(t_{n-4k-3} + 1) + t_{n-8k-4}(t_{n-8k-4} + 1)\right) \bmod 3,$$

with initial data $(t_1, t_2, \ldots, t_{8k+3}, t_{8k+4}) = (0, 0, \ldots, 0, 1)$, turns out to be crucial [22] and is related to the Stolarsky–Harborth constant [2.16].

The most famous quadratic recurrence, however, is

$$s_0 = 0, \qquad s_n = s_{n-1}^2 - \mu \quad \text{for } n \geq 1,$$

where μ may be any complex number. The **Mandelbrot set** M is defined to be the set of all such μ for which $s_n \not\to \infty$ (see Figure 6.3). Since the boundary of M is a fractal of Hausdorff dimension 2 [8.20], it has infinite length [23]. However, the area of M has been rigorously bounded between 1.506302 and 1.561303 and has been heuristically estimated as 1.50659177. See [24–29] for details. No one has dared to conjecture an exact formula for the area of M.

Davison & Shallit [30] studied the second-order quadratic recurrence [6.7]

$$q_0 = q_1 = 1, \quad q_{n+2} = q_n(q_{n+1} + 1) \quad \text{for } n \geq 0$$

and determined that $q_n = \left\lfloor \xi^{\varphi^n} \eta^{(1-\varphi)^n} \right\rfloor$, where φ is the Golden mean [1.2],

$\xi = 1.3505061\ldots$, and $\eta = 1.4298155\ldots$. Another such recurrence [31]

$$r_0 = 0, \quad r_1 = 1, \quad r_{n+2} = r_{n+1} + r_n^2 \quad \text{for } n \geq 0$$

satisfies

$$r_{2n} \sim (1.436\ldots)^{\sqrt{2}^{2n}}, \quad r_{2n+1} \sim (1.451\ldots)^{\sqrt{2}^{2n+1}}.$$

The dependence of the growth on the subscript parity is intriguing.

Greenfield & Nussbaum [32] considered the possibility of a bi-infinite sequence $\{z_n : n = \ldots, -2, -1, 0, 1, 2, \ldots\}$ of positive reals satisfying the recurrence

$$z_0 = 1, \quad z_n = z_{n-1} + z_{n-2}^2 \quad \text{for all } n.$$

It turns out that there is exactly one value $z_1 = 1.5078747554\ldots$ for which this happens.

Stein & Everett [33] and Wright [34] studied the recurrence

$$d_1 = 1, \quad d_{n+1} = (n + \delta) \sum_{k=1}^{n} d_k d_{n-k+1} \quad \text{for } n \geq 1$$

for various values of δ. For $\delta = 0$ and $\delta = -1/3$, they obtained

$$d_n \sim \frac{1}{e} \prod_{j=2}^{n} (2j - 1), \quad d_n \sim (0.35129898\ldots) \prod_{j=2}^{n} (2j - 2),$$

respectively, where e is the natural logarithmic base [1.3]. Both cases possess combinatorial interpretations.

Lenstra [12] and Zagier [35] examined **Göbel's sequence**

$$f_0 = 1, \quad f_n = \frac{1}{n} \left(1 + \sum_{k=0}^{n-1} f_k^2 \right) \quad \text{for } n \geq 1$$

and determined that the first non-integer term is $f_{43} > 10^{178485291567}$; further,

$$f_n \sim (1.0478314475\ldots)^{2^n} \left(n + 2 - n^{-1} + 4n^{-2} - 21n^{-3} + 137n^{-4} - + \cdots \right).$$

Somos [36] examined a related sequence

$$g_0 = 1, \quad g_n = n g_{n-1}^2 \quad \text{for } n \geq 1$$

and found that

$$g_n \sim \gamma^{2^n} \left(n + 2 - n^{-1} + 4n^{-2} - 21n^{-3} + 137n^{-4} - + \cdots \right)^{-1},$$

where the constant γ has an infinite radical expansion

$$\gamma = 1.6616879496\ldots = \sqrt{1 \cdot \sqrt{2 \cdot \sqrt{3 \cdot \sqrt{4 \cdots}}}} = \prod_{j=1}^{\infty} j^{2^{-j}}.$$

Another Somos constant $\lambda = 0.3995246670\ldots$ arises as follows: If $\kappa < \lambda$, then the sequence

$$h_0 = 0, \quad h_1 = \kappa, \quad h_n = h_{n-1}(1 + h_{n-1} - h_{n-2}) \quad \text{for } n \geq 2$$

converges to a limit less than 1; if $\kappa > \lambda$, then the sequence diverges to infinity. This is similar to Grossman's constant [6.4].

[1] A. V. Aho and N. J. A. Sloane, Some doubly exponential sequences, *Fibonacci Quart.* 11 (1973) 429–437; MR 49 #209.

[2] D. H. Greene and D. E. Knuth, *Mathematics for the Analysis of Algorithms*, Birkhäuser, 1982, pp. 31–34; MR 92c:68067.

[3] O. D. Kellogg, On a Diophantine problem, *Amer. Math. Monthly* 28 (1921) 300–303.

[4] T. Takenouchi, On an indeterminate equation, *Proc. Physico-Math. Soc. Japan* 3 (1921) 78–92.

[5] D. R. Curtiss, On Kellogg's Diophantine problem, *Amer. Math. Monthly* 29 (1922) 380–387.

[6] H. E. Salzer, The approximation of numbers as sums of reciprocals, *Amer. Math. Monthly* 54 (1947) 135–142; 55 (1948) 350–356; MR 8,534e and MR 10,18c.

[7] S. W. Golomb, On certain nonlinear recurring sequences, *Amer. Math. Monthly* 70 (1963) 403–405; MR 26 #6112.

[8] S. W. Golomb, On the sum of the reciprocals of the Fermat numbers and related irrationalities, *Canad. J. Math.* 15 (1963) 475–478; MR 27 #105.

[9] J. N. Franklin and S. W. Golomb, A function-theoretic approach to the study of nonlinear recurring sequences, *Pacific J. Math.* 56 (1975) 455–468; MR 51 #10212.

[10] P. Erdös and R. Graham, *Old and New Problems and Results in Combinatorial Number Theory*, Enseignement Math. Monogr. 28, 1980, pp. 30–32, 41; MR 82j:10001.

[11] R. L. Graham, D. E. Knuth, and O. Patashnik, *Concrete Mathematics*, 2nd ed., Addison-Wesley, 1994, pp. 109, 147, 518; MR 97d:68003.

[12] R. K. Guy, *Unsolved Problems in Number Theory*, 2nd ed., Springer-Verlag, 1994; sect. D11, E15; MR 96e:11002.

[13] L. Brenton and R. R. Bruner, On recursive solutions of a unit fraction equation, *J. Austral. Math. Soc.* 57 (1994) 341–356; MR 95i:11024.

[14] T. W. Chaundy and E. Phillips, The convergence of sequences defined by quadratic recurrence-formulae, *Quart. J. Math.* 7 (1936) 74–80.

[15] G. H. Hardy and E. M. Wright, *An Introduction to the Theory of Numbers*, 5th ed., Oxford Univ. Press, 1985, pp. 148–149, 223–225; MR 81i:10002.

[16] F. Lazebnik and Y. Pilipenko, Convergence of $a_{n+1} = a_n^2 - 2$, *Amer. Math. Monthly* 94 (1987) 789–793.

[17] R. André-Jeannin, H. Kappus, and I. Sadoveanu, A radical limit, *Fibonacci Quart.* 30 (1992) 369–371.

[18] F. S. Pirvanescu, G. Williams, and H.-J. Seiffert, A dynamical system recursion, *Math. Mag.* 66 (1993) 127–129.

[19] J. L. King, Y. L. Wong, R. J. Chapman, and C. Cooper, A mean limit, *Amer. Math. Monthly* 102 (1995) 556–557.

[20] P. Flajolet, J.-C. Raoult, and J. Vuillemin, The number of registers required for evaluating arithmetic expressions, *Theoret. Comput. Sci.* 9 (1979) 99–125; MR 80e:68101.

[21] R. Sedgewick and P. Flajolet, *Introduction to the Analysis of Algorithms*, Addison-Wesley, 1996, p. 55.

[22] J. Cassaigne and S. R. Finch, A class of 1-additive sequences and quadratic recurrences, *Experim. Math.* 4 (1995) 49–60; MR 96g:11007.

[23] M. Shishikura, The Hausdorff dimension of the boundary of the Mandelbrot set and Julia sets, *Annals of Math.* 147 (1998) 225–267; MR 2000f:37056.

[24] B. Branner, The Mandelbrot set, *Chaos and Fractals: The Mathematics Behind the Computer Graphics*, ed. R. L. Devaney and L. Keen, Proc. Symp. Appl. Math. 39, Amer. Math. Soc., 1989, pp. 75–106; MR 91a:58130.

[25] J. H. Ewing and G. Schober, The area of the Mandelbrot set, *Numer. Math.* 61 (1992) 59–72; MR 93e:30006.

[26] R. Munafo, The area of the Mandelbrot set via pixel counting, unpublished note (1997).

[27]   J. R. Hill, Fractals and the grand Internet parallel processing project, *Fractal Horizons: The Future Use of Fractals*, ed. C. Pickover, St. Martins Press, 1996, pp. 299–324.

[28]   Y. Fisher and J. Hill, Bounding the area of the Mandelbrot set, unpublished note (1997).

[29]   J. R. Hill, Area of Mandelbrot set components and clusters, unpublished note (1998).

[30]   J. L. Davison and J. O. Shallit, Continued fractions for some alternating series, *Monatsh. Math.* 111 (1991) 119–126; MR 92f:11094.

[31]   W. Duke, S. J. Greenfield, and E. R. Speer, Properties of a quadratic Fibonacci recurrence, *J. Integer Seq.* 1 (1998) 98.1.8; MR 99k:11024.

[32]   S. J. Greenfield and R. D. Nussbaum, Dynamics of a quadratic map in two complex variables, *J. Differ. Eq.* 169 (2001) 57–141; MR 2002b:39013.

[33]   P. R. Stein and C. J. Everett, On a quadratic recurrence rule of Faltung type, *J. Combin. Inform. Sys. Sci.* 3 (1978) 1–10; MR 58 #10704.

[34]   E. M. Wright, A quadratic recurrence of Faltung type, *Math. Proc. Cambridge Philos. Soc.* 88 (1980) 193–197; corrigenda 92 (1982) 379; MR 81i:10016 and MR 83k:10024.

[35]   D. Zagier, Problems posed at the St. Andrews Colloquium, day 5, problem 3 (1996).

[36]   M. Somos, Several constants related to quadratic recurrences, unpublished note (1999).

6.11 Iterated Exponential Constants

Given $y > 0$, what numbers $x > 0$ satisfy $y = x^x$? The answer is more complicated than one might expect. For example,

- $x = 3$ is the unique solution of $x^x = 27$,
- $x = 2$ is the unique solution of $x^x = 4$,
- $x = 1/2$ and $x = 1/4$ are both solutions of $x^x = 2^{-1/2}$, and there are no others.

More generally [1–3],

- $x = \left(\cdots \log_{\frac{1}{y}} \log_{\frac{1}{y}} \frac{1}{e} \right)^{-1}$ is the unique solution of $x^x = y$ for $y \geq e^e = 15.154\ldots$,

- $x = y^{\frac{1}{y}^{\frac{1}{y}^{\cdots}}}$ is the unique solution of $x^x = y$ for $1 \leq y \leq e^e$,

- $x = y^{\frac{1}{y}^{\frac{1}{y}^{\cdots}}}$ and $x = \left(\cdots \log_{\frac{1}{y}} \log_{\frac{1}{y}} e \right)^{-1}$ are both solutions of $x^x = y$ for $0.692\ldots = e^{-1/e} \leq y < 1$, and there are no others.

This is a consequence, in part, of the fact that the **iterated exponential** $\xi^{\xi^{\xi^{\cdots}}}$ converges for $0.065\ldots = e^{-e} \leq \xi \leq e^{1/e} = 1.444\ldots$ and diverges for positive ξ outside this interval. Other phrases for the same type of function include **hyperpower sequence** and **tower of exponents**.

An alternative representation of x as a function of y is $\exp(W(\ln(y)))$, where the **Lambert W function** [3, 4] is

$$
W(\eta) = \begin{cases} -\ln\left(\cdots \log_{e^{-\eta}} \log_{e^{-\eta}} \frac{1}{e} \right) & \text{if } \eta \geq e = 2.718\ldots, \\ \eta \, (e^{-\eta})^{(e^{-\eta})^{\cdots}} & \text{if } -0.367\ldots = -e^{-1} \leq \eta \leq e \end{cases}
$$

and satisfies $W(\eta)\exp(W(\eta)) = \eta$. In particular, $W(\ln(27)) = \ln(3)$, $W(\ln(4)) = \ln(2)$, and $W(-\ln(2)/2) = -\ln(2)$. We will refer to Lambert's function throughout the remainder of this essay.

Consider the equation $x^2 = 2^x$, which has three real roots including 2 and 4. The third root can be written as

$$x = -1 \cdot 2^{-\frac{1}{2} \cdot 2^{-\frac{1}{2} \cdot 2^{\cdot^{\cdot^{\cdot}}}}} = -\frac{2}{\ln(2)} W\left(\frac{\ln(2)}{2}\right) = -0.7666646959\ldots$$

and is known to be transcendental [5]. It is interesting that $W(-\ln(2)/2)$ is elementary but $W(\ln(2)/2)$ is not. Consider instead the equation $x + e^x = 0$, which possesses a unique real root:

$$x = -1 \cdot e^{-1 \cdot e^{-1 \cdot e^{\cdot^{\cdot^{\cdot}}}}} = -W(1) = -0.5671432904\ldots = -\ln(1.7632228343\ldots).$$

Other examples suggest themselves.

The hyperpower analog of the harmonic series

$$H_n = \left(\frac{1}{2}\right)^{\left(\frac{1}{3}\right)^{\cdot^{\cdot^{\left(\frac{1}{n}\right)}}}}$$

is divergent in the sense that even and odd partial exponentials converge to distinct limits [6–8]:

$$\lim_{n\to\infty} H_{2n} = 0.6583655992\ldots < 0.6903471261\ldots = \lim_{n\to\infty} H_{2n+1}.$$

No alternative expressions for these constants are known.

Let i denote the imaginary unit; then the multivalued expression i^i is always real:

$$i^i = \exp\left(-\frac{\pi}{2}(4n+1)\right),$$

which, when $n = 0$, gives $i^i = \exp(-\pi/2) = 0.2078795764\ldots$. If we restrict attention to the principal branch of the logarithm ($n = 0$), iterating the exponential can be proved [9–13] to converge to

$$\frac{2}{\pi} i\, W\left(-\frac{\pi}{2}i\right) = 0.4382829367\ldots + (0.3605924718\ldots)i.$$

Here are two striking integrals: [14–16]

$$\int_0^1 x^x dx = \sum_{n=1}^\infty \frac{(-1)^{n+1}}{n^n} = 0.7834305107\ldots,$$

$$\int_0^1 \frac{1}{x^x} dx = \sum_{n=1}^\infty \frac{1}{n^n} = 1.2912859970\ldots.$$

These are easily proved via term-by-term integration of Maclaurin series expansions. A more difficult evaluation concerns the series [17]

$$\lim_{N\to\infty}\sum_{n=1}^{2N}(-1)^n n^{\frac{1}{n}} = \sum_{k=1}^{\infty}\left((2k)^{\frac{1}{2k}} - (2k-1)^{\frac{1}{2k-1}}\right) = \sum_{m=1}^{\infty}(-1)^m\left(m^{\frac{1}{m}} - 1\right)$$

$$= 1 + \lim_{N\to\infty}\sum_{n=1}^{2N+1}(-1)^n n^{\frac{1}{n}} = 0.1878596424\ldots,$$

which is slowly convergent. No exact formulas are known, although the series bear some resemblance to expressions mentioned in [2.15]. Cesàro summation and Cohen–Villegas–Zagier acceleration [18] are two techniques available to compute the sum.

Long ago, Poisson [19] discovered a remarkable identity:

$$-\frac{\pi}{2}W(-x) = \int_0^{\pi} \frac{\sin(\frac{3}{2}\theta) - x\,e^{\cos(\theta)}\sin(\frac{5}{2}\theta - \sin(\theta))}{1 - 2x\,e^{\cos(\theta)}\cos(\theta - \sin(\theta)) + x^2 e^{2\cos(\theta)}}\sin(\tfrac{1}{2}\theta)\,d\theta,$$

valid for $|x| < e^{-1}$. We wonder if his theory might someday lead to the solution, in terms of a "compact" definite integral, of other transcendental equations (e.g., Kepler's equation [4.8]).

6.11.1 Exponential Recurrences

There is not as much to say about exponential recurrences as about quadratic recurrences [6.10]. The simplest example is [20]

$$c_0 = 0, \qquad c_n = 2^{c_{n-1}} \quad \text{for } n \geq 1.$$

If $\emptyset$ denotes the empty set, then $c_1 = 1$ is the cardinality of the power set $P(\emptyset)$ of $\emptyset$, $c_2 = 2$ is the cardinality of $P(P(\emptyset))$, $c_3 = 4$ is the cardinality of $P(P(P(\emptyset)))$, etc. The Ackermann-like growth of $\{c_n\}$ greatly exceeds that of any exponential function.

Another occurrence of $\{c_n\}$ is as follows. A **rooted identity tree** is a rooted tree for which the only automorphism fixing the root is the identity map [5.6]. Fix an integer $h > 0$. An identity tree of height h consists of a root, a nonempty set of identity trees (all different) of height $h - 1$, and a (possibly empty) set of identity trees (all different) of height $< h - 1$. (See Figure 6.4.) The cardinality of all such identity trees is therefore

$$\left(2^{c_h - c_{h-1}} - 1\right)2^{c_{h-1}} = c_{h+1} - c_h$$

since repetitions are not allowed. These are equivalent to what are called *ranked sets* in set theory.

A variation of this,

$$\gamma_0 = 0.1490279983\ldots, \qquad \gamma_n = 2^{\gamma_{n-1}} \quad \text{for } n \geq 1,$$

arises in combinatorial game theory [21,22]. The number of *impartial misère games* at day n is $g_n = \lceil \gamma_n \rceil$, and each such game can be thought of as a rooted identity tree t satisfying special conditions. Let $S(t)$ denote the set of (distinct) identity subtrees

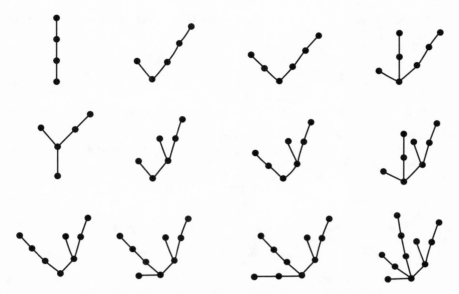

Figure 6.4. There exist twelve rooted identity trees of height 3.

of t with roots adjacent to the root of t. The **outcome** $O(t)$ of t is N if $O(s) = P$ for some $s \in S(t)$ or if t is a single vertex; otherwise $O(t) = P$. A tree t is **reversible** if, for some tree u, $S(u)$ is a proper subset of $S(t)$ and, if $v \in S(t) - S(u)$, then $u \in S(v)$; further, if u is a single vertex, then $O(w) = P$ for some $w \in S(t)$. Finally, a tree t is **canonical** if t is not reversible and if each $s \in S(t)$ is canonical. The number g_n of canonical trees of height $\leq n$ is 1, 2, 3, 5, 22, and 4171780 for $0 \leq n \leq 5$; a corrected value of $g_6 \approx 2^{4171780}$ appears in [23–25]. Conway [21] claimed that constructing an existence proof for the constant γ_0, valid for all n, is not difficult.

[1] R. A. Knoebel, Exponentials reiterated, *Amer. Math. Monthly* 88 (1981) 235–252; MR 82e:26004.
[2] J. M. de Villiers and P. N. Robinson, The interval of convergence and limiting functions of a hyperpower sequence, *Amer. Math. Monthly* 93 (1986) 13–23; MR 87d:26005.
[3] Y. Cho and K. Park, Inverse functions of $y = x^{1/x}$, *Amer. Math. Monthly* 108 (2001) 963–967.
[4] R. M. Corless, G. H. Gonnet, D. E. G. Hare, D. J. Jeffrey, and D. E. Knuth, On the Lambert W function, *Adv. Comput. Math.* 5 (1996) 329–359; MR 98j:33015.
[5] P. Pollack, The intersection of $y = x^2$ and $y = 2^x$, unpublished note (1998).
[6] D. F. Barrow, Infinite exponentials, *Amer. Math. Monthly* 43 (1936) 150–160.
[7] M. Creutz and R. M. Sternheimer, On the convergence of iterated exponentiation, *Fibonacci Quart.* 18 (1980) 341–347; 19 (1981) 326–335; 20 (1982) 7–12; MR 82b:26006, MR 83b:26006, and MR 83i:26002.
[8] L. Baxter, Divergence of an iterated exponential, unpublished note (1996).
[9] W. J. Thron, Convergence of infinite exponentials with complex elements, *Proc. Amer. Math. Soc.* 8 (1957) 1040–1043; MR 20 #2552.
[10] D. L. Shell, On the convergence of infinite exponentials, *Proc. Amer. Math. Soc.* 13 (1962) 678–681; MR 25 #5307.
[11] A. J. Macintyre, Convergence of $i^{i^{i^{\cdot^{\cdot}}}}$, *Proc. Amer. Math. Soc.* 17 (1966) 67; MR 32 #5855.

[12] I. N. Baker and P. J. Rippon, A note on complex iteration, *Amer. Math. Monthly* 92 (1985) 501–504; MR 86m:30024.

[13] I. N. Baker and P. J. Rippon, Towers of exponentials and other composite maps, *Complex Variables Theory Appl.* 12 (1989) 181–200; MR 91b:30068.

[14] Putnam Competition Problem A-4, *Amer. Math. Monthly* 77 (1970) 723, 725.

[15] M. S. Klamkin, R. A. Groeneveld, and C. D. Olds, A comparison of integrals, *Amer. Math. Monthly* 77 (1970) 1114; 78 (1971) 675–676.

[16] B. C. Berndt, *Ramanujan's Notebooks: Part IV*, Springer-Verlag, 1994, p. 308; MR 95e:11028.

[17] M. R. Burns, An alternating series involving n^{th} roots, unpublished note (1999).

[18] H. Cohen, F. Rodriguez Villegas, and D. Zagier, Convergence acceleration of alternating series, *Experim. Math.* 9 (2000) 3–12; MR 2001m:11222.

[19] S. D. Poisson, Suite du memoire sur les integrales definies, *Journal de l'École Royale Polytechnique*, t. 12, c. 19 (1823) 404–509.

[20] R. C. Buck, Mathematical induction and recursive definitions, *Amer. Math. Monthly* 70 (1963) 128–135.

[21] J. H. Conway, *On Numbers and Games*, Academic Press, 1976, pp. 139–141; MR 56 #8365.

[22] S. Plouffe, γ_0 of Conway (Plouffe's Tables).

[23] C. Thompson, Count of day 6 misère-inequivalent impartial games, unpublished note (1999).

[24] D. Hoey and S. Huddleston, Confirmation of C. Thompson's corrected g_6, unpublished note (1999).

[25] N. J. A. Sloane, On-Line Encyclopedia of Integer Sequences, A014221, A038081, A038093, A047995, and A048828.

6.12 Conway's Constant

Suppose we start with a string of digits, for example, 13. We might describe this as "one one, one three" and thus write the **derived string**, 1113. This in turn we describe as "three ones, one three," giving 3113. Continuing, the following sequence of strings are obtained [1]:

$$132113,$$

$$1113122113,$$

$$311311222113,$$

$$13211321322113,$$

$$1113122113121113222113,$$

$$31131122211311123113322113,$$

$$132113213221133112132123222113,$$

$$11131221131211132221232112111312111213322113,$$

$$31131122211311123113321112131221123113111231121123222113.$$

We have given the first twelve strings of this sequence ($k = 1$ to $k = 12$). It can be proved that only the digits 1, 2, and 3 appear at any step, so the process can be continued indefinitely. What can be said about the length of the kth string? Its growth appears to be exponential and at first glance one would anticipate this to be impossibly difficult to characterize more precisely. Conway [2–5], defying expectation, proved that the growth is asymptotic to $C\lambda^k$, where $\lambda = 1.3035772690\ldots = (0.7671198507\ldots)^{-1}$ is the largest zero of the polynomial

$$
\begin{aligned}
&x^{71} - x^{69} - 2x^{68} - x^{67} + 2x^{66} + 2x^{65} + x^{64} - x^{63} - x^{62} - x^{61} - x^{60} \\
&- x^{59} + 2x^{58} + 5x^{57} + 3x^{56} - 2x^{55} - 10x^{54} - 3x^{53} - 2x^{52} + 6x^{51} + 6x^{50} \\
&+ x^{49} + 9x^{48} - 3x^{47} - 7x^{46} - 8x^{45} - 8x^{44} + 10x^{43} + 6x^{42} + 8x^{41} - 5x^{40} \\
&- 12x^{39} + 7x^{38} - 7x^{37} + 7x^{36} + x^{35} - 3x^{34} + 10x^{33} + x^{32} - 6x^{31} - 2x^{30} \\
&- 10x^{29} - 3x^{28} + 2x^{27} + 9x^{26} - 3x^{25} + 14x^{24} - 8x^{23} - 7x^{21} + 9x^{20} \\
&+ 3x^{19} - 4x^{18} - 10x^{17} - 7x^{16} + 12x^{15} + 7x^{14} + 2x^{13} - 12x^{12} - 4x^{11} \\
&- 2x^{10} + 5x^{9} + x^{7} - 7x^{6} + 7x^{5} - 4x^{4} + 12x^{3} - 6x^{2} + 3x - 6.
\end{aligned}
$$

This polynomial and λ were first computed by Atkin; Vardi [6] noticed a typographical error (the x^{35} term was off by a sign in [4]).

Moreover, the same constant λ applies to the growth rates of *all* such sequences, regardless of the starting string, with two trivial exceptions. We started with the string 13 earlier; the constant λ is *universally applicable* except for the empty initial string and the string 22. This astonishing fact is a consequence of what is known as the **Cosmological Theorem**, the proof of which was lost until recently [7]. Ekhad & Zeilberger's tour-de-force is a splendid illustration of the use of software in proving theorems.

Even more can be said. Sometimes a string factors as the concatenation of two strings L and R whose descendents never interfere with each other. We say that the string LR **splits** as $L.R$ and LR is called a **compound**. A string with no nontrivial splittings is called an **element** or **atom**. It turns out that there are ninety-two special atoms (named after the chemical elements Hydrogen, Helium, . . . , Uranium). *Every* string of 1s, 2s, and/or 3s eventually decays into a compound of these elements. Additionally, the relative abundances of the elements approach fixed positive limits, independent of the initial string. Thus, of every million atoms, about 91790 on average will be of Hydrogen (the most common) whereas only about 27 will be of Arsenic (the least common).

Conway's Periodic Table of Elements [3, 4] traces the evolution of the string 13 as previously, but indicates the evolution in terms of elements rather than long ternary strings. For example, when $k = 1$ to $k = 6$, the strings are the elements Pa, Th, Ac, Ra, Fr, and Rn, but when $k = 7$, the first compound emerges: 13211321322113, which may be rewritten as Ho.At because Ho is 1321132 and At is 1322113. As another example, when $k = 91$, Helium derives to the compound Hf.Pa.H.Ca.Li because H is 22.

Let us illustrate further. If we start with 11, we obtain 21, then 1211, and then

$$111221,$$
$$312211,$$
$$13112221,$$
$$1113213211 = 11132.13211 = \text{Hf.Sn}.$$

If we start with 12, the first string is already an element: $12 = \text{Ca}$, while starting with 32 or 23 gives

$$1312, \quad 1213,$$
$$11131112 = 1113.1112 = \text{Th.K}, \quad 11121113 = 1112.1113 = \text{K.Th}.$$

There is also the more general case of strings containing digits other than 1, 2, or 3. If we start with, say, 14 or 55, the theorem regarding relative abundances still applies, but we allow just two additional elements (**isotopes** of Plutonium and Neptunium)

$$Pu_4 = 3122113222122211211123222114,$$
$$Np_4 = 1311222113321132211221123322114,$$

$$Pu_5 = 3122113222122211211123222115,$$
$$Np_5 = 1311222113321132211221123322115,$$

the relative abundances of which tend to 0. This is true for strings with digits 6, 7, 8, 9, ... as well.

We return finally to Conway's constant λ. It is the (unique) largest eigenvalue (in modulus) of the 92×92 transition matrix M whose $(i, j)^{\text{th}}$ element is the number of atoms of element j resulting from the decay of one atom of element i. The relative abundances also arise in a careful eigenanalysis of M. We know that Conway's 71st degree polynomial has Galois group S_{71}, and hence λ cannot be expressed in terms of radicals [8]. See [9–12] as well.

[1] N. J. A. Sloane, On-Line Encyclopedia of Integer Sequences, A001140, A001141, A001143, A001145, A001151, A001154, A001155, A005150, A005341 A006751, and A006715.

[2] M. Mowbray, R. Pennington, and E. Welbourne, Prelude to Professor Conway's article, *Eureka* 46 (1986) 4.

[3] J. H. Conway, The weird and wonderful chemistry of audioactive decay, *Eureka* 46 (1986) 5–16.

[4] J. H. Conway, The weird and wonderful chemistry of audioactive decay, *Open Problems in Communication and Computation*, ed. T. M. Cover and B. Gopinath, Springer-Verlag, 1987, pp. 173–188.

[5] J. H. Conway and R. K. Guy, *The Book of Numbers*, Springer-Verlag, 1996, pp. 208–209; MR 98g:00004.

[6] I. Vardi, *Computational Recreations in Mathematica*, Addison-Wesley, 1991; MR 93e:00002.

[7] S. B. Ekhad and D. Zeilberger, Proof of Conway's lost cosmological theorem, *Elec. Res. Announce. Amer. Math. Soc.* 3 (1997) 78–82; MR 98i:05010.

[8] J. H. Conway, Comments on the "Look and Say sequence," unpublished note (1997).

[9] X. Gourdon and B. Salvy, Effective asymptotics of linear recurrences with rational coefficients, *Discrete Math.* 153 (1996) 145–163; MR 97c:11013.

[10] M. Hilgemeier, One metaphor fits all: A fractal voyage with Conway's audioactive decay, *Fractal Horizons: The Future Use of Fractals*, ed. C. Pickover, St. Martins Press, 1996, pp. 137–162.

[11] J. Sauerberg and L. Shu, The long and the short on counting sequences, *Amer. Math. Monthly* 104 (1997) 306–317; MR 98i:11013.

[12] N. J. A. Sloane, My favorite integer sequences, *Sequences and Their Applications (SETA)*, Proc. 1998 Singapore conf., ed. C. Ding, T. Helleseth, and H. Niederreiter, Springer-Verlag, 1999, pp. 103–130; math.CO/0207175.

7

Constants Associated with Complex Analysis

7.1 Bloch–Landau Constants

Let F denote the set of all complex analytic functions f defined on an open region containing the closure of the unit disk D, centered at the origin, and satisfying $f(0) = 0$, $f'(0) = 1$.

For each $f \in F$, let $b(f)$ be the supremum of all numbers r such that there is a subregion S of D on which f is one-to-one and such that $f(S)$ contains a disk of radius r. Bloch [1–7] showed that $b(f)$ is at least $1/12$. **Bloch's constant** B is defined to be $\inf\{b(f) : f \in F\}$. The precise value of B is unknown, but the following bounds were established by Ahlfors & Grunsky [8] and Heins [9]:

$$0.433 < \frac{\sqrt{3}}{4} < B \le \frac{1}{\sqrt{1 + \sqrt{3}}} \frac{\Gamma(\frac{1}{3})\Gamma(\frac{11}{12})}{\Gamma(\frac{1}{4})} = 0.4718616534\ldots.$$

Ahlfors & Grunsky further conjectured that B is equal to its upper bound.

A related constant is defined as follows: For each $f \in F$, let $l(f)$ be the supremum of all numbers r such that $f(D)$ contains a disk of radius r. **Landau's constant** L [3, 5, 7, 10] is defined to be $\inf\{l(f) : f \in F\}$. It is clear that L is at least as large as B. Like B, we do not know the value of L exactly. The following bounds were determined by Robinson [11] and, independently, by Rademacher [12]:

$$0.5 = \frac{1}{2} < L \le \frac{\Gamma(\frac{1}{3})\Gamma(\frac{5}{6})}{\Gamma(\frac{1}{6})} = 0.5432589653\ldots.$$

Rademacher also conjectured that L is equal to its upper bound.

Both of these conjectures remain unproven to this day [13–17]. The form of the conjectured exact expressions, ratios of gamma function values [1.5.4], are fascinating.

Bonk [18] proved in 1990 that a lower bound for B is $\sqrt{3}/4 + 10^{-14}$, which Minda [19] called the first quantitative improvement in estimating B in a half century. Chen & Gauthier [20, 21] adapted Bonk's method to replace 10^{-14} by 2×10^{-4}, and Yanagihara [22] improved the lower bound for L to $1/2 + 10^{-335}$.

Let G denote the subset of F consisting of one-to-one functions. Such functions are said to be **univalent** (or **schlicht**). Over G, the notions of Bloch constant and Landau constant obviously coincide. Define the **univalent Bloch–Landau constant** K (or **schlicht Bloch–Landau constant**) to be $\inf\{l(f) : f \in G\}$. The most current bounds on K are $0.57088 < K < 0.6564155$ [23–28]. No one has yet hypothesized an exact expression for K.

There are various extensions of these ideas, for example, to a domain D that is not a disk but an annulus [29], or to functions f of not one but several complex variables [30, 31]. To discuss these would take us far afield.

MacGregor [32] raised some interesting questions concerning other geometrical properties of $f(D)$. If $f \in F$, it can be shown that the **diameter** of $f(D)$, defined to be $\sup\{|f(z) - f(w)| : z, w \in D\}$, is at least 2. See [33] for a proof. What else can be said? If $f \in G$, let $a(f)$ denote the area of the intersection of $f(D)$ with the unit disk. The work of Goodman, Jenkins & Reich [34–36] yields that $0.62\pi < A = \inf\{a(f) : f \in G\} < 0.7728\pi$. What is the precise value of the constant A? Also, Strohhäcker [37] showed that, given $f \in G$, there is a line segment in $f(D)$ with one endpoint at the origin and possessing length greater than 0.73. What is the largest number 0.73 can be replaced by? Conceivably this question is related to what is known as the Hayman-Wu constant [7.5]. See also [8.19] for other relevant material.

For each $f \in G$, let $m(f)$ be the supremum of all numbers r such that $f(D)$ contains the disk of radius r, centered at the origin. Note the final hypothesis. Define the **Koebe constant** M [38, 39] to be $M = \inf\{m(f) : f \in G\}$. Koebe [40] proved the existence of M and Bieberbach [41] established Koebe's conjecture that $M = 1/4$. The extremal functions consist of precisely the mapping

$$f(z) = \frac{z}{(1 - z)^2}$$

and its rotations. Observe that there is no nonzero analog of M for the set F. For arbitrarily large integer n, $f(z) = (\exp(nz) - 1)/n$ is in F, but it omits the value $-1/n$ since the exponential function is never zero. Hence no disk, centered at the origin, is contained in $f(D)$ for suitably large n.

[1] A. Bloch, Les théorèmes M. Valiron sur les fonctions entières et la théorie de l'uniformisation, *Annales Faculté Sciences Toulouse* 17 (1925) 1–22.
[2] M. Heins, *Selected Topics in the Classical Theory of Functions of a Complex Variable*, Holt, Rinehart, and Winston, 1962, pp. 45–47, 83–86; MR 29 #217.
[3] E. Hille, *Analytic Function Theory*, v. 2, Ginn, 1962, pp. 382–389; MR 34 #1490.
[4] L. V. Ahlfors, *Conformal Invariants: Topics in Geometric Function Theory*, McGraw-Hill, 1973, pp. 14–15; MR 50 #10211.
[5] J. B. Conway, *Functions of One Complex Variable*, 2nd ed., Springer-Verlag, 1978, pp. 292–296; MR 80c:30003.
[6] W. K. Hayman, *Multivalent Functions*, 2nd ed., Cambridge Univ. Press, 1994, pp. 136–140; MR 96f:30003.
[7] R. Remmert, *Classical Topics in Complex Function Theory*, Springer-Verlag, 1998, pp. 225–242; MR 98g:30002.
[8] L. V. Ahlfors and H. Grunsky, Über die Blochsche Konstante, *Math. Z.* 42 (1937) 671–673.
[9] M. Heins, On a class of conformal metrics, *Nagoya Math. J.* 21 (1962) 1–60; MR 26 #1451.

[10] E. Landau, Über die Blochsche Konstante und zwei verwandte Weltkonstanten, *Math. Z.*
      30 (1929) 608–634.
[11] L. V. Ahlfors, An extension of Schwarz's lemma, *Trans. Amer. Math. Soc.* 43 (1938) 359–
      364 (footnote, p. 364).
[12] H. Rademacher, On the Bloch-Landau constant, *Amer. J. Math.* 65 (1943) 387–390; MR
      4,270d.
[13] G. M. Goluzin, *Geometric Theory of Functions of a Complex Variable* (in Russian), 2nd
      ed., Izdat. Akad. Nauk SSSR, 1966; Engl. transl. in *Amer. Math. Soc. Transl.*, v. 26, 1969;
      MR 36 #2793 and MR 40 #308.
[14] C. D. Minda, Bloch constants, *J. d'Analyse Math.* 41 (1982) 54–84; MR 85e:30013.
[15] A. Baernstein and J. P. Vinson, Local minimality results related to the Bloch and Landau
      constants, *Quasiconformal Mappings and Analysis: A Collection of Papers Honoring F. W.
      Gehring*, ed. P. L. Duren, J. M. Heinonen, B. G. Osgood, and B. P. Palka, Springer-Verlag,
      1998, pp. 55–89; MR 99m:30036.
[16] A. Baernstein, Landau's constant, and extremal problems involving discrete subsets of $\mathbb{C}$,
      Linear and Complex Analysis Problem Book 3, Part II, ed. V. P. Havin and N. K Nikolski,
      Lect. Notes in Math. 1543, Springer-Verlag, 1994, pp. 404–407.
[17] A. Baernstein, A minimum problem for heat kernels of flat tori, *Extremal Riemann Surfaces*,
      ed. J. R. Quine and P. Sarnak, Contemp. Math. 201, Amer. Math. Soc., 1998, pp. 227–243;
      MR 98a:58153.
[18] M. Bonk, On Bloch's constant, *Proc. Amer. Math. Soc.* 110 (1990) 889–894; MR 91c:30011.
[19] D. Minda, The Bloch and Marden constants, *Computational Methods and Function The-
      ory*, Proc. 1989 Valparáiso conf., ed. St. Ruscheweyh, E. B. Saff, L. C. Salinas, and
      R. S. Varga, Lect. Notes in Math. 1435, Springer-Verlag, 1990, pp. 131–142; MR 91k:
      30060.
[20] H. Chen and P. M. Gauthier, On Bloch's constant, *J. d'Analyse Math.* 69 (1996) 275–291;
      MR 97j:30002.
[21] C. Xiong, Lower bound of Bloch's constant, *Nanjing Daxue Xuebao Shuxue Bannian Kan*
      15 (1998) 174–179; MR 2000c:30011.
[22] H. Yanagihara, On the locally univalent Bloch constant, *J. d'Analyse Math.* 65 (1995) 1–17;
      MR 96e:30041.
[23] R. E. Goodman, On the Bloch-Landau constant for schlicht functions, *Bull. Amer. Math.
      Soc.* 51 (1945) 234–239; MR 6,262a.
[24] E. Reich, On a Bloch-Landau constant, *Proc. Amer. Math. Soc.* 7 (1956) 75–76; MR
      17,1066g.
[25] J. A. Jenkins, On the schlicht Bloch constant, *J. Math. Mech.* 10 (1961) 729–734; MR 23
      #A1804.
[26] S. Y. Zhang, On the schlicht Bloch constant, *Beijing Daxue Xuebao* 25 (1989) 537–540
      (in Chinese); MR 91a:30014.
[27] E. Beller and J. A. Hummel, On the univalent Bloch constant, *Complex Variables Theory
      Appl.* 4 (1985) 243–252; MR 86i:30005.
[28] J. A. Jenkins, On the schlicht Bloch constant. II, *Indiana Math. J.* 47 (1998) 1059–1063;
      MR 99m:30071.
[29] P.-S. Chiang and A. J. Macintyre, Upper bounds for a Bloch constant, *Proc. Amer. Math.
      Soc.* 17 (1966) 26–31; MR 32 #5883.
[30] H. Chen and P. M. Gauthier, Bloch constants in several variables, *Trans. Amer. Math. Soc.*
      353 (2001) 1371–1386; MR 2001m:32035.
[31] H. Chen, P. M. Gauthier, and W. Hengartner, Bloch constants for planar harmonic mappings,
      Proc. Amer. Math. Soc. 128 (2000) 3231–3240; MR 2001b:30027.
[32] T. H. MacGregor, Geometric problems in complex analysis, *Amer. Math. Monthly* 79 (1972)
      447–468; MR 45 #7034.
[33] G. Pólya and G. Szegö, *Problems and Theorems in Analysis*, v. 1, Springer-Verlag, 1972,
      ex. 239; MR 81e:00002.
[34] A. W. Goodman, Note on regions omitted by univalent functions, *Bull. Amer. Math. Soc.*
      55 (1949) 363–369; MR 10,601f.

[35] J. A. Jenkins, On values omitted by univalent functions, *Amer. J. Math.* 75 (1953) 406–408; MR 14,967a.
[36] A. W. Goodman and E. Reich, On regions omitted by univalent functions. II, *Canad. J. Math.* 7 (1955) 83–88; MR 16,579e.
[37] E. Strohhäcker, Beiträge zur Theorie der schlichten Funktionen, *Math. Z.* 37 (1933) 356–380.
[38] P. L. Duren, *Univalent Functions*, Springer-Verlag, 1983, pp. 26–31; MR 85j:30034.
[39] J. B. Conway, *Functions of One Complex Variable II*, Springer-Verlag, 1995, pp. 61–67; MR 96i:30001.
[40] P. Koebe, Über die Uniformisierung beliebiger analytischer Kurven, *Nachr. Königlichen Ges. Wiss. Göttingen, Math.-Phys. Klasse* (1907) 191–210.
[41] L. Bieberbach, Über die Koeffizienten derjenigen Potenzreihen welche eine schlichte Abbildungen des Einheitskreises vermitteln, *Sitzungsber. Preuss. Akad. Wiss.* (1916) 940–955.

7.2 Masser–Gramain Constant

Suppose $f(z)$ is an entire function such that $f(n)$ is an integer for each positive integer n. Under what circumstances can we conclude that f is a polynomial? Pólya [1] proved that if

$$\limsup_{r \to \infty} \frac{\ln(M_r)}{r} < \ln(2) = 0.6931471805\ldots, \quad \text{where } M_r = \sup_{|z| \le r} |f(z)|,$$

then the conclusion follows. Moreover, the special case $f(z) = 2^z$ demonstrates that $\ln(2)$ is the largest constant (or "best constant") for which this line of reasoning holds [2–4].

Here is a more difficult but related problem. It involves the Gaussian integers, which constitute the set of all complex numbers with integer real parts and integer imaginary parts. Suppose $f(z)$ is an entire function such that $f(n)$ is a Gaussian integer for each Gaussian integer n. Under what circumstances, again, can we conclude that f is a polynomial? Gel'fond [5], building upon the work of Fukasawa [6], proved that there exists a positive constant α such that

$$\limsup_{r \to \infty} \frac{\ln(M_r)}{r^2} < \alpha$$

implies the conclusion. Not surprisingly, a stronger limiting condition (involving r^2 in the denominator instead of r) is needed to force f to be a polynomial. We will discuss the best constant α later. Our focus is on a different constant δ that arose in one attempt to identify α.

Masser [7] proved that α could be no larger than $\pi/(2e) = 0.5778636748\ldots$ and believed α to be equal to $\pi/(2e)$. He also proved the following weaker result: f must be a polynomial if the following holds:

$$\limsup_{r \to \infty} \frac{\ln(M_r)}{r^2} < \alpha_0 = \frac{1}{2} \exp\left(-\delta + \frac{4c}{\pi}\right),$$

where

$$c = \gamma \beta(1) + \beta'(1) = \frac{\pi}{4}\left(-\ln(2) + 2\ln(\pi) + 2\gamma - 2\ln(L)\right) = 0.6462454398\ldots,$$

γ is the Euler–Mascheroni constant [1.5], $\beta(x)$ is the Dirichlet beta function [1.7], L is Gauss' lemniscate constant [6.1], and δ will be defined shortly. Expressions similar to this appear in our essays on the Landau–Ramanujan constant [2.3] and Sierpinski's constant S [2.10]; in fact, $c = \pi S/4$.

Define δ as a natural two-dimensional generalization of the Euler–Mascheroni constant:

$$\delta = \lim_{n \to \infty} \left(\sum_{k=2}^{n} \frac{1}{\pi\, r_k^2} - \ln(n) \right),$$

where r_k is the minimum over all $r \geq 0$ such that there exists a complex number z for which the closed disk with center z and radius r contains at least k distinct Gaussian integers.

The computation of δ is exceedingly difficult. Gramain & Weber [8] determined bounds $1.811447299 < \delta < 1.897327117$, which imply that $0.1707339 < \alpha_0 < 0.1860446$. It turns out that α_0 is the largest constant that Gel'fond's technique (known as the method of series interpolation) can give. Certainly α_0 is far away from the conjectured best constant $\pi/(2e)$, but it is interesting that α_0 is close to $1/(2e) = 0.1839397205\ldots$. Gramain [9, 10] conjectured that $\alpha_0 = 1/(2e)$, which would imply $\delta = 1 + 4c/\pi = 1.8228252496\ldots$, but no one knows whether this is true.

How would one calculate the Masser–Gramain constant δ to, for example, four decimal places? No formula for r_k is known, so Gramain & Weber [8] had no choice but to evaluate r_k for large k via its definition. One has, for example [7], $r_2 = 1/2$, $r_3 = r_4 = 1/\sqrt{2}$, and bounds [9]

$$\frac{\sqrt{\pi\, (k-1) + 4} - 2}{\pi} < r_k < \sqrt{\frac{k-1}{\pi}}.$$

The upper bound is quite good, but the lower bound must be improved for the sake of accurate estimation of δ. One has

$$\frac{\sqrt{\pi\, (k-6) + 2} - \sqrt{2}}{\pi} \leq r_k$$

for $k \geq 6$, but required further improvements [9, 10] are too complicated to present here. To obtain δ to four decimal places would necessitate computing r_k for k up to 5×10^{13} according to [8]. Unless the algorithm for calculating r_k is made more efficient, the bounds for r_k are improved, another procedure for computing δ is found, or a breakthrough in computer hardware occurs, the identity of δ will remain unknown.

A completely different n-dimensional lattice sum generalization of Euler's constant is discussed in [1.10.1].

Finally, let us resolve a remaining issue. Gramain [9, 10], building upon the work of Gruman [11], proved Masser's conjecture that the best constant α is $\pi/(2e)$. This achievement does not, however, shed any light on the value of δ or α_0.

[1] G. Pólya, Über ganzwertige ganze Funktionen, *Rend. Circ. Mat. Palmero* 40 (1915) 1–16; also in *Collected Papers*, v. 1, ed. R. P. Boas, MIT Press, 1974, pp. 1–16, 771–773.

[2] R. C. Buck, Integral valued entire functions, *Duke Math. J.* 15 (1948) 879–891; MR 10,693c.

[3] R. P. Boas, *Entire Functions*, Academic Press, 1954; MR 16,914f.

[4] L. A. Rubel, *Entire and Meromorphic Functions*, Springer-Verlag, 1996; MR 97c:30001.

[5] A. Gel'fond, Sur les propriétés arithmétiques des fonctions entières, *Tôhoku Math. J.* 30 (1929) 280–285.

[6] S. Fukawawa, Über ganzwertige ganze Funktionen, *Tôhoku Math. J.* 27 (1926) 41–52.

[7] D. W. Masser, Sur les fonctions entières à valeurs entières, *C. R. Acad. Sci. Paris Sér. A-B* 291 (1980) 1–4; MR 81i:10048.

[8] F. Gramain and M. Weber, Computing an arithmetic constant related to the ring of Gaussian integers, *Math. Comp.* 44 (1985) 241–245; corrigendum 48 (1987) 854; MR 87a:11028 and MR 88a:11034.

[9] F. Gramain, Sur le théorème de Fukasawa-Gel'fond-Gruman-Masser, *Séminaire Delange-Pisot-Poitou, Théorie des Nombres, 1980-1981*, Birkhäuser, 1982, pp. 67–86; MR 85d:11071.

[10] F. Gramain, Sur le théorème de Fukasawa-Gel'fond, *Invent. Math.* 63 (1981) 495–506; MR 83g:30028.

[11] L. Gruman, Propriétés arithmétiques des fonctions entières, *Bull. Soc. Math. France* 108 (1980) 421–440; MR 82g:10072.

7.3 Whittaker–Goncharov Constants

Suppose f is an entire function such that f and its derivatives $f^{(n)}, n = 1, 2, 3, \ldots$, each have at least one zero z_n in the unit disk. Under what circumstances can we conclude that f is identically zero? It is not difficult [1–5] to prove that if

$$\limsup_{r \to \infty} \frac{\ln(M_r)}{r} < \ln(2), \quad \text{where } M_r = \sup_{|z| \leq r} |f(z)|,$$

then the conclusion $f = 0$ follows. This bound is not the best possible. Define **Whittaker's constant** W to be the largest number for which

$$\limsup_{r \to \infty} \frac{\ln(M_r)}{r} < W \quad \text{implies} \quad f = 0.$$

Then the previous result plus the example $f(z) = \sin(z) + \cos(z)$ show that $\ln(2) = 0.693\ldots \leq W \leq 0.785\ldots = \pi/4$. We alternatively have the identity

$$\limsup_{n \to \infty} \left| f^{(n)}(z) \right|^{\frac{1}{n}} = \limsup_{r \to \infty} \frac{\ln(M_r)}{r}$$

for any choice of complex number z. In words, the asymptotic local behavior of $f^{(n)}$ is governed by the global nature of the maximum modulus function M.

Other formulations exist for W in terms of Maclaurin series coefficients, as well as conditions involving the behavior of the sequence $\{z_n\}$ or the possible univalence of f. We do not discuss these except to mention that **Goncharov's constant** G arises in a such a way [6,7] and $W = G$ was later proved by Buckholtz [8,9]. A formulation involving what are known as Goncharov polynomials is discussed later [7.3.1].

The best-known rigorous bounds on W are due to Macintyre [10–12]:

$$0.7259\ldots < W < 0.7378\ldots,$$

building upon earlier work by Pólya, Boas, and Levinson. The upper bound arises from a study of entire solutions of the functional differential equation

$$\frac{d}{dz}\varphi(z, q) = \varphi(q\,z, q),$$

that is,

$$\varphi(z, q) = \sum_{n=0}^{\infty} \frac{1}{n!} q^{\frac{n(n-1)}{2}} z^n, \quad |q| \le 1.$$

More precisely, W is no greater than the smallest moduli of zeros of $\varphi(z, q)$, considered over all q. The lower bound for W comes about in a different way.

Numerical heuristics allowed Varga & Wang [12, 13] to deduce that $0.7360 < W$, hence disproving Boas' conjecture [14, 15] that $W = 2/e$. More computations led Waldvogel [16] to deduce that $0.73775075 < W$, but we emphasize that rigorous theoretical support for this work has not been finalized. However, refined estimates of Macintyre's upper bound [12, 13, 16] give $W < 0.7377507574\ldots$ Thus Varga & Waldvogel have conjectured that W is equal to its upper bound. No amount of floating point calculations will suffice to prove an exact equality as such!

Some generalizations of W were defined in [4, 17–22]. Oskolkov [23] claimed to possess a new method for computing an arbitrarily close lower bound to W.

Here is a related topic. Differentiating a power series

$$\sum_{n=0}^{\infty} a_n z^n \rightarrow \sum_{n=1}^{\infty} n\,a_n z^{n-1}$$

and *shifting* a power series (i.e., forming a normalized remainder)

$$\sum_{n=0}^{\infty} a_n z^n \rightarrow \sum_{n=1}^{\infty} a_n z^{n-1}$$

are somewhat similar operations. The aforementioned theory involving W, Goncharov polynomials, and differentiation has an analog for shifting. We will take an alternative viewpoint, for the sake of both simplicity and variety.

Let f be an analytic function whose Maclaurin series

$$f(z) = \sum_{k=0}^{\infty} a_k z^k$$

has radius of convergence exactly equal to 1. Let

$$S_n(z, f) = \sum_{k=0}^{n} a_k z^k, \quad n = 1, 2, 3, \ldots,$$

be the nth partial sum of f and define $\rho_n(f)$ to be the largest moduli of the zeros of the polynomial S_n. Let

$$\rho(f) = \liminf_{n \to \infty} \rho_n(f)$$

and define the **power series constant**

$$P = \sup_f \rho(f).$$

Porter [24] and Kakeya [25, 26] showed that $P \leq 2$. Clunie & Erdös [25] demonstrated that $\sqrt{2} < P < 2$. Buckholtz [27] improved this to $1.7 < P < 1.862$ and Frank [27] improved this to $1.7818 < P < 1.82$. Independent work in estimating $1/P$ was done by Pommiez [28–30]. Just as Whittaker's constant W has formulation in terms of Goncharov polynomials, the power series constant P has formulation in terms of what are called remainder polynomials [7.3.2].

In this case, we consider not a functional differential equation, but rather a functional equation involving shifting. The zeros of the solution

$$\psi(z, q) = \sum_{n=0}^{\infty} q^{\frac{n(n-1)}{2}} z^n, \quad |q| \leq 1,$$

are again studied, yielding a lower bound $P \geq 1.7818046151\ldots$. Waldvogel [16] conjectured that the lower bound is, in fact, the true value of P. This is analogous to before, although the analysis is more complicated.

A third constant, examined in [16], involves certain Padé approximants. Relevant material includes [31–33].

7.3.1 Goncharov Polynomials

Bounds for the Whittaker–Goncharov constant W can theoretically be determined via the **Goncharov polynomials** [7]:

$$G_0(z) = 1, \quad G_n(z, z_0, z_1, \ldots, z_{n-1}) = \int_{z_0}^{z} \int_{z_1}^{t_1} \cdots \int_{z_{n-2}}^{t_{n-2}} \int_{z_{n-1}}^{t_{n-1}} 1 \, dt_n \, dt_{n-1} \ldots dt_2 \, dt_1$$

for $n \geq 1$. An equivalent recursive definition is

$$G_n(z, z_0, z_1, \ldots, z_{n-1}) = \frac{z^n}{n!} - \sum_{k=0}^{n-1} \frac{z_k^{n-k}}{(n-k)!} G_k(z, z_0, z_1, \ldots, z_{k-1}).$$

Evgrafov [34] proved that

$$\left(\limsup_{n \to \infty} g_n^{\frac{1}{n}} \right)^{-1} = W,$$

where

$$g_n = \max_{\substack{|z_k|=1 \\ 0 \leq k \leq n-1}} |G_n(0, z_0, z_1, \ldots, z_{n-1})|.$$

Buckholtz [35] further showed that

$$\left(\frac{2}{5} \right)^{\frac{1}{n}} g_n^{-\frac{1}{n}} < W \leq g_n^{-\frac{1}{n}},$$

and hence the limit superior can be replaced by a limit. Unfortunately, the convergence rate using these formulas is much too slow for accurate estimation of W [12]. Other techniques must be used.

7.3.2 Remainder Polynomials

A lower bound for the power series constant P can theoretically be determined via the **remainder polynomials** [30, 36, 37]:

$$B_0(z) = 1, \quad B_n(z, z_0, z_1, \ldots, z_{n-1}) = z^n - \sum_{k=0}^{n-1} z_k^{n-k} B_k(z, z_0, z_1, \ldots, z_{k-1})$$

for $n \geq 1$. Buckholtz [36] proved that

$$\lim_{n \to \infty} b_n^{\frac{1}{n}} = P,$$

where

$$b_n = \max_{\substack{|z_k|=1 \\ 0 \leq k \leq n-1}} |B_n(0, z_0, z_1, \ldots, z_{n-1})|.$$

Unfortunately, as with the Goncharov polynomials, the convergence rate using these formulas is much too slow for accurate estimation of P.

[1] S. Kakeya, An extension of power series, *Proc. Physico-Math. Soc. Japan* 14 (1932) 125–138.
[2] S. Takenaka, On the expansion of integral transcendental functions in generalized Taylor's series, *Proc. Physico-Math. Soc. Japan* 14 (1932) 529–542.
[3] J. M. Whittaker, *Interpolatory Function Theory*, Cambridge Univ. Press, 1935, pp. 44–45.
[4] R. P. Boas, Entire functions of exponential type, *Bull. Amer. Math. Soc.* 48 (1942) 839–849; MR 4,136c.
[5] R. P. Boas, *Entire Functions*, Academic Press, 1954, pp. 8–13, 172–177; MR 16,914f.
[6] R. P. Boas, An upper bound for the Gontcharoff constant, *Duke Math. J.* 15 (1948) 953–954; MR 10,443c.
[7] W. Goncharov, Recherches sur les dérivées successives des fonctions analytiques, *Annales Sci. École Norm. Sup.* 47 (1930) 1–78.
[8] J. D. Buckholtz, Successive derivatives of analytic functions, *Indian J. Math.* 13 (1971) 83–88; MR 48 #11501.
[9] J. D. Buckholtz and J. L. Frank, Whittaker constants. II, *J. Approx. Theory* 10 (1974) 112–122; MR 50 #2490.
[10] S. S. Macintyre, An upper bound for the Whittaker constant W, *J. London Math. Soc.* 22 (1947) 305–311; MR 10,27a.
[11] S. S. Macintyre, On the zeros of successive derivatives of integral functions, *Trans. Amer. Math. Soc.* 67 (1949) 241–251; MR 11,340b.
[12] R. S. Varga, *Topics in Polynomial and Rational Interpolation and Approximation*, Les Presses de l'Université de Montréal, 1982, pp. 120–129; MR 83h:30041.
[13] R. S. Varga and P. S. Wang, Improved bounds for the Whittaker constant using MACSYMA, *Proc. 1979 MACSYMA Users Conf.*, Washington DC, pp. 121–125.
[14] R. P. Boas, Functions of exponential type. II, *Duke Math. J.* 11 (1944) 17–22; MR 5,175h.
[15] R. P. Boas, Functions of exponential type. IV, *Duke Math. J.* 11 (1944) 799; MR 6,123a.

[16] J. Waldvogel, Zero-free disks in families of analytic functions, *Approximation Theory, Tampa*, ed. E. B. Saff, Lect. Notes in Math. 1287, Springer-Verlag, 1987, pp. 209–228; MR 89g:30012.

[17] R. P. Boas, Expansions of analytic functions, *Trans. Amer. Math. Soc.* 48 (1940) 467–487; MR 2,80e.

[18] V. Ganapathy Iyer, A property of the zeros of the successive derivatives of integral functions, *J. Indian Math. Soc.* 2 (1937) 289–294.

[19] H. S. Wilf, Whittaker's constant for lacunary entire functions, *Proc. Amer. Math. Soc.* 14 (1963) 238–242; MR 26 #2611.

[20] J. L. Frank and J. K. Shaw, Univalence of odd derivatives of even entire functions, *J. Reine Angew. Math.* 277 (1975) 1–4; MR 52 #11039.

[21] J. L. Frank and J. K. Shaw, On analytic functions with gaps, *J. London Math. Soc.* 6 (1973) 577–582; MR 54 #13041.

[22] J. L. Frank and J. K. Shaw, On analytic functions with gaps. II, *Acta Math. Acad. Sci. Hungar.* 27 (1976) 37–42; MR 54 #13042.

[23] V. A. Oskolkov, On a lower bound on the Whittaker constant, *Current Problems in Function Theory*, Proc. 1985 Teberda conf., ed. Yu. F. Korobeinik, Rostov. Gos. Univ., 1987, pp. 34–39, 177; MR 91b:30084.

[24] M. B. Porter, On the polynomial convergents of a power series, *Annals of Math.* 8 (1906-1907) 189–192.

[25] J. Clunie and P. Erdös, On the partial sums of power series, *Proc. Royal Irish Acad. Sect. A* 65 (1967) 113–123; MR 36 #5314.

[26] W. K. Hayman, *Research Problems in Function Theory*, Athlone Press, Univ. of London, 1967, problem 7.7; MR 36 #359.

[27] J. D. Buckholtz, Zeros of partial sums of power series, *Michigan Math. J.* 15 (1968) 481–484; MR 38 #3409.

[28] M. Pommiez, Sur les restes successifs des séries de Taylor, *Annales Faculté Sciences Toulouse* 24 (1960) 77–165; MR 27 #2614.

[29] M. Pommiez, Sur les différénces divisées successives et les restes des séries de Newton généralisées, *Annales Faculté Sciences Toulouse* 28 (1964) 101–110; MR 33 #7559b.

[30] J. D. Buckholtz and J. L. Frank, Whittaker constants, *Proc. London Math. Soc.* 23 (1971) 348–370; MR 45 #5358.

[31] G. W. Crofts and J. K. Shaw, Successive remainders of the Newton series, *Trans. Amer. Math. Soc.* 181 (1973) 369–383; MR 47 #8825.

[32] D. S. Lubinsky and E. B. Saff, Convergence of Padé approximants of partial theta functions and the Rogers-Szegö polynomials, *Constr. Approx.* 3 (1987) 331–361; MR 88m:30092.

[33] G. Szegö, Ein Beitrag zur Theorie der Thetafunktionen, *Sitzungsber. Preuss. Akad. Wiss.* (1926) 242–252; also in *Collected Papers*, v. 1, ed. R. Askey, Birkhäuser, 1982, pp. 795–805.

[34] M. A. Evgrafov, *The Abel-Goncarov Interpolation Problem* (in Russian), Gosudarstv. Izdat. Tehn.-Teor. Lit., 1954; MR 16,1104a.

[35] J. D. Buckholtz, The Whittaker constant and successive derivatives of entire functions, *J. Approx. Theory* 3 (1970) 194–212; MR 41 #5618.

[36] J. D. Buckholtz, Zeros of partial sums of power series. II, *Michigan Math. J.* 17 (1970) 5–14; MR 41 #3718.

[37] J. D. Buckholtz and J. K. Shaw, Zeros of partial sums and remainders of power series, *Trans. Amer. Math. Soc.* 166 (1972) 269–284; MR 45 #8810.

7.4 John Constant

Let X and Y be real Banach spaces (for example, X and Y may be taken to be finite-dimensional Euclidean spaces) and let D be an open subset of X. Suppose two numbers m, M are given with $0 < m \leq M < \infty$. Define a mapping $f : D \to Y$ to be an

(m, M)-**isometry** if it is continuous, open, locally one-to-one, and additionally satisfies

$$m \leq \liminf_{y \to x} \frac{|f(y) - f(x)|}{|y - x|}, \quad \limsup_{y \to x} \frac{|f(y) - f(x)|}{|y - x|} \leq M$$

for all $x \in D$.

What does the last part of this definition mean? If we picture f as deforming the domain D, then it does so in such a manner that lengths of line elements in D are altered by factors constrained to lie between m and M. Such a mapping f is also known as a **quasi-isometry** or a **bi-Lipschitz map**.

John [1–3] proved that, if $m = M$, then f must obey $|f(y) - f(x)|/|y - x| = m$ for all $x, y \in D$ and thus f is a rigid motion, scaled by m. In particular, f is (globally) one-to-one on D.

With this result in mind, it is natural to ask for the largest number $\mu = \mu(D)$ with the property that $M/m < \mu$ implies that all (m, M)-isometries of D are one-to-one. Henceforth assume D is an open ball in X. Gevirtz [4] proved that $\mu \geq r = 1.114305\ldots$, where r is the unique real root of the equation

$$r = \frac{r + \sqrt{25r^2 - 8r}}{2r(3r - 1)}.$$

A numerically sharp lower bound is not known. A few words about upper bounds for μ appear at the end of this essay.

If X is, moreover, a Hilbert space (hence angles can be measured in X), then the additional structure permits improved bounds. Gevirtz [4, 5], extending a result by John [3], showed that $\mu \geq \sqrt{2} = 1.414213\ldots$ If *both* X and Y are Hilbert spaces, then Gevirtz [4], sharpening John [3], demonstrated that $\mu \geq \sqrt{1 + \sqrt{2}} = 1.553773\ldots$ and in [5] showed that in fact $\mu \geq s = 1.65743\ldots$, where s is the minimum value for $t > 0$ of the function

$$s = s(t) = \frac{\pi + 2\sqrt{1 + t^2}}{1 + \frac{\pi}{2} + t}.$$

The proofs of these lower bounds entail fairly complicated arguments that use the basic principles for quasi-isometries established by John. Such lines of attack, however, are not powerful enough to produce numerically sharp results.

John [6] considered the special case in which the mapping is effected by an analytic function of one complex variable. That is, he considered analytic functions f defined on the unit disk D in the z-plane that satisfy $m \leq |f'(z)| \leq M$ at all points $z \in D$. As before, what is the largest number γ such that $M/m \leq \gamma$ implies that f is univalent (in the disk)? The value γ is called the **John constant** for D. Since this is a special case of the preceding, we may expect γ to be larger than μ.

Several researchers, including Avhadiev & Aksentev [7], John [6], Yamashita [8], and Gevirtz [9, 10], worked to determine γ. The best-known bounds [6, 9] are

$$4.810477\ldots \leq \exp(\tfrac{1}{2}\pi) \leq \gamma \leq \exp(\lambda\pi) = 7.1879033516\ldots,$$

where $\lambda = 0.6278342677\ldots$ satisfies the transcendental equation

$$\frac{\pi}{\exp(2\pi\lambda) - 1} = \sum_{k=1}^{\infty} \frac{k}{k^2 + \lambda^2} \exp\left(-\frac{k\pi}{2\lambda}\right).$$

Gevirtz [10] conjectured that, in fact, $\gamma = \exp(\lambda\pi)$ and gave compelling reasons for why this equality might hold. A rigorous proof is not known.

Again, if we picture f as deforming the disk D, a helpful physical interpretation emerges. If D is made of a hypothetical material that offers no resistance to infinitesimal contractions and stretchings by factors between m and M, and infinite resistance beyond these bounds, then how large must the ratio M/m be for one to bend D in such a way to make D touch itself? For analytic functions f, the answer would appear to be $7.1879033516\ldots$.

John constants can be defined for domains D in the complex plane other than the unit disk. A variational approach initiated in this setting [10, 11] provides evidence for the truth of Gevirtz's conjecture.

As a postlude, let us return to the more general conditions of the beginning. If $X = Y$ and X is the one-dimensional real line, then $\mu = \infty$ since a real-valued local homeomorphism of an interval must be a global homeomorphism (since it is monotonic). If $X = Y$ and the dimension of X is at least two, then upper bounds can be placed on μ. For example, if X is a Hilbert space, then $2 \geq \mu \geq 1.65743\ldots$. This is an outgrowth of a simple two-dimensional example by John [3]. If X is only a Banach space, then all that can be said is $64 \geq \mu \geq 1.114305\ldots$. The proof of these bounds appears in [5].

This essay is partly based on a letter from Julian Gevirtz. He also mentioned his long personal association with Fritz John. For this reason, we offer this essay as a small tribute to John's memory [12].

[1] F. John, Rotation and strain, *Commun. Pure. Appl. Math.* 14 (1961) 391–413; also in *Collected Papers*, v. 2, ed. J. Moser, Birkhäuser, 1985, pp. 643–665, 703; MR 25 #1672.

[2] F. John, On quasi-isometric mappings. I, *Commun. Pure. Appl. Math.* 21 (1968) 77–110; note 25 (1972) 497; also in *Collected Papers*, v. 2, ed. J. Moser, Birkhäuser, 1985, pp. 568–602, 636; MR 36 #5716 and MR 46 #715.

[3] F. John, On quasi-isometric mappings. II, *Commun. Pure. Appl. Math.* 22 (1969) 265–278; also in *Collected Papers*, v. 2, ed. J. Moser, Birkhäuser, 1985, pp. 603–616, 637.

[4] J. Gevirtz, Injectivity of quasi-isometric mappings of balls, *Proc. Amer. Math. Soc.* 85 (1982) 345–349; MR 84h:47072.

[5] J. Gevirtz, Upper and lower bounds in injectivity criteria for quasi-isometries, unpublished note (1997).

[6] F. John, A criterion for univalency brought up to date, *Commun. Pure. Appl. Math.* 29 (1976) 293–295; also in *Collected Papers*, v. 2, ed. J. Moser, Birkhäuser, 1985, pp. 633–635, 637; MR 54 #10592.

[7] F. G. Avhadiev and L. A. Aksentev, Sufficient conditions for univalence of analytic functions (in Russian), *Dokl. Akad. Nauk SSSR* 198 (1971) 743–746; Engl. transl. in *Soviet Math. Dokl.* 12 (1971) 859–863; MR 44 #2916.

[8] S. Yamashita, On the John constant, *Math. Z.* 161 (1978) 185–188; MR 58 #22516.

[9] J. Gevirtz, An upper bound for the John constant, *Proc. Amer. Math. Soc.* 83 (1981) 476–478; MR 82j:30026.

[10] J. Gevirtz, On extremal functions for John constants, *J. London Math. Soc.* 39 (1989) 285–298; MR 90h:30049.

[11] J. Gevirtz, The theory of sharp first-order univalence criteria, *J. d'Analyse Math.* 64 (1994) 173–202; MR 96d:30017.
[12] S. Hildebrandt, Remarks on the life and work of Fritz John, *Commun. Pure Appl. Math.* 51 (1998) 971–989; MR 99i:01033.

7.5 Hayman Constants

7.5.1 Hayman–Kjellberg

Let f be a transcendental entire function. That is, f is analytic on the whole complex plane but is not a polynomial. For each $r > 0$, define

$$M(r) = \max_{|z|=r} |f(z)|,$$

the maximum modulus of f over the circle of radius r centered at the origin. Consider the function

$$a(r) = \frac{d^2}{d \ln(r)^2} \ln(M(r)) = \left(r \frac{d}{dr} \right)^2 \ln(M(r)),$$

which exists and is continuous except at isolated points. Hadamard's three circles theorem [1] asserts that $a(r) \geq 0$. What else can be said about $a(r)$?

Hayman [2] proved that there is a constant $A > 0.18$ such that

$$\limsup_{r \to \infty} a(r) \geq A$$

for all f. He conjectured that $A = 1/4$, but this was disproved by Kjellberg [3], who demonstrated that $0.24 < A < 0.25$. Kjellberg mentioned that Richardson might have a proof that $A < 0.245$. More accurate, computer-based estimates of A are still unknown.

7.5.2 Hayman–Korenblum

Let p be a real number with $p \geq 1$. Define $c(p)$ to be the largest real number < 1 so that the following holds: For any functions f and g analytic on the unit disk, if $|f(z)| \leq |g(z)|$ for all z satisfying $c(p) < |z| < 1$, then

$$\int_{|z| \leq 1} |f(z)|^p dx\, dy \leq \int_{|z| \leq 1} |g(z)|^p dx\, dy,$$

where $z = x + i y$.

Hayman [4] proved that $c(2)$ exists and $0.04 = 1/25 \leq c(2) \leq 1/\sqrt{2} = 0.7071\ldots$, confirming a conjecture of Korenblum [5]. (More precisely, Korenblum conjectured the existence of $c(2)$ and conditionally demonstrated that the upper bound holds.) In a significant extension, Hinkkanen [6] proved that $c(p)$ exists and $0.15724 \leq c(p)$, and he asked whether $c(p) \to 1$ as $p \to \infty$. No conjectures have been made about the exact value of $c(2)$, let alone $c(p)$.

7.5.3 Hayman–Stewart

Let f be a meromorphic function. That is, f is analytic on the whole complex plane except for (isolated) poles. It can be proved that f is a quotient of two entire functions. One customarily views f as a map to the Riemann sphere S, because where f has poles it can be considered to take the value ∞. For every $r > 0$ and every point $a \in S$, define

$$n(r, a) = \text{ the number of roots of the equation } f(z) = a \text{ in}$$
$$\text{the disk } |z| \le r, \text{ with due count of multiplicity,}$$

the counting function of a-points of f. Now define two related quantities:

$$n(r) = \max_{a \in S} n(r, a),$$

$$A(r) = \operatorname*{mean}_{a \in S} n(r, a) = \frac{1}{\pi} \int_{S} n(r, a)\, da = \frac{1}{\pi} \int_{|z| \le r} \frac{|f'(z)|^2}{\left(1 + |f(z)|^2\right)^2}\, dx\, dy,$$

where $z = x + i\, y$. It is natural to compare these quantities as $r \to \infty$. Both $A(r) \to \infty$ and $n(r) \to \infty$, except in the case where f is a rational function (quotient of two polynomials), which does not interest us.

Clearly $n(r) \ge A(r)$ for all r since a maximum always exceeds an average. Certain meromorphic functions f can be constructed for which $\limsup_{r \to \infty} n(r)/A(r) = \infty$. Hence we turn attention to the ratio

$$H(f) = \liminf_{r \to \infty} \frac{n(r)}{A(r)}.$$

Hayman & Stewart [7–9] proved that $1 \le H(f) \le e$ for all f. The first example of a meromorphic function with $H(f) > 1$ was constructed by Toppila [10]; in fact, in his example $H(f)$ is at least $80/79$. However, Miles [11] proved that $H(f)$ is no larger than $e - 10^{-28}$ for all f. Thus if we define a constant $h = \sup_f H(f)$, where the supremum is over all nonconstant meromorphic functions f, we have $80/79 \le h \le e - 10^{-28}$.

Here is an interesting variation. Define

$$n_T(r) = \max_{a \in T} n(r, a)$$

for each finite subset T of S. For fixed T, clearly $n_T(r) \le n(r)$. Gary [12] proved that

$$\liminf_{r \to \infty} \frac{n_T(r)}{A(r)} \le 2.65$$

for all f, which contrasts nicely against Miles' more elaborate result. Dare we hope for greater accuracy in estimating any of these constants any time soon?

In a letter, Alexandre Eremenko wrote: "Hayman's constants are all defined as solutions of some complicated extremal problems (extremum over a class of meromorphic functions). It seems that none of these extremal problems has a nice symmetric solution. So one cannot hope for more than finding good numerical bounds for them. Another constant of this type is the univalent Bloch–Landau constant [7.1] By contrast, the ordinary Bloch–Landau constants are (presumably) of a different nature: They are related to some beautiful symmetric extremal configuration (if the conjectured values are correct). Carleson & Jones, by conjecturing that the Clunie–Pommerenke constant β is $1/4$ [7.6], believe that β is of this second kind. Of course, $\beta = 1/4$ cannot happen by accident: Some hidden symmetry should be responsible for this."

7.5.4 Hayman–Wu

Hayman & Wu [13] proved that there is a constant C such that if $f(z)$ is univalent on the open unit disk and L is any line in the plane, then the preimage $f^{-1}(L)$ has length $|f^{-1}(L)| \leq C$. Øyma [14, 15] has proved that the least possible value of C satisfies $\pi^2 \leq C < 4\pi$ and further conjectured that C is equal to the lower limit here.

[1]   J. B. Conway, *Functions of One Complex Variable*, 2nd ed., Springer-Verlag, 1978, p. 137; MR 80c:30003.

[2]   W. K. Hayman, Note on Hadamard's convexity theorem, *Entire Functions and Related Parts of Analysis*, ed. J. Korevaar, S. S. Chern, L. Ehrenpreis, W. H. J. Fuchs, and L. A. Rubel, Proc. Symp. Pure Math. 11, Amer. Math. Soc., 1968, pp. 210–213; MR 40 #5858 and MR 41 errata/addenda, p. 1965.

[3]   B. Kjellberg, The convexity theorem of Hadamard-Hayman, *Proc. Symp. Math.*, Royal Institute of Technology, Stockholm, 1973, pp. 87–114.

[4]   W. K. Hayman, On a conjecture of Korenblum, *Analysis* 19 (1999) 195–205; MR 2000e:30041.

[5]   B. Korenblum, A maximum principle for the Bergman space, *Publicacions Matèmatiques* 35 (1991) 479–486; MR 93j:30018.

[6]   A. Hinkkanen, On a maximum principle in Bergman space, *J. d'Analyse Math.* 79 (1999) 335–344; MR 2000m:30033.

[7]   W. K. Hayman and F. M. Stewart, Real inequalities with applications to function theory, *Proc. Cambridge Philos. Soc.* 50 (1954) 250–260; MR 15,857g.

[8]   W. K. Hayman, *Meromorphic Functions*, Oxford Univ. Press, 1964, pp. 1–20; MR 29 #1337.

[9]   W. K. Hayman, *Research Problems in Function Theory*, Athlone Press, Univ. of London, 1967, problem 1.16; MR 36 #359.

[10] S. Toppila, On the counting function for the a-values of a meromorphic function, *Annales Acad. Sci. Fenn. Ser. A I Math.* 2 (1976) 565–572; MR 58 #22563.

[11] J. Miles, On a theorem of Hayman and Stewart, *Complex Variables* 37 (1998) 425–455; MR 2000a:30062.

[12] J. D. Gary, *On the Supremum of the Counting Function for the a-Values of a Meromorphic Function*, Ph.D. thesis, Univ. of Illinois, 1984.

[13] W. K. Hayman and J. M. G. Wu, Level sets of univalent functions, *Comment. Math. Helv.* 56 (1981) 366–403; MR 83b:30008.

[14] K. Øyma, Harmonic measure and conformal length. *Proc. Amer. Math. Soc.* 115 (1992) 687–689; MR 92i:30007.

[15] K. Øyma, The Hayman-Wu constant, *Proc. Amer. Math. Soc.* 119 (1993) 337–338; MR 93k:30031.

7.6 Littlewood–Clunie–Pommerenke Constants

7.6.1 Alpha

Let $p(z)$ be a polynomial of degree n. The expression $|p'(z)|/(1 + |p(z)|^2)$ is called the **spherical derivative** of $p(z)$, in the sense that it measures how p changes with z, regarded as a map into the Riemann sphere [1]. Define

$$P(p) = \int\limits_{|z| \leq 1} \frac{|p'(z)|}{1 + |p(z)|^2} dx\, dy,$$

where $z = x + i\, y$. This double integral is proportional to the mean spherical derivative of $p(z)$ over the unit disk. We ask about the maximal value

$$F(n) = \sup\{P(p) : \ p \text{ is a polynomial of degree } n\}$$

and the superior limit

$$\alpha = \limsup_{n \to \infty} \frac{\ln(F(n))}{\ln(n)}.$$

Littlewood [2] proved that $F(n)$ is finite and $F(n) \leq \pi \sqrt{n}$, that is, $\alpha \leq 1/2$. He conjectured that $\alpha < 1/2$. Eremenko & Sodin [3,4] proved that $F(n) = o(\sqrt{n})$ as $n \to \infty$. Soon afterward, Lewis & Wu [5] proved that $\alpha \leq 1/2 - 2^{-264}$, thus confirming Littlewood's conjecture. However, Eremenko [6] demonstrated that $\alpha > 0$ and Baker & Stallard [7] improved this to $\alpha \geq 1.11 \times 10^{-5}$.

For rational functions (as opposed to polynomials), the analog of α has value $1/2$ [2, 8, 9]. Littlewood [2] also provided several alternative definitions of α not involving the spherical derivative. The definition of α as given here was provided by Eremenko [10].

7.6.2 Beta and Gamma

A complex analytic function f defined on an open planar region is **univalent** (or **schlicht**) if f is one-to-one; that is, $f(z) = f(w)$ if and only if $z = w$. Let

$$D = \{z : |z| < 1\} \ \text{(the open disk)}, \ E = \{z : |z| > 1\} \ \text{(an open annulus)},$$

$$S = \left\{ \text{univalent } f \text{ on } D \text{ with } f(z) = z + \sum_{n=2}^{\infty} c_n z^n \right\},$$

$$S_1 = \left\{ \text{bounded univalent } f \text{ on } D \text{ with } f(z) = \sum_{n=1}^{\infty} a_n z^n \text{ and } \sup_{z \in D} |f(z)| \leq 1 \right\},$$

$$S_2 = \left\{ \text{univalent } f \text{ on } E \text{ with } f(z) = z + \sum_{n=1}^{\infty} b_n z^{-n} \right\}.$$

For the class S, de Branges [11, 12] proved that $|c_n| \leq n$, confirming Bieberbach's famous conjecture [13]. This inequality is sharp. For S_1 and S_2, analogous sharp inequalities are unknown. It turns out that estimating coefficient decay rates for S_1 and

S_2 are closely related: Let

$$A_n = \sup_{f \in S_1} |a_n|, \qquad B_n = \sup_{f \in S_2} |b_n|,$$

$$-\gamma_1 = \lim_{n \to \infty} \frac{\ln(A_n)}{\ln(n)}, \quad -\gamma_2 = \lim_{n \to \infty} \frac{\ln(B_n)}{\ln(n)}.$$

For each $k = 1, 2$, we have relatively simple bounds $1/2 \leq \gamma_k \leq 1$. Building upon earlier work by Littlewood [14], Clunie & Pommerenke [15–18] showed that

$$0.503125 = \frac{1}{2} + \frac{1}{320} < \gamma_k < 0.803,$$

and Carleson & Jones [19] improved the upper bound to $\gamma_k < 0.76$.

Here is an alternative, more geometric formulation. For $\varepsilon > 0$ and $f \in S_k$, consider the arclength of the image of the circle $|z| = \exp((-1)^k \varepsilon)$ under the map f. Let

$$L_\varepsilon = \sup_{f \in S_1} |\{f(z) : |z| = \exp(-\varepsilon)\}|, \quad M_\varepsilon = \sup_{f \in S_2} |\{f(z) : |z| = \exp(\varepsilon)\}|,$$

$$-\beta_1 = \lim_{\varepsilon \to 0^+} \frac{\ln(L_\varepsilon)}{\ln(\varepsilon)}, \qquad\qquad -\beta_2 = \lim_{\varepsilon \to 0^+} \frac{\ln(M_\varepsilon)}{\ln(\varepsilon)}.$$

Carleson & Jones' arguments show that $0.503 < \gamma_1 = \gamma_2 = 1 - \beta_1 = 1 - \beta_2 < 0.76$ (in fact, they proved more.) The relation $\beta + \gamma = 1$ between power series coefficients and circular image arclengths seemed to be anticipated in earlier papers, but Carleson & Jones proved it explicitly and precisely for the first time.

Eremenko [10] provided a third formulation for these constants in terms of arclengths of Green's function level curves.

7.6.3 Conjectural Relations

Carleson & Jones [19] conjectured that $\gamma = 3/4$ (and hence $\beta = 1/4$) on the basis of numerical experimentation. There may be some skepticism about this belief, but there are no reliable means to confirm it yet.

Eremenko [6, 10] conjectured that $\alpha = \beta$ and further remarked that this can be proved (or disproved) without actual knowledge of α or β. The problem of whether $\alpha = \beta$ is perhaps easier than establishing their actual values.

We close with an unrelated problem. Consider the set of real numbers λ for which

$$\int_{|z| \leq 1} |f'(z)|^\lambda dx \, dy < \infty$$

is true for all $f \in S$. Brennan [20–22] proved that the integral is finite for $-1 - \delta < \lambda < 2/3$ for some $\delta > 0$, but the integral is infinite if $\lambda = 2/3$ or $\lambda = -2$. He conjectured that the integral is finite for $-2 < \lambda < 2/3$, that is, one may take $\delta = 1$. The best value of δ remains an open question.

[1] C. A. Berenstein and R. Gay, *Complex Variables: An Introduction*, Springer-Verlag, 1991, pp. 134–136; MR 92f:30001.

[2] J. E. Littlewood, Some conjectural inequalities with applications to the theory of integral functions, *J. London Math. Soc.* 27 (1952) 387–393; also in *Collected Papers*, v. 2, Oxford Univ. Press, 1982, pp. 1296–1303; MR 14,154f.

[3] A. E. Eremenko and M. L. Sodin, Hypothesis of Littlewood and distribution of values of entire functions, *Funct. Anal. Appl.* 20 (1986) 60–62; MR 87f:30070.

[4] A. E. Eremenko and M. L. Sodin, A proof of the conditional Littlewood theorem on the distribution of the values of entire functions, *Math. USSR-Izv.* 30 (1988) 395–402; MR 88m:30073.

[5] J. L. Lewis and J.-M. Wu, On conjectures of Arakelyan and Littlewood, *J. d'Analyse Math.* 50 (1988) 259–283; MR 89i:30038.

[6] A. E. Eremenko, Lower estimate in Littlewood's conjecture on the mean spherical derivative of a polynomial and iteration theory, *Proc. Amer. Math. Soc.* 112 (1991) 713–715; MR 92k:30008.

[7] I. N. Baker and G. M. Stallard, Error estimates in a calculation of Ruelle, *Complex Variables Theory Appl.* 29 (1996) 141–159; MR 97b:30037.

[8] Y. M. Chen and M. C. Liu, On Littlewood's conjectural inequalities, *J. London Math. Soc.* 1 (1969) 385–397; MR 43 #2192.

[9] W. K. Hayman, On a conjecture of Littlewood, *J. d'Analyse Math.* 36 (1979) 75–95; MR 81j:30042.

[10] A. E. Eremenko, Some constants coming from the work of Littlewood, unpublished note (1999).

[11] L. de Branges, A proof of the Bieberbach conjecture, *Acta Math.* 154 (1985) 137–152; MR 86h:30026.

[12] A. Z. Grinshpan, The Bieberbach conjecture and Milin's functionals, *Amer. Math. Monthly* 106 (1999) 203–214; MR 2000b:30027.

[13] L. Bieberbach, Über die Koeffizienten derjenigen Potenzreihen welche eine schlichte Abbildungen des Einheitskreises vermitteln, *Sitzungsber. Preuss. Akad. Wiss.* (1916) 940–955.

[14] J. E. Littlewood, On the coefficients of schlicht functions, *Quart. J. Math.* 9 (1938) 14–20.

[15] Ch. Pommerenke, On the coefficients of univalent functions, *J. London Math. Soc.* 42 (1967) 471–474; MR 36 #5329.

[16] J. Clunie and Ch. Pommerenke, On the coefficients of univalent functions, *Michigan Math. J.* 14 (1967) 71–78; MR 34 #7786.

[17] Ch. Pommerenke, *Univalent Functions*, Vandenhoeck and Ruprecht, 1975, pp. 125–137; MR 58 #22526.

[18] P. L. Duren, *Univalent Functions*, Springer-Verlag, 1983, pp. 1–40, 234–243; MR 85j:30034.

[19] L. Carleson and P. W. Jones, On coefficient problems for univalent functions and conformal dimension, *Duke Math. J.* 66 (1992) 169–206; MR 93c:30022.

[20] J. E. Brennan, The integrability of the derivative in conformal mapping, *J. London Math. Soc.* 18 (1978) 261–272; MR 80b:30009.

[21] Ch. Pommerenke, On the integral means of the derivative of a univalent function. II, *Bull. London Math. Soc.* 17 (1985) 565–570; MR 87f:30050b.

[22] L. Carleson and N. G. Makarov, Some results connected with Brennan's conjecture, *Ark. Mat.* 32 (1994) 33–62; MR 95g:30030.

7.7 Riesz–Kolmogorov Constants

Let $F(z) = f(z) + i\tilde{f}(z)$ be an analytic function defined on the closed unit disk, with the property that its imaginary part satisfies $\tilde{f}(0) = 0$. Define the p-**Hardy norm** [1,2]

$$\|f\|_p = \left(\frac{1}{2\pi} \int_0^{2\pi} |f(e^{i\theta})|^p \, d\theta \right)^{\frac{1}{p}}, \quad 0 < p < \infty.$$

What can be said about the relative sizes of the conjugate functions f and $\tilde{f}$? Riesz [3] proved that

$$\|\tilde{f}\|_p \leq C_p \cdot \|f\|_p, \quad 1 < p < \infty,$$

and Pichorides [4] and Cole [5] determined the best constant in this inequality to be [6–8]

$$C_p = \begin{cases} \tan\left(\frac{\pi}{2p}\right) & 1 < p \leq 2, \\ \cot\left(\frac{\pi}{2p}\right) & 2 < p < \infty. \end{cases}$$

If $p = 1$, there exist functions F for which $\|f\|_1 < \infty$ but $\|\tilde{f}\|_1 = \infty$. Hence a revised sense of "relative size" becomes necessary in this case.

If S is a measurable subset of the unit circle, let $|S|$ denote its Lebesgue measure, divided by 2π. For $t \geq 0$, define the set

$$S_t(f) = \{z : |f(z)| \geq t \text{ and } |z| = 1\}.$$

Kolmogorov [9] proved the **weak type 1-1 inequality**

$$|S_t(\tilde{f})| \leq C_1 \cdot \frac{1}{t} \cdot \|f\|_1 \quad \text{for all } t > 0$$

and Davis [10] determined the best constant to be

$$C_1 = \frac{\pi^2}{8G} = 1.3468852519\ldots = (0.7424537454\ldots)^{-1},$$

where G is Catalan's constant [1.7]. A corollary of Kolmogorov's theorem is

$$\|\tilde{f}\|_p \leq C_p \cdot \|f\|_1, \quad 0 < p < 1.$$

Davis [11, 12] identified the best constants here to be

$$C_p = \left(\frac{1}{2\pi} \int_0^{2\pi} |\csc(\theta)|^p d\theta\right)^{\frac{1}{p}} = \left(\frac{1}{\sqrt{\pi}} \frac{\Gamma\left(\frac{1-p}{2}\right)}{\Gamma\left(\frac{2-p}{2}\right)}\right)^{\frac{1}{p}},$$

where $\Gamma(x)$ is the gamma function [1.5.4]. There is a related issue of the relative sizes of F and f, which we will not discuss. See also [13–17].

[1] A. G. Zygmund, *Trigonometric Series*, v. 1, 2nd ed., Cambridge Univ. Press, 1959, pp. 131, 252, 377; MR 89c:42001.

[2] P. L. Duren, *Theory of H_p Spaces*, Academic Press, 1970, pp. 53–58; MR 42 #3552.

[3] M. Riesz, Sur les fonctions conjuguées, *Math. Z.* 27 (1927) 218–244.

[4] S. K. Pichorides, On the best values of the constants in the theorems of M. Riesz, Zygmund and Kolmogorov, *Studia Math.* 44 (1972) 165–179 (errata insert); MR 47 #702.

[5] T. W. Gamelin, *Uniform Algebras and Jensen Measures*, Cambridge Univ. Press, 1978, pp. 107–145; MR 81a:46058.

[6] I. E. Verbickii, Estimate of the norm of a function in a Hardy space in terms of the norms of its real and imaginary parts (in Russian), *Mat. Issled.* 54 (1980) 16–20, 164–165; MR 81k:30046.

[7] M. Essén, A superharmonic proof of the M. Riesz conjugate function theorem, *Ark. Mat.* 22 (1984) 241–249; MR 86c:30068.

[8] M. Essén, D. Shea, and C. Stanton, Best constant inequalities for conjugate functions, *J. Comput. Appl. Math.* 105 (1999) 257–264; MR 2000k:42008.

[9] A. N. Kolmogorov, Sur les fonctions harmoniques conjuguées et les séries de Fourier, *Fund. Math.* 7 (1925) 24–29; Engl. transl. in *Selected Works*, v. 1., ed. V. M. Tikhomirov, Kluwer, 1991, pp. 35–40; MR 93d:01096.

[10] B. Davis, On the weak type (1,1) inequality for conjugate functions, *Proc. Amer. Math. Soc.* 44 (1974) 307–311; MR 50 #879.

[11] B. Davis, On Kolmogorov's inequalities $||\tilde{f}||_p \leq C_p \cdot ||f||_1$, $0 < p < 1$, *Trans. Amer. Math. Soc.* 222 (1976) 179–192; MR 54 #10967.

[12] A. Baernstein, Some sharp inequalities for conjugate functions, *Indiana Univ. Math. J.* 27 (1978) 833–852; MR 80g:30022.

[13] C. Bennett, A best constant for Zygmund's conjugate function inequality, *Proc. Amer. Math. Soc.* 56 (1976) 256–260; MR 53 #6214.

[14] S. P. Grushevskii, A generalization of the Kolmogorov inequality, *Soobshch. Akad. Nauk Gruzin. SSR* 103 (1981) 33–36; MR 84h:42020.

[15] C. Choi, A weak-type inequality for differentially subordinate harmonic functions, *Trans. Amer. Math. Soc.* 350 (1998) 2687–2696; MR 99e:31006.

[16] A. B. J. Kuijlaars, Best constants in one-sided weak-type inequalities, *Methods Appl. Anal.* 5 (1998) 95–108; MR 99h:42014.

[17] R. Bañuelos and G. Wang, Davis's inequality for orthogonal martingales under differential subordination, *Michigan Math. J.* 47 (2000) 109–124; MR 2001g:60100.

7.8 Grötzsch Ring Constants

Let R be a planar ring, that is, an open connected subset of the complex plane $\mathbb{C}$. Two regions R_1 and R_2 are **conformally equivalent** if there is an analytic function $f : R_1 \to R_2$ such that f is one-to-one and onto. Clearly this is an equivalence relation. The famous Riemann mapping theorem implies the following:

- Among the simply connected regions, there are exactly two equivalence classes: one consisting of $\mathbb{C}$ alone and the other containing the unit disk (and much more).
- Among the doubly connected regions, there are uncountably many equivalence classes, each containing a circular annulus $A(1, r) = \{z : 1 < |z| < r\}$ for some unique real $r > 1$ (and much more).

In particular, two annuli $A(s, t)$ and $A(u, v)$ are conformally equivalent if and only if $t/s = v/u$, that is, the ratio of outer radius and inner radius is a conformal invariant [1,2].

Let us change the subject slightly for a moment. By a **ring** R in n-dimensional Euclidean space, we mean a region whose complement consists of two components C_0 and C_1, where C_0 is bounded and C_1 is unbounded. Let B_0 and B_1 be the boundary components of R. The **conformal capacity** of R is

$$\text{cap}(R) = \inf_{\varphi} \int_R |\nabla\varphi|^n \, dx,$$

where the infimum is over all real continuously differentiable functions φ on R with values 0 on B_0 and 1 on B_1. The **modulus** of R is

$$\text{mod}(R) = \left(\frac{\sigma}{\text{cap}(R)}\right)^{\frac{1}{n-1}},$$

where $\sigma = n\pi^{n/2}\Gamma(1 + n/2)^{-1}$ is the surface area of the sphere of radius 1 in n-dimensional space. For an n-dimensional spherical annulus $A(s, t)$, we find that [3–8]

$$\text{mod}(A(s, t)) = \ln\left(\frac{t}{s}\right).$$

Therefore, in the case $n = 2$, the modulus of a ring is a conformal invariant. For $n \geq 3$, we lose this nice geometric interpretation since the Riemann mapping theorem no longer applies: The unit n-dimensional ball is conformally equivalent only to another ball or to a half-space. Nevertheless, the modulus is important in other ways (e.g., in distortion theorems associated with quasiconformal mappings).

Let $G(n, a)$ denote the n-dimensional **Grötzsch ring**, that is, the ring whose complementary components are

$$C_0 = \{(x, 0, 0, \ldots, 0) : 0 \leq x \leq a\}, \text{ where } 0 < a < 1;$$

$$C_1 = \left\{(x_1, x_2, \ldots, x_n) : \sum_{i=1}^{n} x_i^2 \geq 1\right\}.$$

In words, $G(n, a)$ is the unit n-ball, slit from 0 to a along a radial vector. It is known that the following limit exists and is finite [7–15]:

$$\ln(\lambda_n) = \lim_{a \to 0^+} (\text{mod}(G(n, a)) + \ln(a));$$

that is, $\text{mod}(G(n, a))$ experiences logarithmic growth as a decreases to 0. In the special case $n = 2$, we have [4, 13, 14]

$$\text{mod}(G(2, a)) = \frac{\pi}{2} \frac{K(\sqrt{1 - a^2})}{K(a)}$$

and hence $\lambda_2 = 4$. K is the complete elliptic integral of the first kind; a similar expression appeared in [4.5]. We also have the interesting asymptotic result [9]

$$\lim_{n \to \infty} \lambda_n^{\frac{1}{n}} = e,$$

where e is the natural logarithmic base [1.3].

No such exact formulas have been found for λ_3 or λ_4. Rigorous lower and upper bounds for λ_n, plus the best-known numerical estimates, are given in Table 7.1 [12, 15]. A table of bounds for $\lambda_n \exp(-n)$ for $3 \leq n \leq 22$ appears in [14], along with a simple inequality

$$2 \exp(0.76(n - 1)) \leq \lambda_n \leq 2 \exp(n - 1).$$

We conclude by returning to the case $n = 2$. What is the formula for the conformal function f that maps $A(1, r)$ onto $G(2, a(r))$, where the slit length $a(r)$ is defined below?

Table 7.1. *Estimates for Parameters λ_n*

n	Lower bound	Best estimate for λ_n	Upper bound
3	9.341	9.37 ± 0.02	9.9002
4	21.85	22.6 ± 0.2	26.046

The mapping turns out to involve the Jacobi elliptic sine function sn [1.4.6]. Higher transcendental functions often occur in this study: The appropriate generalizations for $n \geq 3$ await discovery.

7.8.1 Formula for $a(r)$

The annulus $A(1, r)$ and the Grötzsch ring $G(2, a)$ are conformally equivalent if and only if

$$\ln(r) = \text{mod}(A(1, r)) = \text{mod}(G(2, a)) = \frac{\pi}{2} \frac{K(\sqrt{1 - a^2})}{K(a)}.$$

We wish to solve for a as a function of r. It turns out that $a(r)$ can be written in terms of an infinite product [14, 16]:

$$a(r) = \frac{2b(r)}{1 + b(r)^2}, \text{ where } b(r) = \frac{2}{r} \prod_{j=1}^{\infty} \left(\frac{1 + r^{-8j}}{1 + r^{-8j+4}} \right)^2.$$

Consider the ring $H(n, b)$ whose complementary components are

$$D_0 = \{(x, 0, 0, \ldots, 0) : -b \leq x \leq b\}, \text{ where } 0 < b < 1;$$

$$D_1 = \left\{ (x_1, x_2, \ldots, x_n) : \sum_{i=1}^{n} x_i^2 \geq 1 \right\}.$$

In words, $H(n, b)$ is the unit n-ball, slit symmetrically from $-b$ to b through the origin. Then $H(2, b(r))$, $A(1, r)$, and $G(2, a(r))$ are conformally equivalent. Results for $\text{mod}(G(n, a))$ conceivably have analogs for $\text{mod}(H(n, b))$. See also [17, 18].

[1] J. B. Conway, *Functions of One Complex Variable*, 2nd ed., Springer-Verlag, 1978, pp. 160–164; MR 80c:30003.
[2] P. K. Kythe, *Computational Conformal Mapping*, Birkhäuser, 1998, pp. 295–303; MR 99k:65027.
[3] F. W. Gehring, Symmetrization of rings in space, *Trans. Amer. Math. Soc.* 101 (1961) 499–519; MR 24 #A2677.
[4] O. Lehto and K. I. Virtanen, *Quasiconformal Mappings in the Plane*, Springer-Verlag, 1973, pp. 30–33, 59–62; MR 49 #9202.
[5] G. D. Anderson, Symmetrization and extremal rings in space, *Annales Acad. Sci. Fenn. Ser. A I* 438 (1969) 1–24; MR 41 #465.
[6] G. D. Anderson, Extremal rings in n-space for fixed and varying n, *Annales Acad. Sci. Fenn. Ser. A I* 575 (1974) 1–21; MR 53 #799.
[7] G. D. Anderson, Limit theorems and estimates for extremal rings of high dimension, *Romanian-Finnish Seminar on Complex Analysis*, Proc. 1976 Bucharest conf., ed. C. A.

Cazacu, A. Cornea, M. Jurchescu, and I. Suciu, Lect. Notes in Math. 743, Springer-Verlag, 1979, pp. 10–34; MR 81c:30042.

[8]   P. Caraman, *n-Dimensional Quasiconformal (QCF) Mappings*, Editura Academiei/Abacus Press, 1974, pp. 51–52, 232; MR 50 #10249.

[9]   G. D. Anderson, Dependence on dimension of a constant related to the Grötzsch ring, *Proc. Amer. Math. Soc.* 61 (1976) 77–80; MR 56 #603.

[10] G. D. Anderson and M. K. Vamanamurthy, Estimates for the asymptotic order of a Grötzsch ring constant, *Tôhoku Math. J.* 34 (1982) 133–139; MR 83i:30012.

[11] G. D. Anderson and M. K. Vamanamurthy, Asymptotic estimates for moduli of extremal rings, *Tôhoku Math. J.* 37 (1985) 533–540; MR 87d:30020.

[12] G. D. Anderson and J. S. Frame, Numerical estimates for a Grötzsch ring constant, *Constr. Approx.* 4 (1988) 223–242; MR 89i:30017.

[13] M. Vuorinen, *Conformal Geometry and Quasiregular Mappings*, Lect. Notes in Math. 1319, Springer-Verlag, 1988, pp. 65–67, 88–89; MR 89k:30021.

[14] G. D. Anderson, M. K. Vamanamurthy, and M. Vuorinen, *Conformal Invariants, Inequalities, and Quasiconformal Maps*, Wiley, 1997, pp. 119–120, 149–151, 166–169, 247–264; MR 98h:30033.

[15] K. Samuelsson and M. Vuorinen, Computation of capacity in 3D by means of a posteriori estimates for adaptive FEM, Royal Institute of Technology preprint TRITA-NA-9508 (1995).

[16] Z. Nehari, *Conformal Mapping*, Dover, 1975, pp. 280–296, 333–336; MR 51 #13206.

[17] R. Wegmann, An iterative method for the conformal mapping of doubly connected regions, *J. Comput. Appl. Math.* 14 (1986) 79–98; *Numerical Conformal Mapping*, ed. L. N. Trefethen, North-Holland, 1986, 79–98; MR 87e:30008.

[18] N. Papamichael, I. E. Pritsker, E. B. Saff, and N. S. Stylianopoulos, Approximation of conformal mappings of annular regions, *Numer. Math.* 76 (1997) 489–513; MR 98e:65016.

8

Constants Associated with Geometry

8.1 Geometric Probability Constants

We will only briefly touch the large subject of geometric probability [1] but enough to introduce a few questions.

Suppose a point is randomly selected from the n-dimensional unit cube. The expected Euclidean distance to the cube center, $\delta(n)$, has the following closed-form expressions [2–7]:

$$\delta(1) = \frac{1}{4}, \quad \delta(2) = \frac{1}{6}\left(\sqrt{2} + \ln(1 + \sqrt{2})\right) = 0.3825978582\ldots,$$

$$\delta(3) = \frac{1}{48}\left(6\sqrt{3} + 12\ln(2 + \sqrt{3}) - \pi\right) = 0.4802959782\ldots.$$

It possesses the following bounds (for all n) and asymptotics:

$$\frac{1}{4}n^{\frac{1}{2}} \leq \delta(n) \leq \frac{1}{2}\left(\frac{n}{3}\right)^{\frac{1}{2}}, \quad \delta(n) \sim \frac{1}{2}\left(\frac{n}{3}\right)^{\frac{1}{2}}$$

(in particular, $\delta(n)$ is unbounded). Are closed-form expressions for $\delta(4) = 0.5609498093\ldots$ and $\delta(5) = 0.6312033175\ldots$ possible? Incidently, $2\delta(n)$ is the mean distance from the point to an arbitrary corner of the n-cube. If we examine the analogous problem corresponding to the n-dimensional unit ball [8–14], the expected Euclidean distance is $n/(n + 1)$ (which is bounded, of course).

Suppose two points are independently and uniformly chosen from the unit n-cube. The expected Euclidean distance between them, $\Delta(n)$, is

$$\Delta(1) = \frac{1}{3}, \quad \Delta(2) = \frac{1}{15}\left(\sqrt{2} + 2 + 5\ln(1 + \sqrt{2})\right) = 0.5214054331\ldots,$$

$$\Delta(3) = \frac{1}{105}\left(4 + 17\sqrt{2} - 6\sqrt{3} + 21\ln(1 + \sqrt{2}) + 42\ln(2 + \sqrt{3}) - 7\pi\right)$$

$$= 0.6617071822\ldots$$

and has corresponding bounds and asymptotics:

$$\frac{1}{3}n^{\frac{1}{2}} \le \Delta(n) \le \left(\frac{n}{6}\right)^{\frac{1}{2}}, \quad \Delta(n) \sim \left(\frac{n}{6}\right)^{\frac{1}{2}}.$$

Are closed-form expressions for $\Delta(4) = 0.7776656535\ldots$ and $\Delta(5) = 0.8785309152\ldots$ possible? Much more is known for the unit n-ball analog of this problem: The mean distance in this scenario is a ratio of gamma function values and tends to $\sqrt{2}$ as $n \to \infty$. The fact that, as n grows, the limiting $\Delta(n)$ is finite for n-balls but infinite for n-cubes is very interesting! Additionally, the variance of the distance separating the points in the n-ball tends to zero. Thus, for large n, the separation between two random points is almost always equal to the distance between the extremities of two orthogonal radii [1].

We mention that the expected reciprocal Euclidean distance between two random points in the unit 3-cube is [15, 16]

$$2\left(\frac{\sqrt{2}+1-2\sqrt{3}}{5} - \frac{\pi}{3} - \ln\left[(\sqrt{2}-1)(2-\sqrt{3})\right]\right) = 1.8823126444\ldots,$$

and clearly generalization is possible.

Suppose instead that three (rather than two) points are randomly selected in the unit n-cube. What is the probability, $\Pi(n)$, that the three points form an obtuse triangle? Langford [17, 18] proved that

$$\Pi(2) = \frac{97}{150} + \frac{\pi}{40} = 0.7252064830\ldots,$$

but no one has performed a similar calculation for $\Pi(n)$, $n > 2$. Again, much more is known for the n-ball analog of this problem [19, 20]. Random triangles in the n-ball tend to be acute for large n since most of the volume of the n-ball is near its surface [21]. In fact, such random triangles tend to be approximately equilateral and thus have small probability of being obtuse. See [22–28] for related discussion.

Suppose instead that N points $p_1, p_2, \ldots, p_N$ are randomly selected in the unit n-cube. Let C denote the convex hull of $p_1, p_2, \ldots, p_N$; that is,

$$C = \left\{\sum_{j=1}^{N} \lambda_j p_j : \lambda_j \ge 0 \text{ for all } j \text{ and } \sum_{j=1}^{N} \lambda_j = 1\right\}$$

is the intersection of all convex sets containing $p_1, p_2, \ldots, p_N$. Then,

- the expected n-dimensional volume, $E(V_n(N))$, of C,
- the expected $(n-1)$-dimensional surface area, $E(S_n(N))$, of C, and
- the expected number of vertices, $E(P_n(N))$, on the (polygonal) boundary of C

satisfy

$$\lim_{N\to\infty} \frac{N}{\ln(N)}(1 - E(V_2(N))) = \frac{8}{3},$$

$$\lim_{N\to\infty} \sqrt{N}(4 - E(S_2(N))) = 2\sqrt{\pi}\,M = 4.2472965459\ldots,$$

$$\lim_{N\to\infty} E(P_2(N)) - \frac{8}{3}\ln(N) = \frac{8}{3}(\gamma - \ln(2)) = -0.3091507084\ldots$$

according to Rényi & Sulanke [29–39], where γ denotes the Euler–Mascheroni constant [1.5] and M is Gauss' lemniscate constant [6.1]. Affentranger & Wieacker [40, 41] obtained asymptotics for $V_n(N)$ and $P_n(N)$ for $n \geq 3$. Cabo & Groeneboom [42–45] demonstrated that

$$\lim_{N\to\infty} N\,\mathrm{Var}(S_2(N)) = 4(J - I^2) = 0.9932\ldots,$$

where

$$I = \sqrt{\frac{\pi}{8}}\left[2 - \int_1^\infty \left(\sqrt{1+s^2} - s\right)s^{-3/2}ds\right] = \frac{\sqrt{\pi}}{2}M = 1.0618241364\ldots,$$

$$J = 2 - 4\int_1^\infty \left(\sqrt{1+s^2} - s\right)\varphi(s-1)\,ds + \frac{4}{5}\int_1^\infty \left(\sqrt{1+s^2} - s\right)^2 s^{-2}ds$$

$$+ \frac{1}{4}\int_1^\infty \int_1^t \left(\sqrt{1+s^2} - s\right)\left(\sqrt{1+t^2} - t\right)\psi\left(\frac{t}{s} - 1\right)s^{-3}ds\,dt$$

$$+ \frac{1}{8}\int_1^\infty \int_1^\infty \left(\sqrt{1+s^2} - s\right)\left(\sqrt{1+t^2} - t\right)\psi\left(st - 1\right)\,ds\,dt$$

$$= 1.37575\ldots,$$

and

$$\varphi(s) = \frac{1}{2(s+1)^2} - \frac{1}{4s(s+1)} + \frac{1}{4s}\frac{\arctan(\sqrt{s})}{\sqrt{s}},$$

$$\psi(s) = \frac{15}{s^3} + \frac{1}{s^2} - \left(\frac{15}{s^3} + \frac{6}{s^2} - \frac{1}{s}\right)\frac{\arctan(\sqrt{s})}{\sqrt{s}}.$$

No higher-dimensional analog of this result is known.

Suppose instead that N *lines* are randomly drawn in the square [46, 47]. The average number of regions into which the lines divide the square is given by [48, 49]

$$\frac{N(N-1)\pi}{16} + N + 1,$$

which is another fascinating occurrence of Archimedes' constant π in geometry. The average number of regions into which N random *planes* divide the cube is

$$\frac{(2N + 23)N(N - 1)\pi}{324} + N + 1.$$

What are the higher dimensional analogs of these results? Related material on the maximum possible number of regions appears in [50–52].

We close with a different type of problem (not actually from geometric probability). Here the issue is existence. Is there a positive constant c such that any measurable plane set of area c must contain the vertices of a triangle of area exactly equal to 1? Erdös [53, 54] wondered if c might be as small as $4\pi/(3\sqrt{3})$ but no progress has been made on determining whether c is even finite. A related question, concerning whether every convex region in the Euclidean plane with area 1 can be inscribed in a triangle of area at most equal to 2, was answered long ago [55, 56]. The three-dimensional analog remains unsolved [57].

[1]   L. A. Santaló, *Integral Geometry and Geometric Probability*, Addison-Wesley, 1976, pp. 21–26, 49–58, 212–213, 294–295; MR 55 #6340.

[2]   B. Ghosh, Random distances within a rectangle and between two rectangles, *Bull. Calcutta Math. Soc.* 43 (1951) 17–24; MR 13,475a.

[3]   R. S. Anderssen, R. P. Brent, D. J. Daley, and P. A. P. Moran, Concerning $\int_0^1 \cdots \int_0^1 (x_1^2 + \cdots + x_k^2)^{1/2} dx_1 \ldots dx_k$ and a Taylor series method, *SIAM J. Appl. Math.* 30 (1976) 22–30; MR 52 #15773.

[4]   H. J. Oser and D. J. Daley, An average distance, *SIAM Rev.* 18 (1976) 497–500.

[5]   D. P. Robbins and T. S. Bolis, Average distance between two points in a box, *Amer. Math. Monthly* 85 (1978) 277–278.

[6]   R. E. Pfiefer, A. L. Holshouser, L. R. King, and B. G. Klein, Minimum average distance between points in a rectangle, *Amer. Math. Monthly* 96 (1989) 64–65.

[7]   S. R. Dunbar, The average distance between points in geometric figures, *College Math. J.* 28 (1997) 187–197; MR 98a:52007.

[8]   R. D. Lord, The distribution of distance in a hypersphere, *Annals of Math. Statist.* 25 (1954) 794–798; MR 16,377d.

[9]   J. M. Hammersley, The distribution of distance in a hypersphere, *Annals of Math. Statist.* 21 (1950) 447–452; MR 12,268e.

[10] M. G. Kendall and P. A. P. Moran, *Geometrical Probability*, Hafner, 1963, pp. 41–42, 53–55; MR 30 #4275.

[11] V. S. Alagar, The distribution of the distance between random points, *J. Appl. Probab.* 13 (1976) 558–566; MR 54 #6225.

[12] R. Pinkham and R. Holzsager, A random distance, *Amer. Math. Monthly* 106 (1999) 171–172.

[13] B. Eisenberg and R. Sullivan, Crofton's differential equation, *Amer. Math. Monthly* 107 (2000) 129–139; MR 2001g:60021.

[14] K. Brown, Distances in bounded regions; Distributions of distances (MathPages).

[15] H. Essén and A. Nordmark, Some results on the electrostatic energy of ionic crystals, *Canad. J. Chem.* 74 (1996) 885–891.

[16] Z. F. Seidov and P. I. Skvirsky, Gravitational potential and energy of homogeneous rectangular parallelepiped, astro-ph/0002496.

[17] E. Langford, The probability that a random triangle is obtuse, *Biometrika* 56 (1969) 689–690.

[18] E. Langford, A problem in geometrical probability, *Math Mag.* 43 (1970) 237–244; MR 45 #7774.

[19] G. R. Hall, Acute triangles in the n-ball, *J. Appl. Probab.* 19 (1982) 712–715; MR 83h:60016.

[20] C. Buchta, A note on the volume of a random polytope in a tetrahedron, *Illinois J. Math.* 30 (1986) 653–659; MR 87m:60038.

[21] B. Eisenberg and R. Sullivan, Random triangles in n dimensions, *Amer. Math. Monthly* 103 (1996) 308–318; MR 96m:60025.

[22] V. S. Alagar, On the distribution of a random triangle, *J. Appl. Probab.* 14 (1977) 284–297; MR 55 #9203.

[23] D. G. Kendall, Exact distributions for shapes of random triangles in convex sets, *Adv. Appl. Probab.* 17 (1985) 308–329; MR 86m:60033.

[24] D. G. Kendall and H.-L. Le, Exact shape-densities for random triangles in convex polygons, *Adv. Appl. Probab.* Suppl. (1986) 59–72; MR 88h:60022.

[25] R. K. Guy, There are three times as many obtuse-angled triangles as there are acute-angled ones, *Math. Mag.* 66 (1993) 175–178.

[26] S. Portnoy, A Lewis Carroll pillow problem: Probability of an obtuse triangle, *Statist. Sci.* 9 (1994) 279–284; MR 95h:60003.

[27] D. E. Dobbs and J. L. Zarestky, Acute random triangles, *Nieuw Arch. Wisk.* 15 (1997) 141–162.

[28] Z. F. Seidov, Random triangle in square: Geometrical approach, math.GM/0002134.

[29] A. Rényi and R. Sulanke, Über die konvexe Hülle von n zufällig gewählten Punkten. I, *Z. Wahrsch. Verw. Gebiete* 2 (1963) 75–84; II, 3 (1964) 138–147; also in *Selected Papers of Alfréd Rényi*, v. 3, Akadémiai Kiadó, 1976, pp. 143–152 and 242–251; MR 27 #6190 and MR 29 #6392.

[30] B. Efron, The convex hull of a random set of points, *Biometrika* 52 (1965) 331–343; MR 34 #6820.

[31] H. Raynaud, Sur l'enveloppe convexe des nuages de points aléatoires dans $\mathbb{R}^n$. I, *J. Appl. Probab.* 7 (1970) 35–48; MR 41 #2736.

[32] H. Carnal, Die konvexe Hülle von n rotationssymmetrisch verteilten Punkten, *Z. Wahrsch. Verw. Gebiete* 15 (1970) 168–176; MR 44 #3367.

[33] H. Ziezold, Über die Eckenanzahl zufälliger konvexer Polygone, *Izv. Akad. Nauk Armjan. SSR Ser. Mat.* 5 (1970) 296–312; MR 44 #4800.

[34] C. Buchta, Stochastische Approximation konvexer Polygone, *Z. Wahrsch. Verw. Gebiete* 67 (1984) 283–304; MR 85k:60021.

[35] R. A. Dwyer, Convex hulls of samples from spherically symmetric distributions, *Discrete Appl. Math.* 31 (1991) 113–132; MR 92i:60020.

[36] D. J. Aldous, B. Fristedt, P. S. Griffin, and W. E. Pruitt, The number of extreme points in the convex hull of a random sample, *J. Appl. Probab.* 28 (1991) 287–304; MR 92j:60022.

[37] W. Weil and J. A. Wieacker, Stochastic geometry, *Handbook of Convex Geometry*, v. B, ed. P. M. Gruber and J. M. Wills, North-Holland, 1993, pp. 1391–1431.

[38] R. Schneider, Discrete aspects of stochastic geometry, *Handbook of Discrete and Computational Geometry*, ed. J. E. Goodman and J. O'Rourke, CRC Press, 1997, pp. 167–184.

[39] A. M. Mathai, *An Introduction to Geometrical Probability: Distributional Aspects with Applications*, Gordon and Breach, 1999, pp. 364–383; MR 2001a:60014.

[40] F. Affentranger and J. A. Wieacker, On the convex hull of uniform random points in a simple d-polytope, *Discrete Comput. Geom.* 6 (1991) 291–305; MR 92c:52004.

[41] B. F. van Wel, The convex hull of a uniform sample from the interior of a simple d-polytope, *J. Appl. Probab.* 26 (1989) 259–273; MR 91a:60040.

[42] P. Groeneboom, Limit theorems for convex hulls, *Probab. Theory Relat. Fields* 79 (1988) 327–368; MR 89j:60024.

[43] A. J. Cabo and P. Groeneboom, Limit theorems for functionals of convex hulls, *Probab. Theory Relat. Fields* 100 (1994) 31–55; MR 95g:60017.

[44] I. Hueter, Limit theorems for the convex hull of random points in higher dimensions, *Trans. Amer. Math. Soc.* 351 (1999) 4337–4363; MR 2000a:52008.

[45] J. Keane, Convex hull integrals and the "ubiquitous constant," unpublished note (2000).

[46] S. Goudsmit, Random distribution of lines in a plane, *Rev. Mod. Phys.* 17 (1945) 321–322.

[47]   H. Solomon, *Geometric Probability*, SIAM, 1978, pp. 39–44; MR 58 #7777.

[48]   L. A. Santaló, Valor medio del numero de regiones en que un cuerpo del espacio es dividido por *n* planos arbitrarios, *Rev. Unión Mat. Argentina* 10 (1945) 101–108.

[49]   L. A. Santaló, Sobre la distribucion de planos en el espacio, *Rev. Unión Mat. Argentina* 13 (1948) 120–124.

[50]   A. M. Yaglom and I. M. Yaglom, *Challenging Mathematical Problems with Elementary Solutions*, v. 1, Dover, 1987, pp. 13, 102–106; MR 88m:00012a.

[51]   D. J. Price, Some unusual series occurring in *n*-dimensional geometry, *Math. Gazette* 30 (1946) 149–150.

[52]   H. Dörrie, *100 Great Problems of Elementary Mathematics: Their History and Solution*, Dover, 1965, pp. 283–285; MR 84b:00001.

[53]   P. Erdös, Some combinatorial, geometric and set theoretic problems in measure theory, *Measure Theory*, Proc. 1983 Oberwolfach conf., ed. D. Kölzow and D. Maharam-Stone, Lect. Notes in Math. 1089, Springer-Verlag, 1984, pp. 321–327; MR 85m:28002.

[54]   H. T. Croft, K. J. Falconer, and R. K. Guy, *Unsolved Problems in Geometry*, Springer-Verlag, 1991, sect. G13; MR 95k:52001.

[55]   W. Gross, Über affine Geometrie. XIII: Eine Minimumeigenschaft der Ellipse und des Ellipsoids, *Berichte über die Verhandlungen der Königlich Sächsischen Gesellschaft der Wissenschaften zu Leipzig, Math.-Phys. Klasse* 70 (1918) 38–54.

[56]   H. G. Eggleston, *Problems in Euclidean Space: Applications of Convexity*, Pergamon, 1957, pp. 149–160; MR 23 #A3228.

[57]   E. Calabi, Circumscribing tetrahedron of least volume, unpublished note (1999).

8.2 Circular Coverage Constants

The problem of completely covering the unit interval $[0, 1]$ by N smaller equal subintervals is trivial: Tile the interval with subintervals of length $1/N$. The only necessary overlap occurs at boundary points of the tiling.

The problem of completely covering the planar unit disk D by N smaller equal subdisks is harder. Here overlap is substantial and contributes to the difficulty of solution. Let $r(N)$ denote the minimum radius for which there exists a covering. If D is covered, then in particular its boundary C (the unit circle) must be covered. To cover a unit circular subarc of length $2\pi/N$ requires a disk of radius at least $\sin(\pi/N)$; therefore we have the bound $r(N) \geq \sin(\pi/N)$. Equality occurs, in fact, for $N = 2, 3$, and 4 (see Table 8.1). The case for $N = 7$ is also straightforward: A regular hexagon inscribed in C has edges of length 1, so at least six disks of radius $1/2$ are needed to cover C. A seventh disk of radius $1/2$ is then sufficient to cover the remaining central portion of D.

The case for $N = 5$ is the first nontrivial case. Neville [1,2] provided the first known published solution (see Figure 8.1), although in the last step the value $r(5)$ was given incorrectly. Early editions of [3] repeated his error. One correctly obtains $r(5) = 0.6093828640\ldots$ as the value of $\cos(\theta + \varphi/2)$, where θ and φ are solutions of

Table 8.1. *Minimum Common Radius $r(N)$ of N Subdisks Covering the Unit Disk*

N	1	2	3	4	5	6
$r(N)$	1	1	$\frac{\sqrt{3}}{2} = 0.866025\ldots$	$\frac{\sqrt{2}}{2} = 0.707106\ldots$	$0.609382\ldots$	$0.555905\ldots$
N	7	8	9	10	11	12
$r(N)$	$\frac{1}{2} = 0.5$	$0.445041\ldots$	$0.414213\ldots$	$0.394930\ldots$	$0.380006\ldots$	$0.361103\ldots$

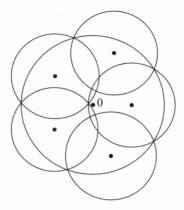

Figure 8.1. Neville's minimal configuration of five circles. It is asymmetric since three disks pass near 0 but two do not.

the following nonlinear system of four equations in four unknowns:

$$2\sin(\theta) - \sin(\theta + \tfrac{1}{2}\varphi + \psi) - \sin(\psi - \theta - \tfrac{1}{2}\varphi) = 0,$$

$$2\sin(\varphi) - \sin(\theta + \tfrac{1}{2}\varphi + \chi) - \sin(\chi - \theta - \tfrac{1}{2}\varphi) = 0,$$

$$2\sin(\theta) + \sin(\chi + \theta) - \sin(\chi - \theta) - \sin(\psi + \varphi) - \sin(\psi - \varphi)$$
$$- 2\sin(\psi - 2\theta) = 0,$$

$$\cos(2\psi - \chi + \varphi) - \cos(2\psi + \chi - \varphi) - 2\cos(\chi) + \cos(2\psi + \chi - 2\theta)$$
$$+ \cos(2\psi - \chi - 2\theta) = 0.$$

A different characterization was provided by Bezdek [4–6]: $r(5)^{-1}$ is the largest real zero of the polynomial

$$a(y)x^6 - b(y)x^5 + c(y)x^4 - d(y)x^3 + e(y)x^2 - f(y)x + g(y)$$

maximized over all y, subject to the constraints $\sqrt{2} < x < 2y + 1$, $-1 < y < 1$, where

$$a(y) = 80y^2 + 64y, \quad b(y) = 416y^3 + 384y^2 + 64y,$$

$$c(y) = 848y^4 + 928y^3 + 352y^2 + 32y,$$

$$d(y) = 768y^5 + 992y^4 + 736y^3 + 288y^2 + 96y,$$

$$e(y) = 256y^6 + 384y^5 + 592y^4 + 480y^3 + 336y^2 + 96y + 16,$$

$$f(y) = 128y^5 + 192y^4 + 256y^3 + 160y^2 + 96y + 32, \quad g(y) = 64y^2 + 64y + 16.$$

Neville [2] knew that $r(5)$ is an algebraic number, for he wrote the following sentence about his system of equations: "It is evident that these particular equations are algebraic and even rational in the tangents of the angles $\theta/2$, $\varphi/4$, $\psi/2$, $\chi/2$, so that an algebraic equation can be found for $\cos(\theta + \varphi/2) \ldots$" Melissen [7] and Zimmermann [8] independently obtained the minimal polynomial of $r(5)$:

$$1296x^8 + 2112x^7 - 3480x^6 + 1360x^5 + 1665x^4 - 1776x^3 + 22x^2 - 800x + 625;$$

however, they may not have been the first to achieve this.

Zahn [9] computed $r(N)$ for $N = 6$ and $8 \leq N \leq 10$ by computer experimentation. Bezdek [10] numerically obtained $r(6) = 0.5559052114\ldots$ as reported in [5–7]; conceivably he may have found a polynomial optimization characterization of $r(6)$ analogous to $r(5)$. Nagy [11] and Krotoszynski [12] conjectured that, for $8 \leq N \leq 10$,

$$r(N) = \left(1 + 2\cos\left(\frac{2\pi}{N-1}\right)\right)^{-1} = \begin{cases} 0.4450418679\ldots & \text{if } N = 8, \\ \sqrt{2} - 1 = 0.4142135623\ldots & \text{if } N = 9, \\ 0.3949308436\ldots & \text{if } N = 10, \end{cases}$$

and Fejes Tóth [13] succeeded in proving the formulas for $r(8)$ and $r(9)$. Evidence for the $r(10)$ formula was given by Melissen [7], who also provided an excellent survey of the subject. More recently, Faugère & Zimmermann [14] discovered the minimal polynomial for $r(6)$:

$$7841367x^{18} - 3344997x^{16} + 62607492x^{14} - 63156942x^{12} + 41451480x^{10}$$
$$- 19376280x^8 + 5156603x^6 - 746832x^4 + 54016x^2 + 3072.$$

All cases $r(N)$ for $N \geq 10$ remain open; we mention that $r(11) < (1 + 2\cos(\pi/5))^{-1}$ and also the conjecture

$$r(12) = \frac{1}{3}\left(1 + (1 + 3\sqrt{57})^{\frac{1}{3}} - 8(1 + 3\sqrt{57})^{-\frac{1}{3}}\right) = 0.3611030805\ldots$$

due to Melissen & Schuur [7].

There are some interesting "inverse" results due to Kerschner [15] and Verblunsky [16]. For example, if we let $N(\varepsilon)$ denote the smallest number of disks of radius ε needed to cover D, the limit of the ratio of the area of D to the total area of the disks,

$$\lim_{\varepsilon \to 0^+} \frac{\pi}{(\pi\varepsilon^2)N(\varepsilon)} = \lim_{\varepsilon \to 0^+} \frac{1}{\varepsilon^2 N(\varepsilon)} = \frac{3\sqrt{3}}{2\pi} = 0.8269933431\ldots,$$

can be thought of as measuring the *asymptotic efficiency* of the covering. If one replaces the unit disk D by a square, one can be even more precise.

Here is a related problem. We can cover the unit interval by intervals of length $1/2$, $1/4$, $1/8$, $1/16$, $1/32$, $\ldots$ in the natural way. Moreover, the common ratio $1/2$ cannot be made smaller. What is the two-dimensional analog of this result? Eppstein [17] found that D could be covered by smaller disks of radii s^k, $k = 1, 2, 3, \ldots$, for $s = 0.77$ but evidently not for $s = 0.765$. A more precise estimate of the smallest $s \leq 0.77$ would be good to see.

The problem of covering a unit square by N smaller equal disks is surveyed in [7, 18]. The dual problem of *packing* disks in a unit disk [1, 7, 19–22] or square [1, 7, 23–28] has attracted much attention, but we will say only a few words. Let $t(N)$ denote the greatest

Table 8.2. *Maximum Common Radius $t(N)$ of N Subdisks Packing the Unit Square*

N	2	3	4	5
$t(N)$	$\sqrt{2} = 1.414213\ldots$	$\sqrt{6} - \sqrt{2} = 1.035276\ldots$	1	$\frac{\sqrt{2}}{2} = 0.707106\ldots$
N	6	7	8	9
$t(N)$	$\frac{\sqrt{13}}{6} = 0.600925\ldots$	$2(2 - \sqrt{3}) = 0.535898\ldots$	$\frac{\sqrt{6}-\sqrt{2}}{2} = 0.517638\ldots$	$\frac{1}{2} = 0.5$

possible minimum distance between N points in the square (see Table 8.2). Computing $t(10) = 0.4212795439\ldots$ was a major obstacle until recently: Schlüter's conjecture [29, 30] has been proven true [31] and here is the minimal polynomial for $t(10)$:

$$1180129x^{18} - 11436428x^{17} + 98015844x^{16} - 462103584x^{15} + 1145811528x^{14}$$
$$- 1398966480x^{13} + 227573920x^{12} + 1526909568x^{11} - 1038261808x^{10}$$
$$- 2960321792x^{9} + 7803109440x^{8} - 9722063488x^{7} + 7918461504x^{6}$$
$$- 4564076288x^{5} + 1899131648x^{4} - 563649536x^{3} + 114038784x^{2}$$
$$- 14172160x + 819200.$$

Here also, as an aside, are two elementary problems involving just two circles.

Imagine two overlapping circles, each of radius 1. If the area A of the inner overlap region is equal to the sum of the areas of the two outer crescents, then clearly $A = 2\pi/3$. What is the distance $2u$ between the centers of the two circles? It can be shown that $u = 0.2649320846\ldots$ is the unique root of the equation

$$u\sqrt{1 - u^2} + \arcsin(u) = \frac{\pi}{6}$$

in the interval $[0, 1]$. Is u transcendental? This is called *Mrs. Miniver's problem* [32, 33].

The second problem is called the *grazing goat problem* [34, 35]. A goat is tethered to a post on the perimeter of a circular field of radius 1. How long should the rope be so that the goat can eat exactly half of the grass in the field? One shows that the length, v, of the rope satisfies

$$v\sqrt{4 - v^2} - 2(v^2 - 2)\arccos\left(\frac{v}{2}\right) = \pi,$$

and hence $v = 1.1587284730\ldots$. Is v transcendental? Are v and u algebraically independent?

[1] H. T. Croft, K. J. Falconer, and R. K. Guy, *Unsolved Problems in Geometry*, Springer-Verlag, 1991, sect. D1, D2, D3; MR 95k:52001.

[2] E. H. Neville, Solutions of numerical functional equations, *Proc. London Math. Soc.* 14 (1915) 308–326.

[3] W. W. Rouse Ball, *Mathematical Recreations and Essays*, 11th ed., MacMillan, 1939, pp. 97–99; MR 88m:00013.

[4] J. Molnár, Über eine elementargeometrische Extremalaufgabe, *Mat. Fiz. Lapok* 49 (1942) 249–253; MR 8,218j.

[5] K. Bezdek, Über einige Kreisüberdeckungen, *Beiträge Algebra Geom.* 14 (1983) 7–13; MR 85a:52012.

[6] K. Bezdek, Über einige optimale Konfigurationen von Kreisen, *Annales Univ. Sci. Budapest Eötvös Sect. Math.* 27 (1984) 143–151; MR 87f:52020.

[7]   J. B. M. Melissen, *Packing and Coverings with Circles*, Ph.D. thesis, Universiteit Utrecht, 1997.

[8]   P. Zimmermann, Computation of the minimal polynomial of Neville's five disc constant, unpublished note (1997).

[9]   C. T. Zahn, Black box maximization of circular coverage, *J. Res. Nat. Bur. Standards B* 66 (1962) 181–216; MR 29 #1583.

[10] K. Bezdek, *Körök optimális fedélsei*, Ph.D. thesis, Eötvös Loránd Univ., Budapest, 1979.

[11] D. Nagy, *Fedések és alkalmazásaik*, M.Sc. thesis, Eötvös Loránd Univ., Budapest, 1974.

[12] S. Krotoszynski, Covering a disk with smaller disks, *Studia Sci. Math. Hungar.* 28 (1993) 277–283; MR 95c:52035.

[13] G. Fejes Tóth, Thinnest covering of a circle by eight or nine congruent circles, unpublished note (1996).

[14] J.-C. Faugère and P. Zimmermann, The minimal polynomial of Bezdek's constant, unpublished note (1998).

[15] R. Kershner, The number of circles covering a set, *Amer. J. Math.* 61 (1939) 665–671; MR 1,8b.

[16] S. Verblunsky, On the least number of unit circles which can cover a square, *J. London Math. Soc.* 24 (1949) 164–170; MR 11,455g.

[17] D. Eppstein, Covering and Packing (Geometry Junkyard).

[18] J. B. M. Melissen and P. C. Schuur, Improved coverings of a square with six and eight equal circles, *Elec. J. Combin.* 3 (1996) R32; MR 97h:52027.

[19] S. Kravitz, Packing cylinders into cylindrical containers, *Math. Mag.* 40 (1967) 65–71.

[20] U. Pirl, Der Mindestabstand von n in der Einheitskreisscheibe gelegenen Punkten, *Math. Nachr.* 40 (1969) 111–124; MR 40 #6379.

[21] H. Melissen, Densest packings of eleven congruent circles in a circle, *Geom. Dedicata* 50 (1994) 15–25; MR 95e:52032.

[22] R. L. Graham, B. D. Lubachevsky, K. J. Nurmela, and P. R. J. Östergård, Dense packings of congruent circles in a circle, *Discrete Math.* 181 (1998) 139–154; MR 99b: 52040.

[23] J. Schaer, The densest packing of 9 circles in a square, *Canad. Math. Bull.* 8 (1965) 273–277; MR 31 #6164.

[24] M. Goldberg, The packing of equal circles in a square, *Math. Mag.* 43 (1970) 24–30.

[25] G. Wengerodt, Die dichteste Packung von 16 Kreisen in einem Quadrat, *Beiträge Algebra Geom.* 16 (1983) 173–190; 25 (1987) 25–46; MR 85j:52024 and MR 88g:52014.

[26] K. J. Nurmela, Packing up to 50 equal circles in a square, *Discrete Comput. Geom.* 18 (1997) 111–120; MR 98e:52020.

[27] K. J. Nurmela and P. R. J. Östergård, More optimal packings of equal circles in a square, *Discrete Comput. Geom.* 22 (1999) 439–457; MR 2000h:05052.

[28] K. J. Nurmela, P. R. J. Östergård, and R. aus dem Spring, Asymptotic behavior of optimal circle packings in a square, *Canad. Math. Bull.* 42 (1999) 380–385; MR 2000g: 52012.

[29] K. Schlüter, Kreispackung in Quadraten, *Elem. Math.* 34 (1979) 12–14; MR 80c:52014.

[30] M. Mollard and C. Payan, Some progress in the packing of equal circles in a square, *Discrete Math.* 84 (1990) 303–307; MR 92d:52043.

[31] R. Peikert, D. Würtz, M. Monagan, and C. de Groot, Packing circles in a square: A review and new results, *System Modelling and Optimization*, Proc 1991 Zurich conf., ed. P. Kall, Lect. Notes in Control and Inform. Sci. 180, Springer-Verlag, 1992, pp. 45–54.

[32] J. Struther, *Mrs. Miniver*, Harcourt Brace, 1940, ch. 12, pp. 94–95.

[33] L. A. Graham, *Ingenious Mathematical Problems and Methods*, Dover, 1959, pp. 6, 64–66; MR 22 #1.

[34] M. Fraser, A tale of two goats, *Math. Mag.* 55 (1982) 221–227.

[35] M. Fraser, The grazing goat in n dimensions, *College Math. J.* 15 (1984) 126–134; MR 85k:00001.

8.3 Universal Coverage Constants

Let U denote the class of all sets in the plane of unit diameter. A planar region R is called a **displacement cover** (or **universal cover**) **for** U if it contains a congruent copy of every set in U. That is, each set of unit diameter can be covered by R after suitable translation and rotation [1–6].

Let S denote a class of specified regions in the plane (e.g., the class of all circular disks). Does there exist an element of S that is both a displacement cover for U and has area as small as possible? If yes, define $A(S)$ to be the area of such an element.

For example, if we focus on the class of all circular disks [3, 4], then

$$A(\text{circles}) = \frac{\pi}{3} = 1.0471975511\ldots,$$

the area of a circle of radius $1/\sqrt{3}$. A similar line of reasoning gives that a square region of side 1 will also suffice:

$$A(\text{squares}) = 1.$$

Better still is the class of regular hexagonal regions:

$$A(\text{regular hexagons}) = \frac{\sqrt{3}}{2} = 0.8660254037\ldots.$$

Consider now the class C of all *convex* planar regions. Lebesgue [7] asked about the value of $\mu = A(C)$, that is, the area of the smallest possible convex blanket that covers all sets of unit diameter. The best-known bounds are

$$0.8257117836\ldots = \frac{\pi}{8} + \frac{\sqrt{3}}{4} \leq \mu \leq \frac{\sqrt{3}}{2} - 2\varepsilon_P - \varepsilon_S - \varepsilon_H \leq 0.84413770$$

due to Pál [7], Sprague [8], and Hansen [9, 10]. The lower bound is the area of the convex hull of a circle and an equilateral triangle, both of unit diameter, with the circle centered at the triangle centroid. The upper bound estimates, incrementally improving on each other, are based on cutting corners off Pál's original regular hexagonal cover:

$$\varepsilon_P = \frac{7\sqrt{3}}{12} - 1 \sim 10^{-2}, \quad \varepsilon_S \sim 10^{-3}.$$

Hansen's two improvements on Sprague's upper bound estimate are tiny: $\sim 10^{-19}$ and 10^{-11}. A more dramatic improvement, in [11], from 0.8441 to 0.8430, was conjectural only. One interesting aspect about Hansen's work is his use of computer simulation. For example, he ruled out certain types of configurations by simulation in [10]; it is not clear whether he has withdrawn his 1981 conjecture. As Klee & Wagon [5] wrote, "Progress on this problem, which has been painfully slow in the past, may be even more painfully slow in the future."

For nonconvex covers, Duff [12, 13] constructed a region with area $0.84413570\ldots$, which is smaller than all known convex examples. It is not surprising that nonconvexity can improve matters; see the related discussion in [8.4] and [8.17].

There are many variations on these problems. If we restrict the meaning of *cover* to encompass only translations (rather than displacements, i.e., translations and rotations,

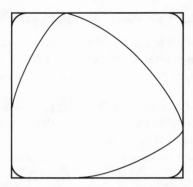

Figure 8.2. A truncated unit square obtained by revolving an inscribed Reuleaux triangle completely within the square and removing the four corner sets not touched.

as we have assumed so far), then the various outcomes are given in [8.3.1]. Also, one can minimize the cover perimeter or mean width rather than area [14–16]. A different sense of minimality – namely, a cover for which no proper subset is a cover – was studied by Eggleston [17] in n dimensions.

There is a discrepancy in the reporting of the upper bound estimate for μ. Meschkowski [2] and Hansen [9] reported Sprague's estimate to be 0.844144, whereas Duff [12] and Klee & Wagon [5] reported the estimate to be 0.84413770. No explanation can be found for this discrepancy.

Finally, we note that early papers on this subject often mistakenly refer to this as *Besicovitch's problem* [18–20].

8.3.1 Translation Covers

A planar region R is called a **translation cover** (or **strong universal cover**) for U if each set of unit diameter can be covered by R after suitable translation [5, 14, 21]. No rotations are allowed. Using notation similar to before, $\tilde{A}(\text{circles}) = \pi/3$ by the obvious rotational symmetry of a disk and $\tilde{A}(\text{squares}) = 1$, but the regular hexagon of Pál is *not* a translation cover [21, 22]. What, therefore, is the value of $\tilde{A}(\text{regular hexagons})$?

If C denotes the class of all convex planar regions, then there is a conjecture [5, 15, 16] that

$$\tilde{A}(C) = \frac{\pi}{6} + 2\sqrt{3} - 3 = 0.9877003907\ldots,$$

which is the area of the truncated unit square in Figure 8.2. No rigorous tight bounds on $\tilde{A}(C)$ seem to appear in the literature. See [23] for a curious connection to the Watts square drill bit. More constants associated with Reuleaux triangles are found in [8.10].

[1] H. T. Croft, K. J. Falconer, and R. K. Guy, *Unsolved Problems in Geometry*, Springer-Verlag, 1991, sect. D15; MR 95k:52001.

[2]   H. Meschkowski, *Unsolved and Unsolvable Problems in Geometry*, Oliver and Boyd, 1966; MR 35 #7206.

[3]   S. R. Lay, *Convex Sets and Their Applications*, Wiley, 1972; MR 93g:52001.

[4]   I. M. Yaglom and V. G. Boltyanskii, *Convex Figures*, Holt, Rinehart and Winston, 1961, pp. 18, 31–33, 122–125, 140–156; MR 14,197d.

[5]   V. Klee and S. Wagon, *Old and New Unsolved Problems in Plane Geometry and Number Theory*, Math. Assoc. Amer., 1991, pp. 23, 92–93; MR 92k:00014.

[6]   C. S. Ogilvy, *Excursions in Geometry*, Dover, 1969, pp. 142–144.

[7]   J. Pál, Über ein elementares Variationsproblem, *Mathematisk-Fysiske Meddelelser, Kongelige Danske Videnskabernes Selskabs*, v. 3 (1920) n. 2, 1–35.

[8]   R. Sprague, Über ein elementares Variationsproblem, *Mathematisk Tidsskrift B* (1936) 96–99.

[9]   H. C. Hansen, A small universal cover of figures of unit diameter, *Geom. Dedicata* 4 (1975) 165–172; MR 53 #1423.

[10] H. C. Hansen, Small universal covers for sets of unit diameter, *Geom. Dedicata* 42 (1992) 205–213; MR 93c:52018.

[11] H. C. Hansen, Towards the minimal universal cover, *Normat* 29 (1981) 115–119, 148; MR 83g:52011.

[12] G. F. D. Duff, A smaller universal cover for sets of unit diameter, *C. R. Math. Rep. Acad. Sci. Canada* 2 (1980) 37–42; MR 81k:52025.

[13] M. D. Kovalev, A minimal Lebesgue covering exists (in Russian), *Mat. Zametki* 40 (1986) 401–406, 430; Engl. transl. in *Math. Notes* 40 (1986) 736–739; MR 88h:52008.

[14] K. Bezdek and R. Connelly, Covering curves by translates of a convex set, *Amer. Math. Monthly* 96 (1989) 789–806; MR 90k:52020.

[15] K. Bezdek and R. Connelly, Minimal translation covers for sets of diameter 1, *Period. Math. Hungar.* 34 (1997) 23–27; MR 98k:52042.

[16] K. Bezdek and R. Connelly, The minimum mean width translation cover for sets of diameter one, *Beiträge Algebra Geom.* 39 (1998) 473–479; MR 99i:52021.

[17] H. G. Eggleston, Minimal universal covers in $\mathbb{E}^n$, *Israel J. Math.* 1 (1963) 149–155; MR 28 #4432.

[18] W. W. Rouse Ball and H. S. M. Coxeter, *Mathematical Recreations and Essays*, MacMillan, 1944, p. 99; MR 88m:00013.

[19] A. Edwards, Professor Besicovitch's minimal problem: A challenge, *Eureka* 20 (1957) 26–27.

[20] H. S. M. Coxeter, Lebesgue's minimal problem, *Eureka* 21 (1958) 13.

[21] G. D. Chakerian, Intersection and covering properties of convex sets, *Amer. Math. Monthly* 76 (1969) 753–766; MR 40 #3433.

[22] D. Chakerian and D. Logothetti, Minimal regular polygons serving as universal covers in $\mathbb{R}^2$, *Geom. Dedicata* 26 (1988) 281–297; MR 89f:52035.

[23] M. Gardner, Curves of constant width, one of which makes it possible to drill square holes, *Sci. Amer.*, v. 208 (1963) n. 2, 148–156 and v. 208 (1963) n. 3, 154; also in *Mathematics: An Introduction to Its Spirit and Use*, W. H. Freeman, 1979, pp. 107–111 and 238–239.

8.4 Moser's Worm Constant

A **worm** is a continuous rectifiable arc of unit length contained in the plane. Let W denote the class of all worms. A planar region R is called a **displacement cover** (or **universal cover**) for W if it contains a congruent copy of every worm in W. That is, each arc of unit length can be covered by R after suitable translation and rotation [1, 2].

Let S denote a class of specified regions in the plane (e.g., the class of all circular disks). Does there exist an element of S that is both a displacement cover for W and has area as small as possible? If yes, define $A(S)$ to be the area of such an element.

For example, if we focus on the class of all circular disks [3], then

$$A(\text{circles}) = \frac{\pi}{4} = 0.7853981633\ldots,$$

the area of a circle of diameter 1. It is somewhat more difficult to prove [4, 5] that a square region of diagonal 1 will also suffice:

$$A(\text{squares}) = \frac{1}{2} = 0.5.$$

Over the larger class of rectangular regions [4, 5],

$$A(\text{rectangles}) = \beta\sqrt{1 - \beta^2} = 0.3943847688\ldots,$$

the area of a rectangle with sides β and $\sqrt{1 - \beta^2}$, where β arises with regard to the broadest curve of unit length [8.4.1]. Better still is the class of semicircular regions [6]:

$$A(\text{semicircles}) = \frac{\pi}{8} = 0.3926990816\ldots,$$

as proved by Meir. Interestingly, the class of equilateral triangular regions remains a mystery. Besicovitch [7] proved that

$$A(\text{equilateral triangles}) \geq \frac{7\sqrt{3}}{27} = 0.4490502094\ldots,$$

the area of the triangle with side $2\sqrt{21}/9$, and thought it likely that equality holds. The conjectured exact expression for A was found by Knox [8]. Any counterexample to this claim, if such a worm exists, must be **zig-zag** in the sense that the worm meets the line segment joining its two endpoints at a third point (possibly more) [9].

Consider now the class C of all *convex* planar regions. **Moser's worm constant** μ is defined to be the value of $A(C)$, that is, the area of the smallest possible convex blanket that covers all worms. The best-known bounds are

$$0.2194626846\ldots = \frac{\beta}{2} \leq \mu \leq 0.27524\ldots$$

as found by Schaer & Wetzel [5, 6] and Poole, Gerriets, Norwood & Laidacker [10–12]. The upper bound is the area of a certain rhombus with portions of two adjacent sides replaced by a circular arc. Some recent unsuccessful attempts have been made to improve the upper bound [13, 14]. Of many conjectures, we mention one in [6, 11, 12]: The circular sector of radius 1 and angle $\pi/6$ covers all possible worms. If true, this would reduce the upper bound on μ to $\pi/12 = 0.261799\ldots$.

There are many variations on these problems. If we restrict worms to be *closed*, that is, with initial point coincident with terminal point, then the results are given in [8.4.2]. If we restrict the meaning of *cover* to encompass only translations (rather than displacements, i.e., translations and rotations, as we have assumed so far), then the various outcomes are given in [8.4.3]. One can minimize the cover perimeter rather than area [15]. Also, one can ask how efficient the cover is, for example, whether the worm is necessarily close to the boundary of the cover, and such an inquiry leads naturally to Bellman's "lost in a forest" problem [16–19].

Here is a related problem [20]: Prove that any worm can be covered by some rectangular blanket of area $1/4$, and that this is the best possible. The question (given a worm, find an element of S that covers it) is similar to the foregoing (find an element of S that covers all worms) but has not received the same amount of attention. Another problem is as follows: Given a worm, show that the maximum possible area of its smallest convex cover is $1/(2\pi) = 0.159154\ldots$. This is attained for a semicircle of unit length [21]. What is the three dimensional analog of this result?

Interesting things happen if we drop the convexity requirement [1,2]. Hansen [22] proposed (without proof) a nonconvex universal cover of area $0.246\ldots$, which is less than the best-known convex cover, but his claim remains unconfirmed. The smallest provable upper bound in this case is $0.26044\ldots$ [23]. Davies [24] constructed nonconvex sets of measure zero that are translation covers for the class of all polygonal arcs in the plane. This is closely allied with the Kakeya–Besicovitch problem [8.17]. Marstrand [25,26], however, proved that any displacement cover for the class of all rectifiable arcs must have positive measure.

8.4.1 Broadest Curve of Unit Length

What is the minimum width of an infinitely long planar strip that contains a congruent copy of every worm in W? Equivalently, fix a worm w for consideration and, for $0 \leq \theta \leq \pi$, let $d(w, \theta)$ denote the distance between supporting parallel lines at angle θ to the x-axis. Define the **breadth** of w to be the minimum value of $d(w, \theta)$ taken over all θ. Our question becomes: What is the worm of largest breadth?

The answer is a **broadworm** or **caliper**, as first discovered by Zalgaller [17,27,28]. See Figure 8.3. This curve has breadth given exactly by

$$\beta = \sup_w \min_\theta d(w, \theta) = \frac{1}{2} \left(\frac{\pi}{2} - \varphi - 2\psi + \tan(\varphi) + \tan(\psi) \right)^{-1}$$
$$= 0.4389253692\ldots = (2.2782916414\ldots)^{-1},$$

where the angles φ and ψ are defined by

$$\varphi = \arcsin\left[\tfrac{1}{6} + \tfrac{4}{3} \sin\left(\tfrac{1}{3} \arcsin(\tfrac{17}{64}) \right) \right], \quad \psi = \arctan\left(\tfrac{1}{2} \sec(\varphi) \right).$$

It follows immediately that any universal rectangular cover must have both sides $\geq \beta$ (to accommodate the caliper) and diagonal ≥ 1 (to accommodate the unit line segment); proving that the $\beta \times \sqrt{1 - \beta^2}$ rectangle is indeed universal requires more work.

Zalgaller [29] also examined the three-dimensional analog of this problem and conjectured that the broadest curve in three-space of unit length has breadth $1/3.921545\ldots = 0.255001\ldots$.

8.4.2 Closed Worms

A **closed worm** is a continuous rectifiable closed curve (with initial point coincident with terminal point) of unit length contained in the plane. As before, we are interested

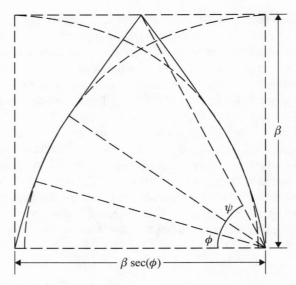

Figure 8.3. A caliper consists of two circular arcs with four tangent segments, configured in a very precise fashion.

in displacement covers of least area. In this more restrictive scenario, we have

$$A'(\text{circles}) = \frac{\pi}{16} = 0.1963495408\ldots,$$

the area of a circle [3, 30, 31] of diameter $1/2$,

$$A'(\text{squares}) = \frac{1}{8} = 0.125,$$

the area of a square [5, 31] of diagonal $1/2$,

$$A'(\text{rectangles}) = \frac{\sqrt{\pi^2 - 4}}{2\pi^2} = 0.1227367657\ldots,$$

the area of a rectangle [5, 31] of sides $1/\pi$ and $\sqrt{\pi^2 - 4}/(2\pi)$, and

$$A'(\text{general triangles}) = \frac{3\sqrt{3}}{4\pi^2} = 0.1316200785\ldots,$$

the area of an equilateral triangle [32, 33] with side $\sqrt{3}/\pi$.

It is curious that so much more is known about the general triangular case for covering closed worms than for covering arbitrary worms (arcs). Here is a related result [34]. The smallest equilateral triangle that can cover every triangle of perimeter 2 has side not 1, but $s = 2/y = 1.0028514266\ldots$, where y is the global minimum of the trigonometric function

$$f(x) = \sqrt{3}\left(1 + \sin\left(\frac{x}{2}\right)\right)\sec\left(\frac{\pi}{6} - x\right)$$

on the interval $[0, \pi/6]$. The constant s also appears in [35] in connection with a more expansive problem.

What can be said about the analog of Moser's worm constant here, that is, the area $\mu' = A'(C)$ of the smallest possible convex blanket that covers all closed worms? Schaer & Wetzel [5] and Chakerian & Klamkin [31] proposed a lower bound equal to the area of the convex hull of a circle of circumference 1 and a line segment of length $1/2$ with midpoint at the circle center:

$$\mu' \geq \frac{1}{4\pi^2} \left(\sqrt{\pi^2 - 4} + \pi - 2 \arccos\left(\frac{2}{\pi} \right) \right) = 0.0963296165\ldots.$$

More recently, Füredi & Wetzel [35] gave improved bounds $0.09666 \leq \mu' \leq 0.11754$, where the upper bound comes from the area of the best rectangle (mentioned earlier) with one small corner clipped off.

Here is a related problem from [31] due to Schaer: Prove that any closed worm can be covered by some rectangular blanket of area $1/\pi^2$, and that this is the best possible. The question (given a worm, find an element of S that covers it) is similar to the foregoing (find an element of S that covers all worms).

8.4.3 Translation Covers

A planar region R is called a **translation cover** (or **strong universal cover**) for W if each worm in W can be covered by R after suitable translation. No rotations are allowed. Since there are two types of worms, we study these separately. For arbitrary worms (arcs), let us consider only the class C of all convex planar regions. In this scenario, we have a complete solution due to Pál [36]:

$$\tilde{\mu} = \tilde{A}(C) = \frac{\sqrt{3}}{3} = 0.5773502692\ldots,$$

the area of an equilateral triangle of height 1. This scenario is perhaps the simplest of all.

For closed worms, we have

$$\hat{A}(\text{circles}) = \frac{\pi}{16} = 0.1963495408\ldots$$

by the obvious rotational symmetry of a disk [3, 30, 31],

$$\hat{A}(\text{general triangles}) = \frac{\sqrt{3}}{9} = 0.1924500897\ldots,$$

the area of an equilateral triangle [32, 33] with side $2/3$,

$$\hat{A}(\text{rectangles}) = \frac{1}{4} = 0.25,$$

the area of a square with side $1/2$, and

$$0.1554479088\ldots \leq \hat{\mu} = \hat{A}(C) \leq 0.16526\ldots,$$

for the convex case, owing to Wetzel [6] and Bezdek & Connelly [15].

[1]   H. T. Croft, K. J. Falconer, and R. K. Guy, *Unsolved Problems in Geometry*, Springer-Verlag, 1991, sect. D18, G6; MR 95k:52001.

[2]   V. Klee and S. Wagon, *Old and New Unsolved Problems in Plane Geometry and Number Theory*, Math. Assoc. Amer., 1991, pp. 23, 92–93; MR 92k:00014.

[3]   J. E. Wetzel, Covering balls for curves of constant length, *Enseign. Math.* 17 (1971) 275–277; MR 48 #12315.

[4]   J. P. Jones and J. Schaer, The worm problem, Univ. of Calgary research paper 100, 1970.

[5]   J. Schaer and J. E. Wetzel, Boxes for curves of constant length, *Israel J. Math.* 12 (1972) 257–265; MR 47 #5726.

[6]   J. E. Wetzel, Sectorial covers for curves of constant length, *Canad. Math. Bull.* 16 (1973) 367–375; MR 50 #14451.

[7]   A. S. Besicovitch, On arcs that cannot be covered by an open equilateral triangle of side 1, *Math. Gazette* 49 (1965) 286–288; MR 32 #6320.

[8]   S. Knox, Calculating the length of Besicovitch's short arc, unpublished note (1994).

[9]   J. E. Wetzel, On Besicovitch's problem, unpublished note (2000).

[10] G. Poole and J. Gerriets, Minimum covers for arcs of constant length, *Bull. Amer. Math. Soc.* 79 (1973) 462–463; MR 47 #4150.

[11] J. Gerriets and G. Poole, Convex regions which cover arcs of constant length, *Amer. Math. Monthly* 81 (1974) 36–41; MR 48 #12310.

[12] R. Norwood, G. Poole, and M. Laidacker, The worm problem of Leo Moser, *Discrete Comput. Geom.* 7 (1992) 153–162; MR 92j:52014.

[13] D. Reynolds, The worm's patchwork quilt, unpublished note (1994).

[14] I. Stewart, Mother Worm's blanket, *Sci. Amer.*, v. 274 (1996) n. 1, 98–99; errata, v. 274 (1996) n. 6, 103.

[15] K. Bezdek and R. Connelly, Covering curves by translates of a convex set, *Amer. Math. Monthly* 96 (1989) 789–806; MR 90k:52020.

[16] R. Bellman, Minimization problem, *Bull. Amer. Math. Soc.* 62 (1956) 270.

[17] V. A. Zalgaller, How to get out of the woods? On a problem of Bellman (in Russian), *Matematicheskoe Prosveshchenie* 6 (1961) 191–195.

[18] H. Joris, Le chasseur perdu dans la forêt, *Elem. Math.* 35 (1980) 1–14; MR 81d:52001.

[19] S. R. Finch and J. E. Wetzel, Lost in a forest, unpublished note (2002).

[20] Putnam Competition Problem B-4, *Amer. Math. Monthly* 77 (1970) 723, 727.

[21] P. A. P. Moran, On a problem of S. Ulam, *J. London Math. Soc.* 21 (1946) 175–179; MR 8,597n.

[22] H. C. Hansen, Ormeproblemet, *Normat* 40 (1992) 119–123, 143; MR 93h:52025.

[23] G. Poole and R. Norwood, An improved upper bound to Leo Moser's worm problem, *Discrete Comput. Geom.*, to appear.

[24] R. O. Davies, Some remarks on the Kakeya problem, *Proc. Cambridge Philos. Soc.* 69 (1971) 417–421; MR 42 #7869.

[25] J. M. Marstrand, Packing smooth curves in $\mathbb{R}^q$, *Mathematica* 26 (1979) 1–12; MR 81d:52009.

[26] J. M. Marstrand, Packing planes in $\mathbb{R}^q$, *Mathematica* 26 (1979) 180–183; MR 81f:2800.

[27] J. Schaer, The broadest curve of length 1, Univ. of Calgary research paper 52, 1968.

[28] A. Adhikari and J. Pitman, The shortest planar arc of width 1, *Amer. Math. Monthly* 96 (1989) 309–327; MR 90d:52016.

[29] V. A. Zalgaller, The problem of the shortest space curve of unit width (in Russian), *Mat. Fiz. Anal. Geom.* 1 (1994) 454–461; MR 98i:52012.

[30] J. C. C. Nitsche, The smallest sphere containing a rectifiable curve, *Amer. Math. Monthly* 78 (1971) 881–882; MR 45 #480.

[31] G. D. Chakerian and M. S. Klamkin, Minimal covers for closed curves, *Math. Mag.* 46 (1973) 55–61; MR 47 #2496.

[32] J. E. Wetzel, Triangular covers for closed curves of constant length, *Elem. Math.* 25 (1970) 78–81; MR 42 #960.

[33] J. E. Wetzel, On Moser's problem of accommodating closed curves in triangles, *Elem. Math.* 27 (1972) 35–36; MR 45 #4282.

[34] J. E. Wetzel, The smallest equilateral cover for triangles of perimeter two, *Math. Mag.* 70 (1997) 125–130.

[35] Z. Füredi and J. E. Wetzel, The smallest convex cover for triangles of perimeter two, *Geom. Dedicata* 81 (2000) 285–293; MR 2001c:52001.

[36] J. Pál, Ein minimumprobleme für ovale, *Math. Annalen* 83 (1921) 311–319.

8.5 Traveling Salesman Constants

Consider n distinct points in the d-dimensional unit cube. Of all $(n-1)!/2$ closed paths (or **tours**) passing through each point precisely once, what is the length $L_d(n)$ of the shortest such path?

Determining $L_d(n)$, the minimum tour-length, is known as the **traveling salesman problem** (TSP). This is one of the best-known combinatorial optimization problems, dominating fields such as operations research, algorithm development, and complexity theory. Its solution is difficult because it cannot be computed in polynomial time, that is, the problem is NP-hard.

We nevertheless encounter some interesting asymptotics: There is a smallest constant α_d such that

$$\limsup_{n \to \infty} \frac{L_d(n)}{n^{(d-1)/d}} \leq \alpha_d, \quad \alpha_d' = \frac{\alpha_d}{\sqrt{d}}$$

for all optimal tours in the cube, and there is another constant β_d such that

$$\lim_{n \to \infty} \frac{L_d(n)}{n^{(d-1)/d}} = \beta_d, \quad \beta_d' = \frac{\beta_d}{\sqrt{d}}$$

for *almost all* optimal tours in the cube, in the sense that the limit fails only for a negligible (measure-zero) subset of the tours. These constants were first examined by Beardwood, Halton & Hammersley [1, 2]. Rigorous bounds are listed in Table 8.3 [3–9].

It is known that [10–14]

$$\lim_{d \to \infty} \beta_d' = \frac{1}{\sqrt{2\pi e}} = 0.2419707245\ldots,$$

$$\frac{1}{\sqrt{2\pi e}} \leq \lim_{d \to \infty} \alpha_d' \leq \frac{2(3 - \sqrt{3})\theta}{\sqrt{2\pi e}} = 0.40509\ldots,$$

where

$$\frac{1}{2} \leq \theta = \lim_{d \to \infty} \theta_d^{\frac{1}{d}} \leq 0.66019$$

Table 8.3. *Bounds on Traveling Salesman Constants α_d' and β_d'*

d	Lower Bound for β_d'	Upper Bound for β_d'	Lower Bound for α_d'	Upper Bound for α_d'
2	0.44194	0.6508	0.75983	0.98398
3	0.37313	0.61772	0.64805	0.90422
4	0.34207	0.55696	0.5946	0.8364

and θ_d is the best sphere packing density in d-space [8.7]. Even if someday the upper bound $2^{-0.59905d+o(d)}$ for θ_d is improved to $2^{-d+o(d)}$, as is believed to be true [15], the upper bound for $\lim_{d\to\infty} \alpha_d'$ will be reduced only to 0.30681. New insights will be required to evaluate this limit exactly [13].

Nonrigorous numerical estimates of β_d, due to Johnson, McGeoch & Rothberg [16] and Percus & Martin [17, 18], give

$$\beta_2 = 0.7124\ldots, \quad \beta_3 = 0.6979\ldots, \quad \beta_4 = 0.7234\ldots.$$

The fact that earlier estimates of β_2 do not agree well may be connected with finite size effects associated with the different experimental methods of computation. Another recent estimate of β_2 is $0.714\ldots$, due to Applegate, Cook & Rohe [19]. This might indicate that Norman & Moscato's [20] conjectured expression for β_2 (based on a fractal space-filling curve),

$$\beta_2 = \frac{4(1+2\sqrt{2})\sqrt{51}}{153} = 0.7147827007\ldots,$$

is justified; it surely indicates the need to assess the quality of random generations underlying TSP simulations.

If the n points are independently and uniformly distributed in the unit square, then the length $\Lambda_2(n)$ of a *random* (not necessarily optimal) tour satisfies [21]

$$\lim_{n\to\infty} \frac{E(\Lambda_2(n))}{n} = \frac{1}{15}\left(\sqrt{2}+2+5\ln(1+\sqrt{2})\right) = 0.521405433\ldots,$$

where E denotes both the average over all tours and the average over all point sets. The exact expression for $0.5214\ldots$ is due to Ghosh [22] and is discussed further in [8.1]. Note that $E(\Lambda_2(n))$ increases on the order of n whereas $L_2(n)$ typically increases on the order of $\sqrt{n}$.

A more precise version of $\lim_{d\to\infty} \beta_d'$ has been conjectured [18]:

$$\beta_d = \sqrt{\frac{d}{2\pi e}}(\pi d)^{\frac{1}{2d}}\left[1 + \frac{2-\ln(2)-2\gamma}{d} + O\left(\frac{1}{d^2}\right)\right],$$

where γ denotes the Euler–Mascheroni constant [1.5]. The basis for this formula is known as the random links TSP, a special case of which we will discuss momentarily.

8.5.1 Random Links TSP

Let K_n be the complete graph on n vertices, that is, every pair of distinct vertices determines an edge. We have removed the ambient d-dimensional space and hence any metric from this setting. Assign independently to each edge a Uniform $[0, 1]$ random variable called a **length**. Observe that lengths are not distances in the usual sense since the triangle inequality is not satisfied. Of all $(n-1)!/2$ tours passing through each vertex precisely once, we can determine the shortest such path, with minimum sum of lengths $L(n)$, and define

$$\lim_{n\to\infty} L(n) = \beta \quad \text{with probability 1.}$$

Krauth & Mézard [23] nonrigorously obtained an analytical expression for β via the cavity method:

$$\beta = \frac{1}{2} \int_{-\infty}^{\infty} f(x)(1 + f(x)) \exp(-f(x))\, dx = 2.0415\ldots = 2(1.0208\ldots),$$

where $f(x)$ is the solution of the integral equation

$$f(x) = \int_{-x}^{\infty} (1 + f(y)) \exp(-f(y))\, dy.$$

In actuality, this is just one scenario (corresponding to $d = 1$) of a d-parametrized family of random link approximations to the d-dimensional Euclidean TSP [16–18, 24].

8.5.2 Minimum Spanning Trees

Let us return to the familiar setting of n distinct points in the unit d-cube. Denote the set of points by V. A **minimum spanning tree** (MST) is a connected graph [5.6] with vertex-set V that has smallest possible length $L_d(n)$ (meaning the sum of edge-lengths in the usual Euclidean sense). Define

$$\lim_{n \to \infty} \frac{L_d(n)}{n^{(d-1)/d}} = \beta_d \quad \text{with probability 1.}$$

Numerical estimates [25, 26] and theoretical results [11] include

$$\beta_2 = 0.6331\ldots, \quad \beta_3 = 0.6232\ldots, \quad \beta_d \sim \sqrt{\frac{d}{2\pi e}} \text{ as } d \to \infty.$$

It is remarkable that an exact (but complicated) expression for β_d exists [27, 28]. We give the formula only for the case $d = 2$. Let Δ_i denote the set of all points $\{x_1, x_2, \ldots, x_{i-1}\}$ in the plane such that the disks D_j of center x_j and radius $1/2$, $0 \le j \le i - 1$, form a connected set, where $x_0 = 0$. Define $g_i(x_1, x_2, \ldots, x_{i-1})$ to be the area of $\bigcup_{j=0}^{i-1} D_j$; then

$$\beta_2 = \frac{1}{2} + \frac{1}{2} \sum_{i=2}^{\infty} \frac{\Gamma(i - \frac{1}{2})}{i!} \int_{\Delta_i} g_i(x_1, x_2, \ldots, x_{i-1})^{-i+\frac{1}{2}}\, dx_1\, dx_2 \ldots dx_{i-1}.$$

Using the first five terms of this series, we can obtain a rigorous lower bound $\beta_2 \ge 0.600822$ [27].

Given a minimum spanning tree, we can study characteristics other than $L_d(n)$. Consider as an example $\tilde{L}_d(n)$, the sum of squared edge-lengths, and define

$$\lim_{n \to \infty} \frac{\tilde{L}_d(n)}{n^{(d-1)/d}} = \tilde{\beta}_d \quad \text{with probability 1.}$$

The existence of $\tilde{\beta}_d$ was proved by Aldous & Steele [29, 30]; numerical estimates include $\tilde{\beta}_2 = 0.4769\ldots$ (which is often called **Bland's constant**) and $\tilde{\beta}_3 = 0.4194\ldots$

[26]. An exact expression for $\tilde{\beta}_d$ can be found as previously [27], with a rigorous lower bound $\tilde{\beta}_2 \geq 0.401 \ldots$.

The sum of squared edge-lengths parameter $\tilde{L}_d(n)$ is also interesting for TSP, given an optimal tour. Although an existence proof for $\tilde{\beta}_d$ is not known, specific point configurations can be constructed so that [31–33]

$$\frac{\tilde{L}_d(n)}{n^{(d-1)/d}} > c_d \ln(n)$$

as $n \to \infty$ for some $c_d > 0$; hence $\tilde{\alpha}_d$ definitely does *not* exist. Other variations abound. If we minimize $\tilde{L}_d(n)$ rather than $L_d(n)$ when computing optimal tours, a different path is often determined (because of the power weighting) and the worst-case constant [34–37]

$$\limsup_{n \to \infty} \frac{\tilde{L}_d(n)}{n^{(d-2)/d}} \leq \hat{\alpha}_d$$

is 4 when $d = 2$. Yukich [38, 39] proved that the corresponding average-case constant $\hat{\beta}_d$ exists as well, but the value of $\hat{\beta}_2$ is open.

For K_n, the complete graph on n vertices with independent Uniform [0, 1] random edge-lengths, consider the MST with sum of lengths $L(n)$. Frieze [40–42] demonstrated that

$$\lim_{n \to \infty} L(n) = \zeta(3) = 1.2020569031 \ldots \text{ in probability}$$

where $\zeta(3)$ is Apéry's constant [1.6], a beautiful result! Janson [43] showed that $\sqrt{n}(L(n) - \zeta(3))$ is asymptotically Normal $(0, \sigma^2)$ with

$$\sigma^2 = \frac{\pi^4}{45} - 2 \sum_{i=0}^{\infty} \sum_{j=1}^{\infty} \sum_{k=1}^{\infty} \frac{(i+k-1)! k^k (i+j)^{i-2} j}{i! k! (i+j+k)^{i+k+2}} = 1.6857 \ldots$$

but no simplification of this constant seems possible. Another relevant occurrence of $\zeta(3)$ is in [44].

8.5.3 Minimum Matching

Again, we consider n distinct points in the unit d-cube, with the additional assumption that n is even. A **matching** is a (disconnected) graph consisting of $n/2$ edges such that each of the n points is met by exactly one edge. A **minimum matching** (MM) is a matching of smallest possible length $L_d(n)$ (meaning the sum of edge-lengths in the usual Euclidean sense). Define β_d as before; the planar case β_2 is often called **Papadimitriou's constant** [45, 46]. Numerical estimates [47–54] and theoretical results [11] include

$$\beta_2 = 0.3104 \ldots, \quad \beta_3 = 0.3172 \ldots, \quad \beta_d \sim \frac{1}{2} \sqrt{\frac{d}{2\pi e}} \text{ as } d \to \infty.$$

The corresponding worst-case constant α_2 satisfies $0.537 \leq \alpha_2 \leq 0.707$ [47].

For K_n, the complete graph on n vertices with independent Uniform $[0, 1]$ random edge-lengths, consider the MM with sum of lengths $L(n)$. Mézard & Parisi [55–57] identified $\beta = \pi^2/12 = 0.8224670334\ldots$ via the replica method (plus an integral equation simpler than that for $f(x)$ earlier), and Aldous [58] found a rigorous proof. Experimental verification appears in [53, 54]. As before, this is just one scenario (corresponding to $d = 1$) of a d-parametrized family of random link approximations to the d-dimensional Euclidean MM problem.

[1]   J. Beardwood, J. H. Halton, and J. M. Hammersley, The shortest path through many points, *Proc. Cambridge Philos. Soc.* 55 (1959) 299–327; MR 22 #202.

[2]   R. M. Karp and J. M. Steele, Probabilistic analysis of heuristics, *The Traveling Salesman Problem: A Guided Tour of Combinatorial Optimization*, ed. E. L. Lawler, J. K. Lenstra, A. H. G. Rinnoov Kan, and D. B. Shmoys, Wiley, 1985, pp. 181–205; MR 87f: 90057.

[3]   J. M. Steele, *Probability Theory and Combinatorial Optimization*, SIAM, 1997, pp. 30–51; MR 99d:60002.

[4]   L. Fejes Toth, Über einen geometrischen Satz, *Math. Z.* 46 (1940) 83–85; MR 1,263g.

[5]   S. Verblunsky, On the shortest path through a number of points, *Proc. Amer. Math. Soc.* 2 (1951) 904–913; MR 13,577c.

[6]   L. Few, The shortest path and the shortest road through n points, *Mathematika* 2 (1955) 141–144; MR 17,1235f.

[7]   H. J. Karloff, How long can a Euclidean traveling salesman tour be?, *SIAM J. Discrete Math.* 2 (1989) 91–99; MR 89m:90063.

[8]   S. Moran, On the length of optimal TSP circuits in sets of bounded diameter, *J. Combin. Theory Ser. B* 37 (1984) 113–141; MR 86i:05087.

[9]   L. A. Goddyn, Quantizers and the worst case Euclidean traveling salesman problem, *J. Combin. Theory Ser. B* 50 (1990) 65–81; MR 91k:90121.

[10] W. D. Smith, *Studies in Computational Geometry Motivated by Mesh Generation*, Ph.D. thesis, Princeton Univ., 1988.

[11] D. Bertsimas and G. Van Ryzin, An asymptotic determination of the minimum spanning tree and minimum matching constants in geometrical probability, *Oper. Res. Lett.* 9 (1990) 223–231; MR 92b:90172.

[12] W. T. Rhee, On the travelling salesperson problem in many dimensions, *Random Structures Algorithms* 3 (1992) 227–233; MR 93d:90053.

[13] J. M. Steele and T. L. Snyder, Worst-case growth rates of some classical problems of combinatorial optimization, *SIAM J. Comput.* 18 (1989) 278–287; MR 90k:90131.

[14] G. A. Kabatyanskii and V. I. Levenshtein, Bounds for packings on a sphere and in space (in Russian), *Problemy Peredachi Informatsii* 14 (1978) 3–25; Engl. transl. in *Problems Information Transmission* 14 (1978) 1–17.

[15] P. M. Gruber, Geometry of numbers, *Handbook of Convex Geometry*, v. B, ed. P. M. Gruber and J. M. Wills, North-Holland, 1993, pp. 739–763; MR 94k:11074.

[16] D. S. Johnson, L. A. McGeoch, and E. E. Rothberg, Asymptotic experimental analysis for the Held-Karp traveling salesman bound, *Proc. 7th ACM-SIAM Symp. on Discrete Algorithms (SODA)*, Atlanta, ACM, 1996, pp. 341–350; MR 96j:68007.

[17] A. G. Percus and O. C. Martin, Finite size and dimensional dependence in the Euclidean traveling salesman problem, *Phys. Rev. Lett.* 76 (1996) 1188–1191; MR 96k: 90057.

[18] N. J. Cerf, J. Boutet de Monvel, O. Bohigas, O.C. Martin, and A. G. Percus, The random link approximation for the Euclidean traveling salesman problem, *J. Physique I* 7 (1997) 117–136; cond-mat/9607080.

[19] D. Applegate, W. Cook, and A. Rohe, Chained Lin-Kernighan for large traveling salesman problems, *INFORMS J. Comput.*, to appear; Forschungsinstitut für Diskrete Mathematik report 99887, Universität Bonn.

[20] M. G. Norman and P. Moscato, The Euclidean traveling salesman problem and a space-filling curve, *Chaos Solitons Fractals* 6 (1995) 389–397.

[21] E. Bonomi and J.-L. Lutton, The *n*-city travelling salesman problem: Statistical mechanics and the Metropolis algorithm, *SIAM Rev.* 26 (1984) 551–568; MR 86e:90041.

[22] B. Ghosh, Random distances within a rectangle and between two rectangles, *Bull. Calcutta Math. Soc.* 43 (1951) 17–24; MR 13,475a.

[23] W. Krauth and M. Mézard, The cavity method and the travelling salesman problem, *Europhys. Lett.* 8 (1989) 213–218.

[24] A. G. Percus and O. C. Martin, The stochastic traveling salesman problem: Finite size scaling and the cavity prediction, *J. Stat. Phys.* 94 (1999) 739–758; MR 2000b:82027.

[25] F. D. K. Roberts, Random minimal trees, *Biometrika* 55 (1968) 255–258; MR 37 #6210.

[26] M. Cortina-Borja and T. Robinson, Estimating the asymptotic constants of the total length of Euclidean minimal spanning trees with power-weighted edges, *Statist. Probab. Lett.* 47 (2000) 125–128; MR 2000k:90060.

[27] F. Avram and D. Bertsimas, The minimum spanning tree constant in geometrical probability and under the independent model: A unified approach, *Annals of Appl. Probab.* 2 (1992) 113–130; MR 93b:60027.

[28] P. Jaillet, Cube versus torus models and the Euclidean minimum spanning tree constant, *Annals of Appl. Probab.* 3 (1993) 582–592; MR 94d:60018.

[29] J. M. Steele, Growth rates of Euclidean minimal spanning trees with power weighted edges, *Annals of Probab.* 16 (1988) 1767–1787; MR 89j:60049.

[30] D. Aldous and J. M. Steele, Asymptotics for Euclidean minimal spanning trees on random points, *Probab. Theory Relat. Fields* 92 (1992) 247–258; MR 93c:60007.

[31] J. Gao and J. M. Steele, Sums of squares of edge lengths and spacefilling curve heuristics for the traveling salesman problem, *SIAM J. Discrete Math.* 7 (1994) 314–324; MR 95a:90083.

[32] T. L. Snyder and J. M. Steele, A priori bounds on the Euclidean traveling salesman, *SIAM J. Comput.* 24 (1995) 665–671; MR 96d:90109.

[33] M. Bern and D. Eppstein, Worst case bounds for subadditive geometric graphs, *Proc. 9th ACM Symp. on Computational Geometry (SCG),* San Diego, ACM, 1993, pp. 183–188.

[34] D. J. Newman, *A Problem Seminar,* Springer-Verlag, 1982, pp. 9–10, 74–75; MR 84d:00004.

[35] B. Bollobás and A. Meir, A travelling salesman problem in the *k*-dimensional unit cube, *Oper. Res. Lett.* 11 (1992) 19–21; MR 93c:90046.

[36] J. E. Yukich, Worst case asymptotics for some classical optimization problems, *Combinatorica* 16 (1996) 575–586; MR 97i:90061.

[37] S. Lee, Worst case asymptotics of power-weighted Euclidean functionals, *Discrete Math.,* to appear.

[38] J. E. Yukich, Asymptotics for the Euclidean TSP with power weighted edges, *Probab. Theory Relat. Fields* 102 (1995) 203–220; MR 96d:60022.

[39] J. E. Yukich, *Probability Theory of Classical Euclidean Optimization Problems,* Lect. Notes in Math. 1675, Springer-Verlag, 1998; MR 2000d:60018.

[40] A. M. Frieze, On the value of a random minimum spanning tree problem, *Discrete Appl. Math.* 10 (1985) 47–56; MR 86d:05103.

[41] J. M. Steele, On Frieze's $\zeta(3)$ limit for lengths of minimal spanning trees, *Discrete Appl. Math.* 18 (1987) 99–103; MR 88i:05063.

[42] B. Bollobás, *Random Graphs,* Academic Press, 1985, pp. 141–144; MR 87f:05152.

[43] S. Janson, The minimal spanning tree in a complete graph and a functional limit theorem for trees in a random graph, *Random Structures Algorithms* 7 (1995) 337–355; MR 97d:05244.

[44] M. D. Penrose, Random minimal spanning tree and percolation on the *N*-cube, *Random Structures Algorithms* 12 (1998) 63–82; MR 99g:60024.

[45] C. H. Papadimitriou, The probabilistic analysis of matching heuristics, *Proc. 15th Allerton Conf. on Communication, Control, and Computing,* Univ. of Illinois, 1978, pp. 368–378.

[46] J. M. Steele, Subadditive Euclidean functionals and nonlinear growth in geometric probability, *Annals of Probab.* 9 (1981) 365–376; MR 82j:60049.

[47] K. J. Supowit, E. M. Reingold, and D. A. Plaisted, The travelling salesman problem and minimum matching in the unit square, *SIAM J. Comput.* 12 (1983) 144–156; MR 84f:90032b.

[48] M. Iri, K. Murota, and S. Matsui, Heuristics for planar minimum-weight perfect matchings, *Networks* 13 (1983) 67–92; MR 84e:90029.

[49] M. Weber and Th. M. Liebling, Euclidean matching problems and the Metropolis algorithm, *Z. Oper. Res. Ser. A-B* 30 (1986) A85–A110; MR 87i:90174.

[50] P. Grassberger and H. Freund, An efficient heuristic algorithm for minimum matching, *Z. Oper. Res.* 34 (1990) 239–253; MR 91e:90088.

[51] D. P. Williamson and M. X. Goemans, Computational experience with an approximation algorithm on large-scale Euclidean matching instances, *INFORMS J. Comput.* 8 (1996) 29–40; MR 95b:68018.

[52] W. Cook and A. Rohe, Computing minimum-weight perfect matchings, *INFORMS J. Comput.* 11 (1999) 138–148.

[53] J. H. Boutet de Monvel and O. C. Martin, Mean field and corrections for the Euclidean minimum matching problem, *Phys. Rev. Lett.* 79 (1997) 167–170; cond-mat/9701182.

[54] J. Houdayer, J. H. Boutet de Monvel, and O. C. Martin, Comparing mean field and Euclidean matching problems, *Europ. Phys. J. B* 6 (1998) 383–393; cond-mat/9803195; MR 99i:82023.

[55] M. Mézard and G. Parisi, On the solution of the random link matching problems, *J. Physique* 48 (1987) 1451–1459.

[56] M. Mézard and G. Parisi, The Euclidean matching problem, *J. Physique* 49 (1988) 2019–2025; MR 90e:90048.

[57] R. Brunetti, W. Krauth, M. Mézard, and G. Parisi, Extensive numerical simulations of weighted matchings: Total length and distribution of links in the optimal solution, *Europhys. Lett.* 14 (1991) 295–301.

[58] D. J. Aldous, The $\zeta(2)$ limit in the random assignment problem, *Random Structures Algorithms* 18 (2001) 381–418; MR 2002f:60015.

8.6 Steiner Tree Constants

Let P denote a set of n points in d-dimensional space. Define

- the **Steiner minimal tree** (SMT) of P to be the shortest connected graph [5.6] that connects P, and
- the **minimum spanning tree** (MST) of P to be the shortest connected graph with vertex-set P that connects P.

Let P_n denote the n vertices of a regular planar polygon with n sides. Figures 8.4 and 8.5 show that, for MSTs, only inter-vertex line segments are permitted, whereas for SMTs,

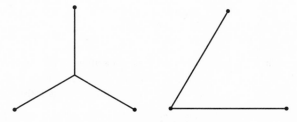

Figure 8.4. The SMT and MST of P_3.

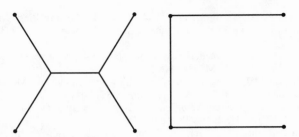

Figure 8.5. The SMT and MST of P_4.

additional vertices can be added to optimize the tree (hence the latter are more difficult to compute, because infinitely many vertex locations are available). If $|G|$ denotes the total edge length of a graph G, then clearly

$$\frac{|\operatorname{SMT}(P_3)|}{|\operatorname{MST}(P_3)|} = \frac{\sqrt{3}}{2} = 0.866\ldots, \quad \frac{|\operatorname{SMT}(P_4)|}{|\operatorname{MST}(P_4)|} = \frac{1+\sqrt{3}}{3} = 0.910\ldots.$$

Incidently, $\operatorname{SMT}(P_5)$ similarly consists of three additional vertices (called **Torricelli** or **Steiner** points), each the intersection of three edges meeting at $120°$, but $\operatorname{SMT}(P_n) = \operatorname{MST}(P_n)$ for $n \geq 6$. This can be confirmed by soap-film experiments as with minimum area solutions of *Plateau's problem* [1].

For an arbitrary set P, it is relatively easy to determine $\operatorname{MST}(P)$; therefore we are interested in the value

$$\rho_d = \inf_{n,\,P} \frac{|\operatorname{SMT}(P)|}{|\operatorname{MST}(P)|},$$

the infimum being over all n-point sets in d-dimensional space, over all positive integers n. The **Steiner ratio** ρ_d indicates how much the total length of an MST can be decreased by allowing Steiner points. Point sets achieving this infimum may be regarded as "possessing the most shortcuts" [2–5].

Du & Hwang [6] proved Gilbert & Pollak's [7] conjecture that

$$\rho_2 = \frac{\sqrt{3}}{2} = 0.8660254037\ldots,$$

and Smith & Smith [8, 9] proved that

$$\rho_3 \leq s_3 = \frac{3\sqrt{3} + \sqrt{7}}{10} = 0.7841903733\ldots$$

by use of a set P called the **3-sausage** (whose points are evenly spaced along a circular helix; see [10–13]). They provided extensive heuristic evidence that $\rho_3 = s_3$, but a rigorous proof is not known. The best lower bound for ρ_3, in fact, for any ρ_d, is [14, 15]

$$\rho_d \geq \frac{2 + x - \sqrt{x^2 + x + 1}}{\sqrt{3}} = 0.6158277481\ldots,$$

where x is the unique positive root of

$$128x^6 + 456x^5 + 783x^4 + 764x^3 + 408x^2 + 108x - 28 = 0.$$

Let us discuss upper bounds in more detail. Define the d-**simplex** to be the natural generalization of the equilateral triangle for $d = 2$ and the regular tetrahedron for $d = 3$. Chung & Gilbert [16] computed bounds for the Steiner ratio r_d in this case and showed that

$$\limsup_{d\to\infty} r_d \leq \frac{\sqrt{3}}{4 - \sqrt{2}} = 0.6698352124\ldots.$$

Smith [15, 17] conjectured that *limit supremum* can be replaced here by *limit* and that this inequality is in fact equality. It is known that $r_d > \rho_d$ if $d \geq 3$ and, for example,

$$r_3 = \frac{1 + \sqrt{6}}{3\sqrt{2}} = 0.813053\ldots, \quad r_4 = \frac{\sqrt{3} + \sqrt{5} + 2\sqrt{6}}{8\sqrt{2}} = 0.783748\ldots.$$

The Steiner ratios s_d corresponding to analogous higher-dimensional d-**sausages** are also known to satisfy $s_d < r_d$ for $d \geq 3$. s_d is strictly decreasing as a function of d. We do not, however, know the numerical value of $\lim_{d\to\infty} s_d$ nor whether $\rho_d = s_d$ for any $d \geq 3$. Du & Smith [15] thought that equality might possibly be true for small d but not for large $d \geq 15$. For example, $s_4 = 0.7439856178\ldots$ has the minimal polynomial [18]

$$900s^8 - 1863s^6 + 2950s^4 - 1511s^2 + 164,$$

and similar progress on evaluating $s_5 = 0.7218106748\ldots$ is perhaps not faraway.

Here is a different viewpoint (similar to our discussion of MSTs in [8.5]). If the n points of P are all constrained to fall within the unit square, then there exist constants c and C for which

$$0.930\sqrt{n} + c < (\tfrac{3}{4})^{\frac{1}{4}}\sqrt{n} + c \leq |\,\mathrm{SMT}(P)\,| < 0.995\sqrt{n} + C$$

for all n, as found by Chung & Graham [19–21]. If the points are instead constrained to fall within the unit d-cube, then

$$|\,\mathrm{SMT}(P)\,| \leq \sqrt{\frac{d}{2\pi e}} n^{1-\frac{1}{d}}$$

as $n \to \infty$, where d is sufficiently large [2, 22]. Improvements of both asymptotic results would be good to see.

[1] R. Courant and H. Robbins, *What Is Mathematics?*, Oxford Univ. Press, 1941; MR 80i:00001.

[2] F. K. Hwang, D. S. Richards, and P. Winter, *The Steiner Tree Problem*, North-Holland, 1992; MR 94a:05051.

[3] A. O. Ivanov and A. A. Tuzhilin, *Minimal Networks: The Steiner Problem and Its Generalizations*, CRC Press, 1994; MR 95h:05050.

[4] D.-Z. Du and F. K. Hwang, The state of art on Steiner ratio problems, *Computing in Euclidean Geometry*, 2nd ed., ed. D.-Z. Du and F. K. Hwang, World Scientific, 1995, pp. 163–191; MR 94i:68304.

[5] D. Cieslik, *Steiner Minimal Trees*, Kluwer, 1998; MR 99i:05062.

[6] D.-Z. Du and F. K. Hwang, A proof of the Gilbert-Pollak conjecture on the Steiner ratio, *Algorithmica* 7 (1992) 121–135; MR 92m:05060.

[7] E. N. Gilbert and H. O. Pollak, Steiner minimal trees, *SIAM J. Appl. Math.* 16 (1968) 1–29; MR 36 #6317.

[8] W. D. Smith and J. M. Smith, On the Steiner ratio in 3-space, *J. Combin. Theory Ser. A* 69 (1995) 301–332; MR 95k:05053.

[9] J. Keane, Simplifying the 3-sausage constant s_3, unpublished note (1999).

[10] A. H. Boerdijk, Some remarks concerning close-packing of equal spheres, *Philips Res. Rep.* 7 (1952) 303–313; MR 14,310b.

[11] H. S. M. Coxeter, *Introduction to Geometry*, 2nd ed., Wiley, 1969, p. 412; MR 90a:51001.

[12] R. Buckminster Fuller, *Synergetics*, MacMillan, 1975, pp. 520–524.

[13] H. S. M. Coxeter, The simplicial helix and the equation $\tan n\theta = n \tan \theta$, *Canad. Math. Bull.* 28 (1985) 385–393; MR 87b:51018.

[14] D.-Z. Du, On Steiner ratio conjectures, *Annals Oper. Res.* 33 (1991) 437–451; MR 92m:90053.

[15] D.-Z. Du and W. D. Smith, Disproofs of generalized Gilbert-Pollak conjecture on the Steiner ratio in three or more dimensions, *J. Combin. Theory Ser. A* 74 (1996) 115–130; MR 97h:05044.

[16] F. R. K. Chung and E. N. Gilbert, Steiner trees for the regular simplex, *Bull. Inst. Math. Acad. Sinica* 4 (1976) 313–325; MR 58 #21738.

[17] W. D. Smith, How to find Steiner minimal trees in Euclidean d-space, *Algorithmica* 7 (1992) 137–177; MR 93a:68064.

[18] J. Keane and G. Niklasch, Evaluating the 4-sausage constant s_4, unpublished note (1999).

[19] F. R. K. Chung and R. L. Graham, On Steiner trees for bounded point sets, *Geom. Dedicata* 11 (1981) 353–361; MR 82j:05072.

[20] H. T. Croft, K. J. Falconer, and R. K. Guy, *Unsolved Problems in Geometry*, Springer-Verlag, 1991, sect. F15; MR 95k:52001.

[21] T. L. Snyder, Worst-case minimum rectilinear Steiner trees in all dimensions, *Discrete Comput. Geom.* 8 (1992) 73–92; MR 93c:90067.

[22] W. D. Smith, *Studies in Computational Geometry Motivated by Mesh Generation*, Ph.D. thesis, Princeton Univ., 1988.

8.7 Hermite's Constants

What is the densest (lattice or non-lattice) packing of equal, non-overlapping spheres in n-dimensional space [1,2]? For $n = 1$, this corresponds to tiling the line with segments of equal length; hence the maximum density Δ_n clearly satisfies $\Delta_1 = 1$. For $n = 2$, the hexagonal lattice packing of circles in the plane gives $\Delta_2 = \pi/\sqrt{12} = 0.9068996821\ldots$, which was first proved by Thue [3,4]. Subsequent proofs were found by Fejes Tóth [5,6] and Segre & Mahler [7]. For $n = 3$, the face-centered cubic packing of spheres in 3-space gives $\Delta_3 = \pi/\sqrt{18} = 0.7404804896\ldots$. This was a well-known conjecture, attributed to Kepler, until it was first proved by Hales [8–10]. What can be said about Δ_n for $n \geq 4$? Can non-lattice packings in 4-space improve upon lattice packings?

If we restrict attention to only lattice packings, then the maximum density δ_n is known for all $n \leq 8$. Let $\omega_n = \pi^{n/2}\Gamma(n/2 + 1)^{-1}$ be the volume of the unit sphere in n-dimensional space and let

$$\gamma_n = 4\left(\frac{\delta_n}{\omega_n}\right)^{\frac{2}{n}}$$

Table 8.4. *Hermite's Constants δ_n and γ_n^n*

n	δ_n	γ_n^n
1	1	1
2	$\frac{\pi}{2\sqrt{3}} = 0.9068996821\ldots$	$\frac{4}{3}$
3	$\frac{\pi}{3\sqrt{2}} = 0.7404804896\ldots$	2
4	$\frac{\pi^2}{16} = 0.6168502750\ldots$	4
5	$\frac{\pi^2}{15\sqrt{2}} = 0.4652576133\ldots$	8
6	$\frac{\pi^3}{48\sqrt{3}} = 0.3729475455\ldots$	$\frac{64}{3}$
7	$\frac{\pi^3}{105} = 0.2952978731\ldots$	64
8	$\frac{\pi^4}{384} = 0.2536695079\ldots$	256

denote **Hermite's constant** of order n. Table 8.4 summarizes what is known for small n [3, 11, 12]. Also, for sufficiently large n, it can be proved that

$$-1 \leq \frac{\log_2(\delta_n)}{n} \leq \frac{\log_2(\Delta_n)}{n} \leq -0.59905\ldots, \quad \frac{1}{2\pi e} \leq \frac{\gamma_n}{n} \leq \frac{1.74338\ldots}{2\pi e}.$$

The expressions for the bounds $c = -0.59905\ldots$ and $4^{1+c} = 1.74338\ldots$ are complicated and are due to Kabatyanskii & Levenshtein [1, 13, 14]. It is believed that $c = -1$ [15], which would imply that $\gamma_n/n \to 1/(2\pi e)$ as $n \to \infty$, but we do not even know whether the limit exists [11]. Need γ_n^n be rational for all n? The Hermite constants γ_n are important as well in the study of quadratic forms and in coding theory.

[1] J. H. Conway and N. J. A. Sloane, *Sphere Packings, Lattices and Groups*, Springer-Verlag, 1988, pp. 1–21; MR 2000b:11077.
[2] H. T. Croft, K. J. Falconer, and R. K. Guy, *Unsolved Problems in Geometry*, Springer-Verlag, 1991, sect. D10, D11; MR 95k:52001.
[3] C. A. Rogers, *Packing and Covering*, Cambridge Univ. Press, 1964, pp. 1–11, 80–85; MR 30 #2405.
[4] A. Thue, Über die dichteste Zusammenstellung von kongruenten Kreisen in einer Ebene, *Videnskapsselskapets Skrifter I, Matematisk-Naturvidenskapelig Klasse, Kristiania*, n. 1, Dybwad, 1910, pp. 1–9; also in *Selected Mathematical Papers*, ed. T. Nagell, A. Selberg, S. Selberg, and K. Thalberg, Universitetsforlaget, 1977, pp. 257–263; MR 57 #46.
[5] L. Fejes Tóth, Über einen geometrischen Satz, *Math. Z.* 46 (1940) 83–85; MR 1,263g.
[6] L. Fejes Tóth, *Lagerungen in der Ebene, auf der Kugel und im Raum*, Springer-Verlag, 1953, pp. 58–61; MR 15,248b.
[7] B. Segre and K. Mahler, On the densest packing of circles, *Amer. Math. Monthly* 51 (1944) 261–270; MR 6,16c.
[8] T. C. Hales, Cannonballs and honeycombs, *Notices Amer. Math. Soc.* 47 (2000) 440–449; MR 2000m:52027.
[9] T. C. Hales, An overview of the Kepler conjecture, math.MG/9811071.
[10] N. J. A. Sloane, Kepler confirmed, *Nature* 395 (1998) 435–436.
[11] P. M. Gruber and C. G. Lekkerkerker, *Geometry of Numbers*, North-Holland, 1987, pp. 385–392, 409–410; MR 88j:11034.
[12] J. C. Lagarias, Point lattices, *Handbook of Combinatorics*, v. I, ed. R. Graham, M. Grötschel, and L. Lovász, MIT Press, 1995, pp. 919–966; MR 96m:11051.

[13]	G. A. Kabatyanskii and V. I. Levenshtein, Bounds for packings on a sphere and in space (in Russian), *Problemy Peredachi Informatsii* 14 (1978) 3–25; Engl. transl. in *Problems Information Transmission* 14 (1978) 1–17.

[14]	W. D. Smith, *Studies in Computational Geometry Motivated by Mesh Generation*, Ph.D. thesis, Princeton Univ., 1988.

[15]	P. M. Gruber, Geometry of numbers, *Handbook of Convex Geometry*, v. B, ed. P. M. Gruber and J. M. Wills, North-Holland, 1993, pp. 739–763; MR 94k:11074.

8.8 Tammes' Constants

Let $S = \{(u, v, w) : u^2 + v^2 + w^2 = 1\}$ denote the unit sphere in three-dimensional space and $|p - q|$ denote Euclidean distance between two points p and q. Let $N \geq 2$ be an integer and α be a real number. The α-**energy** associated with a finite subset $\omega_N = \{x_1, x_2, \ldots, x_N\}$ of points on S is

$$
\varepsilon(\alpha, \omega_N) = \begin{cases} \displaystyle\sum_{i<j} |x_i - x_j|^\alpha & \text{if } \alpha \neq 0, \\ \displaystyle\sum_{i<j} \ln\left(\frac{1}{|x_i - x_j|}\right) & \text{if } \alpha = 0. \end{cases}
$$

Define the **extremal energy** for N points on S by

$$
E(\alpha, N) = \begin{cases} \displaystyle\min_{\omega_N \subseteq S} \varepsilon(\alpha, \omega_N) & \text{if } \alpha \leq 0, \\ \displaystyle\max_{\omega_N \subseteq S} \varepsilon(\alpha, \omega_N) & \text{if } \alpha > 0. \end{cases}
$$

There is tremendous interest in the value of $E(\alpha, N)$ and a representative configuration of points ω_N at which the minimum or maximum energy occurs. The applications include coding theory, electrostatics, crystallography, botany, geometry, and computational complexity. We will mention only a few results here.

Maximizing 1-energy is the same as maximizing the average distance between all pairs of points [1–5]. One can prove that

$$
\lim_{N \to \infty} \frac{1}{N^2} E(1, N) = \frac{2}{3},
$$

and it is known that

$$
\lim_{N \to \infty} \frac{E(1, N) - \frac{2}{3} N^2}{N^{1/2}} = \lambda,
$$

where we have rigorous bounds $-2.5066282746\ldots = -\sqrt{2\pi} \leq \lambda < 0$ and an estimate $\lambda = -0.40096\ldots$ [6,7].

Determining $E(-1, N)$ corresponds to locating identical point electrical charges on the sphere so that they are in equilibrium (assuming the particles repel each other according to the *Coulomb potential*). This is known as **Thomson's electron problem** and the optimizing point configurations are called **Fekete points** [8–13]. One can prove that

$$
\lim_{N \to \infty} \frac{1}{N^2} E(-1, N) = \frac{1}{2},
$$

and, building upon the work of Wagner [14, 15], Kuijlaars & Saff [16, 17] conjectured that

$$\lim_{N \to \infty} \frac{E(-1, N) - \frac{1}{2}N^2}{N^{3/2}} = \sqrt{3} \left(\frac{\sqrt{3}}{8\pi} \right)^{1/2} \zeta\left(\frac{1}{2} \right) \left(\zeta\left(\frac{1}{2}, \frac{1}{3} \right) - \zeta\left(\frac{1}{2}, \frac{2}{3} \right) \right)$$

$$= -0.5530512933\ldots,$$

where $\zeta(s)$ is the usual Riemann zeta function and

$$\zeta(s, a) = \sum_{\substack{k=0 \\ k+a \neq 0}}^{\infty} \frac{1}{(k+a)^s}$$

is the Hurwitz zeta function (with analytic continuation). There is considerable theoretical and empirical evidence that this conjecture is true.

Minimizing 0-energy is equivalent to maximizing the product of distances $\prod_{i<j} |x_i - x_j|$, and it is known that

$$\lim_{N \to \infty} \frac{E(0, N) - \left(-\frac{1}{4}\ln(\frac{4}{e})N^2 - \frac{1}{4}N\ln(N) \right)}{N} = \mu,$$

where we have rigorous bounds $-0.1127687700\ldots \leq \mu \leq -0.0234972918\ldots$ and an estimate $\mu = -0.026422\ldots$ [6, 7, 18, 19].

As $\alpha \to -\infty$, the α-energy is increasingly dominated by the term involving the smallest of the distances, that is,

$$\lim_{\alpha \to -\infty} \varepsilon(\alpha, \omega_N)^{\frac{1}{\alpha}} = \min_{i<j} |x_i - x_j|.$$

Therefore, the minimal energy problem reduces to calculating

$$d_N = \max_{\omega_N} \min_{i<j} |x_i - x_j|,$$

which is the answer to Tammes' 1930 question about pollen grains [8, 21–28]. Equivalently, what is the largest diameter of N congruent circles that can be packed on S (without overlap)? It is known that

$$d_N = \left(\frac{8\pi}{\sqrt{3}} \right)^{\frac{1}{2}} N^{-\frac{1}{2}} + O\left(N^{-\frac{2}{3}} \right)$$

as $N \to \infty$. A more precise estimate of the error term evidently has not been made. Bounds were determined by Fejes Tóth [26, 29, 30] and van der Waerden [26, 31]:

$$2 \left[\frac{\sqrt{3}}{2\pi}N + 3\left(\frac{N}{4\pi} \right)^{\frac{2}{3}} + 3\left(\frac{N}{4\pi} \right)^{\frac{1}{3}} \right]^{-\frac{1}{2}} \leq d_N \leq \left[4 - \csc\left(\frac{\pi}{6} \frac{N}{N-2} \right)^2 \right]^{\frac{1}{2}}.$$

Related questions ask for the smallest diameter of N congruent circles that can *cover* S [32] and for N-point charge configurations on the unit *disk* that achieve equilibrium [33].

[1] L. Fejes Tóth, On the sum of distances determined by a pointset, *Acta Math. Acad. Sci. Hungar.* 7 (1956) 397–401; MR 21 #5937.

[2] R. Alexander, On the sum of distances between *n* points on a sphere, *Acta Math. Acad. Sci. Hungar.* 23 (1972) 443–448; MR 47 #957.

[3] K. B. Stolarsky, Sum of distances between *n* points on a sphere. II, *Proc. Amer. Math. Soc.* 41 (1973) 575–582; MR 48 #12314.

[4] J. Berman and K. Hanes, Optimizing the arrangement of points on the unit sphere, *Math. Comp.* 31 (1977) 1006–1008; MR 57 #17502.

[5] J. Beck, Sums of distances between points on a sphere - An application of the theory of irregularities of distribution to discrete geometry, *Mathematica* 31 (1984) 33–31; MR 86d:52004.

[6] Y. M. Zhou, *Arrangements of Points on the Sphere*, Ph.D. thesis, Univ. of South Florida, 1995.

[7] E. A. Rakhmanov, E. B. Saff, and Y. M. Zhou, Minimal discrete energy on the sphere, *Math. Res. Lett.* 1 (1994) 647–662; MR 96e:78011.

[8] L. L. Whyte, Unique arrangements of points on a sphere, *Amer. Math. Monthly* 59 (1952) 606–611; MR 14,310c.

[9] T. Erber and G. M. Hockney, Equilibrium configurations of *N* equal charges on a sphere, *J. Phys. A* 24 (1991) L1369–L1377.

[10] L. Glasser and A. G. Every, Energies and spacings of point charges on a sphere, *J. Phys. A* 25 (1992) 2473–2482.

[11] K. S. Brown, Min-energy configurations of electrons on a sphere (MathPages).

[12] R. H. Hardin, N. J. A. Sloane, and W. D. Smith, Minimal energy arrangements of points on a sphere (AT&T Labs Research).

[13] T. Erber and G. M. Hockney, Complex systems: Equilibrium configurations of *N* equal charges on a sphere ($2 \leq N \leq 112$), *Advances in Chemical Physics*, v. 98, ed. I. Prigogine and S. A. Rice, Wiley, 1997, pp. 495–594; MR 98e:78002.

[14] G. Wagner, On means of distances on the surface of a sphere (lower bounds), *Pacific J. Math.* 144 (1990) 389–398; MR 91e:52014.

[15] G. Wagner, On means of distances on the surface of a sphere (upper bounds), *Pacific J. Math.* 154 (1992) 381–396; MR 93b:52007.

[16] A. B. J. Kuijlaars and E. B. Saff, Asymptotics for minimal discrete energy on the sphere, *Trans. Amer. Math. Soc.* 350 (1998) 523–538; MR 98e:11092.

[17] E. B. Saff and A. B. J. Kuijlaars, Distributing many points on a sphere, *Math. Intellig.* 19 (1997) 5–11; MR 98h:70011.

[18] G. Wagner, On the product of distances to a point set on a sphere, *J. Austral. Math. Soc. A* (1989) 466–482; MR 90j:11080.

[19] B. Bergersen, D. Boal, and P. Palffy-Muhoray, Equilibrium configurations of particles on a sphere: The case of logarithmic interactions, *J. Phys. A* 27 (1994) 2579–2568.

[20] S. Smale, Mathematical problems for the next century, *Math. Intellig.*, v. 20 (1998) n. 2, 7–15; MR 99h:01033.

[21] J. H. Conway and N. J. A. Sloane, *Sphere Packings, Lattices and Groups*, Springer-Verlag, 1988; MR 2000b:11077.

[22] H. T. Croft, K. J. Falconer, and R. K. Guy, *Unsolved Problems in Geometry*, Springer-Verlag, 1991, sect. D7; MR 95k:52001.

[23] B. W. Clare and D. L. Kepert, The closest packing of equal circles on a sphere, *Proc. Royal Soc. London A* 405 (1986) 329–344; MR 87i:52024.

[24] T. Tarnai and Zs. Gáspár, Arrangement of 23 points on a sphere (on a conjecture of R. M. Robinson), *Proc. Royal Soc. London A* 433 (1991) 257–267; MR 92m:52043.

[25] D. A. Kottwitz, The densest packing of equal circles on a sphere, *Acta Cryst.* A47 (1991) 158–165; errata A47 (1991) 851; MR 92m:52042.

[26] J. B. M. Melissen, *Packing and Coverings with Circles*, Ph.D. thesis, 1997, Universiteit Utrecht.

[27] K. J. Nurmela, Constructing spherical codes by global optimization methods, research report A32, Helsinki Univ. of Technol.

[28] R. H. Hardin, N. J. A. Sloane, and W. D. Smith, Spherical codes (packings) (AT&T Labs Research).

[29] L. Fejes Tóth, On the densest packing of spherical caps, *Amer. Math. Monthly* 56 (1949) 330–331; MR 10,731b and MR 11,870 errata/addenda.

[30] L. Fejes Tóth, *Regular Figures*, MacMillan, 1964; MR 29 #2705.

[31] B. L. van der Waerden, Punkte auf der Kugel. Drei Zusätze, *Math. Annalen* 125 (1952) 213–222; corrigendum 152 (1963) 94; MR 14,401c.

[32] R. H. Hardin, N. J. A. Sloane, and W. D. Smith, Spherical coverings (AT&T Labs Research).

[33] K. J. Nurmela, Minimum-energy point charge configurations on a circular disk, *J. Phys. A* 31 (1998) 1035–1047.

8.9 Hyperbolic Volume Constants

We first describe a certain enumeration problem. Let n be a positive integer. An n-**simplex** is the convex hull of $n + 1$ points in n-dimensional Euclidean space, which are assumed to be in general position. For example, a 1-simplex is a line segment, a 2-simplex is a triangle (with its interior), and a 3-simplex is a tetrahedron (with its interior).

An n-cube is **triangulated** (or, more precisely, **face-to-face vertex triangulated**) if it is partitioned into finitely many n-simplices with disjoint interiors, subject to the constraints that

- the vertices of any n-simplex are also vertices of the cube, and
- the intersection of any two n-simplices is a face of each of them.

Define the **simplexity** $f(n)$ of the n-cube to be the minimum number of n-simplices required to triangulate it (see Figure 8.6). An enormous amount of computation leads to the values of $f(n)$ listed in Table 8.5 and bounds for $f(n)$ listed in Table 8.6 [1–7]. An unsolved problem is to determine a tight lower bound for $f(n)$, valid for all n. We will describe an attempt to do this shortly.

The **standard** n-**simplex** S_n is the regular n-simplex inscribed in the unit n-sphere (e.g., S_2 is the equilateral triangle of area $3\sqrt{3}/4$). The **standard** n-**cube** C_n is the n-cube of side $2/\sqrt{n}$, centered at the origin. Clearly

$$\text{volume of } S_n = \frac{\sqrt{n+1}}{n!}\left(1 + \frac{1}{n}\right)^{\frac{n}{2}}, \quad \text{volume of } C_n = \left(\frac{4}{n}\right)^{\frac{n}{2}}.$$

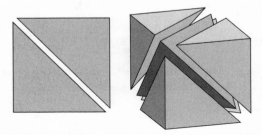

Figure 8.6. Triangulation of the n-cube: $f(2) = 2$ and $f(3) = 5$.

Table 8.5. *Simplexity Values*

n	1	2	3	4	5	6	7
$f(n)$	1	2	5	16	67	308	1493

The best-known attempt to minorize $f(n)$ involves the integrals

$$\xi_n = \text{volume of ideal hyperbolic } n\text{-cube} = \int_{C_n} \left(1 - \sum_{k=1}^{n} x_k^2\right)^{-\frac{n+1}{2}} dx_1 \, dx_2 \ldots dx_n,$$

$$\eta_n = \text{volume of regular ideal hyperbolic } n\text{-simplex}$$

$$= \int_{S_n} \left(1 - \sum_{k=1}^{n} x_k^2\right)^{-\frac{n+1}{2}} dx_1 \, dx_2 \ldots dx_n.$$

More precisely,

$$f(n) \geq \frac{\xi_n}{\eta_n} \geq \frac{1}{2} 6^{\frac{n}{2}} (n+1)^{-\frac{n+1}{2}} n!,$$

as shown by Smith [8] and, independently, Marshall. There is considerable room for improvement – the gap between $f(n)$ and its bounds is huge – but the occurrence of the constants ξ_n and η_n is interesting to us.

It can be demonstrated that $\eta_2 = \pi$, $\eta_3 = \pi \ln(\beta) = 1.0149416064\ldots$, where β is defined in [3.10], and [9–11]

$$\eta_4 = \frac{10\pi}{3} \arcsin\left(\frac{1}{3}\right) - \frac{\pi^2}{3} = 0.2688956601\ldots, \quad \eta_5 = 0.05756\ldots.$$

Also, $\xi_2 = 2\pi$, $\xi_3 = 5\eta_3 = 5.0747080320\ldots$, $\xi_4 = 3.92259368\ldots$, and $\xi_5 = 2.75861972\ldots$ [11, 12]. Asymptotically, we have [8, 9, 12]

$$\eta_n \sim e\frac{\sqrt{n}}{n!}, \quad \xi_n \sim 2\sqrt{\pi}\frac{c^n}{\Gamma\left(\frac{n+1}{2}\right)}$$

as $n \to \infty$, where e is the natural logarithmic base [1.3] and $c = 1.0820884492\ldots$ is twice the maximum of **Dawson's integral** [13, 14]:

$$D(x) = \exp(-x^2) \int_0^x \exp(t^2)\, dt, \quad \frac{c}{2} = 0.5410442246\ldots = \frac{1.2615225101\ldots}{\sqrt{2e}},$$

which occurs uniquely when $x = 0.9241388730\ldots = 1/c$.

Table 8.6. *Bounds for Simplexity $f(n)$*

n	8	9	10
Lower Bound	5522	26593	131269
Upper Bound	13136	105341	928780

In spite of this detailed asymptotic information, it remains open whether $f(n) \geq \gamma^n n!$ for some constant $\gamma > 0$ [15].

[1] R. K. Guy, A couple of cubic conundrums, *Amer. Math. Monthly* 91 (1984) 624–629.

[2] P. S. Mara, Triangulations for the cube, *J. Combin. Theory Ser. A* 20 (1976) 170–177; MR 53 #10624.

[3] J. F. Sallee, A triangulation of the *n*-cube, *Discrete Math.* 40 (1982) 81–86; MR 84d:05065b.

[4] J. F. Sallee, A note on minimal triangulation of the *n*-cube, *Discrete Appl. Math.* 4 (1982) 211–215; MR 84g:52019.

[5] J. F. Sallee, The middle-cut triangulations of the *n*-cube, *SIAM J. Algebraic Discrete Methods* 5 (1984) 407–419; MR 86c:05054.

[6] R. B. Hughes and M. R. Anderson, Simplexity of the cube, *Discrete Math.* 158 (1996) 99–150; MR 97g:90083.

[7] D. Eppstein, How many tetrahedra? (Geometry Junkyard).

[8] W. D. Smith, A lower bound for the simplexity of the *N*-cube via hyperbolic volumes, *Europ. J. Combin.* 21 (2000) 131–137; MR 2001c:52004.

[9] U. Haagerup and H. J. Munkholm, Simplices of maximal volume in hyperbolic *n*-space, *Acta Math.* 147 (1981) 1–11; MR 82j:53116.

[10] J. J. Seidel, On the volume of a hyperbolic simplex, *Studia Sci. Math. Hungar.* 21 (1986) 243–249; MR 88k:51040.

[11] W. D. Smith, *Studies in Computational Geometry Motivated by Mesh Generation*, Ph.D. thesis, Princeton Univ., 1988.

[12] J. Keane, Volumes of ideal hyperbolic cubes, unpublished note (1996).

[13] M. Abramowitz and I. A. Stegun, *Handbook of Mathematical Functions*, Dover, 1972, p. 298; MR 94b:00012.

[14] J. Spanier and K. B. Oldham, *An Atlas of Functions*, Hemisphere, 1987, pp. 405–409.

[15] J. A. De Loera, F. Santos, and F. Takeuchi, Extremal properties for dissections of convex 3-polytopes, *SIAM J. Discrete Math.* 14 (2001) 143–161; MR 2002g:52014.

8.10 Reuleaux Triangle Constants

Of all planar sets of constant width 1, the **Reuleaux triangle** (see Figure 8.7) possesses the least area [1–11] and is the most asymmetric [12–15]. Let us examine certain key phrases in the statement of this theorem more carefully, so that we may introduce several related constants.

A compact convex set $C \subseteq \mathbb{R}^2$ is of **constant width** w if all orthogonal projections of C onto lines have the same length w. More generally, for $C \subseteq \mathbb{R}^d, d > 2$, the required condition becomes that every pair of parallel supporting $(d - 1)$-dimensional planes are at the same distance w apart. (The word *breadth* was used in [8.4.1] for reasons of convention.) For simplicity, set $w = 1$. The first part of the theorem is that the area, $\mu(C)$, of $C \subseteq \mathbb{R}^2$ satisfies

$$\mu(C) \geq \frac{\pi - \sqrt{3}}{2} = 0.7047709230\ldots.$$

It is believed that the volume, $\mu(C)$, of $C \subseteq \mathbb{R}^3$ satisfies

$$\mu(C) \geq \left(\frac{2}{3} - \frac{\sqrt{3}}{4} \arccos\left(\frac{1}{3} \right) \right) \pi = 0.4198600459\ldots,$$

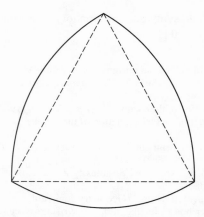

Figure 8.7. The Reuleaux triangle (solid curves) consists of the vertices of an equilateral triangle (dotted lines) together with three arcs of circles, each circle having a center at one of the vertices and endpoints at the other two vertices.

which corresponds to Meisser's tetrahedral analog of the Reuleaux triangle [1, 16]. The best-known lower bound thus far is $(3\sqrt{6} - 7)\pi/3 = 0.3649161225\ldots$; hence there is considerable room for improvement [8, 11].

Asymmetry is more difficult to define, primarily because there are competing notions of it! We focus on just two measures of symmetry, called the Kovner–Besicovitch (inner) and Estermann (outer) measures, respectively [14]:

$$\sigma(C) = \frac{\mu(A)}{\mu(C)}, \quad \tau(C) = \frac{\mu(C)}{\mu(B)},$$

where A is the largest convex centrally symmetric subset of C and B is the smallest convex centrally symmetric superset of C. The second part of the theorem is that, for $C \subseteq \mathbb{R}^2$ [8, 12],

$$\sigma(C) \geq \frac{6\arccos(\frac{5+\sqrt{33}}{12}) + \sqrt{3} - \sqrt{11}}{\pi - \sqrt{3}} = 0.8403426028\ldots$$
$$= 1 - 0.1596573971\ldots,$$

$$\tau(C) \geq \frac{\pi - \sqrt{3}}{\sqrt{3}} = 0.8137993642 = 1 - 0.1862006357\ldots.$$

The corresponding superset B is a regular hexagon circumscribed about the minimizing Reuleaux triangle C; the subset A is a circular hexagon obtained by reflecting C across its center, calling this new subset C', and then forming $C \cap C'$. A higher-dimensional analog of this bound is not known.

Here is one more result. What is the set $C \subseteq \mathbb{R}^2$ of maximal constant width w that avoids all vertices of the integer square lattice? The answer is a Reuleaux triangle, oriented so that one axis of symmetry lies midway between two parallel lattice edges.

Its width $w = 1.5449417003\ldots$ has minimal polynomial [9]

$$4x^6 - 12x^5 + x^4 + 22x^3 - 14x^2 - 4x + 4.$$

We mention that the Reuleaux triangle also appears in conjectures surrounding planar convex translations [8.3.1], maximal planar rendezvous constants [8.21], and exact values of the Bloch–Landau constants [7.1].

[1] T. Bonnesen and W. Fenchel, *Theory of Convex Bodies*, BCS Associates, 1987, pp. 135–149; MR 49 #9736.

[2] W. Blaschke, Konvexe Bereiche gegebener konstanter Breite und kleinsten Inhalts, *Math. Annalen* 76 (1915) 81–93.

[3] M. Fujiwara, Analytic proof of Blaschke's theorem on the curve of constant breadth with minimum area, *Proc. Imperial Akad. Japan* 3 (1927) 307–309; 7 (1931) 300–302.

[4] A. E. Mayer, Der Inhalt der Gleichdicke, *Math. Annalen* 110 (1934–35) 97–127.

[5] H. G. Eggleston, A proof of Blaschke's theorem on the Reuleaux triangle, *Quart. J. Math.* 3 (1952) 296–297; MR 14,496a.

[6] H. G. Eggleston, *Convexity*, Cambridge Univ. Press, 1958, pp. 122–131; MR 23 #A2123.

[7] A. S. Besicovitch, Minimum area of a set of constant width, *Convexity*, ed. V. L. Klee, Proc. Symp. Pure Math. 7, Amer. Math. Soc., 1963, pp. 13–14; MR 27 #1878.

[8] G. D. Chakerian, Sets of constant width, *Pacific J. Math.* 19 (1966) 13–21; MR 34 #4986.

[9] G. T. Sallee, The maximal set of constant width in a lattice, *Pacific J. Math.* 28 (1969) 669–674; MR 39 #2069.

[10] M. Gardner, Curves of constant width, one of which makes it possible to drill square holes, *Sci. Amer.*, v. 208 (1963) n. 2, 148–156 and v. 208 (1963) n. 3, 154; also in *Mathematics: An Introduction to Its Spirit and Use*, W. H. Freeman, 1979, pp. 107–111 and 238–239.

[11] G. D. Chakerian and H. Groemer, Convex bodies of constant width, *Convexity and Its Applications*, ed. P. M. Gruber and J. M. Wills, Birkhäuser, 1983, pp. 49–96; MR 85f:52001.

[12] A. S. Besicovitch, Measure of asymmetry of convex curves. II: Curves of constant width, *J. London Math. Soc.* 26 (1951) 81–93; MR 12,850g.

[13] H. G. Eggleston, Measure of asymmetry of convex curves of constant width and restricted radii of curvature, *Quart. J. Math.* 3 (1952) 63–72; MR 13,768d.

[14] B. Grünbaum, Measures of symmetry for convex sets, *Convexity*, ed. V. L. Klee, Proc. Symp. Pure Math. 7, Amer. Math. Soc., 1963, pp. 233–270; MR 27 #6187.

[15] H. Groemer and L. J. Wallen, A measure of asymmetry for domains of constant width, *Beiträge Algebra Geom.* 42 (2001) 517–521.

[16] I. M. Yaglom and V. G. Boltyanskii, *Convex Figures*, Holt, Rinehart and Winston, 1961, pp. 70–82, 242–264; MR 14,197d.

8.11 Beam Detection Constant

A **beam detector** for the unit circle C is a set of points that intercepts all lines (i.e., **beams**) crossing C. Clearly C is itself a beam detector for C, although it is inefficient. There exist shorter curves that meet the required condition [1, 2]. We need to explain what we mean by *curve* before continuing.

A **path** is a continuous image of an interval in the plane, and an **arc** is a path with no self-intersections. If this is the sense in which we interpret the word *curve*, then there is a complete solution. Joris [3] and Faber, Mycielski & Pedersen [4, 5] proved that a bow-shaped arc (see Figure 8.8) is the shortest path that meets all lines meeting the unit circle.

If we loosen the notion of *curve* then the length can be reduced substantially. An **n-arc** is a union of n (possibly disconnected) arcs. Makai [6, 7] found the 2-arc of

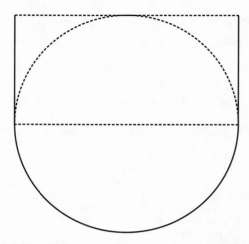

Figure 8.8. Bow-shaped arc of length $\pi + 2 = 5.1415926535\ldots$.

smallest known length, called a **bow-and-arrow** configuration by Thurston [1] (see Figure 8.9). Faber & Mycielski [5] improved on this and found the 3-arc of smallest known length (see Figure 8.10). These examples were rediscovered by Day [8]. For the 2-arc case, the solutions of the simultaneous equations

$$2\cos(\theta_1) - \sin(\tfrac{\theta_2}{2}) = 0, \quad \tan(\tfrac{\theta_1}{2})\cos(\tfrac{\theta_2}{2}) + \sin(\tfrac{\theta_2}{2})\left(\sec(\tfrac{\theta_2}{2})^2 + 1\right) = 2, \quad \theta_3 = \theta_1,$$

give the angles

$$\theta_1 = \theta_3 = 1.2865112676\ldots \approx 73.71°, \quad \theta_2 = 1.1910478286\ldots \approx 68.24°,$$

yielding an upper bound on length for 2-arcs:

$$L_2 \leq 2\pi - 2\theta_1 - \theta_2 + 2\tan(\tfrac{\theta_1}{2}) + \sec(\tfrac{\theta_2}{2}) - \cos(\tfrac{\theta_2}{2}) + \tan(\tfrac{\theta_1}{2})\sin(\tfrac{\theta_2}{2})$$
$$= 4.8189264563\ldots.$$

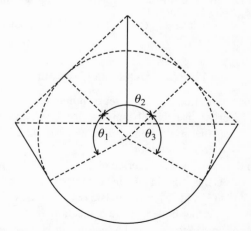

Figure 8.9. The length of a 2-arc is $4.8189264563\ldots$, where $\theta_1 = 1.2865\ldots, \theta_2 = 1.1910\ldots$, and $\theta_3 = 1.2865\ldots$; the name "bow-and-arrow" is well justified.

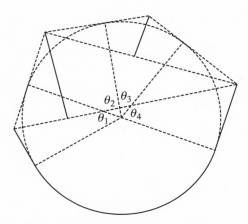

Figure 8.10. The length of a 3-arc is $4.799891547\ldots$, where $\theta_1 = 0.96\ldots$, $\theta_2 = 1.04\ldots$, $\theta_3 = 0.7\ldots$, and $\theta_4 = 1.2\ldots$.

Similar equations give rise to an upper bound on length for 3-arcs:

$$L_3 \leq 4.799891547\ldots$$

but nothing is known corresponding to 4-arcs or 5-arcs. Define the **beam detection constant** to be

$$L = \inf_{n \geq 1} L_n \geq \pi,$$

where the lower bound is due to Croft [9] and Thurston [1]. Some people presume that the sequence $\{L_n\}$ is strictly decreasing, but others believe that n-arcs, $n \geq 4$, cannot improve on 3-arcs.

One could equally well call L the **trench diggers' constant**. Suppose a straight cable of unknown direction is buried underground and all we know is that the cable passes within one unit of a given marker. There is a strategy for digging (highly disconnected) trenches, guaranteed to locate the cable, of total length $L + \varepsilon$ for any $\varepsilon > 0$. Related strategies include escape trajectories for a hunter lost in a dense jungle or a swimmer at sea in a thick fog, who know they are within one unit of a straight boundary [5]. These are special cases of what is known as the "lost in a forest" problem [3, 10–12].

A different generalization of *path* is possible. Instead of the continuous image of an interval, consider any connected closed set in the plane. Instead of ordinary length, consider one-dimensional Hausdorff measure. Eggleston [9, 13] determined that, even for this extended class of curves, the optimal beam detector for C is the bow-shaped arc of length $\pi + 2$. Curiously, if we replace the unit circle C by an equilateral triangle or a square, the optimal known connected beam detector is tree-like, with several branches, called the *Steiner span* of the vertices [8.6]. For the square, as for the circle, we do better still if we discard connectivity [5, 14–19]. The conjectured optimal beam detector for the unit square has two components (as shown in Figure 8.11) and length $(2 + \sqrt{3})/\sqrt{2} = 2.6389584337\ldots = 4(0.6597396084\ldots)$.

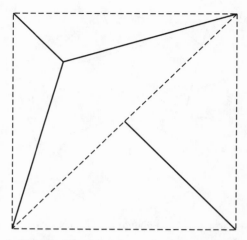

Figure 8.11. The length of the conjectured shortest opaque square fence is 2.6389584337....

Eppstein [1] pointed out an interesting connection with the design of algorithms for computing a minimal *opaque forest* of a convex polygon [20–22]. Other variations of beam detection appear in [23–25].

Zalgaller [26] reformulated the first problem as follows: What is the shortest connected curve in the plane outside an open unit disk such that, moving along this curve, we can see all points of the unit circle C? He then examined the three-dimensional analog: What is the shortest connected curve in 3-space outside an open unit ball such that, moving along this curve, we can see all the points of the unit sphere S? By a nonrigorous argument, Zalgaller obtained an *inspection trajectory* of length 9.576778....

[1] D. Eppstein, Building a better beam detector? (Geometry Junkyard).

[2] H. T. Croft, K. J. Falconer, and R. K. Guy, *Unsolved Problems in Geometry*, Springer-Verlag, 1991, sect. A30; MR 95k:52001.

[3] H. Joris, Le chasseur perdu dans la forêt, *Elem. Math.* 35 (1980) 1–14; MR 81d:52001.

[4] V. Faber, J. Mycielski, and P. Pedersen, On the shortest curve which meets all the lines which meet a circle, *Annales Polonici Math.* 44 (1984) 249–266; MR 87b:52023.

[5] V. Faber and J. Mycielski, The shortest curve that meets all the lines that meet a convex body, *Amer. Math. Monthly* 93 (1986) 796–801; MR 87m:52017.

[6] L. Fejes Tóth, Remarks on the dual to Tarski's plank problem (in Hungarian), *Mat. Lapok* 25 (1974) 13–20 (1977); MR 56 #1204.

[7] E. Makai, On a dual of Tarski's plank problem, *Diskrete Geometrie*, 2 Kolloq., Inst. Math. Univ. Salzburg, 1980, pp. 127–132; Zbl. 459/52005.

[8] I. Stewart, The great drain robbery, *Sci. Amer.*, v. 273 (1995) n. 3, 206–207; supplement, v. 273 (1995) n. 6, 106 and v. 274 (1996) n. 2, 125.

[9] H. T. Croft, Curves intersecting certain sets of great circles on the sphere, *J. London Math. Soc.* 1 (1969) 461–469; MR 40 #865.

[10] R. Bellman, Minimization problem, *Bull. Amer. Math. Soc.* 62 (1956) 270.

[11] J. R. Isbell, An optimal search pattern, *Naval Res. Logist. Quart.* 4 (1957) 357–359; MR 19,820a.

[12] S. R. Finch and J. E. Wetzel, Lost in a forest, unpublished note (2002).

[13] H. G. Eggleston, The maximal inradius of the convex cover of a plane connected set of given length, *Proc. London Math. Soc.* 45 (1982) 456–478; MR 84e:52004.

[14] R. E. D. Jones, Opaque sets of degree α, *Amer. Math. Monthly* 71 (1964) 535–537; MR 29 #2189.

[15] R. Honsberger, *Mathematical Morsels*, Math. Assoc. Amer., 1978, pp. 22–25; MR 58 #9950.

[16] K. A. Brakke, The opaque cube problem, *Amer. Math. Monthly* 99 (1992) 866–871; MR 94b:51025.

[17] B. Kawohl, The opaque square and the opaque cube, *General Inequalities 7*, ed. C. Bandle, W. N. Everitt, L. Losonczi, and W. Walter, Birkhäuser, 1997, pp. 339–346; MR 98f:52006.

[18] B. Kawohl, Symmetry or not?, *Math. Intellig.*, v. 20 (1998) n. 2, 16–22; MR 99e:00010.

[19] B. Kawohl, Some nonconvex shape optimization problems, *Optimal Shape Design*, Proc. 1998 Tróia conf., ed. A. Cellina and A. Ornelas, Lect. Notes in Math. 1740, Springer-Verlag, 2000, pp. 7–46.

[20] V. Akman, An algorithm for determining an opaque minimal forest of a convex polygon, *Inform. Process. Lett.* 24 (1987) 193–198; MR 88d:68094.

[21] P. Dublish, An $O(n^3)$ algorithm for finding the minimal opaque forest of a convex polygon, *Inform. Process. Lett.* 29 (1988) 275–276; MR 90a:68079.

[22] T. Shermer, A counterexample to the algorithms for determining opaque minimal forests, *Inform. Process. Lett.* 40 (1991) 41–42; MR 93e:68134.

[23] I. Bárány and Z. Füredi, Covering all secants of a square, *Intuitive Geometry*, Proc. 1985 Siófok conf., ed. K. Böröczky and G. Fejes Tóth, Colloq. Math. Soc. János Bolyai 48, North-Holland, 1987, pp. 19–27; MR 88h:52020.

[24] W. Kern and A. Wanka, On a problem about covering lines by squares, *Discrete Comput. Geom.* 5 (1990) 77–82; MR 90i:52016.

[25] T. J. Richardson and L. Shepp, The 'point' goalie problem, unpublished note (1997).

[26] V. A. Zalgaller, Shortest inspection lines for a sphere (in Russian), unpublished note (1992).

8.12 Moving Sofa Constant

What is the longest ladder L that can be moved around a right-angled corner in a hallway of unit width? We assume that the ladder is straight and rigid, and that it must remain entirely within the hallway as it is passed through the turn. (All discussion throughout this essay will be constrained to the two-dimensional setting; see Figure 8.12.) The answer to the question is easy: L has the same length as the shortest line segment ab intersecting the point c, which is clearly $2\sqrt{2}$ [1].

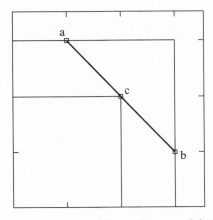

Figure 8.12. This is the optimal ladder passing around the hallway corner.

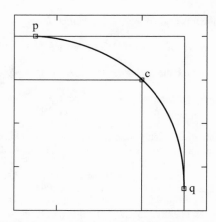

Figure 8.13. This is the optimal wire passing around the hallway corner.

Here is another question: If W is a connected, rigid piece of wire that can be moved around the corner, how large can the diameter of W be? The **diameter** of any continuously differentiable curve is defined to be the maximum of all distances $|x - y|$ between points x and y on the curve. If W is not at all bent, then this reduces to the ladder problem. The largest diameter turns out to be $2(1 + \sqrt{2})$ (see Figure 8.13). The best curve W is the unique quarter-circle pq intersecting the point c [2].

Here is a more difficult problem: What is the greatest possible area for a sofa S that can be moved around the corner [3–5]? We assume only that S is a connected region of the plane. Hammersley [6] showed that the largest area is at least $\pi/2 + 2/\pi = 2.2074\ldots$ (see Figure 8.14) but, contrary to intuition, his region is not optimal.

Gerver (and, independently, Logan) constructed a certain sofa, with complicated boundaries, that possesses a larger area than any other so far examined [7, 8]. (See

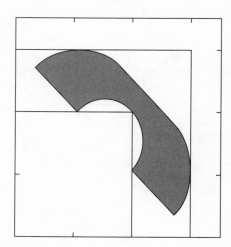

Figure 8.14. Hammersley's sofa consists of two quarter-circles on either side of a $1 \times 4/\pi$ rectangle from which a semicircle of radius $2/\pi$ has been removed.

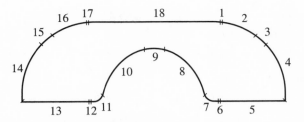

Figure 8.15. The boundary of Gerver's conjectured optimal sofa has eighteen separate pieces.

Figure 8.15.) Further, his sofa is *provably* optimal within the class Σ of all sofas S that

- rotate 90° as S moves around the corner, and
- touch the wall first at two points as S starts to rotate, then at four points, then at three points (when S has rotated 45°), then at four points again, and then at two points again as S finishes rotating.

It would be very surprising if a larger sofa could be found, because it could not be in Σ.

What is the area of Gerver's sofa? To answer this question, first compute constants A, B, φ, and θ via the simultaneous set of four equations

$$A\left(\cos(\theta) - \cos(\varphi)\right) - 2B\sin(\varphi) + (\theta - \varphi - 1)\cos(\theta) - \sin(\theta)$$
$$+ \cos(\varphi) + \sin(\varphi) = 0,$$

$$A\left(3\sin(\theta) + \sin(\varphi)\right) - 2B\cos(\varphi) + 3(\theta - \varphi - 1)\sin(\theta) + 3\cos(\theta)$$
$$- \sin(\varphi) + \cos(\varphi) = 0,$$

$$A\cos(\varphi) - \left(\sin(\varphi) + \frac{1}{2} - \frac{1}{2}\cos(\varphi) + B\sin(\varphi)\right) = 0,$$

$$\left(A + \frac{\pi}{2} - \varphi - \theta\right) - \left(B - \frac{1}{2}(\theta - \varphi)(1 + A) - \frac{1}{4}(\theta - \varphi)^2\right) = 0,$$

obtaining $A = 0.0944265608\ldots$, $B = 1.3992037273\ldots$, $\varphi = 0.0391773647\ldots$, and $\theta = 0.6813015093\ldots$. Next, let

$$r(\alpha) = \begin{cases} \frac{1}{2} & \text{if } 0 \leq \alpha < \varphi, \\ \frac{1}{2}(1 + A + \alpha - \varphi) & \text{if } \varphi \leq \alpha < \theta, \\ A + \alpha - \varphi & \text{if } \theta \leq \alpha < \frac{\pi}{2} - \theta, \\ B - \frac{1}{2}(\frac{\pi}{2} - \alpha - \varphi)(1 + A) - \frac{1}{4}(\frac{\pi}{2} - \alpha - \varphi)^2 & \text{if } \frac{\pi}{2} - \theta \leq \alpha < \frac{\pi}{2} - \varphi, \end{cases}$$

$$s(\alpha) = 1 - r(\alpha),$$

$$u(\alpha) = \begin{cases} B - \frac{1}{2}(\alpha - \varphi)(1 + A) - \frac{1}{4}(\alpha - \varphi)^2 & \text{if } \varphi \leq \alpha < \theta, \\ A + \frac{\pi}{2} - \varphi - \alpha & \text{if } \theta \leq \alpha < \frac{\pi}{4}, \end{cases}$$

and let u' denote the derivative of u. Define three functions y_1, y_2, y_3 by

$$y_1(\alpha) = 1 - \int_0^\alpha r(t)\sin(t)\,dt, \quad y_2(\alpha) = 1 - \int_0^\alpha s(t)\sin(t)\,dt,$$

$$y_3(\alpha) = y_2(\alpha) - u(\alpha)\sin(\alpha).$$

Then the area of the optimal sofa is $2.2195316688\ldots$, that is,

$$2\int_0^{\frac{\pi}{2}-\varphi} y_1(\alpha)r(\alpha)\cos(\alpha)\,d\alpha + 2\int_0^\theta y_2(\alpha)s(\alpha)\cos(\alpha)\,d\alpha$$

$$+ 2\int_\varphi^{\frac{\pi}{4}} y_3(\alpha)\left(u(\alpha)\sin(\alpha) - u'(\alpha)\cos(\alpha) - s(\alpha)\cos(\alpha)\right)\,d\alpha.$$

The three integrals represent, respectively, the area under the convex part of the outer boundary, the area over the convex part of the inside boundary, and the area over the concave part of the inside boundary (where the corner of the hallway scrapes against the sofa).

Sommers [9] examined the problem with the additional condition that S is convex, and he numerically determined the optimal area to be $\geq 1.644703\ldots$. Much more is known if S is rectangular, even if the hallway corner is not right-angled and the two corridors are of different widths [10].

This subject is related to motion planning in robotics, specifically, what is known as the piano mover's problem [11]. Given an open subset U in n-dimensional space and two compact subsets C_0 and C_1 of U, where C_1 is derived from C_0 by a continuous motion, is it possible to move C_0 to C_1 while remaining entirely inside U [12–15]?

[1] G. P. Vennebush, Move that sofa!, *Math. Teacher*, v. 95 (2002) n. 2, 92–97.
[2] P. E. Manne and S. R. Finch, A solution to the bent wire problem, *Amer. Math. Monthly* 109 (2002) 750–752.
[3] L. Moser, Moving furniture through a hallway, Problem 66–11, *SIAM Rev.* 8 (1966) 381–382.
[4] N. R. Wagner, The sofa problem, *Amer. Math. Monthly* 83 (1976) 188–189; MR 53 #1422.
[5] H. T. Croft, K. J. Falconer, and R. K. Guy, *Unsolved Problems in Geometry*, Springer-Verlag, 1991, sect. G5; MR 95k:5200.
[6] J. M. Hammersley, On the emfeeblement of mathematical skills by "Modern Mathematics" and by similar soft intellectual trash in schools and universities, *Bull. Inst. Math. Appl.* 4 (1968) 66–85.
[7] J. L. Gerver, On moving a sofa around a corner, *Geom. Dedicata* 42 (1992) 267–283; MR 93d:51040.
[8] I. Stewart, *Another Fine Math You've Got Me Into...*, W. H. Freeman, 1992, pp. 255–269; MR 93i:00003.
[9] J. A. Sommers, The convex sofa problem, unpublished note (2001).
[10] G. Eriksson, H. Eriksson, and K. Eriksson, Moving a food trolley around a corner, *Theoret. Comput. Sci.* 191 (1998) 193–203; MR 98k:68164.

[11] J. H. Davenport, A "piano movers" problem, *SIGSAM Bull.*, v. 20 (1986) n. 1, 15–17.

[12] B. Buchberger, G. E. Collins, and B. Kutzler, Algebraic methods in geometry, *Annual Review of Computer Science*, v. 3, ed. J. F. Traub, B. J. Grosz, B. W. Lampson, and N. J. Nilsson, Annual Reviews Inc., 1988, pp. 85–119; MR 91g:68156.

[13] D. Leven and M. Sharir, An efficient and simple motion planning algorithm for a ladder moving in two-dimensional space amidst polygonal barriers, *J. Algorithms* 8 (1987) 192–215; MR 88h:68035.

[14] E. B. Feinberg and C. H. Papadimitriou, Finding feasible points for a two-point body, *J. Algorithms* 10 (1989) 109–119; MR 90b:68099.

[15] M.-F. Roy, Géométrie algébrique réelle et robotique: La complexité du déménagement des pianos, *Gazette Math. (Paris)* 51 (1992) 75–96; MR 93f:93090.

8.13 Calabi's Triangle Constant

Let T denote an equilateral triangle. There are clearly three congruent largest squares that can be wedged within T (see Figure 8.16). Do there exist non-equilateral triangles with this property? One would at first expect the answer to be no; for example, a right triangle U always has a unique largest square wedged within U, namely, the square with sides aligned with the perpendicular legs of U.

Calabi examined the question and found an answer defying expectation [1, 2]: A non-equilateral triangle with three congruent largest squares *does* exist and is unique (see Figure 8.17). It is an isosceles triangle and, if AB is the triangular base and $AC = BC$, then the ratio

$$\frac{AB}{AC} = 2\cos(\alpha) = 1.5513875245\ldots$$

is algebraic with minimal polynomial $2x^3 - 2x^2 - 3x + 2$. Also, the angle α at vertex A is given by

$$\alpha = 0.6829826991\ldots \sim 39.13°.$$

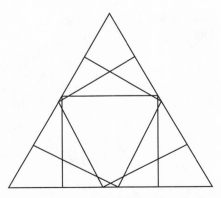

Figure 8.16. An equilateral triangle with three distinct inscribed squares of maximal size.

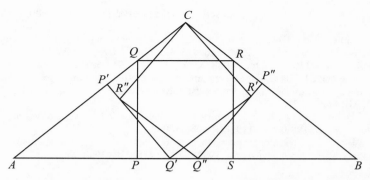

Figure 8.17. A non-equilateral triangle with three distinct inscribed squares of maximal size.

Further related research was conducted by Wetzel [3,4]. Here is an unresolved issue: What is the three-dimensional tetrahedral analog of this result?

[1] J. H. Conway and R. K. Guy, *The Book of Numbers*, Springer-Verlag, 1996, p. 206; MR 98g:00004.
[2] E. Calabi, Outline of proof regarding squares wedged in triangle, unpublished note (1997).
[3] J. E. Wetzel, Squares in triangles, *Math. Gazette* 86 (2002) 28–34.
[4] J. E. Wetzel, Rectangles in triangles, submitted (2001).

8.14 DeVicci's Tesseract Constant

How large a square can be inscribed within a unit cube? This is known as **Prince Rupert's problem**. More generally, how large an m-dimensional cube can be inscribed within a unit n-dimensional cube, where $m < n$?

Let $f(m, n)$ be the edge-length of the optimal m-cube. Clearly $f(1, n) = \sqrt{n}$ for all n. Figure 8.18 suggests that

$$f(2, 3) = \frac{3}{4}\sqrt{2} = 1.0606601717\ldots,$$

and this result has been known for a long time to be true [1–4].

DeVicci [5] proved that

$$f(m, n) = \sqrt{\frac{n}{m}} \text{ if } m \text{ divides } n, \quad f(2, n) = \begin{cases} \sqrt{\dfrac{n}{2}} & \text{if } n \text{ is even,} \\[2mm] \sqrt{\dfrac{4n - 3}{8}} & \text{if } n \text{ is odd.} \end{cases}$$

An elaborate argument gives that [5]

$$f(3, 4) = 1.0074347569\ldots,$$

which has minimal polynomial $4x^8 - 28x^6 - 7x^4 + 16x^2 + 16$. In fact, $f(3, 4)$ is solvable in radicals. Since the name *tesseract* is often used [7] to refer to the 4-cube, we call

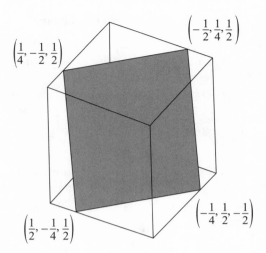

Figure 8.18. The 3-cube with corners at $(\pm 1/2, \pm 1/2, \pm 1/2)$, along with the largest inscribed square.

$f(3, 4)$ **DeVicci's tesseract constant**. According to Gardner [8, 9], the list of people who numerically anticipated this result includes Baer, Bosch, and de Josselin de Jong.

Huber [10] determined more exact evaluations of $f(m, n)$, for example,

$$f(3, 5) = \sqrt{11 - 4\sqrt{6}} = 1.0963763171\ldots.$$

It is known that $f(m, n)$ is always an algebraic number [6]. Might the degree of the corresponding minimal polynomial follow some recognizable function of m and n?

The same problem for maximal rectangles with fixed aspect ratio (instead of squares) in cubes has been comparatively neglected until recently [11].

[1] H. T. Croft, K. J. Falconer, and R. K. Guy, *Unsolved Problems in Geometry*, Springer-Verlag, 1991, sect. B4; MR 95k:52001.
[2] D. J. E. Schrek, Prince Rupert's problem and its extension by Pieter Nieuwland, *Scripta Math.* 16 (1950) 73–80, 261–267.
[3] D. Wells, *The Penguin Dictionary of Curious and Interesting Numbers*, Penguin, 1986, p. 33.
[4] J. G. Mauldon and R. J. Chapman, A variant of Prince Rupert's problem, *Amer. Math. Monthly* 102 (1995) 465–467.
[5] K. R. DeVicci, Largest m-cube in an n-cube, unpublished manuscript (1996).
[6] R. K. Guy and R. J. Nowakowski, Monthly unsolved problems, 1969-1997, *Amer. Math. Monthly* 104 (1997) 967–968.
[7] M. L'Engle, *A Wrinkle in Time*, Dell, 1962.
[8] M. Gardner, Hypercubes, *Sci. Amer.*, v. 215 (1966) n. 5, 138–145 and v. 215 (1966) n. 6, 131–132.
[9] M. Gardner, *The Colossal Book of Mathematics*, W. W. Norton, 2001, pp. 162–174.
[10] G. Huber, Cubing the square: A progress report on the Rupert problems, unpublished note (1999).
[11] R. P. Jerrard and J. E. Wetzel, Prince Rupert's rectangles, submitted (2002).

8.15 Graham's Hexagon Constant

Let P denote an n-sided convex polygon in the plane. Assume that P is of unit diameter, equivalently, that the maximum distance between any two vertices of P is 1. What is the largest possible area, F_n, enclosed by P?

Clearly $F_3 = \sqrt{3}/4 = 0.4330127018\ldots$ and this is achieved uniquely by the equilateral triangle with unit sides. More generally, we have upper and lower bounds

$$\frac{n}{8} \sin\left(\frac{2\pi}{n}\right) \le F_n \le \frac{n}{2} \cos\left(\frac{\pi}{n}\right) \tan\left(\frac{\pi}{2n}\right)$$

valid for all n. Reinhardt [1] proved that the right-hand inequality becomes equality for all odd n, and that this is achieved uniquely by the regular n-gon of unit diameter. One would naively expect the left-hand inequality to become equality for even n, with a similar uniqueness result.

If $n = 4$, the left-hand inequality becomes equality. In all other respects, the situation for even n is unexpected. $F_4 = 1/2$ is achieved not only by the unit square, but by an infinite family of quadrilaterals of unit diameter. So uniqueness fails for $n = 4$. Interestingly, uniqueness holds for $n = 6$. It is not known whether uniqueness also holds for $n = 8, 10, 12, \ldots$.

Let us focus on the case $n = 6$. The regular hexagon of unit diameter has area

$$\frac{n}{8} \sin\left(\frac{2\pi}{n}\right)\bigg|_{n=6} = \frac{3\sqrt{3}}{8} = 0.6495190528\ldots.$$

Graham [2–5] proved the surprising result that this is *not* optimal. He constructed a hexagon of unit diameter that has area $F_6 = 0.6749814429\ldots$, an algebraic number with minimal polynomial

$$4096x^{10} + 8192x^9 - 3008x^8 - 30848x^7 + 21056x^6 + 146496x^5$$
$$- 221360x^4 + 1232x^3 + 144464x^2 - 78488x + 11993$$

(see Figure 8.19).

What can be said about the maximum area for a unit-diameter octagon ($n = 8$)? Briggs, Prieto, Vanderbei, Wright, Gay, and others obtained $F_8 = 0.726868\ldots$ via numerical global optimization techniques. More recently, Audet et al. [6] proved a conjecture of Graham's on the shape of the optimal octagon via a quadratic programming scheme; the corresponding minimal polynomial still remains an open question.

No exact results are known for the decagon ($n = 10$) or the dodecagon ($n = 12$), but numerical estimates are $F_{10} = 0.749137\ldots$ and $F_{12} = 0.760729\ldots$, respectively. Perimeters can be maximized rather than areas [7]. Not much is known about higher dimensions: We know the largest volumes of d-dimensional convex polyhedra with $d + 2$ vertices [8], but cases involving $> d + 2$ vertices evidently remain unsolved.

[1] K. Reinhardt, Extremale Polygone gegebenen Durchmessers, *Jahresbericht Deutsch. Math.-Verein.* 31 (1922) 251–270.
[2] R. L. Graham, The largest small hexagon, *J. Combin. Theory Ser. A* 18 (1975) 165–170; MR 50 #12803.

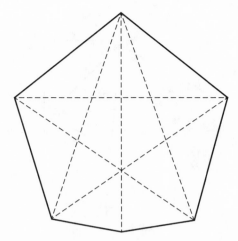

Figure 8.19. Graham's hexagon is the optimal hexagon (meaning it has maximum area) of unit diameter.

[3] J. H. Conway and R. K. Guy, *The Book of Numbers*, Springer-Verlag, 1996, pp. 206–207; MR 98g:00004.
[4] R. K. Guy and J. L. Selfridge, Optimal coverings of the square, *Infinite and Finite Sets*, Proc. 1973 Keszthely conf., ed. A. Hajnal, R. Rado, and V. T. Sós, Colloq. Math. Soc. János Bolyai 10, North-Holland, 1975, pp. 745–799; MR 51 #13873.
[5] H. T. Croft, K. J. Falconer, and R. K. Guy, *Unsolved Problems in Geometry*, Springer-Verlag, 1991, sect. B6; MR 95k:52001.
[6] C. Audet, P. Hansen, F. Messine, and J. Xiong, The largest small octagon, *J. Combin. Theory Ser. A* 98 (2002) 46–59.
[7] N. K. Tamvakis, On the perimeter and the area of the convex polygons of a given diameter, *Bull. Soc. Math. Grèce* 28 A (1987) 115–132; MR 89g:52008.
[8] B. Kind and P. Kleinschmidt, On the maximal volume of convex bodies with few vertices, *J. Combin. Theory Ser. A* 21 (1976) 124–128; MR 53 #11500.

8.16 Heilbronn Triangle Constants

The nth **Heilbronn triangle constant** is the infimum of all numbers H_n for which the following holds [1]: Given any arrangement of n points in the unit square, the smallest triangle formed by any three of the points has area $\leq H_n$.

Goldberg [2] considered the exact values of the first several Heilbronn constants, including $H_3 = H_4 = 1/2 = 0.5$ and made several conjectures. Yang, Zhang & Zeng [3,4] disproved one of the conjectures by showing that $H_5 = \sqrt{3}/9 = 0.1924500897\ldots$ but confirmed Goldberg's assertion that $H_6 = 1/8 = 0.125$. See Figures 8.20 and 8.21. It is also known that $H_7 \geq 0.0838590090\ldots$, where the lower bound has minimal polynomial $152x^3 + 12x^2 - 14x + 1 = 0$, and [5]

$$H_8 \geq \frac{\sqrt{13}-1}{36} = 0.0723764243\ldots, \quad H_9 \geq \frac{9\sqrt{65}-55}{320} = 0.0548759991\ldots.$$

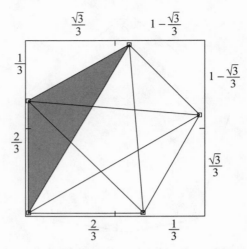

Figure 8.20. The best arrangement of points corresponding to $n = 5$.

Comellas & Yebra [5] expressed confidence that these bounds very likely are optimal, but acknowledged that there is (as yet) no proof of this.

What can be said about the asymptotics of H_n? Heilbronn conjectured in 1950 that $H_n = O(n^{-2})$ as $n \to \infty$. Roth, Schmidt, and others made progress toward proving this by showing that [6, 7]

$$H_n = O(n^{-\frac{8}{7}+\varepsilon})$$

for all sufficiently large n, for any $\varepsilon > 0$. Komlós, Pintz & Szemerédi, however, disproved Heilbronn's conjecture by demonstrating that there exists a constant $c > 0$ for

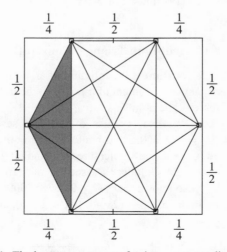

Figure 8.21. The best arrangement of points corresponding to $n = 6$.

which [8]

$$\frac{c \ln(n)}{n^2} \leq H_n$$

for large enough n. Their proof was highly nonconstructive. A recent alternative proof of the lower bound [9] gives a polynomial-time algorithm for finding a configuration of n points where all triangles have area $\geq c \ln(n)/n^2$, for each n. With regard to the upper bound, can the exponent $8/7$ be replaced by 2? This is a difficult question and no one expects a complete answer soon.

Jiang, Li & Vitányi [10, 11] analyzed the average-case scenario (rather than the worst-case one), given n uniformly distributed points in the unit square, and found that the smallest triangle has expected area between $a\,n^{-3}$ and $b\,n^{-3}$ for some constants $0 < a < b$. A study of a higher dimensional analog of Heilbronn's problem was undertaken in [12, 13].

If we replace the unit square in the definition of H_n by an equilateral triangle of unit area, then $\tilde{H}_3 = 1$, $\tilde{H}_4 = 1/3$, $\tilde{H}_5 = 3 - 2\sqrt{2}$, and $\tilde{H}_6 = 1/8$ [14]. In fact, we need not specify that the domain be equilateral, since $\tilde{H}_n$ is independent of the shape of the unit triangle under consideration [6]. Moreover, the asymptotics discussed earlier actually apply (within a constant factor) to the general case of n points sitting in a compact convex domain in the plane.

Here is a vaguely related problem. Suppose the unit square is partitioned into m connected sets. Let d be the maximum of the diameters of the m sets. What is the minimum possible value of d [15–19]? For example, if $m = 3$, then $d = \sqrt{65}/8 = 1.0077822185\ldots$.

Another problem is reminiscent of Dirichlet–Voronoi cells and other geometric close-proximity questions. How should k points be arranged inside a unit square to minimize the average distance in the square to the nearest of the k points [20–26]? As $k \to \infty$, the k points approach the vertices of a regular hexagonal lattice. There are many variations. We mention finally that the problem of packing l disks in a unit square is the same as determining the greatest possible minimum distance between l points in the square [8.2].

[1] R. K. Guy, *Unsolved Problems in Number Theory*, 2nd ed., Springer-Verlag, 1994, sect. F4; MR 96e:11002.

[2] M. Goldberg, Maximizing the smallest triangle made by N points in a square, *Math. Mag.* 45 (1972) 135–144; MR 45 #5875.

[3] L. Yang, J. Z. Zhang, and Z. B. Zeng, Heilbronn problem for five points, Int. Centre Theoret. Physics preprint IC/91/252 (1991).

[4] L. Yang, J. Z. Zhang, and Z. B. Zeng, A conjecture on the first several Heilbronn numbers and a computation (in Chinese), *Chinese Annals Math. Ser. A* 13 (1992) 503–515; MR 93i:51045.

[5] F. Comellas and J. L. A. Yebra, New lower bounds for Heilbronn numbers, *Elec. J. Combin.* 9 (2002) R6.

[6] K. F. Roth, Developments in Heilbronn's triangle problem, *Adv. Math.* 22 (1976) 364–385; MR 55 #2771.

[7] J. Komlós, J. Pintz, and E. Szemerédi, On Heilbronn's triangle problem, *J. London Math. Soc.* 24 (1981) 385–396; MR 82m:10051.

[8]   J. Komlós, J. Pintz, and E. Szemerédi, A lower bound for Heilbronn's problem, *J. London Math. Soc.* 25 (1982) 13–24; MR 83i:10042.

[9]   C. Bertram-Kretzberg, T. Hofmeister, and H. Lefmann, An algorithm for Heilbronn's problem, *SIAM J. Comput.* 30 (2000) 383–390; also in *Proc. 3rd Computing and Combinatorics Conf.* (COCOON), Shanghai, 1997, ed. T. Jiang and D. T. Lee, Lect. Notes in Comp. Sci. 1276, Springer-Verlag, 1997, pp. 23–31; MR 2001b:05200.

[10] T. Jiang, M. Li, and P. Vitányi, The expected size of Heilbronn's triangles, *Proc. 14th IEEE Conf. on Computational Complexity (CCC)*, Atlanta, 1999, IEEE, pp. 105–113; math.CO/9902043.

[11] T. Jiang, M. Li, and P. Vitányi, The average-case area of Heilbronn-type triangles, *Random Structures Algorithms* 20 (2002) 206–219.

[12] G. Barequet, A lower bound for Heilbronn's triangle problem in *d* dimensions, *SIAM J. Discrete Math.* 14 (2001) 230–236; also in *Proc. 10th ACM-SIAM Symp. on Discrete Algorithms (SODA)*, Baltimore, ACM, 1999, pp. 76–81; MR 2002h:05159.

[13] G. Barequet, A duality between small-face problems in arrangements of lines and Heilbronn-type problems, *Discrete Math.* 237 (2001) 1–12; MR 2002c:52032.

[14] L. Yang, J. Z. Zhang, and Z. B. Zeng, On the Heilbronn numbers of triangular regions (in Chinese), *Acta Math. Sinica* 37 (1994) 678–689; MR 95k:52014.

[15] J. Lipman, Covering a square, *Amer. Math. Monthly* 65 (1958) 775.

[16] C. S. Ogilvy, *Tomorrow's Math: Unsolved Problems for the Amateur*, Oxford Univ. Press, 1962, pp. 20–21, 146–147.

[17] R. Honsberger, On sets of points in the plane, *Two Year College Math. J.* 11 (1980) 116–117.

[18] C. H. Jepsen, Coloring points in the unit square, *College Math. J.* 17 (1986) 231–237.

[19] R. K. Guy and J. L. Selfridge, Optimal coverings of the square, *Infinite and Finite Sets*, Proc. 1973 Keszthely conf., ed. A. Hajnal, R. Rado, and V. T. Sós, Colloq. Math. Soc. János Bolyai 10, North-Holland, 1975, pp. 745–799; MR 51 #13873.

[20] L. Fejes Tóth, The isepiphan problem for *n*-hedra, *Amer. J. Math.* 70 (1948) 174–180; MR 9,460f.

[21] L. Fejes Tóth, *Lagerungen in der Ebene auf der Kugel und im Raum*, Springer-Verlag, 1972; MR 50 #5603.

[22] B. Bollobás and N. Stern, The optimal structure of market areas, *J. Econom. Theory* 4 (1972) 174–179; MR 57 #8996.

[23] C. H. Papadimitriou, Worst-case and probabilistic analysis of a geometric location problem, *SIAM J. Comput.* 10 (1981) 542–557; MR 82h:90039.

[24] P. M. Gruber, A short analytic proof of Fejes Tóth's theorem on sums of moments, *Aequationes Math.* 58 (1999) 291–295; MR 2000j:52012.

[25] P. M. Gruber, Optimal configurations of finite sets in Riemannian 2-manifolds, *Geom. Dedicata* 84 (2001) 271–320; MR 2002f:52017.

[26] F. Morgan and R. Bolton, Hexagonal economic regions solve the location problem, *Amer. Math. Monthly* 109 (2002) 165–172.

8.17 Kakeya–Besicovitch Constants

A region R in the plane is a **Kakeya region** if, inside R, a line segment of unit length can be **reversed**, that is, maneuvered continuously and without leaving R to reach its original position but rotated through $180°$. Kakeya [1] asked what the least possible area of such a region R might be.

Let

$$K = \inf_{R \text{ Kakeya}} \text{area}(R),$$

where the infimum extends over all Kakeya regions. Besicovitch [2, 3] proved the astonishing result that $K = 0$, which is to say that unit line segments can be reversed within regions of arbitrarily small area. His proof used highly multiply connected regions (i.e., with many holes) that are unbounded (i.e., with large diameters). People wondered if such complicated regions were truly necessary and what the effect of further restrictions on R might be [4–7].

Van Alphen [8] proved that $K = 0$ if R is restricted to fall within a circle of radius $2 + \varepsilon$, for any $\varepsilon > 0$. So boundedness is not an issue. Later, Cunningham [9] proved that $K = 0$ even if R is simply connected (i.e., with no holes) and falls within a circle of radius 1. So even the absence of holes is not an issue. These are remarkably intricate results and explanations of their significance outside geometry may be found in [10–13].

Different restrictions give rise to different results. Let

$$K_c = \inf_{\substack{R \text{ convex} \\ \text{Kakeya}}} \text{area}(R)$$

(meaning that, for any two points $P, Q \in R$, the line segment $PQ \subseteq R$) and

$$K_s = \inf_{\substack{R \text{ star-shaped} \\ \text{Kakeya}}} \text{area}(R)$$

(meaning that there is a point $O \in R$ such that, for any point $P \in R$, the line segment $OP \subseteq R$). Pál [14] proved that

$$K_c = \frac{\sqrt{3}}{3} = 0.5773502691\ldots,$$

which corresponds to the equilateral triangle of height 1.

In contrast, Bloom, Schoenberg & Cunningham [6, 9, 15] proved that

$$0.0290888208\ldots = \frac{\pi}{108} \le K_s \le \frac{5 - 2\sqrt{2}}{24}\pi = 0.2842582246\ldots$$
$$= (0.0904822031\ldots)\pi,$$

and Schoenberg further conjectured that K_s is equal to its upper bound. This evidently remains an open problem.

[1] S. Kakeya, Some problems on maxima and minima regarding ovals, *Science Reports, Tôhoku Imperial Univ.* 6 (1917) 71–88.

[2] A. S. Besicovitch, On Kakeya's problem and a similar one, *Math. Z.* 27 (1928) 312–320.

[3] A. S. Besicovitch, The Kakeya problem, *Amer. Math. Monthly* 70 (1963) 697–706; MR 28 #502.

[4] H. T. Croft, K. J. Falconer, and R. K. Guy, *Unsolved Problems in Geometry*, Springer-Verlag, 1991, sect. G6; MR 95k:52001.

[5] H. Meschkowski, *Unsolved and Unsolvable Problems in Geometry*, Oliver and Boyd, 1966, pp. 103–109; MR 35 #7206.

[6] I. J. Schoenberg, On the Kakeya-Besicovitch problem, *Mathematical Time Exposures*, Math. Assoc. Amer., 1982, pp. 168–184; MR 85b:00001.

[7] K. J. Falconer, *The Geometry of Fractal Sets*, Cambridge Univ. Press, 1985, pp. 95–109; MR 88d:28001.

[8]   H. J. van Alphen, Generalization of a theorem of Besicovitsch (in Dutch), *Mathematica, Zutphen B* 10 (1942) 144–157; MR 7,320b.

[9]   F. Cunningham, The Kakeya problem for simply connected and for star-shaped sets, *Amer. Math. Monthly* 78 (1971) 114–129; MR 43 #1044.

[10] T. Wolff, Recent work connected with the Kakeya problem, *Prospects in Mathematics*, Proc. 1996 Princeton conf., ed. H. Rossi, Amer. Math. Soc., 1999, pp. 129–162; MR 2000d:42010.

[11] J. Bourgain, Harmonic analysis and combinatorics: How much may they contribute to each other?, *Mathematics: Frontiers and Perspectives*, ed. V. Arnold, M. Atiyah, P. Lax, and B. Mazur, Amer. Math. Soc., 2000, pp. 13–32; MR 2001c:42009.

[12] T. Tao, From rotating needles to stability of waves: Emerging connections between combinatorics, analysis, and PDE, *Notices Amer. Math. Soc.* 48 (2001) 294–303; amplification 566; commentary 678; MR 2002b:42021.

[13] N. Katz and T. Tao, Recent progress on the Kakeya conjecture, *Proc. 6th Conf. on Harmonic Analysis and Partial Differential Equations*, El Escorial, *Publicacions Matèmatiques* Extra Volume (2002) 161–179; math.CA/0010069.

[14] J. Pál, Ein minimumprobleme für ovale, *Math. Annalen* 83 (1921) 311–319.

[15] F. Cunningham and I. J. Schoenberg, On the Kakeya constant, *Canad. J. Math.* 17 (1965) 946–956; MR 31 #6163.

8.18 Rectilinear Crossing Constant

Let G be a graph [5.6]. A **rectilinear drawing** is a mapping of G into the plane with the property that vertices go to distinct points and edges go to straight line segments. Over all possible such drawings of G, determine one with the minimum number, $\bar{v}(G)$, of crossings of edges in the plane. Call $\bar{v}(G)$ the **rectilinear crossing number** of G [1–4].

For the complete graph K_n, with n vertices and all $\binom{n}{2}$ possible edges, the known values of and bounds on $\bar{v}(K_n)$ are listed in Tables 8.7 and 8.8 [5–8].

Asymptotically, we have [8,9]

$$0.311507 < \rho = \lim_{n \to \infty} \frac{\bar{v}(K_n)}{\binom{n}{4}} = \sup_n \frac{\bar{v}(K_n)}{\binom{n}{4}} \le \frac{6467}{16848} < 0.383844.$$

An exact value for ρ is unknown.

Here is a seemingly unconnected problem, due to Sylvester [10], from geometric probability. Let R be an open convex set in the plane with finite area. Randomly choose four points independently and uniformly in R. With probability 1, no three of the points are collinear, so the convex hull of the four points is either a triangle (one point in the convex hull of the other three) or a quadrilateral. Let $q(R)$ denote the probability that the convex hull is a quadrilateral. Sylvester asked for the minimum and maximum values of $q(R)$ over all convex sets R in the plane.

Table 8.7.   *Values of* $\bar{v}(K_n)$

n	4	5	6	7	8	9	10	11	12
$\bar{v}(K_n)$	0	1	3	9	19	36	62	102	153

Table 8.8. *Bounds on $\bar{v}(K_n)$*

n	13	14	15
Upper Bound	229	324	447
Lower Bound	221	310	423

Blaschke [11, 12] proved that the maximum of $q(R)$ is

$$1 - \frac{35}{12\pi^2} = 0.7044798810\ldots,$$

which is achieved when R is an ellipse, and the minimum is $2/3$, attained when R is a triangle. See [13–21] for details and related problems.

If we relax the conditions on R, what corresponding results hold? Let R be an open set in the plane with finite area (i.e., convexity is no longer required). Define $q(R)$ as before. Then clearly $\sup_R q(R) = 1$ since we may take R to be a very thin annulus, in which four randomly selected points will almost surely span a quadrilateral.

The infimum of $q(R)$ is more difficult to study. Scheinerman & Wilf [22, 23] proved the remarkable fact that

$$\inf_R q(R) = \rho,$$

thus relating two seemingly unconnected constants. With its heightened status, ρ perhaps will attract the attention necessary for it someday to be computed.

We have discussed rectilinear drawings; by way of contrast, **ordinary drawings** permit curved edges that lead to the **ordinary crossing number** $v(G)$. In this case, Guy [1] conjectured that

$$v(K_n) = \frac{1}{4} \left\lfloor \frac{n}{2} \right\rfloor \left\lfloor \frac{n-1}{2} \right\rfloor \left\lfloor \frac{n-2}{2} \right\rfloor \left\lfloor \frac{n-3}{2} \right\rfloor,$$

and this has been confirmed for $n \leq 12$ [24]. No analogous conjectured formula is known for $\bar{v}(K_n)$. It is believed that $\bar{v}(K_n) > v(K_n)$ for sufficiently large n [25].

There are several related notions of the *thickness* of a graph; see [25, 26] for definitions and references. Many fundamental constants like ρ apparently exist in geometric probability (in the older literature, under what was once called *integral geometry*), yet are extremely difficult to calculate.

[1] P. Erdös and R. K. Guy, Crossing number problems, *Amer. Math. Monthly* 80 (1973) 52–57; MR 52 #2894.
[2] A. T. White and L. W. Beineke, Topological graph theory, *Selected Topics in Graph Theory*, ed. L. W. Beineke and R. J. Wilson, Academic Press, 1978, pp. 15–49; MR 81e:05059.
[3] M. Gardner, *Knotted Doughnuts and Other Mathematical Entertainments*, W. H. Freeman, 1986, pp. 133–144; MR 87g:00007.
[4] N. J. A. Sloane, On-Line Encyclopedia of Integer Sequences, A000241 and A014540.
[5] D. Singer, The rectilinear crossing number of certain graphs, unpublished manuscript (1971).
[6] W. D. Smith, *Studies in Computational Geometry Motivated by Mesh Generation*, Ph.D. thesis, Princeton Univ., 1988.

[7] A. Brodsky, S. Durocher, and E. Gethner, The rectilinear crossing number of K_{10} is 62, *Elec. J. Combin.* 8 (2001) R23; cs.DM/0009023; MR 2002f:05058.

[8] O. Aichholzer, F. Aurenhammer, and H. Krasser, Progress on rectilinear crossing numbers, Institut für Grundlagen der Informationsverarbeitung report, Technische Universität Graz (2002).

[9] A. Brodsky, S. Durocher, and E. Gethner, Toward the rectilinear crossing number of K_n: New drawings, upper bounds, and asymptotics, *Discrete Math.* to appear; cs.DM/0009028.

[10] J. J. Sylvester, On a special class of questions on the theory of probabilities, *Birmingham British Assoc. Report* 35 (1865) 8–9; also in *Collected Mathematical Papers*, v. 2, ed. H. F. Baker, Cambridge Univ. Press, 1904, pp. 480–481.

[11] W. J. E. Blaschke, Über affine Geometrie. XI: Lösung des Vierpunktproblems von Sylvester aus der Theorie der geometrischen Wahrscheinlichkeiten, *Berichte über die Verhandlungen der Königlich Sächsischen Gesellschaft der Wissenschaften zu Leipzig, Math.-Phys. Klasse* 69 (1917) 436–453.

[12] W. J. E. Blaschke, *Vorlesungen über Differential-geometrie. II: Affine Differential-geometrie*, Springer-Verlag, 1923.

[13] M. G. Kendall and P. A. P. Moran, *Geometrical Probability*, Hafner, 1963, pp. 42–46; MR 30 #4275.

[14] V. Klee, What is the expected volume of a simplex whose vertices are chosen at random from a given convex body?, *Amer. Math. Monthly* 76 (1969) 286–288.

[15] W. J. Reeds, Random points in a simplex, *Pacific J. Math.* 54 (1974) 183–198; MR 51 #8959.

[16] L. A. Santaló, *Integral Geometry and Geometric Probability*, Addison-Wesley, 1976, pp. 63–65; MR 55 #6340.

[17] H. Solomon, *Geometric Probability*, SIAM, 1978, pp. 101–125; MR 58 #7777.

[18] R. E. Pfiefer, The historical development of J. J. Sylvester's problem, *Math. Mag.* 62 (1989) 309–317.

[19] H. T. Croft, K. J. Falconer, and R. K. Guy, *Unsolved Problems in Geometry*, Springer-Verlag, 1991, sect. B5; MR 95k:52001.

[20] N. Peyerimhoff, Areas and intersections in convex domains, *Amer. Math. Monthly* 104 (1997) 697–704; MR 98g:52009.

[21] A. M. Mathai, *An Introduction to Geometrical Probability: Distributional Aspects with Applications*, Gordon and Breach, 1999, pp. 159–171; MR 2001a:60014.

[22] E. R. Scheinerman and H. S. Wilf, The rectilinear crossing number of a complete graph and Sylvester's "Four Point Problem" of geometric probability, *Amer. Math. Monthly* 101 (1994) 939–943; MR 95k:52006.

[23] H. S. Wilf, Some crossing numbers, and some unsolved problems, *Combinatorics, Geometry and Probability: A Tribute to Paul Erdös*, Proc. 1993 Trinity College conf., ed. B. Bollobás and A. Thomason, Cambridge Univ. Press, 1997; MR 98d:00027.

[24] D. Applegate, W. Cook, S. Dash, and N. Dean, Ordinary crossing numbers for K_{11} and K_{12}, unpublished note (2001).

[25] C. Thomassen, Embeddings and minors, *Handbook of Combinatorics*, v. I, ed. R. Graham, M. Grötschel, and L. Lovász, MIT Press, 1995, pp. 301–349; MR 97a:05075.

[26] M. B. Dillencourt, D. Eppstein, and D. S. Hirschberg, Geometric thickness of complete graphs, *Graph Drawing*, Proc. 1998 Montréal conf., ed. S. H. Whitesides, Lect. Notes in Comp. Sci. 1547, Springer-Verlag, 1998, pp. 102–110; math.CO/9910185; MR 2000g:68118.

8.19 Circumradius-Inradius Constants

The **circumradius** $R(K)$ of a planar compact convex set K is the radius of the smallest disk that contains K, and the **inradius** $r(K)$ is the radius of the largest disk contained by K. Formulas for R and r corresponding to well-known sets appear in [1–3]. Interesting constants involving R or r emerge in various geometric optimization problems over families of sets; we will give three examples out of potentially many.

Consider all triangles Δ that lie in a compact convex set F of width 1. (The **width** of F is the minimum over lengths of all orthogonal projections of F onto lines.) Let us examine the maximum inradius $a(F) = \max_\Delta r(\Delta)$ over all such triangles for several special sets F:

- If F_4 is the square of width 1 (i.e., of side 1), then [4, 5]

$$a(F_4) = \frac{-1 + \sqrt{5}}{4} = 0.3090169943\ldots.$$

- If F_5 is the regular pentagon of width 1 (i.e., of side $2\cot(2\pi)/5$), then

$$a(F_5) = 0.2440155280\ldots,$$

which has minimal polynomial [6, 7]

$$5x^9 - 170x^8 + 436x^7 - 205x^6 - 96x^5 + 440x^4 - 120x^3 + 64x^2 - 80x + 16.$$

- If F_6 is the regular hexagon of width 1 (i.e., of side $1/\sqrt{3}$), then

$$a(F_6) = \frac{1}{4} = 0.25.$$

Note that $a(F_5) < \min\{a(F_4), a(F_6)\}$. In fact, it is known that [8]

$$0.166 < \frac{1}{6} \leq \inf_F a(F) \leq a(F_5),$$

where the infimum is taken over arbitrary F. Might this infimum actually be equal to its upper bound? This is an unsolved problem.

For the following, we require some notation. Let S denote the square with vertices $(\pm 1, \pm 1)$ and let $h_1, h_2, \ldots, h_8$ denote its half-edges (proceeding counterclockwise). Given a nonvertical line L passing through $(0, 0)$, let L^+ denote the half-line in the right half-plane and let L^- denote the half-line in the left half-plane. Let us agree that L^+ intercepts h_i and L^- intercepts h_j, where $i \equiv j \bmod 4$. Define M^+ to be a third half-line passing through $(0, 0)$ that intercepts h_k, where $k \neq i$ and $k \neq j$; we say that M^+ is **suitably distinct** from L. Finally, let Z denote the standard integer lattice in the plane, that is, with basis vectors $(1, 0)$ and $(0, 1)$.

Consider all compact convex sets G whose interiors contain the origin but no other lattice points. (In the language of [2.23], G is Z-**allowable**.) Assume further that the circumcenter of G is at the origin, that its corresponding circumcircle is C, and that for any line L passing through $(0, 0)$, we cannot have both $G \cap L^+ \cap C \neq \emptyset$ and $G \cap L^- \cap C \neq \emptyset$ unless there exists a suitably distinct half-line M^+ for which $G \cap M^+ \cap C \neq \emptyset$. (In words, G does not protrude outside S simultaneously in opposite directions unless it protrudes significantly elsewhere too.) Then [9]

$$\sup_G R(G) = 1.6847127097\ldots,$$

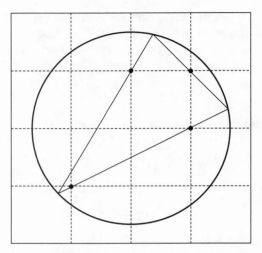

Figure 8.22. This Z-admissible triangle T has maximal circumradius $R(T) = 1.6847127097\ldots$.

which has minimal polynomial $5x^6 - 15x^4 + 3x^2 - 2$. A set with maximal circumradius is the non-isosceles triangle T shown in Figure 8.22. If we did not impose the technical condition regarding L^+, L^-, and M^+, then the supremum would be infinite (imagine a thin plank of width ε and length $1/\varepsilon$, passing through the origin and avoiding all nonzero lattice points).

Here is a result that relates the circumcenter of a compact convex set K with its centroid (i.e., center of gravity). Let $b(K)$ denote the distance between the circumcenter and the centroid, divided by $R(K)$. Clearly $\inf_K b(K) = 0$, for consider a disk or an equilateral triangle. It is known that [10]

$$\sup_K b(K) = \frac{2}{3}x = 0.4278733971\ldots,$$

where x is the unique solution of the transcendental equation

$$x^2 + 2\sqrt{1 - x^2} = 2x(x + \arccos(x)), \quad -1 \leq x \leq 1.$$

The extremal set is, in this case, a certain symmetric trapezoid with one of its parallel edges replaced by a circular arc.

Inradii are involved in the formulation of certain problems far removed from geometry, for example, Bloch–Landau constants [7.1] and the eigenanalysis of vibrating membranes [11–13].

[1] H. S. M. Coxeter, *Regular Polytopes*, Methuen, 1948, pp. 2–3, 20–23; MR 51 #6554.
[2] H. S. M. Coxeter, *Introduction to Geometry*, Wiley, 1964, pp. 10–16; MR 90a:51001.
[3] M. Berger, *Geometry I*, Springer-Verlag, 1987, pp. 280–287; MR 95g:51001.
[4] L. Funar and A. Bondesen, Circles, triangles, squares and the Golden mean, *Amer. Math. Monthly* 96 (1989) 945–946.
[5] F. F. Abi-Khuzam and R. Barbara, A sharp inequality and the inradius conjecture, *Math. Inequal. Appl.* 4 (2001) 323–326; MR 2002a:51021.

[6]   R. Stong, A pentagonal maximum problem, *Amer. Math. Monthly* 104 (1997) 169–171.

[7]   W. Li and Y. Cheng, Solution to the regular pentagon problem, unpublished note (1991).

[8]   L. Funar and C. A. Rogers, Inradii and width, *Amer. Math. Monthly* 97 (1990) 858.

[9]   P. W. Awyong and P. R. Scott, On the maximal circumradius of a planar convex set containing one lattice point, *Bull. Austral. Math. Soc.* 52 (1995) 137–151; MR 96g:52030.

[10] P. R. Scott, Centre of gravity and circumcentre of a convex body in the plane, *Quart. J. Math.* 40 (1989) 111–117; MR 89m:52017.

[11] R. Bañuelos and T. Carroll, Brownian motion and the fundamental frequency of a drum, *Duke Math. J.* 75 (1994) 575–602; addendum 82 (1996) 227; MR 96m:31003 and MR 97f:31004.

[12] R. Bañuelos, T. Carroll, and E. Housworth, Inradius and integral means for Green's functions and conformal mappings, *Proc. Amer. Math. Soc.* 126 (1998) 577–585; MR 98g:30016.

[13] D. Betsakos, Harmonic measure on simply connected domains of fixed inradius, *Ark. Mat.* 36 (1998) 275–306; MR 2000a:30048.

8.20 Apollonian Packing Constant

Consider the two pictures in Figure 8.23. The left starts with a large circular boundary and three inner disks; the right starts with a curvilinear triangular boundary and a single disk. Both packings are obtained by inscribing a disk D_i of maximal radius in each gap left uncovered by previous iterations. Every new disk is tangent to all existing disks it touches and, clearly, the resulting configuration has three-fold rotational symmetry.

What can be said about the **residual set** E of the packing, that is, the points not covered by a disk? The set E can be shown to be of Lebesgue measure zero. One important quantity is the **packing exponent** ε, defined to be the infimum value of e for which [1, 2]

$$\sum_{i=1}^{\infty} |D_i|^e < \infty,$$

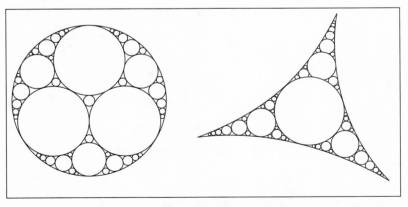

Figure 8.23. Apollonian packing illustrated with initial circle and inital curvilinear triangle.

Table 8.9. *Estimates of Packing Constant ε*

Estimate	Source
1.306951	Melzak [2]
1.3058	Boyd, as reported by Mandelbrot [11]
1.305636	Boyd [12]
1.305684	Manna & Herrmann [13]
1.305686729	Thomas & Dhar [14]
1.305688	McMullen [15]

where $|D|$ denotes the diameter of D. Another important quantity is the **Hausdorff dimension** $\dim(E)$, defined to be the unique value for which [1, 3]

$$\sup_{\delta > 0} \inf_{\substack{\text{countable} \\ \delta\text{-covers} \\ U_i}} \sum_{i=1}^{\infty} |U_i|^s = \begin{cases} \infty & \text{if } 0 \leq s < \dim(E), \\ 0 & \text{if } s > \dim(E), \end{cases}$$

where, by a δ-**cover** U_i, we mean $E \subseteq \bigcup_{i=1}^{\infty} U_i$, where each U_i is an open set and $0 < |U_i| \leq \delta$ for all i. It turns out that

$$\varepsilon = \dim(E),$$

as shown by Larman [4] and Boyd [5–7]. Further work by Boyd [8–10] and others yielded rigorous bounds

$$1.300197 < \varepsilon < 1.314534.$$

We also have numerical estimates from various sources (see Table 8.9).

Is $\dim(E)$ minimal, considered against all other disk packing strategies? Boyd [6] answered that this is a difficult question. Whether any progress has been made in resolving this is not known. See [2.16], which makes reference to Sierpinski's gasket, that is, to the packing of similarly-oriented equilateral triangles in an oppositely-oriented triangle (for which $\dim(E)$ is known to be exactly $\ln(3)/\ln(2)$). The subject has also recently become interesting to number theorists [16].

[1] K. J. Falconer, *The Geometry of Fractal Sets*, Cambridge Univ. Press, 1985, pp. 7–9, 14–15, 125–131; MR 88d:28001.
[2] Z. A. Melzak, On the solid-packing constant for circles, *Math. Comp.* 23 (1969) 169–172; MR 39 #6179.
[3] K. E. Hirst, The Apollonian packing of circles, *J. London Math. Soc.* 42 (1967) 281–291; MR 35 #876.
[4] D. G. Larman, On the exponent of convergence of a packing of spheres, *Mathematika* 13 (1966) 57–59; MR 34 #1928.
[5] D. W. Boyd, Osculatory packing by spheres, *Canad. Math. Bull.* 13 (1970) 59–64; MR 41 #4387.
[6] D. W. Boyd, The residual set dimension of the Apollonian packing, *Mathematika* 20 (1973) 170–174; MR 58 #12732.
[7] C. Tricot, A new proof for the residual set dimension of the Apollonian packing, *Math. Proc. Cambridge Philos. Soc.* 96 (1984) 413–423; MR 85j:52022.

[8]   D. W. Boyd, Lower bounds for the disk packing constant, *Math. Comp.* 24 (1970) 697–704; MR 43 #3924.

[9]   D. W. Boyd, The disk-packing constant, *Aequationes Math.* 7 (1971) 182–193; MR 46 #2557.

[10] D. W. Boyd, Improved bounds for the disk-packing constant, *Aequationes Math.* 9 (1973) 99–106; MR 47 #5728.

[11] B. B. Mandelbrot, *The Fractal Geometry of Nature*, W. H. Freeman, 1983, pp. 169–172, 360; MR 84h:00021.

[12] D. W. Boyd, The sequence of radii of the Apollonian packing, *Math. Comp.* 39 (1982) 249–254; MR 83i:52013.

[13] S. S. Manna and H. J. Herrmann, Precise determination of the fractal dimensions of Apollonian packing and space-filling bearings, *J. Phys. A* 24 (1991) L481–L490; MR 92c:52027.

[14] P. B. Thomas and D. Dhar, The Hausdorff dimension of the Apollonian packing of circles, *J. Phys. A* 27 (1994) 2257–2268; MR 95f:28010.

[15] C. T. McMullen, Hausdorff dimension and conformal dynamics. III: Computation of dimension, *Amer. J. Math.* 120 (1998) 691–721; MR 2000d:37055.

[16] R. L. Graham, J. C. Lagarias, C. L. Mallows, A. R. Wilks, and C. H. Yan, Apollonian circle packings: Number theory, *J. Number Theory*, to appear; math.NT/0009113.

8.21 Rendezvous Constants

Let E denote a compact, connected subset of d-dimensional Euclidean space. Gross [1] and Stadje [2] independently proved the following: There is a unique real number $a(E)$ such that, for all (not necessarily distinct) points $x_1, x_2, \ldots, x_n \in E$, there exists $y \in E$ with

$$\frac{1}{n} \sum_{i=1}^{n} |x_i - y| = a(E).$$

In words, there is a point $y \in E$ such that the average distance from y to $x_1, x_2, \ldots, x_n$ is $a(E)$. The constant $a(E)$ works for all collections of n points, for any positive integer n. Moreover, no other constant will work, which is most surprising!

For example, if E is convex, then $a(E)$ is the circumradius of E. We henceforth will focus on nonconvex sets E. If C is a circle of diameter 1, then $a(C) = 2/\pi = 0.6366197723\ldots$ [3,4]. If Δ is an isosceles triangle with baselength 2 and perimeter $2\lambda + 2$, then [5]

$$a(\Delta) = \begin{cases} \dfrac{\lambda^2 + 2\lambda - \sqrt{\lambda^2 - 1} - 2\sqrt{(\lambda - \sqrt{\lambda^2 - 1})\lambda(\lambda + 1)}}{\lambda^2 + 3\lambda - 1 - \lambda\sqrt{\lambda^2 - 1} - 2\sqrt{(\lambda - \sqrt{\lambda^2 - 1})\lambda(\lambda + 1)}} & \text{for } \sqrt{2} \leq \lambda \leq \xi, \\[2ex] \dfrac{\lambda^2 + 1}{2\lambda} & \text{for } \lambda \geq \xi, \end{cases}$$

where $\xi = 2.3212850380\ldots$ has minimal polynomial $2x^5 - 4x^4 - 5x^2 + 4x - 1$. No one has yet found a closed-form expression for $a(E)$ if E is an arbitrary ellipse or acute triangle.

Two alternative definitions of $a(E)$ are as follows:

$$a(E) = \sup_{n \geq 1} \sup_{x_1, x_2, \ldots, x_n \in E} \min_{y \in E} \frac{1}{n} \sum_{i=1}^{n} |x_i - y| = \inf_{n \geq 1} \inf_{x_1, x_2, \ldots, x_n \in E} \max_{y \in E} \frac{1}{n} \sum_{i=1}^{n} |x_i - y|,$$

and its association with the minimax theorem of game theory becomes obvious [1, 3, 6].

Define the **rendezvous constant**, $r(E)$, of E to be the normalized ratio

$$r(E) = \frac{a(E)}{\text{diam}(E)}, \quad \text{diam}(E) = \max_{u,v \in E} |u - v|.$$

For this to make sense, E cannot be a single point p (for the diameter to be nonzero) and cannot be a finite set (by connectedness). With these restrictions, Gross and Stadje proved that $1/2 \le r(E) < 1$. What is the maximum value, R_d, of $r(E)$ considered over all sets E in d-dimensional Euclidean space? Clearly $R_1 = 1/2$. When $d = 2$, it seems likely that the Reuleaux triangle T provides the answer [8.10]. Nickolas & Yost [7] and Wolf [8] rigorously established the bounds

$$\max\left\{\frac{2}{3}, r(T)\right\} \le R_2 \le \frac{1}{2} + \frac{\pi}{16} < 0.69634955,$$

and the best-known numerical estimate of $r(T)$ is $0.6675277360\ldots$ [9]. No closed-form expression for $r(T)$ has been discovered. The conjecture $R_2 = r(T)$ deserves more attention!

For $d > 2$, we have bounds [7]

$$\frac{d}{d+1} \le R_d \le \frac{\Gamma(\frac{d}{2})^2 2^{d-2}\sqrt{2d}}{\Gamma(d-\frac{1}{2})\sqrt{\pi(d+1)}} < \sqrt{\frac{d}{d+1}},$$

where $\Gamma(x)$ is the gamma function [1.5.4]. These bounds are less precise than those for $d = 2$. No one has attempted to guess the higher dimensional shapes that maximize the rendezvous constant, as far as is known.

A second relevant conjecture is that $R_2 = S_2$, where [8–11]

$$S_d = \sup_{n \ge 1} \sup_{\substack{x_1, x_2, \ldots, x_n \\ |x_i - x_j| \le 1}} \frac{1}{n^2} \sum_{i=1}^{n} \sum_{j=1}^{n} |x_i - x_j|.$$

In words, S_d is the average pairwise distance of arbitrary points $x_1, x_2, \ldots, x_n$ in d-dimensional space, where no pair x_i, x_j has separation exceeding 1.

We have more bounds $a(E) \le b(E)$, where [8]

$$b(E) = \sup_{n \ge 1} \sup_{x_1, x_2, \ldots, x_n \in E} \frac{1}{n^2} \sum_{i=1}^{n} \sum_{j=1}^{n} |x_i - x_j|.$$

The study of $b(E)$ begins with a generalization: replacing the summations by integrals and the point masses x_i by a probability density, then applying potential theory [12–16]. A third conjecture is that $a(T) = b(T)$ [9]. Another special case, when E is the two-dimensional sphere, was discussed in [8.8].

The preceding material can be generalized: E may be any compact, connected metric space. In fact, E need not even have a metric: Stadje [2] proved that E need only be a compact, connected Hausdorff space possessing a real-valued continuous symmetric function $f(x, y)$ for $x, y \in E$ (a kind of "weak metric").

Finally, let E be the ellipse with semimajor axis 2 and semiminor axis 1. It is numerically known that $a(E) = 2.1080540666\ldots$ [9]. Although there is no precise formula for $a(E)$, as stated earlier, it would be good nevertheless someday to better understand the nature of this constant.

[1] O. Gross, The rendezvous value of metric space, *Advances in Game Theory*, ed. M. Dresher, L. S. Shapley, and A. W. Tucker, Princeton Univ. Press, 1964, pp. 49–53; MR 28 #5841.

[2] W. Stadje, A property of compact connected spaces, *Arch. Math. (Basel)* 36 (1981) 275–280; MR 83e:54028.

[3] J. Cleary, S. A. Morris, and D. Yost, Numerical geometry – Numbers for shapes, *Amer. Math. Monthly* 93 (1986) 260–275; MR 87h:51043.

[4] H. T. Croft, K. J. Falconer, and R. K. Guy, *Unsolved Problems in Geometry*, Springer-Verlag, 1991, sect. G1; MR 95k:52001.

[5] D. K. Kulshestha, T. W. Sag, and L. Yang, Average distance constants for polygons in spaces with nonpositive curvature, *Bull. Austral. Math. Soc.* 42 (1990) 323–333; MR 92b:51025.

[6] C. Thomassen, The rendezvous number of a symmetric matrix and a compact connected metric space, *Amer. Math. Monthly* 107 (2000) 163–166; MR 2001a:54040.

[7] P. Nickolas and D. Yost, The average distance property for subsets of Euclidean space, *Arch. Math. (Basel)* 50 (1988) 380–384; MR 89d:51026.

[8] R. Wolf, Averaging distances in real quasihypermetric Banach spaces of finite dimension, *Israel J. Math.* 110 (1999) 125–151; MR 2001f:46012.

[9] G. Larcher, W. C. Schmid, and R. Wolf, On the approximation of certain mass distributions appearing in distance geometry, *Acta Math. Hungar.* 87 (2000) 295–316; MR 2001f:65013.

[10] L. Fejes Tóth, Über eine Punktverteilung auf der Kugel, *Acta Math. Acad. Sci. Hungar.* 10 (1959) 13–19; MR 21 #4393.

[11] H. S. Witsenhausen, On the maximum of the sum of squared distances under a diameter constraint, *Amer. Math. Monthly* 81 (1974) 1100–1101; MR 51 #6594.

[12] L. Fejes Tóth, On the sum of distances determined by a pointset, *Acta Math. Acad. Sci. Hungar.* 7 (1956) 397–401; MR 21 #5937.

[13] G. Björck, Distributions of positive mass, which maximize a certain generalized energy integral, *Ark. Mat.* 3 (1956) 255–269; MR 17,1198b.

[14] R. Alexander and K. B. Stolarsky, Extremal problems of distance geometry related to energy integrals, *Trans. Amer. Math. Soc.* 193 (1974) 1–31; MR 50 #3121.

[15] R. Alexander, Generalized sums of distances, *Pacific J. Math.* 56 (1975) 297–304; MR 58 #24005.

[16] G. D. Chakerian and M. S. Klamkin, Inequalities for sums of distances, *Amer. Math. Monthly* 80 (1973) 1009–1017; MR 48 #9558.

Table of Constants

0.0255369745 . . .	c_0^-; with Lenz–Ising constants [5.22]
0.0261074464 . . .	4th Matthews constant [2.4]
0.026422 . . .	With Tammes' constants [8.8]
0.0275981 . . .	$\kappa_S(p_c)$; with percolation cluster density constants [5.18]
0.0282517642 . . .	3rd Du Bois Reymond constant [3.12]
0.0333810598 . . .	One of the Feigenbaum–Coullet–Tresser constants [1.9]
0.0354961590 . . .	$-\lambda_4$; with Gauss–Kuzmin–Wirsing constant [2.17]
0.0355762113 . . .	$-41/16 + 3\sqrt{3}/2$; with percolation cluster density [5.18]
0.0369078300 . . .	With Golomb–Dickman constant [5.4]
0.0370072165 . . .	With Golomb–Dickman constant [5.4]
0.0381563991 . . .	One of Rényi's parking constants [5.3]
0.0403255003 . . .	e_0; with Lenz–Ising constants [5.22]
0.0461543172 . . .	With Stieltjes constants [2.21]
0.0482392690 . . .	$m_{3,4}$; with Meissel–Mertens constants [2.2]
0.0484808014 . . .	p_2; with Vallée's constant [2.19]
0.0494698522 . . .	With Golomb–Dickman constant [5.4]
0.0504137604 . . .	With Euler–Gompertz constant [6.2]
0.0548759991 . . .	Conjectured value of H_9, Heilbronn triangle constants [8.16]
0.05756 . . .	With hyperbolic volume constants [8.9]
0.0585498315 . . .	$1/(2\pi e)$; with Hermite's constants [8.7]
0.0605742294 . . .	One of the Euler totient constants [2.7]
0.0608216553 . . .	3rd Matthews constant [2.4]
0.0648447153 . . .	One of Pólya's random walk constants [5.9]
0.0653514259 . . .	Norton's constant [2.18]
0.0653725925 . . .	With Stieltjes constants [2.21]
0.065770 . . .	$\kappa_S(1/2)$; with percolation cluster density constants [5.18]
0.0657838882 . . .	With Gibbs–Wilbraham constant [4.1]
0.0659880358 . . .	e^{-e}; one of the iterated exponential constants [6.11]
0.0723764243 . . .	Conjectured value of H_8, Heilbronn triangle constants [8.16]
0.0728158454 . . .	Negative of 1st Stieltjes constant [2.21]
0.0729126499 . . .	One of Pólya's random walk constants [5.9]
0.0757395140 . . .	With Vallée's constant [2.19]
0.0773853773 . . .	With Vallée's constant [2.19]
0.0810614667 . . .	With Stieltjes constants [2.21]
0.0838590090 . . .	Conjectured value of H_7, Heilbronn triangle constants [8.16]
0.0858449341 . . .	One of Pólya's random walk constants [5.9]
0.0883160988 . . .	With Golomb–Dickman constant [5.4]
0.0894898722 . . .	$G/\pi - 1/2$; with Gibbs–Wilbraham constant [4.1]
0.0904822031 . . .	Conjectured value of K_s/π, with Kakeya–Besicovitch [8.17]
0.0923457352 . . .	With de Bruijn–Newman constant [2.32]
0.0931878229 . . .	$\exp(-\pi^2/(6\ln(2)))$; with Khintchine–Lévy constants [1.8]
0.0946198928 . . .	With Meissel–Mertens constants [2.2]
0.0948154165 . . .	With Otter's tree enumeration constants [5.6]
0.097 . . .	Base-10 self-numbers density constant [2.24]

0.1878596424...	With iterated exponential constants [6.11]
0.1895600483...	Triangular entropy of folding, with Lieb's square ice [5.24]
0.1924225474...	With Otter's tree enumeration constants [5.6]
0.1924500897...	$\sqrt{3}/9$; value of H_5, Heilbronn triangle constant [8.16]
0.1932016732...	One of Pólya's random walk constants [5.9]
0.1945280495...	2nd Du Bois Reymond constant [3.12]
0.1994588183...	Vallée's constant [2.19]
0.1996805161...	Conjectured value of weakly triple-free set constant [2.26]
0.2007557220...	With Meissel–Mertens constants [2.2]
0.2076389205...	With de Bruijn–Newman constant [2.32]
0.2078795764...	$i^i = \exp(-\pi/2)$; with iterated exponential constants [6.11]
0.209...	Base-4 self-numbers density constant [2.24]
0.2095808742...	With Golomb–Dickman constant [5.4]
0.21...	One of Cameron's sum-free set constants [2.25]
0.2173242870...	Lochs' constant, with Porter–Hensley constants [2.18]
0.218094...	3D critical point, with Lenz–Ising constants [5.22]
0.2183801414...	One of Pólya's random walk constants [5.9]
0.2192505830...	With Glaisher–Kinkelin constant [2.15]
0.221654...	3D inverse critical temperature, with Lenz–Ising [5.22]
0.2221510651...	With Otter's tree enumeration constants [5.6]
0.2265708154...	With hard square entropy constant [5.12]
0.2299...	Square-diagonal entropy of folding, with Lieb's square ice [5.24]
0.2351252848...	Conway–Guy constant, with Erdös' sum-distinct set constant [2.28]
0.2387401436...	With Otter's tree enumeration constants [5.6]
0.24...	One of the Hayman constants [7.5]
0.2419707245...	$1/\sqrt{2\pi e}$; Sobolev isoperimetric [3.6], traveling salesman [8.5]
0.2424079763...	With hard square entropy constant [5.12]
0.2440155280...	One of the circumradius-inradius constants [8.19]
0.247...	Abundant numbers density constant [2.11]
0.25	$1/4$; Koebe's constant, with Bloch–Landau constants [7.1]
0.2503634293...	With Otter's tree enumeration constants [5.6]
0.2526602590...	Binary self-numbers density constant [2.24]
0.2536695079...	δ_8; with Hermite's constants [8.7]
0.2545055235...	With Kalmár's composition constant [5.5]
0.255001...	With Moser's worm constants [8.4]
0.2614972128...	M; one of the Meissel–Mertens constants [2.2]
0.2649320846...	Mrs. Miniver's constant, with circular coverage constants [8.2]
0.2665042887...	With Otter's tree enumeration constants [5.6]
0.2677868402...	Unforgeable word constant, with pattern-free words [5.17]
0.2688956601...	With hyperbolic volume constants [8.9]
0.2696063519...	With Meissel–Mertens constants [2.2]
0.2697318462...	One of the Pell–Stevenhagen constants [2.8]

0.3271293669...   With Landau–Ramanujan constant [2.3]
0.3287096916...   With Kepler–Bouwkamp constant [6.3]
0.3289868133... $30/\pi^2$; with Hafner–Sarnak–McCurley constant [2.5]
0.3332427219...   Hard hexagon entropy constant, with hard square [5.12]
0.3333333333...   1/3; with Rényi's parking constants [5.3]
0.3349813253...   With Meissel–Mertens constants [2.2]
0.3383218568...   With Otter's tree enumeration constants [5.6]
0.3405373295...   One of Pólya's random walk constants [5.9]
0.3472963553... $2\sin(\pi/18)$; with percolation cluster density constants [5.18]
0.35129898...   One of the quadratic recurrence constants [6.10]
0.3522211004...   With Hafner–Sarnak–McCurley constant [2.5]
0.3529622229...   With Otter's tree enumeration constants [5.6]
0.3532363719...   Hafner–Sarnak–McCurley constant [2.5]
0.3551817423...   With Otter's tree enumeration constants [5.6]
0.359072...   With percolation cluster density constants [5.18]
0.3605924718... $\text{Im}(i^{i^{i^{\cdots}}})$; with iterated exponential constants [6.11]
0.3607140971...   With Otter's tree enumeration constants [5.6]
0.3611030805... $r(12)$ conjectured value; with circular coverage constants [8.2]
0.3625364234...   One of Otter's tree enumeration constants [5.6]
0.364132...   One of Rényi's parking constants [5.3]
0.3678794411... $1/e$; natural logarithmic base [1.3], iterated exponentials [6.11]
0.368...   With hard square entropy constant [5.12]
0.3694375103... C_7; one of the Hardy–Littlewood constants [2.1]
0.3720486812...   With digital search tree constants [5.14]
0.3728971438...   One of the extreme value constants [5.16]
0.3729475455... δ_6; with Hermite's constants [8.7]
0.3733646177...   One of the binary search tree constants [5.13]
0.3739558136...   Artin's constant [2.4]
0.3790522777...   One of the self-avoiding walk constants [5.10]
0.380006... $r(11)$ conjectured value; with circular coverage constants [8.2]
0.3825978582...   One of the geometric probability constants [8.1]
0.3919177761...   One of the extreme value constants [5.16]
0.3926990816... $\pi/8$; with Moser's worm constants [8.4]
0.3943847688...   One of Moser's worm constants [8.4]
0.3949308436... $r(10)$ conjectured value; with circular coverage constants [8.2]
0.3972130965...   With Otter's tree enumeration constants [5.6]
0.3995246670...   One of the quadratic recurrence constants [6.10]
0.3995352805... α^{-1}; one of the Feigenbaum–Coullet–Tresser constants [1.9]
0.40096...   With Tammes' constants [8.8]
0.402...   With percolation cluster density constants [5.18]
0.4026975036...   With Otter's tree enumeration constants [5.6]
0.4074951009...   Hard square entropy constant [5.12]
0.4080301397... $(2 - e^{-1})/4$; one of Rényi's parking constants [5.3]
0.4097321837...   Conjectured value of Berry–Esseen constant [4.7]

0.4098748850...	C_5; one of the Hardy–Littlewood constants [2.1]
0.412048...	With Lenz–Ising constants [5.22]
0.4124540336...	Prouhet–Thue–Morse constant [6.8]
0.4127732370...	With Kalmár's composition constant [5.5]
0.4142135623...	$\sqrt{2} - 1$; with circular coverage [8.2], Lenz–Ising constants [5.22]
0.4159271089...	One of the extreme value constants [5.16]
0.4194...	One of the traveling salesman constants [8.5]
0.4198600459...	With Reuleaux triangle constants [8.10]
0.4203723394...	Minkowski–Bower constant [6.9]
0.4207263771...	Conjectured value of integer Chebyshev constant [4.9]
0.4212795439...	Schlüter's constant $t(10)$; with circular coverage constants [8.2]
0.4213829566...	$(6\ln(2))/\pi^2$; Lévy's constant [1.8]
0.4217993614...	With Pisot–Vijayaraghavan–Salem constants [2.30]
0.422...	With hard square entropy constant [5.12]
0.4227843351...	$1 - \gamma$; with Euler–Mascheroni [1.5], Stieltjes constants [2.21]
0.4278733971...	With circumradius-inradius constants [8.19]
0.4281657248...	With Euler–Mascheroni constant[1.5]
0.4282495056...	Carefree constant, with Hafner–Sarnak–McCurley constant [2.5]
0.4302966531...	With Young–Fejér–Jackson constants [3.14]
0.4323323583...	$(1 - e^{-2})/2$; one of Rényi's parking constants [5.3]
0.4330619231...	With Klarner's polyomino constant [5.19]
0.434...	With Hardy–Littlewood constants [2.1]
0.4381562356...	With Otter's tree enumeration constants [5.6]
0.4382829367...	$\mathrm{Re}(i^{i^{i^{\cdots}}})$; with iterated exponential constants [6.11]
0.4389253692...	One of Moser's worm constants [8.4]
0.43961...	One of the self-avoiding walk constants [5.10]
0.4399240125...	One of Otter's tree enumeration constants [5.6]
0.4406867935...	$\ln(\sqrt{2} + 1)/2$; with Lenz–Ising constants [5.22]
0.4428767697...	With Otter's tree enumeration constants [5.6]
0.4450418679...	$r(8)$; with circular coverage constants [8.2]
0.4466...	3D dimer constant [5.23]
0.4472135955...	$1/\sqrt{5}$; 1st Diophantine approximation constant [2.23]
0.4490502094...	One of Moser's worm constants [8.4]
0.4522474200...	One of the Meissel–Mertens constants [2.2]
0.4545121805...	With Alladi–Grinstead constant [2.9]
0.4567332095...	With Otter's tree enumeration constants [5.6]
0.461543...	With Stieltjes constants [2.21]
0.4645922709...	With Landau–Ramanujan constant [2.3]
0.4652576133...	δ_5; with Hermite's constants [8.7]
0.4656386467...	With Otter's tree enumeration constants [5.6]
0.4702505696...	2·(Conway–Guy constant), with Erdös' sum-distinct set [2.28]
0.4718616534...	Conjectured value of Bloch's constant [7.1]

0.4749493799...	Weierstrass constant, with Gauss' lemniscate constant [6.1]
0.4756260767...	With Plouffe's constant [6.5]
0.4769...	Bland's constant, with traveling salesman constants [8.5]
0.4802959782...	One of the geometric probability constants [8.1]
0.4834983471...	With Golomb–Dickman constant [5.4]
0.4865198884...	With Landau–Ramanujan constant [2.3]
0.4876227781...	Gaussian twin prime constant, with Hardy–Littlewood constants [2.1]
0.4906940504...	With Landau–Ramanujan constant [2.3]
0.4945668172...	Shapiro–Drinfeld constant [3.1]
0.4956001805...	$1 - \gamma_0 - \gamma_1$; with [2.21] Stieltjes constants
0.5	$1/2$; with percolation cluster density [5.18], Landau–Ramanujan [2.3]
0.5163359762...	With Kepler–Bouwkamp constant [6.3]
0.5178759064...	With Otter's tree enumeration constants [5.6]
0.5212516264...	With Lebesgue constants [4.2]
0.5214054331...	Ghosh's constant, with geometric probability [8.1], traveling salesman [8.5]
0.5235987755...	$\pi/6$; with Archimedes [1.4], Madelung's constant [1.10]
0.531280...	With Gauss–Kuzmin–Wirsing constant [2.17]
0.5313399499...	One of the Pythagorean triple constants [5.2]
0.5341...	With Lenz–Ising constants [5.22]
0.5349496061...	One of Otter's tree enumeration constants [5.6]
0.5351070126...	With Artin's constant [2.4]
0.5392381750...	One of Pólya's random walk constants [5.9]
0.5396454911...	$\zeta(1/2) + 2$; with Euler–Mascheroni constant [1.5]
0.5405...	One of the longest subsequence constants [5.20]
0.5410442246...	With hyperbolic volume constants [8.9]
0.5432589653...	Conjectured value of Landau's constant [7.1]
0.5530512933...	Kuijlaars–Saff constant, with Tammes' constants [8.8]
0.5559052114...	Bezdek's constant $r(6)$; with circular coverage constants [8.2]
0.5598656169...	With Alladi–Grinstead constant [2.9]
0.5609498093...	One of the geometric probability constants [8.1]
0.5614594835...	$e^{-\gamma}$; Euler's constant [1.5], totient [2.7], Golomb–Dickman [5.4]
0.562009...	With Rényi's parking constant [5.3]
0.5671432904...	$W(1)$; solution of $xe^x = 1$, with iterated exponential constants [6.11]
0.5682854937...	With the abundant numbers density constant [2.11]
0.5683000031...	With Euler–Gompertz constant [6.2]
0.5697515829...	Weakly carefree constant, with Hafner–Sarnak–McCurley constant [2.5]
0.5731677401...	$(3/4)\cdot$(Landau–Ramanujan constant) [2.3]
0.57339...	One of the Pell–Stevenhagen constants [2.8]

0.5743623733...	With Otter's tree enumeration constants [5.6]
0.5759599688...	Stephens' constant, with Artin's constant [2.4]
0.5761487691...	With Klarner's polyomino constant [5.18]
0.5767761224...	With Landau–Ramanujan constant [2.3]
0.5772156649...	Euler–Mascheroni constant, γ [1.5]; also Stieltjes constants [2.21]
0.5773502691...	$1/\sqrt{3}$; with Kakeya–Besicovitch constants [8.17]
0.5778636748...	$\pi/(2e)$; with Masser–Gramain constant [7.2]
0.5784167628...	$(8/7)\cos(2\pi/7)\cos(\pi/7)^2$; with Diophantine approximation constants [2.23]
0.5801642239...	One of the optimal stopping constants [5.15]
0.5805775582...	Pell constant [2.8]
0.5817480456...	With Madelung's constant [1.10]
0.5819486593...	With Landau–Ramanujan constant [2.3]
0.5825971579...	ρ; one of Pólya's random walk constants [5.9]
0.5831218080...	$2G/\pi$; 2D dimer constant [5.23]; also Kneser–Mahler [3.10]
0.5851972651...	With Euler–Gompertz constant [6.2]
0.5877...	One of the self-avoiding walk constants [5.10]
0.5878911617...	With hard square entropy constant [5.12]
0.59...	One of the optimal stopping constants [5.15]
0.5926327182...	Lehmer's constant [6.6]
0.5927460...	p_c; with percolation cluster density constants [5.18]
0.5947539639...	With Otter's tree enumeration constants [5.6]
0.5963473623...	Euler–Gompertz constant [6.2]
0.5990701173...	$M/2$; with Gauss' lemniscate constant [6.1]
0.6069...	One of the longest subsequence constants [5.20]
0.6079271018...	$6/\pi^2$; with Archimedes [1.4], Hafner–Sarnak–McCurley [2.5]
0.6083817178...	One of the Euler totient constants [2.7]
0.6093828640...	Neville's constant $r(5)$, with circular coverage constants [8.2]
0.6134752692...	Strongly triple-free set constant [2.26]
0.6168502750...	δ_4; with Hermite's constants [8.7]
0.6168878482...	With Otter's tree enumeration constants [5.6]
0.6180339887...	$\phi - 1$; with [1.2] Golden Mean
0.6194036984...	One of the Lenz–Ising constants [5.22]
0.6223065745...	Backhouse's constant, with Kalmár's constant [5.5]
0.6231198963...	With Otter's tree enumeration constants [5.6]
0.6232...	One of the traveling salesman constants [8.5]
0.6243299885...	Golomb–Dickman constant [5.4]
0.6257358072...	With Glaisher–Kinkelin constant [2.15]
0.6278342677...	With John constant [7.4]
0.6294650204...	Davison–Shallit constant ξ_1; with Cahen's constant [6.7]
0.6312033175...	One of the geometric probability constants [8.1]
0.6321205588...	$1 - 1/e$; with natural logarithmic base [1.3]
0.6331...	One of the traveling salesman constants [8.5]

0.6333683473 ...	2·(Atkinson–Negro–Santoro constant), with Erdös' sum-distinct set [2.28]
0.6351663546 ...	$C_3 = 2D/9$; one of the Hardy–Littlewood constants [2.1]
0.6366197723 ...	$2/\pi$; with Archimedes [1.4], rendezvous constants [8.21]
0.6389094054 ...	With Landau–Ramanujan constant [2.3]
0.6419448385 ...	With Meissel–Mertens constants [2.2]
0.6434105462 ...	Cahen's constant ξ_2 [6.7]
0.6462454398 ...	With Masser–Gramain constant [7.2]
0.6467611227 ...	With Euler–Gompertz constant [6.2]
0.6537 ...	One of the longest subsequence constants [5.20]
0.6539007091 ...	ξ_3; with Cahen's constant [6.7]
0.6556795424 ...	With Euler–Gompertz constant [6.2]
0.6563186958 ...	With Otter's tree enumeration constants [5.6]
0.6569990137 ...	$-\delta_0$; Hall–Montgomery constant [2.33]
0.6583655992 ...	One of the iterated exponential constants [6.11]
0.6594626704 ...	One of Pólya's random walk constants [5.9]
0.6597396084 ...	$(2 + \sqrt{3})/(4\sqrt{2})$; with beam detection constant [8.11]
0.6600049346 ...	ξ_4; with Cahen's constant [6.7]
0.6601618158 ...	Twin prime constant, with Hardy–Littlewood constants [2.1]
0.6613170494 ...	Feller–Tornier constant, with Artin's constant [2.4]
0.6617071822 ...	One of the geometric probability constants [8.1]
0.6627434193 ...	Laplace limit constant [4.8]
0.6632657345 ...	ξ_5; with Cahen's constant [6.7]
0.6672538227 ...	With Feller's coin tossing constants [5.11]
0.6675277360 ...	With rendezvous constants [8.21]
0.6697409699 ...	Shanks' constant, with Hardy–Littlewood constants [2.1]
0.67 ...	Erdös–Lebensold constant [2.27]
0.6709083078 ...	With Madelung's constant [1.10]
0.6749814429 ...	Graham's hexagon constant [8.15]
0.676339 ...	One of the percolation cluster density constants [5.18]
0.6774017761 ...	With Kalmár's constant [5.5]
0.6821555671 ...	With Otter's tree enumeration constants [5.6]
0.6829826991 ...	With Calabi's triangle constant [8.13]
0.6844472720 ...	With Otter's tree enumeration constants [5.6]
0.6864067314 ...	C_{quad}; one of the Hardy–Littlewood constants [2.1]
0.6867778344 ...	With Kalmár's constant [5.5]
0.6903471261 ...	One of the iterated exponential constants [6.11]
0.6922006276 ...	$e^{-1/e}$; one of the iterated exponential constants [6.11]
0.6931471805 ...	ln(2); with natural logarithmic base [1.3]
0.6962 ...	One of the percolation cluster density constants [5.18]
0.6975013584 ...	2nd Pappalardi constant, with Artin's constant [2.4]
0.6977746579 ...	$I_1(2)/I_0(2)$; with Euler–Gompertz constant [6.2]
0.6979 ...	One of the traveling salesman constants [8.5]
0.6995388700 ...	One of Otter's tree enumeration constants [5.6]

0.70258...	Embree–Trefethen constant, with Golden mean [1.2]
0.7041699604...	With Fransén–Robinson constant [4.6]
0.7044798810...	$1 - 35/(12\pi^2)$; with rectilinear crossing constant [8.18]
0.7047534517...	With Landau–Ramanujan constant [2.3]
0.7047709230...	$(\pi - \sqrt{3})/2$; with Reuleaux triangle constants [8.10]
0.7059712461...	With Porter–Hensley constants [2.18]
0.708...	One of Pólya's random walk constants [5.9]
0.7098034428...	Rabbit constant, with Prouhet–Thue–Morse constant [6.8]
0.7124...	One of the traveling salesman constants [8.5]
0.7147827007...	Conjectured value, one of the traveling salesman constants [8.5]
0.7172...	One of the longest subsequence constants [5.20]
0.7213475204...	$1/(2\ln(2))$; with Lengyel's constant [5.7], Feller's coin tossing [5.11]
0.7218106748...	5D Steiner ratio, with Steiner tree constants [8.6]
0.7234...	One of the traveling salesman constants [8.5]
0.7235565167...	One of Pólya's random walk constants [5.9]
0.7236067977...	$(1/2)(1 + 1/\sqrt{5})$; with Diophantine approximation constants [2.23]
0.7252064830...	$97/150 + \pi/40$; Langford's constant, with geometric probability [8.1]
0.7266432468...	With van der Corput's constant [3.15]
0.726868...	With Graham's hexagon constant [8.15]
0.7322131597...	Unforgeable word constant, with pattern-free words [5.17]
0.7326498193...	With Landau–Ramanujan constant [2.3]
0.7373383033...	Grossman's constant [6.4]
0.7377507574...	Conjectured value of Whittaker–Goncharov constant [7.3]
0.7404804896...	$\pi/\sqrt{18}$; densest sphere packing, with Hermite's constants [8.7]
0.7424537454...	One of the Riesz–Kolmogorov constants [7.7]
0.7439711933...	Sarnak's constant, with Artin's constant [2.4]
0.7439856178...	4D Steiner ratio, with Steiner tree constants [8.6]
0.7475979202...	One of Rényi's parking constants [5.3]
0.749137...	With Graham's hexagon constant [8.15]
0.7493060013...	With Kneser–Mahler polynomial constants [3.10]
0.75	$3/4$; one of the self-avoiding walk constants [5.10]
0.7520107423...	One of the abelian group enumeration constants [5.1]
0.7578230112...	Flajolet–Odlyzko constant, with Golomb–Dickman [5.4]
0.760729...	With Graham's hexagon constant [8.15]
0.7608657675...	$(1/2)\cdot$(Bateman–Stemmler constant), with Hardy–Littlewood [2.1]
0.7642236535...	Landau–Ramanujan constant [2.3]
0.7647848097...	With Meissel–Mertens constants [2.2]
0.7656250596...	With Liouville–Roth constants [2.22]
0.7666646959...	With iterated exponential constants [6.11]

0.7669444905...	With Niven's constant [2.6]
0.7671198507...	Conway's constant [6.12]
0.77100...	One of the self-avoiding walk constants [5.10]
0.7711255236...	With Gauss–Kuzmin–Wirsing constant [2.17]
0.7735162909...	Flajolet–Martin constant, with Prouhet–Thue–Morse [6.8]
0.7759021363...	Bender's constant, with Lengyel's constant [5.7]
0.7776656535...	One of the geometric probability constants [8.1]
0.7824816009...	With Golomb–Dickman constant [5.4]
0.7834305107...	One of the iterated exponential constants [6.11]
0.7841903733...	3D Steiner ratio, with Steiner tree constants [8.6]
0.7853805572...	With Kepler–Bouwkamp constant [6.3]
0.7853981633...	$\pi/4$; with Kepler–Bouwkamp [6.3], Moser's worm [8.4]
0.7885305659...	Lüroth analog of Khintchine's constant [1.8]
0.79...	One of the optimal stopping constants [5.15]
0.7916031835...	One of Otter's tree enumeration constants [5.6]
0.7922082381...	Lal's constant, with Hardy–Littlewood constants [2.1]
0.8003194838...	Conjectured value, weakly triple-free set constant [2.26]
0.8008134543...	Bender's constant, with Lengyel's constant [5.7]
0.8019254372...	With Euler–Mascheroni constant [1.5]
0.8043522628...	One of the optimal stopping constants [5.15]
0.8086525183...	Solomon's parking constant, with Rényi's parking [5.3]
0.8093940205...	Alladi–Grinstead constant [2.9]
0.8116869215...	One of Flajolet's constants, with Thue–Morse [6.8]
0.8118...	One of the longest subsequence constants [5.20]
0.8125565590...	Stolarsky–Harborth constant [2.16]
0.8128252421...	With Young–Fejér–Jackson constants [3.14]
0.81318...	c_0; one of the longest subsequence constants [5.20]
0.8137993642...	With Reuleaux triangle constants [8.10]
0.8175121124...	With Shapiro–Drinfeld constant [3.1]
0.82...	With k-satisfiability constants [5.21]
0.822...	One of Pólya's random walk constants [5.9]
0.8224670334...	$\pi^2/12$; with traveling salesman constants [8.5]
0.8247830309...	$(\sqrt{5}-1)/\sqrt{2}$; one of Turán's power sum constants [3.16]
0.8249080672...	2·(Prouhet–Thue–Morse constant) [6.8]
0.8269933431...	$3\sqrt{3}/(2\pi)$; with circular coverage constants [8.2]
0.8319073725...	$1/\zeta(3)$; with Apéry's constant [1.6]
0.8324290656...	Rosser's constant, with Hardy–Littlewood constants [2.1]
0.8346268416...	$1/M$; with Gauss' lemniscate constant [6.1]
0.8351076361...	With Hall–Montgomery constant [2.33]
0.8371132125...	A_3'; with Brun's constant [2.14]
0.8403426028...	With Reuleaux triangle constants [8.10]
0.8427659133...	$(6\ln(2))/\pi^2$; Lévy's constant [1.8]
0.8472130848...	$3M/\sqrt{2}$; ubiquitous constant, with Gauss' lemniscate [6.1]
0.8507361882...	Paper folding constant, with Prouhet–Thue–Morse [6.8]

0.8561089817...	With Landau–Ramanujan constant [2.3]
0.8565404448...	3rd Pappalardi constant, with Artin's constant [2.4]
0.8621470373...	With Gauss–Kuzmin–Wirsing constant [2.17]
0.8636049963...	With Stolarsky–Harborth constant [2.16]
0.8657725922...	Conjectured value of integer Chebyshev constant [4.9]
0.8660254037...	$\sqrt{3}/2$; 2D Steiner ratio [8.6], universal coverage [8.3]
0.8689277682...	With Landau–Ramanujan constant [2.3]
0.8705112052...	With Otter's tree enumeration constants [5.6]
0.8705883800...	A_4; with Brun's constant [2.14]
0.8711570464...	One of Flajolet's constants, with Thue–Morse [6.8]
0.8728875581...	With Landau–Ramanujan constant [2.3]
0.8740191847...	$L/3$; with Landau–Ramanujan [2.3], Gauss' lemniscate [6.1]
0.8740320488...	One of Turán's power sum constants [3.16]
0.8744643684...	With Niven's constant [2.6]
0.8785309152...	One of the geometric probability constants [8.1]
0.8795853862...	With Lenz–Ising constants [5.22]
0.8815138397...	Average class number, with Artin's constant [2.4]
0.8856031944...	Minimum of $\Gamma(x)$, with Euler–Mascheroni constant [1.5.4]
0.8905362089...	$e^{\gamma}/2$; with Hardy–Littlewood constants [2.1]
0.8928945714...	With Niven's constant [2.6]
0.8948412245...	With Landau–Ramanujan constant [2.3]
0.90177...	$\sqrt{c_0}$; one of the longest subsequence constants [5.20]
0.90682...	One of Rényi's parking constants [5.3]
0.9068996821...	$\pi/\sqrt{12}$; densest circle packing, with Hermite's constants [8.7]
0.9089085575...	With "one-ninth" constant [4.5]
0.91556671...	One of Rényi's parking constants [5.3]
0.9159655941...	Catalan's constant, G [1.7]
0.9241388730...	With hyperbolic volume constants [8.9]
0.9285187329...	With Gauss–Kuzmin–Wirsing constant [2.17]
0.9296953983...	$\ln(2)/2 + 2G/\pi$; with Lenz–Ising constants [5.22]
0.9312651841...	4th Pappalardi constant, with Artin's constant [2.4]
0.9375482543...	$-\zeta'(2)$; with Porter's constant [2.18]
0.9468064072...	With Landau–Ramanujan constant [2.3]
0.9625228267...	With Lebesgue constants [4.2]
0.9625817323...	c_0^+; with [5.22] Lenz–Ising constants
0.9730397768...	With Landau–Ramanujan constant [2.3]
0.9780124781...	Elbert's constant, with Shapiro–Drinfeld [3.1]
0.9795555269...	3rd Bendersky constant, with Glaisher–Kinkelin [2.15]
0.9848712825...	One of Rényi's parking constants [5.3]
0.9852475810...	With Landau–Ramanujan constant [2.3]
0.9877003907...	With universal coverage constants [8.3]
0.9878490568...	ln(Khintchine's constant) [1.8]
0.9891336344...	2·(Shapiro–Drinfeld constant) [3.1]
0.9894312738...	With Lebesgue constants [4.2]

0.9920479745...	4th Bendersky constant, with Glaisher–Kinkelin [2.15]
0.9932...	With geometric probability constants [8.1]
1	One; conjectured value of Linnik's constant, Baker's constant [2.12]
1.0028514266...	With Moser's worm constants [8.4]
1.0031782279...	Generalized Stirling constant, with Stieltjes constants [2.21]
1.0074347569...	DeVicci's tesseract constant [8.14]
1.0077822185...	$\sqrt{65}/8$; with Heilbronn triangle constants [8.16]
1.0096803872...	5th Bendersky constant, with Glaisher–Kinkelin [2.15]
1.0149416064...	$\pi \ln(\beta)$; Gieseking's constant, with Kneser–Mahler [3.10]
1.0174087975...	h_3; with Euler–Mascheroni constant [1.5.4]
1.0185012157...	With Porter–Hensley constant [2.18]
1.0208...	One of the traveling salesman constants [8.5]
1.0250590965...	With Lenz–Ising constants [5.22]
1.0306408341...	$\pi^2/(6\ln(2)\ln(10))$; Lévy's constant [1.8]
1.0309167521...	2nd Bendersky constant, with Glaisher–Kinkelin [2.15]
1.0346538818...	One of the Meissel–Mertens constants [2.2]
1.0451637801...	Li(2); with Euler–Gompertz constant [6.2]
1.0471975511...	$\pi/3$; with universal coverage constants [8.3]
1.0478314475...	One of the quadratic recurrence constants [6.10]
1.0544399448...	With Landau–Ramanujan constant [2.3]
1.0547001962...	One of the self-avoiding walk constants [5.10]
1.0606601717...	With DeVicci's tesseract constant [8.14]
1.0662758532...	With Lebesgue constants [4.2]
1.0693411205...	One of Pólya's random walk constants [5.9]
1.0786470120...	One of Pólya's random walk constants [5.9]
1.0786902162...	With Sobolev isoperimetric constants [3.6]
1.0820884492...	With hyperbolic volume constants [8.9]
1.0873780254...	One of Feller's coin tossing constants [5.11]
1.0892214740...	With Vallée's constant [2.19]
1.0894898722...	$1/2 + G/\pi$; with Wilbraham–Gibbs constant [4.1]
1.0939063155...	One of Pólya's random walk constants [5.9]
1.0963763171...	With DeVicci's tesseract constant [8.14]
1.0978510391...	A_3; with Brun's constant [2.14]
1.0986419643...	Paris' constant, with Golden mean [1.2]
1.0986858055...	Lengyel's constant [5.7]
1.1009181908...	With digital search tree constants [5.14]
1.1038396536...	With Gauss–Kuzmin–Wirsing constant [2.17]
1.1061028674...	One of Pólya's random walk constants [5.9]
1.1064957714...	One of the Copson–de Bruijn constants [3.5]
1.1128357889...	$(4L)/(3\pi)$; with Landau–Ramanujan constant [2.3]
1.1169633732...	One of Pólya's random walk constants [5.9]
1.1178641511...	Goh-Schmutz constant, with Golomb–Dickman [5.4]
1.1180339887...	$\sqrt{5}/2$; one of the Steinitz constants [3.13]

1.128057...	One of the percolation cluster density constants [5.18]
1.1289822228...	With Otter's tree enumeration constants [5.6]
1.13198824...	Viswanath's constant, with Golden mean [1.2]
1.1365599187...	With Otter's tree enumeration constants [5.6]
1.1373387363...	One of the digital search tree constants [5.14]
1.1481508398...	With Porter's constant [2.18]
1.1504807723...	Goldbach–Vinogradov constant, with Hardy–Littlewood [2.1]
1.1530805616...	With Landau–Ramanujan constant [2.3]
1.1563081248...	One of Pólya's random walk constants [5.9]
1.1574198038...	With Otter's tree enumeration constants [5.6]
1.1575...	One of the self-avoiding walk constants [5.10]
1.1587284730...	Grazing goat constant, with circular coverage constants [8.2]
1.159...	One of the self-avoiding walk constants [5.10]
1.1662436161...	$4G/\pi$; with Lenz–Ising constants [5.22]
1.1762808182...	Salem constant [2.30]
1.177043...	One of the self-avoiding walk constants [5.10]
1.1789797444...	$2G/\pi$; with Wilbraham–Gibbs constant [4.1]
1.1803405990...	h_1; with Euler–Mascheroni constant [1.5.4]
1.1865691104...	$\pi^2/(12\ln(2))$; Lévy's constant [1.8]
1.1874523511...	Foias' constant, with Grossman's constant [6.4]
1.1981402347...	M; Gauss' lemniscate constant [6.1]
1.1996786402...	With Laplace limit constant [4.8]
1.2013035599...	Rosser's constant, with Hardy–Littlewood constants [2.1]
1.2020569031...	$\zeta(3)$; Apéry's constant [1.6]
1.205...	One of the self-avoiding walk constants [5.10]
1.2087177032...	Baxter's constant, with Lieb's square ice constant [5.24]
1.2160045618...	One of Otter's tree enumeration constants [5.6]
1.21667...	One of the self-avoiding walk constants [5.10]
1.2241663491...	One of Otter's tree enumeration constants [5.6]
1.2267420107...	Fibonacci factorial constant, with Golden mean [1.2]
1.2368398446..	One of Feller's coin tossing constants [5.11]
1.238...	With Lenz–Ising constants [5.22]
1.2394671218...	One of Pólya's random walk constants [5.9]
1.257...	With Prouhet–Thue–Morse constant [6.8]
1.2577468869...	With Alladi–Grinstead [2.9], Khintchine–Lévy [1.8]
1.2599210498...	$\sqrt[3]{2}$; with Pythagoras' constant [1.1]
1.2610704868...	With binary search tree constants [5.13]
1.2615225101...	With hyperbolic volume constants [8.9]
1.2640847353...	One of the quadratic recurrence constants [6.10]
1.2672063606...	μ_6; one of the extreme value constants [5.16]
1.272...	One of the self-avoiding walk constants [5.10]
1.275...	One of the self-avoiding walk constants [5.10]
1.2824271291...	Glaisher–Kinkelin constant [2.15]
1.2885745539...	With Feigenbaum–Coullet–Tresser constants [1.9]

1.2910603681...	With Vallée's constant [2.19]
1.2912859970...	One of the iterated exponential constants [6.11]
1.2923041571...	With Landau–Ramanujan constant [2.3]
1.2940...	One of the self-avoiding walk constants [5.10]
1.2985395575...	Bateman's A constant, with Hardy–Littlewood [2.1]
1.302...	Square-free word constant [5.17]
1.3035772690...	Conway's constant [6.12]
1.30568...	Apollonian packing constant [8.20]
1.3063778838...	Mills' constant [2.13]
1.3110287771...	Quarter-lemniscate arclength $L/2$, Gauss' constant [6.1]
1.3135070786...	K_{-3}; with Khintchine's constant [1.8]
1.3203236316...	$2C_{\text{twin}}$; one of the Hardy–Littlewood constants [2.1]
1.3247179572...	With Golden mean [1.2], Pisot–Vijayaraghavan constants [2.30]
1.3325822757...	With Meissel–Mertens [2.2], totient constants [2.7]
1.3385151519...	$\exp(G/\pi)$; 2D dimer constant [5.23]
1.3426439511...	With hard square entropy constant [5.12]
1.34375	43/32; one of the self-avoiding walk constants [5.10]
1.3468852519...	One of the Riesz–Kolmogorov constants [7.7]
1.3505061...	One of the quadratic recurrence constants [6.10]
1.3511315744...	With Vallée's constant [2.19]
1.3521783756...	μ_7; one of the extreme value constants [5.16]
1.3531302722...	With optimal stopping constants [5.15]
1.3694514039...	Shallit's constant, with Shapiro–Drinfeld constant [3.1]
1.3728134628...	$2C_{\text{quad}}$; one of the Hardy–Littlewood constants [2.1]
1.3750649947...	One of the Meissel–Mertens constants [2.2]
1.37575...	With geometric probability constants [8.1]
1.3813564445...	β; with Kneser–Mahler polynomial constants [3.10]
1.3905439387...	Bateman's B constant, with Hardy–Littlewood [2.1]
1.3932039296...	One of Pólya's random walk constants [5.9]
1.3954859724...	Hard hexagon entropy constant, with hard square [5.12]
1.3994333287...	With Kalmár's composition constant [5.5]
1.4011551890...	Myrberg's constant, with Feigenbaum–Coullet–Tresser [1.9]
1.4045759346...	Conjectured value of complex Grothendieck constant [3.11]
1.4092203477...	With Stolarsky–Harborth constant [2.16]
1.4106861346...	With Euler–Gompertz constant [6.2]
1.4142135623...	$\sqrt{2}$; Pythagoras' constant [1.1]
1.4236003060...	μ_8; one of the extreme value constants [5.16]
1.4298155...	One of the quadratic recurrence constants [6.10]
1.4359911241.....	$1/3 + 2\sqrt{3}/\pi$; 1st Lebesgue constant [4.2]
1.4426950408...	$\ln(2)^{-1}$; with Porter–Hensley constants [2.18]
1.4446678610...	$e^{1/e}$; one of the iterated exponential constants [6.11]
1.4503403284...	K_{-2}; with Khintchine's constant [1.8]
1.4513692348...	Ramanujan–Soldner constant, with Euler–Gompertz [6.2]

1.4560749485...	Backhouse's constant, with [5.5]
1.457...	Cube-free word constant [5.17]
1.4603545088...	$-\zeta(1/2)$; with Apéry's constant [1.6]
1.4609984862...	Baxter's constant, with Lieb's square ice [5.24]
1.4616321449...	x minimizing $\Gamma(x)$, with Euler–Mascheroni constant [1.5.4]
1.4655712318...	Moore's constant, with the Golden mean [1.2]
1.4670780794...	Porter's constant [2.18]
1.4677424503...	One of the Feigenbaum–Coullet–Tresser constants [1.9]
1.4681911223...	With Alladi–Grinstead constant [2.9]
1.4741726868...	One of Otter's tree enumeration constants [5.6]
1.4762287836...	With Kalmár's composition constant [5.5]
1.4767...	One of the self-avoiding walk constants [5.10]
1.4879506635...	$-\zeta(2/3)/\zeta(2)$; with Niven's constant [2.6]
1.4880785456...	One of Otter's tree enumeration constants [5.6]
1.5028368010...	One of the quadratic recurrence constants [6.10]
1.5030480824...	Hard square entropy constant [5.12]
1.50659177...	Area of Mandelbrot set, quadratic recurrence [6.10]
1.50685...	Nagle's constant, with Lieb's square ice constant [5.24]
1.5078747554...	Greenfield–Nussbaum constant, quadratic recurrence [6.10]
1.5163860591...	One of Pólya's random walk constants [5.9]
1.5217315350...	Bateman–Stemmler constant, Hardy–Littlewood [2.1]
1.5299540370...	With Gauss' lemniscate constant [6.1]
1.5353705088...	With digital search tree constants [5.14]
1.5396007178...	$(4/3)^{3/2}$; Lieb's square ice constant [5.24]
1.5422197217...	Madelung constant for planar hexagonal lattice [1.10]
1.5449417003...	With Reuleaux triangle constants [8.10]
1.5464407087...	With hard square entropy constant [5.12]
1.5513875245...	Calabi's triangle constant [8.13]
1.5557712501...	One of the Feigenbaum–Coullet–Tresser constants [1.9]
1.5707963267...	$\pi/2$; with Archimedes' constant [1.4]
1.5849625007...	$\ln(3)/\ln(2)$; with Stolarsky–Harborth constant [2.16]
1.5868266790...	With Feigenbaum–Coullet–Tresser constants [1.9]
1.6066951524...	One of the digital search tree constants [5.14]
1.6153297360...	With Lenz–Ising constants [5.22]
1.6155426267...	Negative of 2D NaCl Madelung constant [1.10]
1.6180339887...	Golden mean, φ [1.2]
1.6222705028...	Odlyzko–Wilf constant, with Mills' constant [2.13]
1.6281601297...	Flajolet–Martin constant, with Prouhet–Thue–Morse [6.8]
1.6366163233...	With Erdös–Lebensold constant [2.27]
1.6421884352...	2nd Lebesgue constant [4.2]
1.644703...	With moving sofa constant [8.12]
1.6449340668...	$\pi^2/6$; with Apéry [1.6], Hafner–Sarnak–McCurley [2.5]
1.6467602581...	With digital search tree constants [5.14]
1.6600...	With Lieb's square ice constant [5.24]

1.9021605831...	Brun's constant [2.14]
1.9081456268...	β^2 ; with Kneser–Mahler polynomial constants [3.10]
1.9093378156...	Negative of 5D NaCl Madelung constant [1.10]
1.9126258077...	One of Otter's tree enumeration constants [5.6]
1.9276909638...	One of the Feigenbaum–Coullet–Tresser constants [1.9]
1.9287800...	Wright's constant, with Mills' constant [2.13]
1.940215351...	2D monomer-dimer constant [5.23]
1.9435964368...	One of the Euler totient constants [2.7]
1.9484547890...	c_4; with Kneser–Mahler polynomial constants [3.10]
1.9504911124...	4·(Gaussian twin prime constant), with Hardy–Littlewood [2.1]
1.9655570390...	Negative of 6D NaCl Madelung constant [1.10]
1.9670449011...	c_5; with Kneser–Mahler polynomial constants [3.10]
1.9771268308...	c_6; with Kneser–Mahler polynomial constants [3.10]
1.9954559575...	With Fransén–Robinson constant [4.6]
2	Two; conjectured value of fast matrix multiplication constant [2.29]
2.006...	With Erdös–Lebensold constant [2.27]
2.0124059897...	Negative of 7D NaCl Madelung constant [1.10]
2.0287578381...	With Du Bois Reymond constants [3.12]
2.0415...	One of the traveling salesman constants [8.5]
2.0462774528...	Lüroth analog of Lévy's constant [1.8]
2.05003...	One of the Whitney–Mikhlin extension constants [3.8]
2.0524668272...	Negative of 8D NaCl Madelung constant [1.10]
2.0531987328...	With self-avoiding walk constants [5.10]
2.0780869212...	$\ln(\varphi)^{-1}$; with Porter–Hensley constants [2.18]
2.1080540666...	With rendezvous constants [8.21]
2.1102339661...	Brown–Wang constant, from Young–Fejér–Jackson [3.14]
2.158...	Mian–Chowla constant, with Erdös' reciprocal sum [2.20]
2.1732543125...	$\zeta(3/2)/\zeta(3)$; with Niven's constant [2.6]
2.1760161352...	With Kneser–Mahler polynomial constants [3.10]
2.1894619856...	One of Otter's tree enumeration constants [5.6]
2.1918374031...	One of Otter's tree enumeration constants [5.6]
2.2001610580...	Lüroth analog of Khintchine's constant [1.8]
2.2038565964...	One of the Euler totient constants [2.7]
2.2195316688...	Moving sofa constant [8.12]
2.2247514809...	Robinson's C constant, with Khintchine's constant [1.8]
2.2394331040...	Takeuchi–Prellberg constant [5.8]
2.2665345077...	With Fransén–Robinson constant [4.6]
2.2782916414...	One of Moser's worm constants [8.4]
2.2948565916...	One of the abelian group enumeration constants [5.1]
2.3...	Estimate of $s_c(3)$, with k-satisfiability constants [5.21]
2.3025661371...	One of Flajolet's constants, with Thue–Morse [6.8]
2.3038421962...	Robinson's A constant, with Khintchine's constant [1.8]
2.3091385933...	With Klarner's polyomino constant [5.19]

2.3136987039...	With Madelung's constant [1.10]
2.3212850380...	With rendezvous constants [8.21]
2.3360...	With Lieb's square ice constant [5.24]
2.3507...	One of the Landau–Kolmogorov constants [3.3]
2.3565273533...	One of the monomer-dimer constants [5.23]
2.3731382208...	$\pi^2/(6\ln(2))$; Lévy's constant [1.8]
2.37597...	With Klarner's polyomino constant [5.19]
2.3768417063...	Conjectured value of integer Chebyshev constant [4.9]
2.3979455861...	With Du Bois Reymond constants [3.12]
2.4048255576...	First zero of $J_0(x)$, with Sobolev isoperimetric constants [3.6]
2.4149010237...	With Golomb–Dickman constant [5.4]
2.4413238136...	With Lebesgue constants [4.2]
2.4725480752...	With Sobolev isoperimetric constants [3.6]
2.4832535361...	One of Otter's tree enumeration constants [5.6]
2.4996161129...	One of the abelian group enumeration constants [5.1]
2.5029078750...	α; one of the Feigenbaum–Coullet–Tresser constants [1.9]
2.5066282746...	$\sqrt{2\pi}$; Stirling's constant; with Archimedes [1.4], Glaisher–Kinkelin [2.15]
2.5175403550...	One of Otter's tree enumeration constants [5.6]
2.5193561520...	With Madelung's constant [1.10]
2.5695443449...	$e^\gamma/\ln(2)$; with Euler–Mascheroni constant [1.5]
2.5849817595...	Sierpinski's constant [2.10]
2.5980762113...	$\sqrt{27/4}$; with Lieb's square ice constant [5.24]
2.6034...	With Lieb's square ice constant [5.24]
2.6180339887...	Golden root $\varphi+1$, with Tutte–Beraha [5.25], Gauss–Kuzmin–Wirsing [2.17]
2.6220575542...	Half-lemniscate arclength L, Gauss' constant [6.1]
2.6381585303...	Estimate of 2D self-avoiding walk constant [5.10]
2.6389584337...	$(2+\sqrt{3})/\sqrt{2}$; with beam detection constant [8.11]
2.67564...	With Klarner's polyomino constant [5.19]
2.6789385347...	$\Gamma(1/3)$; with Euler–Mascheroni constant [1.5.4]
2.6789638796...	4·(Shanks' constant), with Hardy–Littlewood constants [2.1]
2.6811281472...	One of Otter's tree enumeration constants [5.6]
2.6854520010...	Khintchine's constant [1.8]
2.7182818284...	Natural logarithmic base, e [1.3]
2.72062...	One of the self-avoiding walk constants [5.10]
2.7494879027...	One of Otter's tree enumeration constants [5.6]
2.75861972...	With hyperbolic volume constants [8.9]
2.7865848321...	With Fransén–Robinson constant [4.6]
2.8077702420...	Fransén–Robinson constant [4.6]
2.8154600332...	One of Otter's tree enumeration constants [5.6]
2.8264199970...	Murata's constant, with Artin [2.4], totient [2.7]
2.8336106558...	One of the Feigenbaum–Coullet–Tresser constants [1.9]
2.8372974794...	With Madelung's constant [1.10]

2.8582485957...	One of the Hardy–Littlewood constants [2.1]
2.9409823408...	$c_o/\sqrt{2\pi}$; with Lengyel's constant [5.7]
2.9409900447...	$c_e/\sqrt{2\pi}$; with Lengyel's constant [5.7]
2.9557652856...	One of Otter's tree enumeration constants [5.6]
2.9904703993...	Goh–Schmutz constant, with Golomb–Dickman [5.4]
3	Three; with Tutte–Beraha constants [5.25]
3.0079...	With Erdös' reciprocal sum constants [2.20]
3.01...	With Erdös' reciprocal sum constants [2.20]
3.1415926535...	Archimedes' constant, π [1.4]
3.1477551485...	Quadratic residues constant, with Meissel–Mertens [2.2]
3.1704593421...	One of the Euler totient constants [2.7]
3.1962206165...	"Plate" constant, with Sobolev isoperimetric constants [3.6]
3.2099123007...	$\exp(4G/\pi)$; 2D dimer constant [5.23]; also Kneser–Mahler [3.10]
3.2469796037...	Silver root, one of the Tutte–Beraha constants [5.25]
3.2504...	With Lieb's square ice constant [5.24]
3.2659724710...	One of Otter's tree enumeration constants [5.6]
3.2758229187...	$\exp(\pi^2)/(12\ln(2))$; Lévy's constant [1.8]
3.2871120555...	One of Otter's tree enumeration constants [5.6]
3.2907434386...	One of Otter's tree enumeration constants [5.6]
3.3038421963...	Robinson's B constant, with Khintchine's constant [1.8]
3.33437...	Bumby's constant, with Freiman's constant [2.31]
3.3412669407...	With Otter's tree enumeration constants [5.6]
3.3598856662...	With digital search tree constants [5.14]
3.3643175781...	Van der Corput's constant [3.15]
3.4070691656...	Magata's constant, with Kalmár's composition constant [5.5]
3.4201328816...	With self-avoiding walk constants [5.10]
3.4493588902...	Robinson's D constant, with Khintchine's constant [1.8]
3.4627466194...	Q^{-1}; with digital search tree constants [5.14], Lengyel [5.7]
3.501838...	With self-avoiding walk constants [5.10]
3.5070480758...	With Feller's coin tossing constants [5.11]
3.5795...	With Lieb's square ice constant [5.24]
3.6096567319...	Conjectured value of ρ_2, Diophantine approximation [2.23]
3.6180339887...	$\varphi + 2$; one of the Tutte–Beraha constants [5.25]
3.6256099082...	$\Gamma(1/4)$; with Euler–Mascheroni constant [1.5.4]
3.63600703...	One of the Feigenbaum–Coullet–Tresser constants [1.9]
3.6746439660...	Quadratic residues constant, with Meissel–Mertens [2.2]
3.6754...	One of the longest subsequence constants [5.20]
3.7038741039...	2·(Wilbraham–Gibbs constant) [4.1]
3.764435608...	2D monomer-dimer constant [5.23]
3.7962...	z_c; with hard square entropy constant [5.12]
3.8264199970...	Murata's constant + 1, with Artin [2.4], totient [2.7]
3.8695192413...	With optimal stopping constants [5.15]
3.9002649200...	With Madelung's constant [1.10]

3.921545...	With Moser's worm constants [8.4]
3.92259368...	With hyperbolic volume constants [8.9]
4	Four; Tutte–Beraha [5.25], 2D Grötzsch ring constant [7.8]
4.0180767046...	One of the Feigenbaum–Coullet–Tresser constants [1.9]
4.062570...	Klarner's polyomino constant [5.18]
4.121326...	One of the Feigenbaum–Coullet–Tresser constants [1.9]
4.1327313541...	$\sqrt{2\pi e}$; Sobolev isoperimetric [3.6], traveling salesman [8.5]
4.1507951...	One of the self-avoiding walk constants [5.10]
4.1511808632...	One of the Hardy–Littlewood constants [2.1]
4.2001...	With Lieb's square ice constant [5.24]
4.2472965459...	One of the geometric probability constants [8.1]
4.25...	Estimate of $r_c(3)$, with k-satisfiability constants [5.21]
4.3076923076...	56/13; Korn constant for 3D ball [3.7]
4.3110704070...	One of the binary search tree constants [5.13]
4.5278295661...	Freiman's constant [2.31]
4.5651...	With Lieb's square ice constant [5.24]
4.5678018826...	Gasper's constant, with Young–Fejér–Jackson [3.14]
4.5860790989...	One of Pólya's random walk constants [5.9]
4.5908437119...	$\Gamma(1/5)$; with Euler–Mascheroni constant [1.5.4]
4.6592661225...	Bateman–Grosswald c_{03} constant, with Niven's constant [2.6]
4.6692016091...	δ; one of the Feigenbaum–Coullet–Tresser constants [1.9]
4.68404...	Estimate of 3D self-avoiding walk constant [5.10]
4.7300407448...	"Rod" constant, with Sobolev isoperimetric [3.6]
4.799891547...	Three-arc approximation of beam detection constant [8.11]
4.8189264563...	Two-arc approximation of beam detection constant [8.11]
4.8426...	One of the self-avoiding walk constants [5.10]
4.9264...	With Artin's constant [2.4]
5.0747080320...	With hyperbolic volume constants [8.9]
5.1387801326...	With Sobolev isoperimetric constants [3.6]
5.1667...	With Lieb's square ice constant [5.24]
5.2441151086...	Lemniscate arclength $2L$, Gauss' constant [6.1]
5.2569464048...	With Euler–Mascheroni constant [1.5.4]
5.4545172445...	With Khintchine–Lévy constants [1.8]
5.5243079702...	With Khintchine–Lévy constants [1.8]
5.5553...	With Lieb's square ice constant [5.24]
5.5663160017...	$\Gamma(1/6)$; with Euler–Mascheroni constant [1.5.4]
5.6465426162...	One of Otter's tree enumeration constants [5.6]
5.6493764966...	Conjectured value of integer Chebyshev constant [4.9]
5.7831859629...	With Sobolev isoperimetric constants [3.6]
5.8726188208...	Bateman–Grosswald $-c_{13}$ constant, with Niven's constant [2.6]
5.9087...	With Artin's constant [2.4]
5.9679687038...	One of the Feigenbaum–Coullet–Tresser constants [1.9]

6.0 ...	One of Cameron's sum-free set constants [2.25]
6.2831853071 ...	2π; with Archimedes' constant [1.4]
6.3800420942 ...	One of Otter's tree enumeration constants [5.6]
6.77404 ...	Estimate of 4D self-avoiding walk constant [5.10]
6.7992251609 ...	One of the Feigenbaum–Coullet–Tresser constants [1.9]
6.8 ...	One of Cameron's sum-free set constants [2.25]
7.1879033516 ...	Conjectured value of John constant [7.4]
7.2569464048 ...	With Euler–Mascheroni constant [1.5.4]
7.2846862171 ...	One of the Feigenbaum–Coullet–Tresser constants [1.9]
7.3719494907 ...	c_o; with Lengyel's constant [5.7]
7.3719688014 ...	c_e; with Lengyel's constant [5.7]
7.7431319855 ...	One of the digital search tree constants [5.14]
7.7581602911 ...	One of Otter's tree enumeration constants [5.6]
8.3494991320 ...	One of the Feigenbaum–Coullet–Tresser constants [1.9]
8.7000366252 ...	Kepler–Bouwkamp constant [6.3]
8.7210972 ...	One of the Feigenbaum–Coullet–Tresser constants [1.9]
8.83854 ...	Estimate of 5D self-avoiding walk constant [5.10]
9.0803731646 ...	Hensley's constant [2.18]
9.27738 ...	One of the Feigenbaum–Coullet–Tresser constants [1.9]
9.2890254919 ...	Reciprocal of "one-ninth" constant [4.5]
9.2962468327 ...	One of the Feigenbaum–Coullet–Tresser constants [1.9]
9.37 ...	3D Grötzsch ring constant [7.8]
9.576778 ...	With beam detection constant [8.11]
9.6694754843 ...	Bateman–Grosswald c_{04} constant, with Niven's constant [2.6]
9.7 ...	Estimate of $r_c(4)$, with k-satisfiability constants [5.21]
10.5101504239 ...	Zagier's constant, with Freiman's constant [2.31]
10.7310157948 ...	$\exp(\pi^2/(6\ln(2)))$; Lévy's constant [1.8]
10.87809 ...	Estimate of 6D self-avoiding walk constant [5.10]
11.0901699437 ...	$(11 + 5\sqrt{5})/2$; with hard square entropy constant [5.12]
12.262874 ...	With self-avoiding walk constants [5.10]
12.6753318106 ...	16·(Lal's constant), with Hardy–Littlewood constants [2.1]
14.1347251417 ...	1st zeta function zero, with Glaisher–Kinkelin constant [2.15]
14.6475663016 ...	One of the abelian group enumeration constants [5.1]
15.1542622415 ...	e^e; one of the iterated exponential constants [6.11]
16.3638968792 ...	β; one of the Feigenbaum–Coullet–Tresser constants [1.9]
16.9787814834 ...	Bateman–Grosswald c_{14} constant, with Niven's constant [2.6]
19.4455760839 ...	Bateman–Grosswald c_{05} constant, with Niven's constant [2.6]
20.9 ...	Estimate of $r_c(5)$, with k-satisfiability constants [5.21]
21.0220396387 ...	2nd zeta function zero, with Glaisher–Kinkelin constant [2.15]
22.6 ...	4D Grötzsch ring constant [7.8]
25.0108575801 ...	3rd zeta function zero, with Glaisher–Kinkelin constant [2.15]

29.576303 . . .   One of the Feigenbaum–Coullet–Tresser constants [1.9]

39.1320261423 . . .   With Calabi's triangle constant [8.13]

43.2 . . .   Estimate of $r_c(6)$, with k-satisfiability constants [5.21]

55.247 . . .   One of the Feigenbaum–Coullet–Tresser constants [1.9]

118.6924619727 . . .   One of the abelian group enumeration constants [5.1]

137.0359 . . .   Inverse fine structure constant, with Feigenbaum–
                              Coullet–Tresser [1.9]

Author Index

Subject Index

Added in Press

The following results are too beautiful to be overlooked. The **Gaussian integers** $a + bi$, where a, b are integers and $i^2 = -1$, form a unique factorization domain with units $\{\pm 1, \pm i\}$. Suppose two Gaussian integers are chosen at random. The probability that they are coprime, in the limit over large disks, is [1,2]

$$\frac{6}{\pi^2 G} = 0.6637008046\ldots$$

where G is Catalan's constant [1.7]. This is slightly greater than the corresponding probability that two ordinary integers are coprime [1.4].

In the same way, the **Eisenstein–Jacobi integers** $a + b\omega$, where a, b are integers and $\omega = (-1 + i\sqrt{3})/2$, form a unique factorization domain with units $\{\pm 1, \pm i, \pm \omega\}$. The probability that two such randomly chosen integers are coprime, in the limit over large disks, is [1,3]

$$\frac{6}{\pi^2 H} = 0.7780944891\ldots$$

where

$$H = \frac{4\pi}{3\sqrt{3}} \ln(\beta) = \sum_{k=0}^{\infty} \left(\frac{1}{(3k+1)^2} - \frac{1}{(3k+2)^2} \right) = 0.7813024128\ldots$$

and β is discussed extensively in [3.10].

The constants $6/(\pi^2 G)$ and $6/(\pi^2 H)$ are also, respectively, the probabilities that a random Gaussian integer is square-free and a random Eisenstein–Jacobi integer is square-free. As in [2.5], there are related notions of *carefreeness* but the corresponding constants are not yet known.

Incidently, the pairwise coprimality result conjectured at the end of [2.5] has been proved to be true [4].

And, as this book goes to press, it is unclear [5] whether the prime limit infimum problem given at the conclusion of [2.13] is solved (or nearly so).

[1] G. E. Collins and J. R. Johnson, The probability of relative primality of Gaussian integers, *Proc. 1988 Int. Symp. Symbolic and Algebraic Computation (ISSAC)*, Rome, ed. P. Gianni, Lect. Notes in Comp. Sci. 358, Springer-Verlag, 1989, pp. 252–258; MR 90m:11165.

[2] E. Pegg, The neglected Gaussian integers (MathPuzzle).

[3] E. Kowalski, Coprimality and squarefreeness within quadratic fields, unpublished note (2003).

[4] J.-Y. Cai and E. Bach, On testing for zero polynomials by a set of points with bounded precision, *Theoret. Comput. Sci.* 296 (2003) 15–25.

[5] D. Goldston and C. Yildirim, Small gaps between primes, submitted (2003).